KT-478-703

CONTENTS

Stedman's

Pocket

Medical

Dictionary

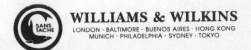

WILLIAMS & WILKINS

LONDON · BALTIMORE · BUENOS AIRES · HONG KONG
MUNICH · PHILADELPHIA · SYDNEY · TOKYO

Publisher: Anne Lenehan
Editor: Harriet Felscher
Consulting Editor: Ruth Koenigsberg
Designer: Daniel Pfisterer
Production Coordinator: Barbara Felton

Copyright © 1993
Williams & Wilkins
Broadway House
2-6 Fulham Broadway
London SW6 1AA
England

telephone (071) 385-2357
telefax (071) 385-2922

9 8 7 6 5 4 3 2

Printed and bound in Great Britain by Cox & Wyman Ltd, Reading, Berks.

A CIP catalogue record for this book is available from the British Library.

ISBN 0-683-14528-2

PUBLISHER'S PREFACE

Since its first appearance in 1911, *Stedman's Medical Dictionary* has gained a worldwide reputation as a scholarly and authoritative source for medical words. *Stedman's* consultants, leaders in their fields, regularly write, review, and rewrite *Stedman's* definitions. *Stedman's* is the parent book to an entire family of books, the newest of which is the English edition of *Stedman's Pocket Medical Dictionary* with British spellings.

Stedman's Pocket Medical Dictionary has been prepared by drawing entries directly from the databank for *Stedman's Medical Dictionary* and revising for spelling. *Stedman's Pocket* is intended to be a concise, easy-to-handle reference in a pocket-sized format that will serve the needs of medical personnel—both student and practitioner. Medical students and students in the fields of nursing, medical secretarial science, physiotherapy, medical technology, or other medically related fields will find *Stedman's Pocket Medical Dictionary* helpful in their studies and in the early stages of their careers. Practitioners at every level should find this dictionary a quick, reliable resource for daily reference.

Because legibility is such an important factor in quick look-ups for spelling and reference, *Stedman's Pocket* has taken its page style from its parent book. It retains the boldface subentries indented and aligned at the left allowing the quickest search for an entry.

We hope our readers are pleased with the results and invite suggestions and comments that will be considered for incorporation into future editions of the dictionary. Please write to Anne Lenehan, Williams & Wilkins Ltd., Broadway House, 2-6 Fulham Broadway, London SW6 1AA, England.

HOW TO USE THIS DICTIONARY

Vocabulary Organization:

MAIN ENTRY
SUBENTRY

STEDMAN'S POCKET MEDICAL DICTIONARY is organized into main entry terms and subentry terms. This organization allows the reader to find the major terms as main entries and then groups terms together that have a noun in common. These groups of terms are indented under the main word, much like an index. For example, the term **disease** is listed as a main entry. All terms that include the word **disease** are grouped together in alphabetic order and indented below it as an index would be. This index-like format provides two advantages: a visual advantage— terms are easy to find and read—and a spatial advantage— related terms are grouped together in one place.

Alphabetization

The vocabulary is ordered letter by letter, not word by word. Disregard only the letter that abbreviates the main word in subentries and any hyphens, numbers, italicized word parts, or Greek letters that are part of a term.

Cross References

Lightface italics are used to alert the reader to a cross reference located as a subentry under a main entry noun. The main noun appears in italics. In cross references where the cross reference term is a single word, no change in typeface is added. In the same way, where subentries cross refer to another subentry in the same group with the main word abbreviated, no change in typeface is added.

Abbreviations
Used in Vocabulary and Etymology

Ar.	Arabic
A.S.	Anglo-Saxon
c., ca.	L. *circa*, about
cf.	L. *confer*, compare
Eng.	English
e.g.	L. *exempli gratia*, for example
Fr.	French
fr.	from
G.	Greek
Gael.	Gaelic
gen.	genitive
Ger.	German
Hind.	Hindu
i.e.	L. *id est*, that is
Ind.	Indian
It.	Italian
Jap.	Japanese
L.	Latin
L.L.	Late Latin
M.E.	Middle English
Mediev. L.	Medieval Latin
Med. L.	Medieval Latin
Mod. L.	Modern Latin
NA	Nomina Anatomica
neut., ntr	neuter
obs.	obsolete
O.E.	Old English
O.Fr.	Old French
Pers.	Persian
Pg.	Portuguese
p.	participle
pl.	plural
pp.	past participle
priv.	privative, negative
q.v.	L. *quod vide*, which see
sing.	singular
Sp.	Spanish
thr.	through
U.S.	United States

A

a-, an- [G. *alpha*, privative or negative, inseparable prefix, usually *an-* before a vowel] Prefix equivalent to the L. *in-* and E. *un-*; not, without, -less.

ab- [L. *ab*, from] Prefix signifying from, away from, off.

abap'ical Opposite the apex.

aba'sia [G. a- priv. + *basis*, step] Inability to walk.

abdo'men [L. *abdomen*, etym. uncertain] [NA] Belly; the part of the trunk that lies between the thorax and the pelvis. The a. does not include the vertebral region posteriorly but is considered by some anatomists to include the pelvis. It contains the greater part of the abdominal cavity, and is divided by arbitrary planes into nine regions.

  acute a., surgical a. any serious intra-abdominal condition attended by pain, tenderness, and muscular rigidity, and implying the need for any emergency operation.

  carinate a., a sloping of the sides with prominence of the central line of the a.

  navicular a., scaphoid a., a condition in which the anterior abdominal wall is sunken and presents a concave contour.

abdom'inal Relating to the abdomen.

abdomino-, abdomin- [L. *abdomen*] Combining forms denoting relationship to the abdomen.

abdom'inoplasty [abdomino- + G. *plassō*, to form] An operation performed on the abdominal wall for aesthetic purposes.

abdom'inoves'ical Relating to the abdomen and urinary bladder, or to the abdomen and gallbladder.

abduce' Abduct.

abdu'cent [L. *abducens*] Abducting; drawing away.

abduct' To move away from the median line.

abduc'tion [L. *abductio*] **1.** Movement away from the median line. **2.** Monocular rotation (duction) of the eye toward the temple. **3.** A position resulting from such movement.

abduc'tor A muscle that draws a part away from the median line.

aber'rancy Aberration.

aber'rant [L. *aberrans*] **1.** Wandering off; said of certain ducts, vessels, or nerves taking an unusual course. **2.** Differing from the normal; in botany or zoology, said of certain atypical individuals in a species. **3.** Ectopic (1).

aberra'tion [L. *aberratio*] **1.** A straying from the normal situation. **2.** Deviant development or growth.

  chromatic a., the difference in focus or magnification of an image arising because of a difference in the refraction of different wavelengths composing white light.

  chromosome a., any deviation from the normal number or morphology of chromosomes.

  optical a., failure of rays from a point source to form a perfect image after traversing an optical system.

abe'talipoproteinae'mia Bassen-Kornzweig syndrome; a disorder characterized by an absence of plasma lipoproteins having a density less than 1.063, presence of acanthocytes in blood, retinal pigmentary degeneration, malabsorption, engorgement of upper intestinal absorptive cells with dietary triglycerides, and neuromuscular abnormalities; autosomal recessive inheritance.

abio'sis [G. a- priv. + *bios*, life] **1.** Nonviability. **2.** Absence of life.

abiot'ic Incompatible with life.

abiot'rophy [G. a- priv. + *bios*, life, + *trophē*, nourishment] Premature loss of vitality or degeneration of certain cells or tissues, usually of genetic aetiology; generic term applied to hereditary degenerative diseases.

abir'ritant 1. Soothing; relieving irritation. **2.** An agent possessing this property.

abirrita'tion [L. *ab*, from, + *irrito*, pp. *-atus*, to irritate] The diminution or abolition of reflex or other irritability in a part.

ablate' [L. *ab-latus*, taking away] To remove, or to destroy the function of.

abla'tion [L. see ablate] Removal of a body part or the destruction of its function, as by a surgical procedure, morbid process, or noxious substance.

ablepha'ria, ableph'aron [G. a- priv. + *blepharon*, eyelid] Congenital absence, partial or complete, of the eyelids.

abnormal'ity [L. *ab*, from, + *norma*, rule] An anomaly, deformity, malformation, or difference from the usual.

abo'rad, abo'ral [L. *ab*, from, + *os* (*or-*), mouth] In a direction away from the mouth; opposite of orad.

abort' [L. *aborto*, to miscarry] **1.** To expel an embryo or fetus before it is viable. **2.** To arrest a disease in its earliest stages. **3.** To arrest in growth or development; to cause to remain rudimentary.

abor'tient Abortifacient (1).

abortifa'cient [L. *abortus*, abortion, + *facio*, to make] **1.** Producing abortion. **2.** An agent that produces abortion.

abor'tion **1.** Expelling an embryo or fetus prior to being viable. **2.** The arrest of any action or process before its normal completion.

criminal a., termination of pregnancy without medical or legal justification.

induced a., a. brought on purposefully by drugs or mechanical means.

septic a., an infectious a. complicated by fever, endometritis, and parametritis.

spontaneous a., a. occurring naturally.

therapeutic a., a. induced because of the mother's physical or mental health, or to prevent birth of a deformed child or a child resulting from rape.

abor'tus [L.] The product of an abortion.

abra'chia [G. *a-* priv. + *brachiōn*, arm] Congenital absence of arms.

abrade' [L. *ab-rado*, to scrape off] **1.** To wear away by mechanical action. **2.** To scrape away the surface layer from a part.

abra'sion [see abrade] **1.** An excoriation or circumscribed removal of the superficial layers of skin or mucous membrane. **2.** A scraping away of a portion of the surface. **3.** Grinding; in dentistry, the wearing away of tooth substance.

abra'sive **1.** Causing abrasion. **2.** Any material used to produce abrasion.

abreac'tion In freudian psychoanalysis, an episode of emotional release or catharsis associated with the bringing into conscious recollection previously repressed unpleasant experiences.

abrup'tio placen'tae [L. to break off] Premature detachment of a normally situated placenta.

ab'scess [L. *abscessus*, a going away] **1.** A circumscribed collection of pus appearing in acute or chronic, localized infection, and associated with tissue destruction and, frequently, swelling. **2.** A cavity formed by liquefaction necrosis within solid tissue.

alveolar a., an a. in the dentoalveolar process, either in a lateral periodontal or periapical periodontal position.

Bezold's a., an a. deep in the neck associated with suppuration in the mastoid tip cells.

Brodie's a., a chronic a. of bone surrounded by dense fibrous tissue and sclerotic bone.

cold a., an a. without heat or other usual signs of inflammation.

dentoalveolar a., an a. confined to the dentoalveolar process investing a tooth root.

dry a., the remains of an a. after the pus is absorbed.

perforating a., an a. that breaks down tissue barriers to enter adjacent areas.

peritonsillar a., quinsy; extension of tonsillar infection beyond the capsule with abscess formation usually above and behind the tonsil.

Pott's a., a tuberculous a. of the spine.

psoas a., an a., usually tuberculous, originating in tuberculous spondylitis and extending through the iliopsoas muscle to the inguinal region.

abscis'sion [L. *ab-scindo*, pp. *-scissus*, to cut away from] Cutting away.

ab'sence [L. *absentia*] Petit mal; paroxysmal attacks of brief clouding of consciousness that may be unaccompanied (simple a.) or accompanied (complex a.) by other abnormalities.

Absid'ia A genus of fungi (family Mucoraceae) commonly found in nature; thermophilic species survive in compost piles at temperatures exceeding 45°C and may cause phycomycosis in humans.

absorb' [L. *ab-sorbeo*, to suck in] **1.** To take in by absorption. **2.** To reduce the intensity of transmitted light.

absorb'ent **1.** Having the power to absorb, soak up, or take into itself a gas, liquid, light rays, or heat. **2.** Any substance possessing such power.

absorp'tion Taking in, incorporation, or reception of gases, liquids, light, or heat.

ab'stinence [L. *abs- tineo*, to hold back] Refraining from indulgence in certain foods, drink, or drugs, or from sexual intercourse.

abter'minal [L. *ab*, from + *terminus*, end] In a direction away from the end and toward the centre; denoting the course of an electrical current in a muscle.

abu'lia [G. a- priv. + boulē, will] Loss or impairment of the ability to perform voluntary actions or to make decisions.

abuse' **1.** Misuse, wrong use, especially excessive use, of anything. **2.** Injurious, harmful, or offensive treatment.

abut'ment In dentistry, a natural tooth or implanted tooth substitute, used for the support or anchorage of a fixed or removable prosthesis.

Acanthamoe'ba [G. akantha, thorn, spine, + Mod. L. amoeba] A free-living amoeba found in soil, sewage, and water, several species of which cause acanthamoeblasis.

acanth'amoebi'asis Infection by amoebae of the genus Acanthamoeba that may result in a necrotizing dermal or tissue invasion, or a fulminating and usually fatal primary amoebic meningoencephalitis.

acantho- [G. akantha, thorn] Combining form denoting relationship to a spinous process, or meaning spiny or thorny.

Acan'thocheilone'ma [acantho- + G. cheilos, lip, + nēma, thread] A genus of filarial worm parasitic in man, now part of the genus Dipetalonema.

acan'thocyte [acantho- + G. kytos, cell] An erythrocyte characterized by multiple spiny cytoplasmic projections and in acanthocytosis.

acan'thocyto'sis. A rare condition in which the majority of erythrocytes are acanthocytes; a regular feature of abetalipoproteinaemia.

acantho'ma [acantho- + G. -oma, tumour] A tumorous hypertrophy of epidermal squamous cells that may be malignant, benign, or even non-neoplastic.

acantho'sis [acantho- + G. -osis, condition] An increase in the thickness of the prickle cell layer of the epidermis.

   a. ni'gricans, an eruption of velvet warty benign growths and hyperpigmentation occurring in the skin of the axillae, neck, anogenital area, and groins; in adults it is associated with internal malignancy or reticulosis; a benign (juvenile) type occurs in children.

acap'nia [G. a- priv. + kapnos, smoke] Absence of carbon dioxide in the blood. See also hypocapnia.

acari'asis Any disease caused by mites, usually a skin infestation. See also mange; scabies.

acar'icide [Mod. L. acarus, a mite, fr. G. akari + L. caedo, to cut, kill] **1.** Destructive to acarids, or mites. **2.** An agent having this property.

Acar'idae A family (order Acarina) of exceptionally small mites, usually 0.5 mm or less, abundant in dried fruits and meats, grain, meal, and flour; frequently a cause of severe dermatitis among persons hypersensitized by frequent handling of infested products.

Acari'na [G. akari, a mite] An order of Arachnida that includes the mites and ticks.

ac'arine A member of the order Acarina.

Ac'arus [G. akari, mite] A genus of mites (family Acaridae).

   A. folliculo'rum, Demodex folliculorum.

   A. scabie'i, Sarcoptes scabiei.

   A. triti'ci, Pediculoides ventricosus.

acatalasae'mia Takahara's disease; hereditary absence or low levels of catalase in the blood, often manifest by recurrent infection or ulceration of the gums and related oral structures.

accel'erant Accelerator.

accel'erator [l. accelerans, pres. part. of ac-celero, to hasten, fr. celer, swift] **1.** Anything that increases rapidity of action or function. **2.** In physiology, a nerve, muscle, or substance that quickens movement or response. **3.** A catalytic agent used to hasten a chemical reaction.

acces'sory [L. accessorius] Supernumerary; auxiliary; denoting certain muscles, nerves, glands, etc.

acclima'tion, acclimatiza'tion Physiological adjustment of an individual to a different climate, especially to a change in environmental temperature or altitude.

accommoda'tion [L. ac-commodo, pp. -atus, to adapt, fr. modus, a measure] The act or state of adjustment or adaptation.

   negative a., adjustment of the lens for distant vision by relaxation of the ciliary muscles.

   positive a., a. for near vision by contraction of the ciliary muscles.

accre'tio cor'dis Adhesion of the pericardium to adjacent extracardiac structures.

accre′tion [L. *accretio*, fr. *ad*, to, + *crescere*, to grow] **1.** Increase by addition to the periphery of material of the same nature as that already present; *e.g.*, the manner of growth of crystals. **2.** In dentistry, foreign material (usually plaque or calculus) collecting on the surface of a tooth or in a cavity. **3.** A growing together.

aceph′aly [G. *a-* priv. + *kephalē*, head] Absence of a head.

acer′vuline [Mod. L. *acervulus*, a little heap] Occurring in clusters; aggregated.

acet-, aceto- Combining forms denoting the two-carbon fragment of acetic acid.

ac′etab′ulec′tomy [acetabulum + G. *ektomē*, excision] Excision of the acetabulum.

ac′etab′uloplas′ty [acetabulum + G. *plassō*, to fashion] Restorative surgery of the acetabulum.

acetab′ulum, gen. **acetab′uli,** pl. **acetab′ula** [L. a shallow vinegar vessel or cup] [NA] A cup-shaped depression on the external surface of the hip bone, in which the head of the femur fits.

acetamin′ophen   *N*-Acetyl-*p*-aminophenol; antipyretic and analgesic.

ac′etate (Ac)   A salt or ester of acetic acid.

ace′tic acid A characteristic component of vinegar; **diluted a. a.** contains 6% w/v of a. a.; **glacial a. a.** contains 99% absolute a. a.

aceto-   See acet-.

acetoace′tic acid   A ketone body formed in excess and appearing in the urine in starvation or diabetes.

acetonae′mia [acetone + G. *haima*, blood] Presence of acetone or ketone bodies in relatively large amounts in the blood.

ac′etone A compound with solvent properties, abnormal amounts of which occur in urine and blood of diabetics, sometimes imparting an ethereal odour to the urine and breath.

acetonu′ria [acetone + G. *ouron*, urine] Excretion in the urine of abnormal amounts of acetone, an indication of incomplete oxidation of large amounts of fat; commonly occurs in diabetic acidosis.

ac′etylcho′line (ACh) The acetic ester of choline, liberated from preganglionic and postganglionic endings of parasympathetic fibres and from preganglionic fibres of the sympathetic nervous system as a result of

nerve injuries, whereupon it acts as a neurotransmitter on the effector organ.

ac′etylsalicyl′ic acid   Aspirin.

achala′sia [G. *a-* priv. + *chalasis*, a slackening] Failure to relax; referring especially to visceral openings or sphincter muscles.

  oesophageal a., cardiospasm; loss of motor innervation causing an obstruction to develop in the terminal oesophagus just proximal to the cardio-oesophageal junction; the upper oesophagus becomes dilated and filled with retained food.

achei′ria, achi′ria [G. *a-* priv. + *cheir*, hand] **1.** Congenital absence of the hands. **2.** Anaesthesia in, with loss of the sense of possession of, one or both hands; a condition sometimes noted in hysteria.

achil′lobursi′tis Inflammation of a bursa beneath the tendo calcaneus.

achillor′rhaphy [Achilles (tendon) + G. *rhaphē*, a sewing] Suture of the tendo calcaneus.

achillot′omy [Achilles (tendon) + G. *tomē*, incision] Division of the tendo calcaneus.

achlorhy′dria [G. *a-* priv. + chlorhydric (acid)] Absence of hydrochloric acid from the gastric juice.

acho′lia [G. *a-* priv. + *cholē*, bile] Suppressed secretion of bile.

acholu′ria [G. *a-* priv. + *cholē*, bile, + *ouron*, urine] Absence of bile pigments from the urine in certain cases of jaundice.

acholu′ric   Without bile in the urine.

achondropla′sia [G. *a-* priv. + *chondros*, cartilage, + *plasis*, a moulding] An abnormality of conversion of cartilage into bone; a type of chondrodystrophy resulting in dwarfism apparent at birth, with short extremities but normal trunk; due to mutation or to autosomal dominant inheritance.

achondroplas′tic   Relating to achondroplasia.

achroma′sia [G. *achrōmos*, colourless] **1.** Pallor associated with the hippocratic facies of extremely severe and chronic illness. **2.** Achromia.

achromatop′sia [G. *a-* priv. + *chrōma*, colour, + *opsis*, vision] A severe congenital deficiency in colour perception, often associated with nystagmus and reduced visual acuity.

achro′mia [G. *a-* priv. + *chrōma*, colour] **1.** Deficiency of natural pigmentation, congenital or acquired. **2.** Lack of capacity to accept stains in cells or tissue.

achy'lia [G. a- priv. + chylos, juice] **1.** Absence of gastric juice or other digestive secretions. **2.** Absence of chyle.

achy'lous [G. achylos, without juice] **1.** Lacking in gastric juice or other digestive secretion. **2.** Having no chyle.

ac'id [L. acidus, sour] **1.** A compound yielding hydrogen ion in a polar solvent (e.g., in water); a.'s form salts by replacing all or part of the hydrogen with an electropositive element or radical. An a. containing one displaceable atom of hydrogen in the molecule is called **monobasic**; one containing two such atoms, **dibasic**; and one containing more than two, **polybasic**. **2.** Sour; sharp to the taste. For individual acids, see specific names.

acidae'mia [acid + G. haima, blood] An increase in the hydrogen ion concentration of the blood or a fall below normal in pH.

acid-fast Denoting bacteria that are not decolorized by acid-alcohol after having been stained.

acid'ify **1.** To render acid. **2.** To become acid.

acid'ity **1.** The state of being acid. **2.** The acid content of a fluid.

acido'sis [acid + G. -ōsis, condition] A state characterized by actual or relative decrease of alkali in body fluids in proportion to the acid content, the pH of body fluids may be normal or decreased.

　　diabetic a., decreased pH and bicarbonate concentration in the body fluids caused by accumulation of ketone bodies in diabetes mellitus.

　　renal tubular a., a clinical syndrome characterized by inability to excrete acid urine and by low plasma bicarbonate and high plasma chloride concentrations, often with hypokalaemia.

acid'ulous Acid or sour.

acidu'ria [acid + G. ouron, urine] **1.** Excretion of an acid urine. **2.** Excretion of an abnormal amount of any specified acid. Individual types of a. are listed by specific name.

ac'inar, acin'ic Pertaining to the acinus.

ac'inous Resembling an acinus or grape-shaped structure.

ac'inus, gen. and pl. **ac'ini** [L. berry, grape] [NA] One of the minute grape-shaped secre-tory portions of an acinous gland. See also alveolus.

ac'ne [probably a corruption (or copyist's error) of G. akmē, point of efflorescence] An inflammatory follicular, papular, and pustular eruption involving the sebaceous apparatus.

　　a. vulga'ris, an eruption, predominantly of the face, upper back, and chest, comprising comedones, cysts, papules, and pustules on an inflammatory base; occurs primarily during puberty and adolescence.

ac'neform, acne'iform Resembling acne.

acous'tic Relating to hearing or the perception of sound.

acous'tics [G. akoustikos, relating to hearing] The science concerned with sounds and their perception.

acquired' [L. ac-quiro (adq-), to obtain] Denoting a disease, predisposition, etc., that is not congenital but has developed after birth.

ac'rid [L. acer (acr-), pungent] Sharp; pungent; biting; irritating.

acrit'ical [G. a- priv. + kritikos, critical] **1.** Not critical; not marked by crisis. **2.** Indeterminate, especially concerning prognosis.

acro- [G. akron, extremity, akros, extreme] A combining form denoting extreme, extremity, tip, end, peak, topmost.

ac'roanaesthe'sia [acro- + G. an- priv. + aisthēsis sensation] Anaesthesia of one or more of the extremities.

acrocepha'lia Oxycephaly.

acrocephal'ic Oxycephalic.

acroceph'alopolysyndac'tyly Carpenter's syndrome; congenital malformation in which oxycephaly, brachysyndactyly of hand, and preaxial polydactyly of feet are associated with mental retardation.

acroceph'alosyndac'tyly [acrocephaly + G. syn, together, + daktylos, finger] A congenital syndrome characterized by peaked head, due to premature closure of skull sutures, associated with fusion or webbing of digits; autosomal dominant inheritance.

　　type I a., Apert's syndrome; a. with the second through fifth digits fused into one mass with a common nail; often accompanied by moderately severe acne vulgaris of the forearms; autosomal dominant inheritance.

　　type II a., Apert-Crouzon syndrome; a. with facial characteristics of Crouzon disease, with extremely hypoplastic maxilla; fusion of digits is less severe, with thumb and fifth finger usually separate; autosomal dominant inheritance.

acroceph'aly [acro- + G. *kephalē*, head] Oxycephaly.

acrocyano'sis [acro- + G. *kyanos*, blue, + -*osis*, condition] A circulatory disorder in which the hands, and less commonly the feet, are persistently cold, blue, and sweaty; milder forms are closely allied to chilblains.

ac'rocyanot'ic. Characterized by acrocyanosis.

ac'rodermati'tis [acro- + G. *derma*, skin, + -*itis*, inflammation] Inflammation of the skin of the extremities.

ac'rodermato'sis [acro- + G. *derma*, skin, + -*osis*, condition] Any cutaneous affection involving the more distal portions of the extremities.

acrodyn'ia [acro- + G. *odynē*, pain] **1.** A disease of infants caused almost exclusively by mercury poisoning and manifested by erythema of the extremities, chest, and nose, polyneuritis, and gastrointestinal symptoms. **2.** In adults, a syndrome comprising anorexia, photophobia, sweating, and tachycardia, associated with mercury ingestion.

ac'romegal'ic Pertaining to acromegaly.

acromeg'aly [acro- + G. *megas*, large] A disorder marked by progressive enlargement of the head and face, hands and feet, and thorax, due to excessive secretion of growth hormone by the anterior lobe of the pituitary gland.

acro'mioclavic'ular Relating to the acromion and the clavicle; denoting the articulation between the clavicle and the scapula and its ligaments.

acro'mion [G. *akrōmion*, fr. *akron*, tip, + *ōmos*, shoulder] [NA] The lateral end of the spine of the scapula which projects as a broad flattened process overhanging the glenoid fossa, articulates with the clavicle, and gives attachment to part of the deltoid and of the trapezius muscles.

ac'roparaesthe'sia [acro- + paraesthesia] **1.** Paraesthesia (numbness, tingling, and other abnormal sensations) of one or more of the extremities. **2.** An extreme degree of paraesthesia.

acrop'athy [acro- + G. *pathos*, disease] Hereditary clubbing of the digits without an associated progressive disease; autosomal dominant inheritance.

acropho'bia [acro- + G. *phobos*, fear] A morbid dread of heights.

acrosclero'sis Stiffness and tightness of the skin of the fingers, with atrophy of the soft tissue and osteoporosis of the distal phalanges of the hands and feet; a form of progressive systemic sclerosis occurring with Raynaud's phenomenon.

acrot'ic [G. *a*- priv. + *krotos*, a striking] Denoting acrotism.

ac'rotism [G. *a*- priv. + *krotos*, a striking] Absence or imperceptibility of the pulse.

ACTH Adrenocorticotropic *hormone*.

ac'tin One of the protein components into which actomyosin can be split; exists in a fibrous form (F-actin) or a globular form (G-actin).

actin'ic [G. *aktis* (*aktin*-), a ray] Relating to the chemically active rays of the electromagnetic spectrum.

actino- [G. *aktis* (*aktin*-), a ray, beam] A combining form meaning a ray, as of light; applied to any form of radiation or to any structure with radiating parts. See also *radio-*.

ac'tinodermati'tis [actino- + G. *derma*, skin, + -itis, inflammation] **1.** Inflammation of the skin produced by exposure to sunlight. **2.** Adverse reaction of skin to radiation therapy.

Ac'tinomy'ces [actino- + G. *mykēs*, fungus] A genus of nonmotile, nonsporeforming, anaerobic to facultatively anaerobic bacteria (family Actinomycetaceae); pathogenic for man and/or other animals; type species is *A. bovis.*

  A. bo'vis, a species causing actinomycosis in cattle.

  A. israe'lii, a species causing human actinomycosis and, occasionally, infections in cattle.

actinomycete A member of the genus *Actinomyces.*

actinomyce'cin A group of antibiotic agents isolated from several species of *Streptomyces* (originally *Actinomyces*) that are active against Gram-positive bacteria, fungi, and neoplasms.

ac'tinomyco'sis [actino- + G. *mykēs*, fungus, + -osis, condition] A disease primarily of cattle and man, caused by *Actinomyces bovis* in cattle and by *A. israelii* and *Arachnia propionica* in man, that produces chronic destructive abscesses or granulomas. In man, a. commonly affects the cervicofacial area, abdomen, or thorax; in cattle, the lesion is commonly found in the mandible.

ac'tinother'apy In dermatology, ultraviolet light therapy.

ac'tivator That which renders another substance active or that accelerates a process or reaction.

ac'tomy'osin A protein complex composed of the globulin myosin and actin in the micellae of the muscle fibre; the essential contractile substance of muscle.

acu'ity [thr. Fr. fr. L. *acuo*, pp. *acutus*, sharpen] Sharpness, clearness, distinctness, especially in vision.

acu'minate [L. *acumino*, pp. *-atus*, to sharpen] Pointed; tapering to a point.

ac'upuncture [L. *acus*, needle, + puncture] An Oriental procedure in which specific areas associated with peripheral nerves are pierced with fine needles to produce surgical anaesthesia, relieve pain, and promote therapy.

acute' [L. *acutus*, sharp] **1.** Of short and sharp course, not chronic; said of a disease. **2.** Sharp; pointed at the end.

acy'clovir A synthetic purine nucleoside analogue used as an antiviral agent in the treatment of genital herpes; the sodium salt is used for parenteral therapy.

ad- [L. *ad*, to] Prefix denoting increase, adherence, or motion toward, and sometimes with an intensive meaning.

-ad [L. *ad*, to] Suffix in anatomical nomenclature having the significance of the English ward; denoting toward or in the direction of.

adactyl'ia, adac'tylism Adactyly.

adac'tylous Without fingers or toes.

adac'tyly [G. *a-* priv. + *daktylos*, digit] Congenital absence of fingers or toes.

Ad'am's apple Laryngeal *prominence*.

adapta'tion [L. *ad-apto*, pp. *-atus*, to adjust] **1.** Acquisition of modifications fitting a plant or animal to life in a new environment or under new conditions. **2.** An advantageous change in function or constitution of an organ or tissue to meet new conditions. **3.** Adjustment of the pupil and retina to varying degrees of illumination. **4.** A property of certain receptors through which they become less responsive or cease to respond to repeated or continued stimuli the intensity of which is kept constant. **5.** The fitting, condensing, or contouring of a restorative material, foil, or shell to a tooth or cast so as to be in close contact.

dark a., scotopic a., the adjustment of the eye occurring under reduced illumination in which the sensitivity to light is greatly increased.

light a., photopic a., the adjustment of the eye occurring under increased illumination in which the sensitivity to light is reduced.

ad'dict A person who is habituated to a substance or practice, especially one considered harmful.

addic'tion [L. *ad-dico*, pp. *-dictus*, consent] Habitual psychological and physiological dependence on a substance or practice which is beyond voluntary control.

adduct' [L. *ad-duco*, pp. *-ductus*, to bring toward] To draw toward the median line.

adduc'tion **1.** Movement of a limb toward the median line, or beyond it. **2.** Monocular rotation (duction) of the eye toward the nose. **3.** A position resulting from such movement.

adduc'tor A muscle that draws a part toward the median line.

aden- See adeno-.

adenec'tomy [aden- + G. *ektomē*, excision] Excision of a gland.

aden'iform Adenoid (1).

ad'enine A major purine found in both RNA and DNA, and also in various free nucleotides of importance to the body.

adeni'tis [aden- + *-itis*, inflammation] Inflammation of a lymph node or of a gland.

adeno-, aden- [G. *aden*, gland] Combining forms denoting relation to a gland.

ad'enocarcino'ma A malignant neoplasm of epithelial cells in glandular or glandlike pattern.

acinic cell a., an a. arising from secreting cells of a racemose gland, particularly the salivary glands.

papillary a., an a. containing finger-like processes of vascular connective tissue covered by neoplastic epithelium, projecting into cysts or the cavity of glands or follicles.

ad'enocyte [adeno- + G. *kytos*, a hollow (cell)] A gland cell.

ad'enofibro'ma A benign neoplasm composed of glandular and fibrous tissues.

ad'enoid [adeno- + G. *eidos*, appearance] **1.** Glandlike; of glandular appearance. **2.** See adenoids.

ad'enoidec'tomy [adenoid + G. *ek-tomē*, excision] Surgical removal of adenoid growths in the nasopharynx.

ad'enoidi'tis Inflammation of nasopharyngeal lymphoid tissue.

ad'enoids Hypertrophy of the pharyngeal tonsil resulting from chronic inflammation.

ad'enolympho'ma A benign glandular tumour usually arising in the parotid gland and composed of two rows of eosinophilic epithelial cells, which are often cystic and papillary, together with a lymphoid stroma.

adeno'ma [adeno- + G. *-oma*, tumour] An ordinarily benign neoplasm of epithelial tissue in which the tumour cells form glands or glandlike structures in the stroma.

adeno'matoid Resembling an adenoma.

adenop'athy [adeno- + G. *pathos*, suffering] Swelling of or abnormal enlargement in the lymph nodes.

ad'enosarco'ma A malignant neoplasm arising simultaneously or consecutively in mesodermal tissue and glandular epithelium of the same part.

aden'osine (A, Ado) A condensation product of adenine and D-ribose; a nucleoside found among the hydrolysis products of all nucleic acids and of the various adenine nucleotides.

adenosine diphosphate (ADP) A condensation product of adenosine with pyrophosphoric acid; formed from ATP by the hydrolysis of the terminal phosphate group of the latter compound.

adenosine triphosphate (ATP) Immediate precursors of adenine nucleotides in RNA.

adeno'sis Any generalized glandular disease.

   sclerosing a., A nodular benign breast lesion occurring most frequently in relatively young women and consisting of hyperplastic distorted lobules of acinar tissue with increased collagenous stroma.

adenot'omy [adeno- + G. *tomē*, a cutting] Incision of a gland.

ad'enotonsillec'tomy Operative removal of tonsils and adenoids.

Ad'enovir'idae A family of double-stranded DNA-containing viruses, of which there are more than 80 antigenic types (species); it develops in nuclei of infected cells and causes diseases of the respiratory tract and conjunctiva.

ad'enovi'rus [G. *adēn*, gland, + virus] Any virus of the family Adenoviridae.

adhe'sion [L. *adhesio*, to stick to] **1.** The process of adhering or uniting of two surfaces or parts, especially the union of the opposing surfaces of a wound. **2.** In the plural, inflammatory bands that connect opposing serous surfaces.

   primary a., *healing* by first intention.

   secondary a., *healing* by second intention.

adhe'sive 1. Relating to, or having the characteristics of, an adhesion. **2.** Any material that adheres to a surface or causes adherence between surfaces.

a'diaphore'sis [G. a- priv. + *diaphorēsis*, perspiration] Anhidrosis.

a'diaphoret'ic Anhidrotic.

adip-, adipo- [L. *adeps*, fat] Combining form relating to fat.

ad'ipocele [adipo- + G. *kēlē*, tumour] Lipocele.

ad'ipocere [adipo- + G. *cera*, wax] A fatty substance of waxy consistency into which dead animal tissues are sometimes converted.

ad'ipoid [adipo- + G. *eidos*, resemblance] Lipoid.

ad'ipose Fatty; relating to fat.

adipo'sis [adipo- + G. *-osis*, condition] An excessive local or general accumulation of fat in the body.

   a. cardia'ca, fatty *heart* (2).

   a. doloro'sa, a condition characterized by a deposit of symmetrical nodular or pendulous masses of fat in various regions of the body, with discomfort or pain.

adipos'ity Obesity.

ad'iposu'ria [adipo- + G. *ouron*, urine] Lipuria.

ad'itus, pl. **ad'itus** [L. access, fr. *ad-eo*, pp. *-itus*, go to] [NA] An entrance to a cavity or channel.

ad'juvant [L. *ad-juvo*, to give aid to] **1.** A substance added to a drug product formulation which affects the action of the active ingredient in a predictable way. **2.** In immunology, a vehicle used to enhance antigenicity; *e.g.*, a suspension of minerals on which antigen is adsorbed; or water-in-oil emulsion in which antigen solution is emulsified in mineral oil (Freund's incomplete a.), sometimes with the inclusion of killed mycobacteria

(Freund's complete a.) to further enhance antigenicity.

adnex'a, sing. **adnex'um** [L. connected parts, appendages] Appendages; parts accessory to the main organ or structure.

adoles'cence [L. *adolescentia*] Period between puberty and attaining complete growth and maturity.

ado'ral [L. *ad*, to, + *os* (*or*-), mouth] Near or directed toward the mouth.

adren-, adrenal-, adreno- [L. *ad*, toward, + *ren*, kidney] Combining forms relating to the adrenal gland.

adre'nal [L. *ad*, to, + *ren*, kidney] **1.** Near or upon the kidney. **2.** An adrenal gland or separate tissue thereof.

adre'nalec'tomy [adrenal + G. *ektomē*, excision] Removal of one or both adrenal glands.

adren'aline Epinephrine; a catecholamine neurohormone of the adrenal medulla that is the most potent stimulant (sympathomimetic) of adrenergic α- and β- receptors, resulting in increased heart rate and force of contraction, vasoconstriction or vasodilation, relaxation of bronchiolar and intestinal smooth muscle, glycogenolysis, lipolysis, and other metabolic effects.

adrener'gic [adren- + G. *ergon*, work] **1.** Relating to nerve cells or fibres of the autonomic nervous system that employ adrenaline as their neurotransmitter. **2.** Relating to drugs that mimic the actions of the sympathetic nervous system.

adreno- See adren-.

adre'nocor'tical Pertaining to adrenal cortex.

adre'nocorticotro'pic, adre'nocorticotro'phic [adrenal cortex + G. *trophē*, nurture; *tropē*, a turning] Affecting growth or activity of adrenal cortex.

adre'nocorticotro'pin, adre'nocorticotro'phin Adrenocorticotropic *hormone*.

adrenolyt'ic [adreno- + G. *lysis*, loosening, dissolution] Denoting antagonism to or inhibition of the action of adrenaline, noradrenaline, and related sympathomimetics.

adrenomeg'aly [adreno- + G. *megas*, big] Enlargement of the adrenal glands.

adsorb' [L. *ad*, to, + *sorbeo*, to suck in] To take up by adsorption.

adsor'bent **1.** A substance that adsorbs. **2.** In pharmacology, a substance endowed

with the property of attaching other substances to its surface without any chemical action.

adsorp'tion [L. *ad*, to, + *sorbeo*, to suck up] The property of a substance to attract and hold to its surface a gas, liquid or a substance in solution or in suspension.

adter'minal In a direction toward the nerve endings, muscular insertions, or the extremity of any structure.

adul'tera'tion. The alteration of any substance by the deliberate addition of a component not ordinarily part of that substance; usually used to imply that the substance is debased as a result.

advance'ment A surgical procedure in which a tendinous insertion or a skin flap is severed from its attachment and sutured to a point farther forward.

adventi'tia [L. *adventicius*, coming from abroad, foreign] The outermost covering of any organ or structure which is properly derived from without and does not form an integral part of such organ or structure; specifically, the outer coat of an artery.

adventi'tial Relating to the adventitia of an organ or structure.

Aё'des [G. *aēdēs*, unpleasant, unfriendly] A widespread genus of small mosquitoes frequently found in tropical and subtropical regions; includes **A. aegyp'ti,** the yellow fever mosquito, a species that is also the vector of dengue viruses.

-aemia [G. *haima*, blood] Suffix meaning blood.

aer-, aero- [G. *aēr* (L. *aer*), air] Combining form denoting relationship to air or gas.

aera'tion **1.** Airing. **2.** Saturating a fluid with air or other gas. **3.** The change of venous into arterial blood in the lungs.

aer'obe [aero- + G. *bios*, life] **1.** An organism that can live and grow in the presence of free oxygen. **2.** An organism that can use oxygen as a final electron acceptor in a respiratory chain.

   obligate a., one that cannot live or grow in the absence of free oxygen.

aero'bic **1.** Relating to an aerobe. **2.** Living in air.

aeropha'gia, aeroph'agy [aero- + G. *phagein*, to eat] The excessive swallowing of air.

aer'osinusi'tis Inflammation of the paranasal sinuses caused by a difference in pressure within the sinus relative to ambient pressure, secondary to obstruction of the sinus orifice.

aer'osol 1. A liquid agent or solution dispersed in air in the form of a fine mist for therapeutic, insecticidal, and other purposes. **2.** A product packaged under pressure and containing therapeutically active ingredients intended for topical application and for introduction into body orifices.

aeroti'tis me'dia [aero- + G. *ous*, ear, + suffix *-itis*, inflammation] An acute or chronic traumatic inflammation of the middle ear caused by a reduction in pressure in the air in the tympanic cavity relative to ambient pressure, secondary to eustachian tube obstruction.

aescula'pian [L. *Aesculapius*, G. *Asklēpios*, the god of medicine] Relating to Aesculapius, the art of medicine, or a medical practitioner.

aesthesio- [G. *aesthēsis*, sensation] Combining form relating to sensation or perception.

aesthesiom'eter [aesthesio- + G. *metron*, measure] An instrument for determining the state of tactile and other forms of sensibility.

aesthe'sioneuro'sis Any sensory neurosis; *e.g.*, anaesthesia, hyperaesthesia, paraesthesia.

aes'tival [L. *aestivus*, summer (adj.)] Relating to or occurring in the summer.

aetiolog'ic Relating to aetiology.

aetiol'ogy [G. *aitia*, cause, + *logos*, treatise, discourse] The science and study of the causes of disease and their mode of operation.

afeb'rile Apyretic.

affect' [L. *affectus*, state of mind] Emotional feeling tone and mood attached to a thought, including its external manifestations.

affec'tion 1. Feeling; love. **2.** A disease; an abnormal condition of body or mind.

af'ferent [L. *afferens*, fr. *af-fero*, to bring to] Toward a centre, denoting certain arteries, veins, lymphatics, and nerves.

affin'ity [L. *affinis*, neighbouring] **1.** In chemistry, the force that impels certain atoms to unite with certain others to form compounds. **2.** The selective staining of a tissue by a dye or the uptake of a dye, chemical, or other substance selectively by a tissue.

afibrin'ogenae'mia The absence of fibrinogen in the plasma.

    congenital a., a rare disorder of blood coagulation in which little or no fibrinogen can be found in plasma; autosomal recessive inheritance.

af'terbirth The placenta and membranes that are extruded from the uterus after birth.

af'terimage Persistence of the image after the object has disappeared or the eyes are closed.

af'terpains Painful cramplike contractions of the uterus occurring after childbirth.

af'tertaste A taste persisting after contact of the tongue with the substance has ceased.

agalac'tia [G. a- priv. + *gala* (*galakt-*), milk] Absence of milk in the breasts after childbirth.

agam'maglob'ulinae'mia Absence of, or extremely low levels of, the gamma fraction of serum globulin; sometimes used loosely to denote absence of immunoglobulins in general.

a'gar [Bengalese] A polysaccharide, derived from various red algae, used as a solidifying agent in culture media.

age [F. *âge*, L. *aetas*] **1.** The period that has elapsed since the birth of a living being. **2.** To grow old; to gradually develop changes in structure which are not due to preventable disease or trauma and which are associated with an increased probability of death.

agen'esis [G. a- priv. + *genesis*, production] Absence, failure of formation, or imperfect development of any part.

a'gent [L. *ago*, pres. p. *agens* (*agent-*), to perform] An active force or substance capable of producing an effect.

    antianxiety a., a functional category of drugs useful in the treatment of anxiety and able to reduce anxiety at doses that do not cause excessive sedation.

    antipsychotic a., a functional category of neuroleptic drugs that are helpful in the treatment of psychosis and have a capacity to ameliorate thought disorder.

    blocking a., a drug that blocks transmission at an autonomic receptor site, autonomic synapse, or neuromuscular junction.

    Eaton a., *Mycoplasma pneumoniae.*

    promoting a., an a., by itself noncarcinogenic, that enhances tumour production in a tissue previously exposed to sub-carcinogenic doses of a carcinogen (the latter then is called an initiating a.).

ageu'sia [G. *a*- priv. + *geusis*, taste] Loss of the sense of taste.

agglutina'tion [L. *ad*, to, + *gluten*, glue] **1.** The process by which suspended bacteria, cells, or other particles of similar size are caused to adhere and form into clumps. **2.** Adhesion of the surfaces of a wound.

 cold a., a. of red blood cells by their own serum or by any other serum when the blood is cooled below body temperature.

 group a., a. by antibodies specific for minor (group) antigens common to several bacteria, each of which possesses its own major specific antigen.

agglu'tinin 1. An antibody that causes clumping or agglutination of the bacteria or other cells which either stimulated the formation of the a., or contain immunologically similar, reactive antigen. **2.** A substance, other than a specific agglutinating antibody, that causes organic particles to agglutinate.

 saline a., an anti-Rh antibody that causes agglutination of Rh+ erythrocytes when they are suspended either in saline or in a protein medium.

 serum a., an anti-Rh antibody which coats Rh+ erythrocytes; the cells do not agglutinate when suspended in saline, but do agglutinate when suspended in serum or other protein media.

agglutin'ogen [agglutinin + G. *-gen*, production] An antigenic substance that stimulates the formation of specific agglutinin.

ag'gregate [L. *ag-grego*, pp. *-atus*, to add to] **1.** To collect together in a mass or cluster. **2.** The total of individual units making up a mass or cluster.

aggres'sion A domineering, forceful, or assaultive verbal or physical action toward another person as the motor component of the affects of anger, hostility, or rage.

ag'ing 1. The process of growing old, especially by failure of replacement of cells in sufficient number to maintain function. **2.** The gradual deterioration of a mature organism resulting from time-dependent, irreversible changes in structure that are intrinsic to the particular species, and which eventually lead to decreased ability to cope with the stresses of the environment, thereby increasing the probability of death.

aglos'sia [G. *a*- priv. + *glossa*, tongue] Congenital absence of the tongue.

agluti'tion Dysphagia.

agna'thia [G. *a*- priv. + *gnathos*, jaw] Congenital absence of the lower jaw, usually accompanied by approximation of the ears.

agna'thous Relating to agnathia.

agno'sia [G. ignorance; from a- priv. + *gnōsis*, knowledge] Lack of sensory-perceptual ability to recognize impressions from one or more of the senses.

-agogue, -agog [G. *agōgos*, leading forth] Suffix indicating a promoter or stimulant of.

ag'onist [G. *agōn*, a contest] **1.** Denoting a muscle in a state of contraction, with reference to its opposing muscle, or antagonist. **2.** A drug capable of combining with receptors to initiate drug actions; possesses affinity and intrinsic activity.

ag'orapho'bia [G. *agora*, marketplace, + *phobos*, fear] An irrational fear of leaving the familiar setting of home.

-agra [G. *agra*, a seizure] Suffix meaning sudden onslaught of acute pain.

agran'ulocyte [G. *a*- priv. + L. *granulum*, granule, + G. *kytos*, cell] A nongranular leucocyte.

agran'ulocyto'sis An acute condition characterized by pronounced leucopenia with great reduction in the number of polymorphonuclear leucocytes; infected ulcers are likely to develop in mucous membranes and in the skin.

agraph'ia [G. *a*- priv. + *graphō*, to write] Loss of the ability to write or express thoughts in writing.

a'gue [Fr. *aigu*, acute] **1.** Archaic term for malarial fever. **2.** A chill.

AIDS Acquired immunodeficiency syndrome; a disease that compromises the competency of the immune system, characterized by persistent lymphadenopathy and various opportunistic infections, such as *Pneumocystis carnii* pneumonia, cytomegalovirus, disseminated histoplasmosis, candidiasis, and isosporiasis, and malignancies such as Kaposi's sarcoma; the aetiologic agent is HIV, transmissible by body fluids such as blood and semen.

air [G. *aēr*; L. *aer*] The atmosphere, a mixture of gases in the following approximate percentages by volume after water vapour has been removed: oxygen, 20.94; nitrogen, 78.03;

argon and other rare gases, 0.99; carbon dioxide, 0.04. Formerly used to mean any respiratory gas, regardless of its composition.

air'way **1.** Any part of the respiratory tract through which air passes during breathing. **2.** In anaesthesia or resuscitation, a device for correcting obstruction to breathing.

akar'yocyte [G. a- priv. + *karyon*, kernel, + *kytos*, a hollow (cell)] A cell without a nucleus (karyon), such as the erythrocyte.

akinaesthe'sia [G. a- priv. + *kinēsis*, motion, + *aisthēsis*, sensation] Absence of the sense of perception of movement; absence of the muscular sense.

akine'sia, akine'sis [G. a- priv. + *kinēsis*, movement] **1.** Absence or loss of the power of voluntary motion. **2.** The postsystolic interval of rest of the heart.

akinet'ic Relating to or suffering from akinesia.

a'la, gen. and pl. **a'lae** [L. wing] [NA] Any winglike or expanded structure.

ala'lia [G. a- priv. + *lalia*, talking] Loss of the power of speech through impairment in the articulatory apparatus.

al'anine (Ala) One of the amino acids occurring widely in proteins.

a'lar **1.** Relating to a wing; winged. **2.** Axillary. **3.** Relating to the ala of such structures as the nose, sphenoid, sacrum.

al'ba [fem. of L. *albus*, white] **1.** White. **2.** *Substantia* alba.

al'binism [L. *albus*, white] Congenital leucoderma or leucopathia; an inherited deficiency or absence of pigment in the skin, hair, and eyes, or eyes only, due to tyrosene abnormality in production of melanin.

albi'no [L. *albus*, white] An individual with albinism.

albu'men [L. the white of egg] Egg *albumin.*

albu'min [L. *albumen* (-*min*-), the white of egg] A type of simple protein widely distributed throughout the tissues and fluids of plants and animals.

  blood a., serum a.

  egg a., albumen; the chief protein occurring in the white of egg, resembling in many respects serum a.

  serum a. the a. present in the blood plasma and in serous fluids; the principal protein in plasma.

albu'minu'ria [albumin + G. *ouron*, urine] The presence of protein in urine, chiefly

albumin but also globulin; usually indicative of disease, but sometimes resulting from a temporary or transient dysfunction, in contrast to a truly pathologic condition.

al'cohol [Ar. *al*, the, + *kohl*, fine antimonial powder, the term being applied first to a fine powder, then, to anything impalpable (spirit)] **1.** One of a series of organic chemical compounds in which a hydrogen (H) attached to carbon is replaced by a hydroxyl (OH). **2.** Ethanol; ethyl alcohol; CH_3CH_2OH; a liquid containing 92.3% by weight, corresponding to 94.9% by volume, at 15.56°, of C_2H_5OH. It has been used in beverages and as a solvent, vehicle, and preservative; externally as a rubefacient, coolant, and disinfectant.

  denatured a., ethyl a. rendered unfit for consumption as a beverage by the addition of one or several chemicals; used in industry.

alcohol'ic **1.** Relating to, containing, or produced by alcohol. **2.** A person addicted to the use of a. beverages in excess.

al'coholism Chronic heavy drinking or intoxication resulting in impairment of health, dependency as a coping mechanism, and increased adaptation to the effects of alcohol requiring increasing doses to achieve and sustain a desired effect.

  acute a., a temporary mental disturbance with muscular incoordination and paresis, induced by the ingestion of alcoholic beverages in toxic amounts.

  chronic a., a pathologic condition, affecting chiefly the nervous and gastroenteric systems, caused by the habitual use of alcoholic beverages in toxic amounts.

al'dehyde A compound containing the radical $-CH=O$, reducible to an alcohol (CH_2OH), oxidizable to an acid (COOH); *e.g.,* acetaldehyde.

aldos'terone A steroid hormone produced by the adrenal cortex; its major action is to facilitate potassium exchange for sodium in the distal renal tubule, causing sodium reabsorption and potassium and hydrogen loss.

aldos'teronism A disorder caused by excessive secretion of aldosterone.

  primary a., Conn's syndrome; an arenocortical disorder caused by excessive secretion of aldosterone and characterized by headaches, nocturia, polyuria, fatigue, hypertension, hypokalaemic alkalosis, potassium depletion, hypervolaemia, and decreased plasma renin activity; may be associated with small benign adrenocortical adenomas.

secondary a., pathological a resulting not from a defect intrinsic to the adrenal cortex but from a stimulation of secretion caused by extra-adrenal disorders; it is associated with increased plasma renin activity and occurs in heart failure, nephrotic syndrome, cirrhosis, and hypoproteinaemia.

aleukae'mia [G. a- priv. + *leukos*, white, + *haima*, blood] **1.** Literally, a lack of leucocytes in the blood. Generally used to indicate varieties of leukaemic disease in which the white blood cell count in circulating blood is normal or even less than normal (*i.e.*, no leucocytosis), but a few young leucocytes are observed; sometimes used more restrictedly for unusual instances of leukaemia with no leucocytosis and no young forms in the blood. **2.** Leukaemic changes in bone marrow associated with a subnormal number of leucocytes in the blood.

al'gae [pl. of L. *alga*, seaweed] A division of cellular cryptogamous plants, including seaweeds.

algaesthe'sia [G. *algos*, pain, + *aisthēsis*, sensation] **1.** The appreciation of pain. **2.** Hypersensitivity to pain.

aige-, aigesi-, aigo- [G. *algos*, pain] Combining forms meaning pain.

alge'sia [G. *algēsis*, a sense of pain] Algaesthesia.

alge'sic Algetic.

algesiom'eter [G. *algēsis*, sense of pain, + *-metron*, measure] An instrument for measuring the degree of sensitivity to a painful stimulus.

alget'ic 1. Painful, or relating to or causing pain. **2.** Relating to hypersensitivity to pain.

-algia [G. *algos*, pain] Suffix meaning pain or painful condition.

algo- See alge-.

al'gorithm The written steps in protocol for management of health care problems.

aliena'tion [L. *alleno*, pp. -*atus*, to make strange] A condition characterized by lack of meaningful relationships to others and sometimes resulting in depersonalization and estrangement from others.

alimen'tary [L. *alimentarius*, fr. *alimentum*, nourishment] Relating to food or nutrition, or to the organs of digestion.

alimenta'tion Providing of nourishment.

alina'sal [L. *ala*, + *nasus*, nose] Relating to the alae nasi, or flaring portions of the nostrils.

al'iquot In chemistry and immunology, pertaining to a portion of the whole; loosely, any one of two or more samples of something, of the same volume or weight.

alisphe'noid [L. *ala*, + *sphēn*, wedge] Relating to the greater wing of the sphenoid bone.

alkalae'mia [alkali + G. *haima*, blood] A decrease in H-ion concentration of the blood or a rise in pH, irrespective of alterations in the level of bicarbonate ion.

al'kali, pl. **al'kalis** or **al'kalies** [Ar., *al*, the, + *qalīy*, soda ash] A strongly basic substance yielding hydroxide ions (OH-) in solution; *e.g.*, sodium hydroxide, potassium hydroxide.

al'kaline Relating to or having the reaction of an alkali.

alkalin'ity The condition of being alkaline.

al'kaloid Any one of hundreds of plant products distinguished by basic reactions, now restricted to heterocyclic nitrogen-containing and often complex structures possessing pharmacological activity; *e.g.*, atropine, nicotine, caffeine, cocaine. For medicinal purposes the salts of a.'s are usually used.

alkalo'sis A pathophysiological disorder characterized by H ion loss or base excess in body fluids (metabolic a.), or caused by CO_2 loss due to hyperventilation (respiratory a.).

alkap'tonu'ria [alkapton + G. *ouron*, urine] The excretion of homogentisic acid (alkapton) in the urine due to an inherited disorder of phenylalanine and tyrosine metabolism; the urine turns dark if allowed to stand or if an alkali is added; autosomal recessive inheritance.

al'kyl 1. A hydrocarbon radical of the general formula C_nH_{2n+1}. **2.** A compound, such as tetraethyl lead, in which a metal is combined with alkyl radicals.

al'kylation Substitution of an alkyl radical for a hydrogen atom.

al'lachaesthe'sia [G. *allachē*, elsewhere, + *aisthēsis*, sensation] A condition in which a sensation is referred to a point other than that to which the stimulus is applied.

allaesthe'sia [G. *allos*, other, + *aisthēsis*, sensation] Allachaesthesia in which the sensation of a stimulus in one limb is referred to the opposite limb.

allanto-, allant- [G. *allas*, sausage] Combining forms for allantois.

allanto'ic Relating to the allantois.

allanto'is [allanto- + G. *eidos*, appearance] In man, a vestigial fetal membrane developing from the yolk sac.

allele' [G. *allelōn*, reciprocally] Any one of a series of two or more different genes that may occupy the same position or locus on a specific chromosome.

alle'lomorph [G. *allelōn*, reciprocally, + *morphē*, shape] Allele.

al'lergen [allergy + G. *-gen*, producing] Antigen.

allergen'ic Antigenic.

aller'gic Relating to any response stimulated by an allergen (antigen).

al'lergist One who specializes in the treatment of allergies.

al'lergy [G. *allos*, other, + *ergon*, work] **1.** Acquired (induced) sensitivity; the immunologic state induced in a susceptible subject by an antigen (allergen), characterized by a marked change in reactivity. On the subject's initial contact with it, the antigen is seemingly inert immunologically, but after a latent period the subject becomes sensitive, even to antigen that persists from the initial inoculation, and thereafter, the specific antigen evokes a reaction within minutes or hours, the severity of which depends upon quantitative relationships and route of entrance of antigen. **2.** An acquired hypersensitivity to certain drugs and biologic preparations.

allo- [G. *allos*, other] Prefix meaning "other," differing from the normal or usual.

allobar'bital A sedative and hypnotic.

allocor'tex [allo- + L. *cortex*, bark (cortex)] See *cortex* cerebri.

al'logene'ic, al'logen'ic Pertaining to different gene constitutions within the same species, in contradistinction to isogeneic and heterogeneic.

al'lograft A graft from an allogeneic donor of the same species as the recipient.

alloker'atoplasty The replacement of opaque corneal tissue with a transparent prosthesis, usually acrylic.

al'loplast [allo- + G. *plastos*, formed] **1.** A graft of an inert metal or plastic material. **2.** An inert foreign body used for implantation into tissues.

al'losome [allo- + G. *sōma*, body] One of the chromosomes differing in appearance or behaviour from the ordinary chromosomes, or autosomes, and sometimes unequally distributed among the germ cells.

al'lotransplanta'tion Removal of tissue from one individual and grafting it into another of the same species.

al'oe Dried juice from the leaves of plants of the genus *Aloe* (family Liliaceae), from which are derived various pharmaceutical preparations.

alope'cia [G. *alōpekia*, a disease like fox mange] Baldness; loss of hair.

   a. area'ta, a. of unknown aetiology characterized by circumscribed, noninflamed areas of baldness on the scalp, eyebrows, and bearded portion of the face.

   cicatricial a., a. cicatrisa'ta, a. produced by scar formation as in certain dermatoses.

   a. heredita'ria, male pattern a., a. resulting from sex-influenced dominant inheritance, with androgen stimulation required to produce hair loss in heterozygous individuals; homozygous females may have minor hair loss without androgen stimulation.

   a. medicamento'sa, diffuse hair loss, most notably of the scalp, caused by administration of various types of drugs.

Al'phavirus A genus of viruses (family Togaviridae) formerly classified as group A arboviruses.

al'ternans [L.] Alternating; often used substantively for alternation of the heart.

al'um A double sulphate of aluminum and of an alkaline earth element or ammonium, markedly astringent and used as a styptic.

alumin'ium [L. *alumen*, alum] A metallic element; symbol Al, atomic no. 13, atomic weight 26.98; in various compounds, used as an astringent, antiperspirant, antiseptic, and antipyretic.

alveoal'gia [alveolus + G. *algos*, pain] Dry socket; sequela to tooth extractions in which the blood clot in the socket disintegrates, leading to an empty socket that becomes secondarily infected.

alveolal'gia Alveoalgia.

alve'olar Relating to an alveolus.

alve'oli Plural of alveolus.

alveoli'tis **1.** Inflammation of alveoli. **2.** Inflammation of a tooth socket (alveolus dentalis).

   acute pulmonary a., acute inflammation involving the pulmonary alveoli, which may result in necrosis with haemorrhage into the lungs; may be associated with glomerulonephritis, in Goodpasture's syndrome.

extrinsic allergic a., pneumoconiosis resulting from hypersensitivity due to repeated inhalation of organic dust, usually specified according to occupational exposure.

alveolo- [L. *alveolus, q.v.*] Combining form denoting relation to an alveolus or to the alveolar process.

alve'oloplas'ty [alveolo- + G. *plassō*, to form] Surgical preparation of the alveolar ridges for the reception of dentures; shaping and smoothing of socket margins after extraction of teeth with subsequent suturing to insure optimal healing.

alve'olus, gen. and pl. **alve'oli** [L. dim. of *alveus*, trough, a hollow sac, cavity] [NA] A small cell or cavity; a sac-like dilation.

a. denta'lis [NA], tooth socket; a socket in the alveolar process of the maxilla or mandible, into which each tooth fits and is attached by means of the periodontal membrane.

a. pulmo'nis [NA], pulmonary alveoli; terminal dilations of the bronchioles where gas exchange is thought to occur.

amal'gam [G. *malagma*, a soft mass] An alloy of an element or a metal with mercury. In dentistry, primarily of two types: silver-tin alloy, containing small amounts of copper and zinc, and a second type containing more copper (12 to 30% by weight); used for filling teeth and making dies.

Amani'ta [G. *amanitai*, fungi] A genus of fungi, many members of which are highly poisonous.

A. musca'ria, a toxic species of mushroom that contains muscarine, which produces psychosis-like states and other symptoms caused by muscarine.

A. phalloi'des, a species of mushroom containing poisonous principles including phalloidine and amanitin, which cause gastroenteritis, hepatic necrosis, and renal necrosis.

amas'tia [G. *a-* priv. + *mastos*, breast] Congenital absence of one or both breasts.

amauro'sis [G. *amauros*, dark, obscure, + *-osis*, condition] Blindness, especially that occurring without apparent change in the eye itself; *e.g.*, from a cortical lesion.

a. congeni'ta of Leber, an autosomal recessive cone-rod abiotrophy causing blindness or severely reduced vision at birth, frequently with keratoconus.

a. fu'gax, a temporary blindness that may result from a transient ischaemia due to carotid artery insufficiency or to centrifugal force.

amaurot'ic Relating to or suffering from amaurosis.

ama'zia Amastia.

ambi- [L. *ambo*, both] Prefix meaning round; all (both) sides.

ambidex'trous [ambi- + L. *dexter*, right] Having equal facility in the use of both hands.

ambly- [G. *amblys*, dull] Combining form denoting dullness, dimness.

Amblyom'ma [ambly- + G. *omma*, eye, vision] A genus of ornate, hard ticks (family Ixodidae). *A. americanum*, the Lone-Star tick, and *A. cajennense* are important pests and vectors of Rocky Mountain spotted fever.

amblyo'pia [G. *amblyōpia*, dimness of vision, fr. *amblys* dull, + *ōps*, eye] Dimness of vision; partial loss of sight.

am'blyoscope [amblyopia + G. *skopeō*, to view] A reflecting stereoscope used for measuring or training binocular vision, and for stimulation of vision in the amblyopic eye.

ambo- [G. *ambo*, both] Prefix meaning round; all (both) sides.

am'bulant Ambulatory.

am'bulatory [L. *ambulo*, p.p. *-atus*, to walk] Walking about or able to walk about; not confined to bed.

amel'ia [G. *a-* priv. + *melos*, a limb] Congenital absence of one or more limbs.

am'elogen'esis The production and development of enamel.

a. imperfec'ta, a group of hereditary defects characterized by faulty metabolism in either of two steps of enamel formation: defective matrix formation leads to enamel hypoplasia; defective maturation leads to enamel hypocalcification.

amenorrhoe'a [G. *a-* priv. + *mēn*, month, + *rhoia*, flow] Absence or abnormal cessation of the menses.

primary a., a. in which the menses have never occurred.

secondary a., any a. in which the menses appeared at puberty but have been suppressed.

amen'tia   [L. madness, fr. *ab*, from, + *mens*, mind] **1.** Mental *retardation*. **2.** Dementia.

ame'tria   [G. a- priv. + *mētra*, uterus] Congenital absence of the uterus.

ametro'pia   [G. *ametros*, disproportionate, fr. a- priv. + *metron*, measure, + *ōps*, eye] A condition in which there is some error of refraction in consequence of which parallel rays, with the eye at rest, are not focused on the retina.

am'inate   To combine with ammonia.

am'ine   A substance that may be derived from ammonia by the replacement of one or more of the hydrogen atoms by hydrocarbon or other radicals.

amino-   A prefix denoting a compound containing the amino group, $-NH_2$.

ami'no ac'id (AA)   An organic acid in which one of the CH hydrogen atoms has been replaced by NH_2.

    essential a. a.'s, α-amino acids required by animals that must be supplied in the diet (*i.e.*, cannot be synthesized by the animal) either as free a. acids or in proteins.

ami'noacidae'mia   [amino acid + G. *haima*, blood] Excessive amounts of specific amino acids in the blood.

ami'noacidu'ria   [amino acid + G. *ouron*, urine] Excretion of amino acids in urine, especially in excessive amounts.

p-am'inobenzo'ic acid (PABA)   A factor (vitamin B_x) in the vitamin B complex, a part of all folic acids and required for its formation; neutralizes the bacteriostatic effects of the sulphonamides.

p-aminosalicylic acid (PAS, PASA)   A bacteriostatic agent against tubercle bacilli, used as an adjunct to streptomycin.

am'inotrans'ferases   Transaminases; enzymes transferring amino groups between an α-amino acid to (usually) a 2-keto acid.

amito'sis   [G. a- priv. + mitosis] Direct division of the nucleus and cell, without the complicated changes in the former that occur in the ordinary process of cell reproduction.

ammo'nia   A volatile gas, NH_3, very soluble in water, forming the base, NH_4OH, combining with acids to form ammonium compounds.

ammonio-   Combining form indicating an ammonium group.

ammo'nium   The radical, $NH_4{}^+$, formed by combination NH_3 and H^+; behaves as a univalent metal in forming ammonium compounds.

amne'sia   [G. *amnēsia*, forgetfulness] Disturbance in memory of information stored in long term memory, in contrast to short term memory, manifested by total or partial inability to recall past experiences.

    anterograde a.,   a. in reference to events occurring after the trauma or disease that caused the condition.

    retrograde a.,   a. in reference to events that occurred before the trauma or disease that caused the condition.

amne'sic   Relating to or affected with amnesia.

amnes'tic   **1.** Amnesic. **2.** Agent causing amnesia.

amnio-   [G. *amnion, q.v.*] Combining form relating to the amnion.

am'niocente'sis   [amnio- + G. *kentēsis*, puncture] Transabdominal aspiration of fluid from the amniotic sac.

amniog'raphy   [amnio- + G. *graphō*, to write] Roentgenography of the amniotic sac after the injection of an opaque, water-soluble solution into the sac.

am'nion   [G. the membrane around the fetus] Amniotic sac; the innermost of the membranes enveloping the embryo *in utero* and filled with the amniotic fluid.

amnion'ic   Relating to the amnion.

amnioni'tis   [amnion + G. *-itis*, inflammation] Inflammation resulting from infection of the amnion, usually resulting from premature rupture of the membranes and often associated with neonatal infection.

amnios'copy   [amnio- + G. *skopeō*, to view] Examination of the amniotic fluid in the lowest part of the sac by means of an endoscope introduced through the cervical canal.

amniot'ic   Amnionic.

amniot'omy   Artificial rupture of the fetal membranes as a means of inducing or expediting labour.

Amoe'ba   [Mod. L. fr. G. *amoibē*, change] A genus of naked, lobose, pseudopod-forming protozoa of the class Sarcodina (or Rhizopoda). The typical parasites of man are now placed in the genera *Entamoeba*, *Endolimax*, *Iodamoeba*, and *Dientamoeba*.

amoe'ba, pl. **amoe'bae, amoe'bas** Common name for *Amoeba* and similar naked, lobose, sarcodine protozoa.

amoebi'asis [amoeba + G. -*iasis*, condition] Infection with *Entamoeba histolytica* or other pathogenic amoebas.

amoe'bic Relating to, resembling, or caused by amoebas.

amoe'bicide [amoeba + L. *caedo*, to kill] Any agent that causes the destruction of amoebas.

amor'phous 1. Without definite shape or visible differentiation in structure. **2.** Not crystallized.

amoxicil'lin A semisynthetic penicillin antibiotic with an antimicrobial spectrum similar to that of ampicillin.

amphet'amine A powerful synthetic CNS stimulant closely related in its structure and action to ephedrine and other sympathomimetic amines; used as the sulphate.

amphi- [G. *amphi*, two-sided] Combining form meaning on both sides, surrounding, double.

amphibar'ic [amphi- + G. *baros*, pressure] Denoting a pharmacologic material that may lower or elevate arterial blood pressure, depending on the dose.

ampho- [G. *amphō*, both] Combining form meaning on both sides, surrounding, double.

amphoter'ic [G. *amphoteroi* (pl.), both, fr. *amphō*, both] Having two opposite characteristics, especially having the capacity or reacting as either an acid or a base.

amphoter'icin B An amphoteric polyene antibiotic prepared from *Streptomyces nodosus;* also a nephrotoxic antifungal agent.

ampicil'lin An acid-stable semisynthetic penicillin derived from 6-aminopenicillanic acid, with a broader spectrum of antimicrobial action than penicillin G, inhibiting the growth of Gram-positive and Gram-negative bacteria; not resistant to penicillinase.

am'poule, am'pule [L. *ampulla*, *q.v.*] A hermetically sealed container, usually made of glass, containing a sterile medicinal solution, or powder to be made up in solution, to be used for subcutaneous, intramuscular, or intravenous injection.

ampul'la, gen. and pl. **ampul'lae** [L. a two-handled bottle] [NA] A saccular dilation of a canal or duct.

ampul'lar Relating in any sense to an ampulla.

amputa'tion [L. *amputatio*, to cut around, prune] The cutting off of a limb or part of a limb, the breast, or a projecting part.

amputee' A person with an amputated limb.

amye'linated Unmyelinated.

amyg'dala, gen. and pl. **amyg'dalae** [L. fr. G. *amygdalē*, almond; in Mediev. & Mod. L. a tonsil] **1.** *Corpus* amygdaloideum. **2.** Denoting the tonsilla cerebelli, as well as the lymphatic tonsils (pharyngeal, palatine, lingual, laryngeal, and tubal).

amyg'daloid [amygdala + G. *eidos*, appearance] Resembling an almond or a tonsil.

amyl- See amylo-.

a'myl The radical formed from a pentane, C_5H_{12}, by removal of one H; several isomeric forms exist.

  a. nitrite, used as a vasodilator in angina pectoris and as an antidote in cyanide poisoning.

amyla'ceous Starchy.

am'ylase One of a group of starch-splitting or amylolytic enzymes that cleave starch, glycogen, and related polysaccharides.

amylo-, [G. *amylon*, starch] Combining form indicating starch or polysaccharide nature or origin.

am'yloid [amylo- + G. *eidos*, resemblance] Any of a group of chemically diverse proteins that appears microscopically homogeneous, but is composed of linear non-branching aggregated fibrils arranged in sheets when seen under the electron microscope, occurs characteristically as pathologic extracellular deposits in the walls of blood vessels (amyloidosis), especially in association with reticuloendothelial tissue; the chemical nature of the proteinaceous fibrils is dependent upon the underlying disease process.

amyloido'sis [amyloid + G. -*osis*, condition] A disease of unknown cause characterized by the extracellular accumulation of amyloid in various organs and tissues of the body.

amylol'ysis [amylo- + G. *lysis*, dissolution] Hydrolysis of starch into sugar.

amyosta'sia [G. a- priv. + *mys*, muscle, + *stasis*, standing] Difficulty in standing, due to muscular tremor or incoordination.

amyosthe'nia [G. a- priv. + *mys*, muscle, + *sthenos*, strength] Muscular weakness.

amyoto'nia [G. a- priv. + *mys*, muscle, + *tonos*, tone] Myatonia.

a. congen'ita, atonic pseudoparalysis of congenital origin observed especially in infants and characterized by absences of muscular tone only in muscles innervated by the spinal nerves.

amyotro'phic Relating to muscular atrophy.

amyot'rophy [G. a- priv. + *mys*, muscle, + *trophē*, nourishment] Muscular wasting or atrophy.

an- See a-.

ana- [G. *ana*, up] Prefix meaning up, toward, apart; distinguished from *an-*, which is a-privative with *n* before a vowel.

anabiot'ic 1. Resuscitating; restorative. **2.** A revivifying remedy; a powerful stimulant.

anabol'ic Relating to or promoting anabolism.

anab'olism [G. *anabolē*, a raising up] The process of assimilation of nutritive matter and its conversion into living substance. This includes synthetic processes and requires energy. *Cf.* catabolism.

anab'olite Any substance formed as a result of anabolic processes.

anaclit'ic [G. *ana*, toward; + *klinein*, to lean] Leaning or depending upon; in psychoanalysis, relating to the dependence of the infant on the mother or mother substitute.

anacrot'ic Referring to the upstroke or ascending limb of the arterial pulse tracing.

anacu'sis [G. *an-* priv. + *akousis*, hearing] Total loss or absence of the ability to perceive sound as such.

anae'mia [G. *anaimia*, fr. *an-* priv. + *haima*, blood] Any condition in which the number of red blood cells per mm³, the amount of haemoglobin in 100 ml of blood, and the volume of packed red blood cells per 100 ml of blood are less than normal; clinically, generally pertaining to the concentration of oxygen-transporting material in a designated volume of blood, in contrast to total quantities.

aplastic a., a. characterized by a greatly decreased formation of erythrocytes and haemoglobin, and usually associated with pronounced granulocytopenia and thrombocytopenia, as a result of hypoplastic or aplastic bone marrow.

Cooley's a., *thalassaemia* major.

Fanconi's a., a type of idiopathic refractory a. characterized by pancytopenia, hy-poplasia of the bone marrow, and congenital anomalies, occurring in members of the same family.

haemolytic a., a. resulting from abnormal destruction of erythrocytes in the body.

pernicious a., a chronic progressive a. of older adults thought to result from a defect of the stomach, with atrophy and associated lack of an "intrinsic" factor, resulting in malabsorption of vitamin B_{12}; characterized by greatly decreased red blood cell counts, low levels of haemoglobin, numerous macrocytic erythrocytes, and hypo- or achlorhydria, in association with a predominant number of megaloblasts and relatively few normoblasts in the bone marrow.

refractory a., any of a group of anaemic conditions in which there is persistent, frequently advanced a. that is not successfully treated by any means except blood transfusions, and that is not associated with another primary disease.

sickle cell a., a. characterized by the presence of crescent- or sickle-shaped erythrocytes in peripheral blood, excessive haemolysis, and active haemopoiesis; haemoglobin is abnormal, up to 85% or more being sickle cell haemoglobin (Hb S) and the remainder fetal haemoglobin (Hb F); individuals are homozygous for the sickle cell gene, whereas those heterozygous for this gene have sickle cell trait.

sideroblastic a., sideroachrestic a., refractory a. characterized by the presence of sideroblasts in the bone marrow.

spherocytic a., hereditary *spherocytosis.*

anae'mic Pertaining to or characterized by anaemia.

an'aphase [G. *ana*, up, + *phasis*, appearance] The stage of mitosis or meiosis in which the chromosomes move from the equatorial plate toward the poles of the cell.

anaer'obe [G. *an-* priv. + *aēr*, air, + *bios*, life] A microorganism that can live and grow in the absence of free oxygen.

facultative a., one able to live or grow in the presence or absence of free oxygen.

obligate a., one that will live or grow only in the absence of free oxygen.

anaero'bic 1. Relating to an anaerobe. **2.** Living without oxygen.

anaesthe'sia [G. *anaisthēsia*, fr. *an-* priv. + *aisthēsis*, sensation] A state characterized by loss of sensation, the result of pharmacological depression of nerve function or of neurological disease.

block a., conduction a.

caudal a., regional a. by injection of local anaesthetic into the epidural space via the sacral hiatus.

conduction a., regional a. in which local anaesthetic solution is injected about nerves to inhibit nerve transmission.

general a., loss of ability to perceive pain associated with loss of consciousness, produced by intravenous or inhalation anaesthetic agents.

regional a., use of local anaesthetic solution(s) to produce circumscribed areas of loss of sensation.

spinal a., (1) sensory denervation produced by injection of local anaesthetic solution(s) into the spinal subarachnoid space; (2) loss of sensation produced by disease of the spinal cord.

an'aesthesiol'ogist A physician specializing solely in anaesthesiology and related areas.

an'aesthesiol'ogy [anaesthesia + G. *logos*, treatise] The medical specialty concerned with the pharmacological, physiological, and clinical basis of anaesthesia and related fields, including resuscitation, intensive respiratory care, and pain.

anaesthet'ic 1. A compound that reversibly depresses neuronal function, producing loss of ability to perceive pain and/or other sensations. 2. Collective designation for anaesthetizing agents administered to an individual subject at a particular time. 3. Characterized by loss of sensation or capable of producing loss of sensation. 4. Associated with or due to the state of anaesthesia.

anaes'thetist One who administers an anaesthetic; *e.g.*, an anaesthesiologist, a physician who is not an anaesthesiologist, a nurse anaesthetist.

a'nal Relating to the anus.

analep'tic [G. *analēptikos*, restorative] 1. Invigorating; restorative. 2. An agent that so acts. 3. A central nervous system stimulant.

analge'sia [G. insensibility, fr. *an*- priv. + *algēsis*, sensation of pain] A condition in which nociceptive stimuli are perceived but are not interpreted as pain; usually accompanied by sedation without loss of consciousness.

analge'sic 1. A compound capable of producing analgesia. 2. Characterized by reduced response to painful stimuli.

analget'ic 1. Analgesic (1). 2. Associated with altered pain perception.

anal'ity Referring to the psychic organization derived from, and characteristic of, the anal period of psychosexual development.

an'alogue [G. *ana-logos*, analogous] 1. One of two organs or parts in different species of animals or plants, that differ in structure or development but are similar in function. 2. A compound that resembles another in structure, such as an isomer.

anal'ysis, pl. **anal'yses** [G. a breaking up, fr. *ana*, up + *lysis*, a loosening] 1. The breaking up of a chemical compound into simpler elements; a process by which the composition of a substance is determined. 2. The separation of any compound substance or concept into the parts composing it. 3. See psychoanalysis. 4. Applied in electroencephalography to the estimation or recording of the components of a complex wave form in terms of their frequency and amplitude.

an'alyst 1. One who makes analytical determinations. 2. Short term for psychoanalyst.

an'aphylac'tic Relating to anaphylaxis; manifesting extremely great sensitivity to foreign protein or other material.

an'aphylax'is [G. *ana*, away from, back from, + *phylaxis*, protection] The immediate transient kind of immunologic (allergic) reaction characterized by contraction of smooth muscle and dilation of capillaries due to release of pharmacologically active substances (histamine, bradykinin, serotonin, and slow-reacting substance).

anapla'sia [G. *ana*, again, + plasis, a moulding] Loss of structural differentiation, especially as seen in most, but not all, malignant neoplasms.

anar'thria [G. fr. *an-arthros*, without joints; (of sound) inarticulate] Loss of the power of articulate speech.

anasar'ca [G. *ana*, through, + *sarx* (sark-), flesh] A generalized infiltration of oedema fluid into subcutaneous connective tissue.

anastomo'sis, pl. **anastomo'ses** [G. *anastomōsis*, from *anastomoō*, to furnish with a mouth] 1. A natural communication, direct or indirect, between two blood vessels or other tubular structures; also incorrectly applied to nerves. **2.** Operative union of two hollow or tubular structures. **3.** An opening created by surgery, trauma, or disease between two or more normally separate spaces or organs.

anastomot'ic Pertaining to an anastomosis.

anatom'ical 1. Relating to anatomy. **2.** Structural.

anat'omist A specialist in the science of a anatomy.

anat'omy [G. *anatomē*, dissection, from *ana*, apart, + *tomē*, a cutting] **1.** The morphologic structure of an organism. **2.** The science of the morphology or structure of organisms.

    comparative a., the comparative study of animal structure in regard to homologous organs or parts.

    gross a., macroscopic a. general a. studied without the use of the microscope.

    microscopic a., the branch of a. in which the structure of cells, tissues, and organs is studied with the light microscope. See histology.

an'conal, anco'neal [G. *ankōn*, elbow] Relating to the elbow.

anconi'tis [G. *ankōn*, elbow, + *-itis*, inflammation] Inflammation of the elbow joint.

ancylo- See ankylo-.

Ancylos'toma [G. *ankylos*, curved, hooked, + *stoma*, mouth] A genus of nematodes that are parasitic in the duodenum, they attach themselves to villi in the mucous membrane, suck blood, and may cause a state of anaemia, especially in cases of malnutrition.

    A. brazilien'se, a species normally an intestinal parasite of dogs and cats but also found in man as a cause of human cutaneous larva migrans.

    A. cani'num, a species common in dogs, but also occurring in human skin as a cause of cutaneous larva migrans.

    A. duodena'le, the Old World hookworm, a species widespread in temperate areas, in contrast to the more tropical distribution of the New World hookworm, *Necator americanus;* the cause of ancylostomiasis.

an'cylostomi'asis Hookworm disease caused by *Ancylostoma duodenale*, producing eosinophilia, anaemia, emaciation, dyspepsia, and, in children with severe long-continued infections, swelling of the abdomen with mental and physical maldevelopment.

andro- [G. *anēr* (gen. *andros*), male] Combining form meaning masculine; pertaining to the male of the species.

an'droblasto'ma 1. A testicular tumour microscopically resembling fetal testis, with varying proportions of tubular and stromal elements; the tubules contain Sertoli cells, which may cause feminization. **2.** Arrhenoblastoma.

an'drogen A generic term for an agent, usually a hormone, that stimulates the activity of the accessory sex organs of the male, encourages the development of male sex characteristics, or prevents the changes in the latter that follow castration; natural a.'s are steroid derivatives of androstane.

androg'yny [andro- + G. *gynē*, woman] Female *pseudohermaphroditism*.

anencephal'ic, anenceph'alous Relating to anencephaly.

anenceph'aly [G. *an-* priv. + *enkepholas*, brain] Markedly defective development of the brain, together with absence of the bones of the cranial vault and the cerebral and cerebellar hemispheres, and with only a rudimentary brainstem and some traces of basal ganglia present.

an'euploid'y State of having an abnormal number of chromosomes not an exact multiple of the haploid number.

an'eurysm [G. *aneurysma* (*mat-*), a dilation, fr. *eurys*, wide] Circumscribed dilation of an artery, or a blood-containing tumour connecting directly with the lumen of an artery.

    arteriosclerotic a., atherosclerotic a., the commonest type of a., occuring in the abdominal aorta and other large arteries in the elderly; due to weakening of the media by severe atherosclerosis.

    cirsoid a., dilation of a group of blood vessels due to congenital malformation with arteriovenous shunting.

    dissecting a., splitting or dissection of an arterial wall by blood entering through an intimal tear or by interstitial haemorrhage.

    false a., (1) pulsating, encapsulated haematoma in communication with the lumen of the ruptured vessel; **(2)** pseudoaneurysm.

    fusiform a., an elongated spindle-shaped dilation of an artery.

    saccular a., sacculated a., a sac-like bulging on one side of an artery.

aneurys'mal, aneurysmat'ic Relating to an aneurysm.

angi- See angio-.

angiecta'sia, angiec'tasis [angio-
+ G. *ektasis*, a stretching] Dilation of a lymphatic or blood vessel.

angiectat'ic [angio- + G. *ektatos*, capable of extension] Marked by the presence of dilated blood vessels.

angii'tis [angio- + G. *-itis*, inflammation] Vasculitis; inflammation of a blood vessel (arteritis, phlebitis) or of a lymphatic vessel (lymphangitis).

angi'na [L. quinsy] **1.** Sore throat from any cause. **2.** A severe constricting pain; commonly referring to a. pectoris.

  Ludwig's a., cellulitis of the submandibular spaces, usually spreading to involve the sublingual and submental spaces.

  a. pec'toris, severe constricting pain in the chest, often radiating from the precordium to the left shoulder and down the arm, due to ischaemia of the heart muscle, usually caused by coronary disease.

  Vincent's a., an ulcerative infection of the tonsils and pharynx caused by fusiform and spirochaetal organisms; usually associated with necrotizing ulcerative gingivitis.

angio-, angi- [G. *angeion*, vessel] Combining forms relating to blood or lymph vessels.

an'giocardi'tis [angio- + G. *kardia*, heart, + *-itis*, inflammation] Inflammation of the heart and blood vessels.

an'giocar'diogram The x-ray image produced by angiocardiography.

an'giocardiog'raphy [angio- + G. *kardia*, heart, + *graphō*, to write] X-ray imaging of the heart and great vessels made visible by the intravenous injection of a radiopaque solution.

an'giofibro'sis Fibrosis of the walls of blood vessels.

angiog'raphy [angio- + G. *graphō*, to write] Radiography of vessels after the injection of a radiopaque material.

angio'ma [angio- + G. *-ōma*, tumour] A swelling or tumour due to proliferation with or without dilation of the blood vessels (haemangioma) or lymphatics (lymphangioma).

  cavernous a., cavernous *haemangioma*.

  cherry a., senile *haemangioma*.

  a. serpigino'sum, the presence of rings of red dots on the skin, which tend to widen peripherially, due to proliferation, with subsequent atrophy, of the superficial capillaries.

  telangiectatic a., a. composed of dilated vessels.

an'giomato'sis A condition characterized by multiple angiomas.

  encephalofacial a., encephalotrigeminal a., Sturge-Weber *syndrome*.

  retinocerebral a., Lindau's *disease*.

angio'matous Relating to or resembling an angioma.

an'gio-oede'ma Angioneurotic *oedema*.

angiop'athy [angio- + G. *pathos*, suffering] Any disease of the blood vessels or lymphatics.

an'gioplasty [angio- + G. *plassō*, to form] Reconstruction of a blood vessel.

  percutaneous transluminal coronary a., an operation for enlarging a narrowed coronary arterial lumen by peripheral introduction of a balloon-tip catheter and dilating the lumen on withdrawal of the inflated catheter tip.

an'glosarco'ma A rare malignant neoplasm occurring most often in the breast and skin, and believed to originate from the endothelial cells of blood vessels.

an'giospasm Vasospasm.

angioten'sin A family of decapeptides with vasoconstrictive activity.

anhedo'nia [G. *an-* priv. + *hedonē*, pleasure] Absence of pleasure from the performance of acts that would ordinarily be pleasurable.

anhidro'sis [G. *an-* priv. + *hidrōs*, sweat] Absence of sweating.

anhidrot'ic 1. Relating to, or characterized by, anhidrosis. **2.** An agent that reduces, prevents, or stops sweating. **3.** Denoting a reduction or absence of sweat glands.

anhydro- [G. *an-* priv., + *hydōr*, water] Prefix denoting the removal of water.

anhy'drous Containing no water, especially water of crystallization.

an'iline [Ar. *an-nil*, indigo] The parent substance of many synthetic dyes; formally derived from benzene by the substitution of $-NH_2$ for one of the hydrogen atoms.

an'ilinism, an'ilism Chronic aniline poisoning characterized by gastric and cardiac weakness, vertigo, muscular depression, intermittent pulse, and cyanosis.

an'ion An ion that carries a negative charge, going therefore to the positively charged anode; in salts, the acid radicals are a.'s.

anion exchange The process by which an anion in a mobile (liquid) phase exchanges with another anion previously bound to a solid, positively charged phase, the latter being an anion exchanger.

aniseiko'nia [G. *anisos*, unequal, + *eikōn*, an image] Unequal retinal image; a relative difference in size or shape of ocular images.

aniso- [G. *anisos*, unequal] Combining form meaning unequal or dissimilar.

anisoco'ria [aniso- + G. *korē*, pupil] Unequal size of the pupils.

anisometro'pia [aniso- + G. *metron*, measure, + *ōps*, sight] Difference in the refractive power of the eyes.

ani'sometrop'ic Relating to anisometropia.

an'kle 1. The joint between the leg and foot in which the tibia and fibula above articulate with the talus below. 2. The region of the a. joint. 3. Talus.

ankylo- [G. *ankylos*, bent, crooked; *ankylōsis*, stiffness or fixation of a joint] Combining form meaning bent, crooked, stiff, or fixed.

an'kylosed Stiffened; bound by adhesions; denoting a joint in a state of ankylosis.

ankylo'sis [G. *ankylōsis*, stiffening of a joint] Stiffening or fixation of a joint as the result of a disease process, with fibrous or bony union across the joint.

an'nular [L. *anulus*, ring] Ring-shaped.

an'nuloplasty [L. *anulus*, ring, + G. *plassō*, to form] Reconstruction of an incompetent (usually mitral) cardiac valve.

annulor'rhaphy [L. *anulus*, ring, + G. *raphē*, seam] Closure of a hernial ring by suture.

an'nulus See anulus.

an'odyne [G. *an-* priv. + *odynē*, pain] A compound less potent than an anaesthetic or a narcotic but capable of relieving pain.

a'nogen'ital. Relating to both the anal and the genital regions.

anom'aly [G. *anōmalia*, irregularity] Deviation from the average or norm; anything structurally unusual or irregular or contrary to a general rule.

anonych'ia [G. *an-* priv. + *onyx (onych-)*, nail] Congenital absence of the nails.

Anoph'eles [G. *anōphelēs*, useless, harmful, fr. *an-* priv. + *ōpheleō*, to be of use] A genus of mosquitoes (family Culicidae, subfamily Anophelinae) containing over 90 species, many of which are vectors of malaria.

anoph'eline Referring to the *Anopheles* mosquito.

anophthal'mia, anophthal'mos, anophthal'mus [G. *an-* priv. + *ophthalmos*, eye] Complete absence of tissues of the eyes.

a'noplasty. Reconstructive surgery on the anus.

anor'chia, anorchidism, anorchism [G. *an-* priv. + *orchis*, testis] Absence of the testes.

anorec'tal Relating to both anus and rectum.

anorec'tic, anoret'ic 1. Causing, or characterized by, anorexia. 2. An agent so acting.

anorex'ia [G. fr. *an-* priv. + *orexis*, appetite] Diminished appetite; aversion to food.

  a. nervo'sa, a personality disorder manifested by extreme aversion to food, usually occurring in young women, resulting in extreme weight loss, amenorrhoea, and constitutional disorders.

anorex'ic Relating to or suffering from anorexia nervosa.

anos'mia [G. *an-* priv. + *osmē*, sense of smell] Loss of the sense of smell.

anov'ular, anov'ulatory Not related to or coincident with ovulation.

anovula'tion Suspension or cessation of ovulation.

anoxae'mia [G. *an-* priv. + oxygen + G. *haima*, blood] Absence of oxygen in arterial blood.

anox'ia [G. *an-* priv. + oxygen + *-ia*, condition] Absence of oxygen in inspired gases, arterial blood, or tissues.

an'sa, gen. and pl. **an'sae** [L. loop, handle] [NA] Any anatomical structure in the form of a loop or an arc.

antac'id Neutralizing an acid.

antag'onism [G. *anti*, against, + *agōnizomai*, to fight] Mutual resistance; denoting mutual opposition in action between muscles, drugs, diseases, or physiologic processes or between drugs and diseases or drugs and physiologic processes.

antag'onist Something opposing or resisting the action of another; denoting certain

muscles, drugs, etc., that tend to neutralize or
impede the action or effect of others.

ante- [L. *ante*, before] Prefix denoting before. See also pre-, pro-.

antebra′chial Relating to the forearm.

anteflex′ion A bending forward; a sharp
forward curve or angulation; denoting especially a forward bend in the uterus at the
junction of corpus and cervix.

antemor′tem [L. acc. case of *mors*
(*mort*-), death] Before death.

antena′tal [ante- + L. *natus*, birth] Prenatal.

antepar′tum [ante- + L. *pario*, pp. *partus*, to bring forth] Before labour or childbirth.

ante′rior [L.] **1.** Before, in relation to time
or space. **2.** [NA] Ventral; in human anatomy,
denoting the front surface of the body; often
used to indicate the position of one structure
relative to another. **3.** Near the head or rostral
end of certain embryos.

antero- A prefix denoting anterior.

an′terograde [L. *gradior*, pp. *gressus*, to
step, go] Moving forward.

an′terolat′eral In front of and away from
the middle line.

an′teroposte′rior Relating to both front
and rear.

antever′sion [ante- + Mediev. L. *versio*,
a turning] Turning forward, inclining forward
as a whole without bending.

anthe′lix [anti- + G. *helix*, coil] [NA] An
elevated ridge of cartilage anterior and
roughly parallel to the posterior portion of the
auricle helix.

anthelmin′tic [anti- + G. *helmins*, worm]
1. Vermifuge; an agent that destroys or ex-
pels intestinal worms. **2.** Having the power to
destroy or expel intestinal worms.

an′thracoid [G. *anthrax*, carbuncle, +
eidos, resemblance] **1.** Resembling a carbuncle or cutaneous anthrax **2.** Resembling
anthrax.

anthraco′sis Accumulation of carbon
from inhaled smoke or coal dust in the lungs.

an′thrax [G. *anthrax* (*anthrak*-), charcoal,
coal, a carbuncle] A disease occurring in man
from infection of subcutaneous tissues with
Bacillus anthracis; marked by haemorrhage
and serous effusions in the organs and cavities in the body and by extreme prostration.
Primary forms are pulmonary, gastroenteric
or intestinal, and cutaneous.

anthropo- [G. *anthrōpos*, man] A combining form meaning human, or denoting some
relationship to man.

an′thropoid [G. *anthrōpo- eidēs*, man-
like] Resembling man in structure and form.

anthropol′ogy [anthropo- + G. *logos*,
treatise] The branch of science concerned
with man's origins and development.

anthropomet′ric Relating to anthro-
pometry.

anthropom′etry [anthropo- + G. *metron*, measure] The branch of anthropology
concerned with comparative measurements
of the human body and its parts.

an′thropomor′phism [anthropo- + G.
morphē, form] Attribution of human characteristics to nonhuman creatures or inanimate
objects.

anti- [G. *anti*, against] Prefix signifying
against, opposing, or, in relation to symptoms
and diseases, curative; also to denote an
antibody (immunoglobulin) specific for the
thing indicated; *e.g.*, antitoxin (antibody specific for a toxin).

antiac′id Antacid.

an′tiadrener′gic Denoting an agent that
annuls or antagonizes the effects of the sympathetic nervous system.

antibacte′rial Destructive to or preventing the growth of bacteria.

antibiot′ic **1.** A chemical substance derived from a mould or bacteria that inhibits the
growth of other microorganisms. **2.** Relating
to such an action.

   broad spectrum a., an a. having a
wide range of activity against both Gram-
positive and Gram-negative organisms.

an′tibody **1.** Generally, any body or substance, soluble or cellular, which is evoked by
the stimulus provided by the introduction of
antigen and which reacts specifically with antigen in some demonstrable way. **2.** One of
the classes of globulins (immunoglobulins)
present in the blood serum or body fluids as a
result of antigenic stimulus or occurring "naturally."

an′ticholiner′gic Antagonistic to the action of parasympathetic or other cholinergic
nerve fibres.

an′ticholines′terase A drug that inhibits or inactivates acetylcholinesterase.

anticoag′ulant Preventing coagulation.

an′ticonvul′sant, an′ticonvul′sive
Preventing or arresting convulsions.

antidepres'sant Counteracting depression.

an'tidiuret'ic An agent that reduces the output of urine.

an'tidote [anti- + G. *dotos*, what is given] An agent that neutralizes a poison or counteracts its effects.

antiemet'ic [anti- + G. *emetikos*, emetic] Preventing or arresting vomiting.

an'tigen'ic Allergenic; having the properties of an antigen (allergen).

an'tigen (Ag) [anti(body) + G. *-gen*, producing] Allergen; any substance that, as a result of coming in contact with appropriate tissues of an animal body, induces a state of sensitivity and/or resistance to infection or toxic substances after a latent period and which reacts in a demonstrable way with tissues and/or antibody of the sensitized subject *in vivo* or *in vitro*.

an'tihaemolyt'ic Preventing haemolysis.

an'tihaemorrhag'ic Arresting haemorrhage.

antihe'lix Anthelix.

antihis'tamines Drugs having an action antagonistic to that of histamine.

an'tihyperten'sive Indicating a drug or mode of treatment that reduces high blood pressure.

anti-inflam'matory Reducing inflammation by acting on body mechanisms, without directly antagonizing the causative agent.

an'timicro'bial Tending to destroy microbes, to prevent their development, or to prevent their pathogenic action.

an'timycot'ic [anti- + G. *mykēs*, fungus] Antagonistic to fungi.

an'tineoplas'tic Preventing the development, maturation, or spread of neoplastic cells.

an'tiperistal'sis Reversed *peristalsis*.

an'tiperistal'tic 1. Relating to antiperistalsis. 2. Impeding or arresting peristalsis.

an'tiprurit'ic Preventing or relieving itching.

an'tipsychot'ic 1. An antipsychotic *agent*. 2. Denoting the actions of such an agent.

an'tipyret'ic [anti- + G. *pyretos*, fever] Antifebrile; reducing fever.

an'tiscorbu'tic Preventing or relieving scurvy.

antisep'sis [anti- + G. *sēpsis*, putrefaction] Prevention of infection by inhibiting the growth of infectious agents.

antisep'tic Relating to or capable of effecting antisepsis.

antise'rum Serum that contains demonstrable antibody or antibodies specific for one (**monovalent a., specific a.**) or more (**polyvalent a.**) antigens.

an'tispasmod'ic Preventing or relieving convulsions or spasms.

antitox'in [anti- + G. *toxicon*, poison] Antibody formed in response to antigenic poisonous substances of biologic origin, such as bacterial exotoxins, phytotoxins, and zootoxins. Generally, a. refers to whole, or globulin fraction, of serum from animals (usually horses) immunized by injections of the specific toxoid.

antitra'gus [G. *anti*, opposite, + *tragos*, a goat, the tragus] [NA] A projection of the auricle posterior to the tragus from which it is separated by the intertragic notch.

α-1-antitryp'sin A glycoprotein that is the major protease inhibitor of human serum; it is synthesized in the liver and is genetically polymorphic due to the presence of over 20 alleles.

antitus'sive [anti- + L. *tussis*, cough] Relieving a cough.

antiven'in An antitoxin specific for an animal or insect venom.

antivi'ral Opposing a virus, weakening or abolishing its action.

an'tra Plural of antrum.

an'tral Relating to an antrum.

antrec'tomy [antrum + G. *ektomē*, excision] 1. Removal of the walls of an antrum. 2. Removal of the antrum (pyloric half) of the stomach.

antro- [L. *antrum*, from G. *antron*, a cave] Combining form denoting relationship to any antrum.

antros'tomy [antro- + G. *stoma*, mouth] Formation of an opening into an antrum.

antrot'omy [antro- + G. *tomē*, incision] Incision through the wall of an antrum.

an'trum, pl. **an'tra** [L. fr. G. *antron*, a cave] 1. [NA] Any nearly closed cavity, particularly one with bony walls. 2. The pyloric end of the stomach, partially shut off, during digestion, from the cardiac end (fundus) by the prepyloric sphincter.

an'ulus, pl. **an'uli** [L.] [NA] A circular or ring-shaped structure.

anure'sis [G. *an-* priv. + *ouresis*, urination] Inability to pass urine.

anuret'ic Relating to anuresis.

anu'ria Absence of urine formation.

a'nus, pl. **a'nus** [L.] [NA] The lower opening of the digestive tract through which faecal matter is expelled.

imperforate a., anal *atresia*.

an'vil Incus.

anxi'ety [L. *anxietas*] In psychoanalysis, apprehension of danger and dread accompanied by restlessness, tension, tachycardia, and dyspnoea unattached to a clearly identifiable stimulus.

aor'ta, pl. **aor'tae** [Mod. L. fr. G. *aorte*, from *aeiro*, to lift up] [NA] A large artery that is the main trunk of the systemic arterial system, arising from the base of the left ventricle and ending at the left side of the body of the fourth lumbar vertebra by dividing to form the right and left common iliac arteries. Its parts are: 1) ascending a., 2) aortic arch; and 3) descending a., which is divided into the thoracic a. and abdominal a.

aor'tic Relating to the aorta or the a. orifice of the left ventricle of the heart.

aortog'raphy [aorta + G. *grapho*, to write] Radiographic visualization of the aorta and its branches by injection of contrast media.

ap'athet'ic Exhibiting apathy; indifferent.

ap'athy [G. *apatheia*, fr. a- priv. + *pathos*, suffering] Absence of emotion; indifference; insensibility.

ap'erture [L. *apertura*, an opening] 1. An opening; orifice. 2. The diameter of the objective of a microscope.

a'pex, pl. **ap'ices** [L. summit or tip] [NA] The extremity of a conical or pyramidal structure.

Ap'gar score Evaluation of a newborn infant's physical status by assigning numerical values (0 to 2) to each of five criteria: heart rate, respiratory effort, muscle tone, response to stimulation, and skin colour.

apha'gia [G. a- priv. + *phagein*, to eat] Dysphagia.

apha'kia [G. a- priv. + *phakos*, lentil, anything shaped like a lentil] Absence of the lens of the eye.

apha'sia [G. speechlessness, fr. a- priv. + *phasis*, speech] Impaired or absent communication by speech, writing, or signs, due to

dysfunction of brain centres in the dominant hemisphere.

Broca's a., motor a.

conduction a., a. in which the subject can speak and write in a way, but skips or repeats words or substitutes one word for another, the lesion being in the association tracts connecting the various language centres.

motor a., a. in which the power of expression by writing, speaking, or signs is lost.

sensory a., receptive a. loss of the ability to comprehend written (or printed) or spoken words.

apha'siac, apha'sic Relating to or suffering from aphasia.

apho'nia [G. a- priv. + *phone*, voice] Loss of the voice in consequence of disease or injury of the organ of speech.

aphra'sia [G. a- priv. + *phrasis*, speaking] Inability to speak, from any cause.

aphrodis'iac 1. Increasing sexual desire. 2. Anything that arouses or increases sexual desire.

aph'tha, pl. **aph'thae** [G. ulceration] 1. In the singular, a minute ulcer on a mucous membrane, often covered by a grey or white exudate. 2. In the plural, small white spots associated with small ulcerations on the mucous membrane of the mouth.

Bednar's aphthae, a traumatic affection of the newborn consisting of two yellow, flattened, slightly elevated patches, often ulcerated, one on either side of the median raphe of the palate.

aph'thous Characterized by or relating to aphthae or aphthosis.

aphylax'is [G. a- priv. + *phylaxis*, a guarding] Nonimmunity; lack of protection against disease.

a'pical 1. Relating to the apex of a pyramidal or pointed structure. 2. Situated nearer to the apex of a structure in relation to a specific reference point.

ap'ices Plural of apex.

apico- [L. *apex*, summit or tip] Combining form relating to any apex.

apicoec'tomy [apico- + G. *ektome*, excision] Root resection; surgical removal of a dental root apex.

apla'sia [G. a- priv. + *plasis*, a molding] 1. Defective development or congenital absence of an organ or tissue. 2. In haematology, incomplete, retarded, or defective development, or a cessation of the usual regenerative process.

aplas'tic Pertaining to aplasia, or conditions characterized by defective regeneration, as in a. anaemia.

ap'noea [G. *apnoia*, want of breath] Absence of breathing.

 sleep-induced a. a. resulting from failure of the respiratory centre to stimulate adequate respiration during sleep.

apo- [G. *apo*, away from, off] Combining form meaning, usually, separated from or derived from.

ap'ocrine [G. *apo-krino̅*, to separate] See apocrine *gland*.

aponeuro'sis, pl. **aponeuro'ses** [G. the end of the muscle where it becomes tendon, fr. *apo*, from, + *neuron*, sinew] [NA] A fibrous sheet or expanded tendon, giving attachment to muscular fibres and serving as the means of origin or insertion of a flat muscle.

ap'oneurot'ic Relating to an aponeurosis.

apoph'ysis, pl. **apoph'yses** [G. an offshoot] An outgrowth or projection, especially one from a bone; bony process or outgrowth that lacks an independent centre of ossification.

apoplec'tic Relating to, suffering from, or predisposed to apoplexy.

ap'oplexy [G. *apople̅xia*] **1.** Classical but obsolete term for stroke. **2.** An effusion of blood into a tissue or organ.

apparat'us, pl. **apparat'us** [L. equipment, fr. *ap-paro*, pp. *-atus*, to prepare] **1.** A collection of instruments adapted for a special purpose or an instrument made up of several parts. **2.** [NA] A system; the group of glands, ducts, blood vessels, muscles, or other anatomical structures concerned in the performance of some function.

ap'pendec'tomy [appendix + G. *ek-tome̅*, excision] Surgical removal of the vermiform appendix.

appen'dicec'tomy Appendectomy.

appendici'tis [appendix + G. *-itis*, inflammation] Inflammation of the vermiform appendix.

ap'pendic'ular 1. Relating to an appendix or appendage. **2.** Relating to the limbs.

appen'dix, pl. **appen'dices** [L. appendage, fr. *ap- pendo* (*adp-*), to hang something on] **1.** [NA] An appendage. **2.** Specifically, the appendix vermiformis.

 a. vermifor'mis, vermiform a., [NA], a wormlike intestinal diverticulum extending from the blind end of the caecum and ending in a blind extremity.

ap'petite [L. *ad-peto*, pp. *-petitus*, to seek after, desire] A desire or longing to satisfy any conscious physical or mental need.

applana'tion [L. *ad*, toward, + *planum*, plane] In tonometry, the flattening of the cornea by pressure.

ap'plicator [L. *ap-plico*, to attach to] A slender rod at one end of which is attached a pledget of cotton or other substance for making local application to any accessible surface.

approx'imate [L. *ad*, to, + *proximus*, nearest] To bring close together. In dentistry: **1.** Proximate, denoting the contact surfaces, either mesial (proximal) or distal, of two adjacent teeth. **2.** Close together; denoting the teeth in the human jaw.

approxima'tion In surgery, bringing tissue edges into desired apposition for suturing.

aprax'ia [G. *a-* priv. + *pratto̅*, to do] **1.** A disorder of voluntary movement, consisting in partial or complete incapacity to execute purposeful movements, without impairment of muscular power, sensibility, and coordination. **2.** A psychomotor defect in which one is unable to properly use a known object.

apty'alism [G. *a-* priv. + *ptyalon*, saliva] Asialism.

apyret'ic Afebrile; nonfebrile; without fever.

aq'ueduct Aqueductus.

aqueduc'tus, pl. **aqueduc'tus** [L. fr. *aqua*, water, + *ductus*, a leading] [NA] A conduit or canal.

aq'ueous Watery; of, like, or containing water.

Arach'nida [G. *arachne*, spider] A class of arthropods consisting of spiders, scorpions, harvestmen, mites, ticks, and allies.

arach'nodac'tyly [G. *arachne̅*, spider, + *daktylos*, finger] Abnormally long and slender hands and fingers, and often feet and toes; a characteristic of Marfan's syndrome.

arach'noid [G. *arachne̅*, spider, cobweb, + *eidos*, resemblance] Resembling a cobweb; denoting specifically the arachnoidea covering the brain and spinal cord.

arachnoi'dea, arachnoi'des [Mod. L. *arachnoideus, -ea*, fr. G. *arachne̅*, spider,

+ *eidos*, resemblance] [NA] A delicate fibrous membrane forming the middle of the three coverings of the brain (**a. enceph'ali**) and spinal cord (**a. spina'lis**) ; it is closely applied to the outer membrane, the dura mater, from which it is separated only by the subdural cleft, but between it and the inner layer, the pia mater, lies the subarachnoid space.

arboriza'tion [L. *arbor*, tree] Ramification, denoting especially: (1) the terminal branching of nerve fibres or blood vessels; (2) the leaflike pattern formed under certain conditions by a dried smear of cervical mucus.

ar'bovi'rus, ar'borvi'rus [*arthropod-borne virus*] A large, heterogenous group of RNA viruses divisible into groups on the basis of characteristics of the virions; most are associated with arthropods which may serve as vectors. Although about 75 species can infect man, only about 45 species produce disease; apparent infections may be separated into three clinical syndromes: undifferentiated type fevers (systemic febrile disease), haemorrhagic fevers, and encephalitides.

arc [L. *arcus*, a bow] A curved line or segment of a circle.

reflex a., the route followed by nerve impulses in the production of a reflex act, from the periphery through the afferent nerve to the nervous system and thence through the efferent nerve to the effector organ.

arch-, arche-, archi-, archo- [G. *arche*, origin, beginning] Combining forms meaning primitive, or ancestral; also first, or chief.

ar'cuate [L. *arcuatus*, bowed] Arched; having the shape of a bow.

a'rea, pl. **a'reae** [L. a courtyard] 1. [NA] Any circumscribed surface or space. 2. All of the part supplied by a given artery or nerve. 3. A part of an organ having a special function.

 Broca's a., Broca's *centre*.

 Brodmann's a.'s, a.'s of the cerebral cortex mapped out on the basis of the cortical cytoarchitectural patterns.

 Wernicke's a., Wernicke's *centre*.

are'ola, pl. **are'olae** [L. dim of *area*] 1. [NA] Any small area. 2. One of the spaces or interstices in areolar tissue. 3. A. mammae. 4. A pigmented, depigmented, or erythematous zone surrounding a papule, pustule, weal, or cutaneous neoplasm.

 a. mam'mae [NA], **a. papillaris,** a circular pigmented area surrounding the nipple which is dotted with little projections due to the presence of glands beneath.

ar'ginine (Arg) One of the amino acids occurring among the hydrolysis products of protein.

arm [L. *armus*, fore-quarter of an animal; G. *harmos*, a shoulder joint] The segment of the superior limb between the shoulder and the elbow; commonly used to mean the whole superior limb.

arrec'tor, pl. **arrecto'res** [L. that which raises] Erector.

arrest' [O.Fr. *arester*, fr. LL. *adresto*, to stop behind] 1. To stop; check; restrain. 2. A stoppage; an interference with or a checking of the regular course of a disease or symptom, or the performance of a function. 3. Inhibition of a developmental process, usually the ultimate stage of development.

 cardiac a., a loss of effective cardiac function, which results in cessation of circulation.

arrhe'noblasto'ma [G. *arrhen*, male, + *blastos*, germ, + *-oma*, tumour] A rare ovarian tumour that produces masculinization and often contains tubules and luteinized cells.

arrhi'nia [G. a- priv. + *rhis* (rhin-), nose] Absence of the nose.

arrhyth'mia [G. a- priv. + *rhythmos*, rhythm] Loss of rhythm; denoting especially an irregularity of the heart beat.

 cardiac a., see cardiac *dysrhythmia*.

 sinus a., irregularity of the heart beat, the beat being under the control of its normal pacemaker, the sinus (S-A) node.

ar'senic [Mod. L. fr. G. *arsenikon*, fr. *arsen*, strong] An element, a steel-grey metal, symbol As, atomic no. 33, atomic weight 74.9; forms a number of poisonous compounds, some of which are used in medicine.

arsen'ical, arsen'ic Relating to or containing arsenic.

ar'tefact [L. *ars*, art, + *facio*, pp. *factus*, to make]. 1. Anything, especially in a histologic specimen or a graphic record, caused by the technique used and not a natural occurrence, but merely incidental. 2. A skin lesion produced or perpetuated by self-inflicted action.

arteri-, See arterio-.

arte'ria, gen. and pl. **arte'riae** [L. from G. *artēria*, the windpipe; later, an artery as distinct from a vein] [NA] Artery; a blood vessel conveying blood in a direction away from the heart. With the exception of the pulmonary and umbilical arteries, the arteries convey red or aerated blood.

arte'rial Relating to one or more arteries or to the entire system of arteries.

arteriec'tasis, arteriecta'sia [L. *arteria*, artery, + G. *ektasis*, distension] Vasodilation of the arteries.

arterio-, arteri- [L. *arteria*, fr. G. *artēria*, artery] Combining forms meaning artery.

arte'riogram [arterio- + G. *gramma*, something written] X-ray image of an artery after injection of contrast medium into it.

arteriog'raphy [arterio- + G. *graphō*, to write] Visualization of an artery or arteries by x-rays after injection of a radiopaque contrast medium.

arterio'la, pl. **arterio'lae** [Mod. L. dim. of *arteria*, artery] [NA] A minute artery with a muscular wall; a terminal artery continuous with the capillary network.

arterio'lar Of or pertaining to an arteriole or the arterioles collectively.

arte'riole Arteriola.

arterioli'tis [L. *arteriola*, arteriole, + G. *-itis*, inflammation] Inflammation of the wall of arterioles.

arteriolo- [L. *arteriola*, arteriole] Combining form relating to arterioles.

arterio'losclero'sis Arteriosclerosis affecting mainly the arterioles.

arteriop'athy [arterio- + G. *pathos*, suffering] Any disease of the arteries.

  hypertensive a., arterial degeneration resulting from hypertension.

arte'rioplasty [arterio- + G. *plassō*, to form] Surgical reconstruction of the wall of an artery.

arterior'rhaphy [arterio- + G. *rhaphē*, seam] Suture of an artery.

arte'riorrhex'is [arterio- + G. *rhēxis*, rupture] Rupture of an artery.

arte'riosclero'sis [arterio- + G. *sklērōsis*, hardness] Arterial sclerosis; hardening of the arteries; types generally recognized are: atherosclerosis, Mönckeberg's a., hypertensive a., and arteriolosclerosis.

  hypertensive a., progressive increase in muscle and elastic tissue of arterial walls, resulting from hypertension.

  Mönckeberg's a., arterial sclerosis involving the peripheral arteries, especially of the legs of older people, with deposition of calcium in the medial coat.

arte'riosclerot'ic Relating to or affected by arteriosclerosis.

arte'riosteno'sis [arterio- + G. *stenōsis*, a narrowing] Narrowing of the calibre of an artery, either temporary, through vasoconstriction, or permanent, through arteriosclerosis.

arte'riove'nous (AV) Relating to both an artery and a vein or to both arteries and veins in general; both arterial and venous.

arteri'tis [L. *arteria*, artery, + G. *-itis*, inflammation] Inflammation involving an artery.

ar'tery [L. *arteria*, fr. G. *artēria*] Arteria.

  collateral a., (1) one that runs parallel with a nerve or other structure; **(2)** one through which a collateral circulation is established.

  communicating a., one that connects two larger a.'s

arthral'gia [G. *arthron*, joint, + *algos*, pain] Severe pain in a joint, especially one not inflammatory in character.

arthrec'tomy [G. *arthron*, joint, + *ektomē*, excision] Exsection of a joint.

arthrit'ic Relating to arthritis.

arthri'tis, pl. **arthrit'ides** [G. fr. *arthron*, joint, + *-itis*, inflammation] Inflammation of one or more joints.

  a. defor'mans, rheumatoid a.

  hypertrophic a., osteoarthritis.

  juvenile rheumatoid a., polyarticular joint disease associated with lymph node and splenic enlargement, occurring in infants and young children.

  rheumatoid a., a chronic and progressive systemic disease, especially common in women, affecting connective tissue; a. is the dominant clinical manifestation, accompanied by thickening of articular soft tissue, with extension of synovial tissue over articular cartilages, which become eroded, leading to deformities and disability.

arthro-, arthr- [G. *arthron*, joint] Combining forms denoting a joint or articulation.

ar'throcele [arthro- + G. *kēlē*, hernia, tumour] **1.** Hernia of the synovial membrane through the capsule of a joint. **2.** Any swelling of a joint.

arthrocente'sis [arthro- + G. *kentēsis*, puncture] Aspiration into a joint; withdrawal of fluid through a puncture needle.

arthrocla'sia [arthro- + G. *klasis*, a breaking] Forcible breaking up of the adhesions in ankylosis.

arthrode'sis [arthro- + G. *desis*, a binding together] Surgical stiffening of a joint.

arthrodyn'ia [arthro- + G. *odynē*, pain] Arthralgia.

ar'throgram An x-ray of a joint; usually implies the introduction of a contrast agent into the joint capsule.

arthrog'raphy [arthro- + G. *graphō*, to describe] Radiography of a joint.

ar'throgrypo'sis [arthro- + G. *gryphōsis*, a crooking] A congenital defect of the limbs characterized by contractures, flexion, and extension.

    a. mul'tiplex congen'ita, limitation of range of joint motion and contractures present at birth, usually involving multiple joints.

arthrop'athy [arthro- + G. *pathos*, suffering] Disease affecting a joint.

    tabetic a., Charcot's joint; a neuropathic joint commonly associated with tabes dorsalis or diabetic neuropathy.

ar'throplasty [arthro- + G. *plassō*, to form] **1.** Creation of an artificial joint **2.** Surgical restoration of the integrity and functional power of a joint.

ar'thropod [arthro- + G. *pous*, foot] A member of the phylum Arthropoda.

Arthrop'oda [arthro- | G. *pous*, foot] A phylum of the Metazoa that includes the classes Crustacea (crabs, shrimps, crayfish, lobsters), Insecta, Arachnida (spiders, scorpions, mites, ticks), Chilopoda (centipedes), Diplopoda (millipedes), Merostomata (horseshoe crabs), and various other groups.

ar'throsclero'sis [arthro- + G. *sklērōsis*, hardening] Stiffness of the joints.

ar'throscope An endoscope for examining joint interiors.

arthros'copy [arthro- + G. *skopeō*, to view] Endoscopic examination of the interior of a joint.

arthro'sis 1. [G. *arthrōsis*, a jointing] A joint. **2.** [arthro- + G. -*osis*, condition] A trophic degenerative affection of a joint.

arthros'tomy [arthro- + G. *stoma*, mouth] Establishment of a temporary opening into a joint cavity.

arthrot'omy [arthro- + G. *tomē*, a cutting] Cutting into a joint.

artic'ular Relating to a joint.

articula'tio, pl. **artic'ulatio'nes** [L. a forming of vines] Joint; in anatomy, the place of union, usually movable, between two or more bones. Joints are classified into three general morphological types: cartilaginous, fibrous, and synovial.

    a. cartilag'inis [NA], cartilaginous joint; a joint in which the apposed bony surfaces are united by cartilage, either a synchondrosis or a symphysis.

    a. fibro'sa [NA], fibrous joint; a union of two bones by fibrous tissue such that there is no joint cavity and little motion possible; types of fibrous joints are sutura, syndesmosis, and gomphosis.

    a. spheroi'dea [NA], ball-and-socket joint; a multiaxial joint in which a sphere on the head of one bone fits into a rounded cavity in the other bone, as in the hip joint.

    a. synovia'lis [NA], synovial joint; a joint in which the opposing bony surfaces are covered with a layer of hyaline cartilage or fibrocartilage; some degree of free movement is possible.

    a. tem'poromandibula'ris [NA], temporomandibular joint; the joint between the head of the mandible and the mandibular fossa and articular tubercle of the temporal bone.

articula'tion [L. *articulatio, q.v.*] **1.** Articulatio. **2.** A joining or connecting together loosely so as to allow motion between the parts. **3.** Distinct connected speech or enunciation.

ar'tifact Artefact.

aryte'noid [G. *arytainoeides*, ladle-shaped] Denoting a cartilage (cartilago arytenoidea) and a muscle (musculus arytenoideus) of the larynx.

asbes'tos [G. unquenchable] A fibrous natural material, composed of calcium and magnesium silicates, used for thermal insulation and fireproofing.

asbesto'sis Pneumoconiosis due to inhalation of asbestos particles; sometimes complicated by pleural mesothelioma or bronchial carcinoma.

ascari'asis [G. *askaris*, an intestinal worm, + -*iasis*, condition] Disease caused by infection with *Ascaris* or related ascarid nematodes.

as'carid 1. Any nematode of the family Ascarididae. **2.** Pertaining to such nematodes.

Ascarid'idae [G. *askaris,* an intestinal worm] A family of large intestinal roundworms (superfamily Ascaridoidea) that includes the genus *Ascaris.*

As'caris [G. *askaris,* an intestinal worm] A genus of large roundworms parasitic in the small intestine of man and many other vertebrates.

 A. lumbricoi'des, one of the commonest human parasites causing symptoms such as restlessness, fever, and sometimes diarrhoea; the similar species, *A. suum* (or *A. lumbricoides suum*) is common in swine.

asci'tes [L. fr. G. *askos,* a bag, + *-ites, q.v.*] Accumulation of serous fluid in the peritoneal cavity.

ascor'bate A salt or ester of ascorbic acid.

ascor'bic acid Vitamin C; the antiscorbutic vitamin, specifically preventing scurvy; a strong reducing agent, also used as an antioxidant in foodstuffs.

-ase Termination denoting an enzyme suffixed to the name of the substance (substrate) upon which the enzyme acts; enzymes named before the convention was established generally have an *-in* ending.

asep'sis [G. a- priv. + *sēpsis,* putrefaction] A condition in which living pathogenic organisms are absent; a state of sterility.

asep'tic Marked by or relating to asepsis.

asex'ual 1. Without sex, as in a. reproduction. **2.** Having no sexual desire or interest.

asi'alism, asia'lia [G. a-priv. + *sialon,* saliva] Diminished or arrested secretion of saliva.

aspar'aginase 1. An enzyme catalysing the hydrolysis of asparagine to aspartic acid and ammonia. **2.** The enzyme from *Escherichia coli,* used in the treatment of acute leukaemia and other neoplastic diseases.

asparagine (Asn) The β-amide of aspartic acid, a nonessential amino acid occurring in proteins.

aspar'tic acid (Asp) One of the amino acids occurring in proteins.

as'pergillo'ma 1. An infectious granuloma caused by *Aspergillus.* **2.** A variety of bronchopulmonary aspergillosis; a ball-like mass of *Aspergillis fumigatus* colonizing an existing cavity in the lung.

as'pergillo'sis Presence of any species of *Aspergillus* in the tissues or on a mucous surface and the symptoms produced thereby.

Aspergil'lus [Mediev. L. a sprinkler] A genus of fungi (class Ascomycetes) that contains many species, a number of them with black, brown, or green spores. Few species are pathogenic; *e.g., A. fumigatus,* a species that is the common cause of aspergillosis.

asper'matism, asper'mia [G. a-priv. + *sperma,* seed] Lack of secretion or of expulsion of semen following ejaculation.

asphyx'ia [G. a- priv. + *sphyzō,* to throb] Impaired or absent exchange of oxygen and carbon dioxide on a ventilatory basis; combined hypercapnia and hypoxia or anoxia.

aspira'tion 1. Removal, by suction, of a gas or fluid. **2.** Inspiratory sucking into the airways of fluid or foreign body, as of vomitus. **3.** Surgical technique for cataract, requiring a small corneal incision, severance of the lens capsule, fragmentation of the lens material, and aspiration with a needle.

as'pirator An apparatus for removing fluid by aspiration from any of the body cavities; consists usually of a hollow needle or trocar and cannula, connected by tubing with a container vacuumized by a syringe or reversed air (suction) pump.

as'pirin Acetylsalicylic acid; a widely used analgesic, antipyretic, and anti-inflammatory agent.

asple'nia Absence of the spleen.

as'say 1. Analysis; test of purity; trial. **2.** To examine; to subject to analysis.

assimila'tion [L. *as-similo,* pp. *-atus,* to make alike] **1.** Incorporation of digested materials from food into the tissues of the organism. **2.** Amalgamation and modification of newly perceived information and experiences into the existing cognitive structure.

asta'sia [G. unsteadiness] Inability, through muscular incoordination, to stand.

asta'sia-aba'sia. Inability to either stand or walk in the normal manner as a symptom of conversion hysteria.

as'teato'sis [G. a- priv. + *stear* (steat-), fat] Diminished or arrested action of the sebaceous glands.

aste'reogno'sis [G. a- priv. + *stereos,* solid, + *gnōsis,* knowledge] Inability to judge the form of an object by touch.

asterix'is [G. a- priv. + *stērixis,* fixed position] An abnormal tremor consisting of involuntary jerking movements, especially in the hands; commonly called a "liver flap" because of its frequent occurrence in patients with impending hepatic coma, although also seen in other forms of metabolic encephalopathy.

asthe'nia [G. *astheneia*, weakness] Weakness or debility.

neurocirculatory a., Da Costa's or effort syndrome; a syndrome of functional nervous and circulatory irregularities characterized by increased susceptibility to fatigue, palpitation, dyspnoea, rapid pulse, precordial pain, and anxiety; observed especially in soldiers on active duty.

astheno'pia [G. *astheneia*, weakness, + *ops*, eye] Eyestrain; subjective symptoms of ocular fatigue, discomfort, lacrimation, and headaches arising from use of the eyes.

asth'ma [G.] Originally, a term used to mean "difficult breathing"; now used to denote bronchial a.

bronchial a., a condition of the lungs in which there is widespread narrowing of airways, varying over short periods of time either spontaneously or as a result of treatment, due in varying degrees to contraction (spasm) of smooth muscle, oedema of the mucosa, and mucus in the lumen of the bronchi and bronchioles; caused by the local release of spasmogens and vasoactive substances in the course of an allergic process.

cardiac a., the bronchoconstriction being secondary to the pulmonary congestion and oedema of left ventricular failure.

asthmat'ic Relating to or suffering from asthma.

astigmat'ic Relating to astigmatism.

astig'matism [G. *a*- priv. + *stigma* (*stigmat*-), a point] **1.** A lens or optical system having different curvatures in different meridians. **2.** A condition of unequal curvatures along the different meridians in one or more of the refractive surfaces of the eye, in consequence of which the rays from a luminous point are not focused at a single point on the retina.

astigmatom'eter, astigmom'eter An instrument for measuring the degree and determining the variety of astigmatism.

astrag'alar Relating to the astragalus or talus.

astrag'alus [G. *astragalos*, ball of the ankle joint] Talus.

astrin'gent [L. *astringens*] Causing contraction of the tissues, arrest of secretion, or control of bleeding.

as'trocyte [G. *astron*, + *kytos*, hollow (cell)] One of the large neuroglia cells of nervous tissue.

fibrous a., stellate cell with long processes found in the white substance of the brain and spinal cord and characterized by having bundles of fine filaments in its cytoplasm.

protoplasmic a., one form of a., found in grey substance, having few fibrils and numerous branching processes.

astrocyto'ma [G. *astron*, star, + *kytos*, cell, + *-oma*, tumour] A relatively well differentiated glioma composed of neoplastic cells that resemble one of the types of astrocytes, with varying amounts of fibrillary stroma.

astrog'lia [G. *astron*, star, + neuroglia] Astrocyte.

asymptomat'ic Without symptoms, or producing no symptoms.

a'syner'gia, asyn'ergy [G. *a*- priv. + *syn*, with, + *ergon*, work] Lack of cooperation or working together of parts that normally act in unison.

asys'tole [G. *a*- priv. + *systolē*, a contracting] Absence of contractions of the heart.

asystol'ic **1.** Relating to asystole. **2.** Not systolic.

atax'ia [G. *a*- priv. + *taxis*, order] Inability to coordinate the muscles in voluntary movement.

Friedreich's a., hereditary cerebellar a.

hereditary cerebellar a., a disease of later childhood and early adult life, marked by ataxic gait, hesitating and explosive speech, nystagmus, and sometimes optic neuritis.

hereditary spinal a., sclerosis of the posterior and lateral columns of the spinal cord, occurring in children and marked by a. in the lower extremities, extending to the upper, followed by paralysis and contractures; autosomal recessive inheritance.

motor a., inability to perform coordinated muscular movements.

a. telangiecta'sia, a familial single-gene autosomal recessive disease characterized by progressive cerebellar a., with oculocutaneous telangiectases, proneness to pulmonary infections, and immunodeficiency.

-ate   Termination used to denote a salt or ester of an "-ic" acid.

atelec'tasis   [G. *ateles*, incomplete, + *ektasis*, extension] Absence of gas from a part or the whole of the lungs, due to failure of expansion or resorption of gas from the alveoli.

atelio'sis   [G. *ateles*, incomplete, + *-osis*, condition] Incomplete development of the body or any of its parts, as in infantilism and dwarfism.

athero-   [G. *athere*, gruel] Combinig form relating to the deposit of gruel-like, soft, pasty materials.

atherogen'esis   Formation of atheroma, important in the pathogenesis of arteriosclerosis.

athero'ma   [G. *athere*, gruel, + *-oma*, tumour] Lipid deposits in the intima of arteries, producing a yellow swelling on the endothelial surface, characteristic of atherosclerosis.

athero'matous   Relating to or affected by atheroma.

ath'eroscle'ro'sis   Arteriosclerosis characterized by irregularly distributed lipid deposits in the intima of large and medium-sized arteries; associated with fibrosis and calcification, and present to some degree in the middle-aged and elderly.

ath'etoid   Resembling athetosis.

atheto'sis   [G. *athetos*, without position or place] A constant succession of slow, writhing, involuntary movements of flexion, extension, pronation, and supination of the fingers and hands, and sometimes of the toes and feet.

athy'mia   [G. a- priv. + *thymos*, mind, also thymus] **1.** Absence of affect or emotivity; morbid impassivity. **2.** Absence of the thymus gland or its secretion.

atlanto-, atlo-   [G. *atlas*, q.v.] Combining forms relating to the atlas.

atlan'toax'ial   Pertaining to the atlas and the axis; denoting the joint between the two vertebrae.

at'las   [*Atlas*, G. myth. char.] [NA] First cervical vertebra, articulating with the occipital bone and rotating around the dens of the axis.

atlo-   See atlanto-.

at'om   [G. *atomos*, indivisible, uncut] The ultimate particle of an element, once believed to be as indivisible as its name indicates; now known to be composed of subatomic particles, notably protons, neutrons and electrons, the first two making up most of the mass of the atomic nucleus.

atom'ic   Relating to an atom.

at'omizer   A device used to reduce liquid medication to a spray or aerosol.

aton'ic   Relaxed; without normal tone or tension.

at'ony, ato'nia   [G. *atonia*, languor] Relaxation, flaccidity, or lack of tone or tension.

atop'ic   Relating to or marked by atopy.

at'opy   [G. *atopia*, strangeness, fr. a- priv. + *topos*, a place] Type I allergic reaction, specifically one with strong familial tendencies, caused by allergens such as pollens, foods, dander, and insect venoms.

atre'sia   [G. a- priv. + *tresis*, a hole] Absence of a normal opening or normally patent lumen.

    anal a., a. a'ni,   imperforate anus; congenital absence of an anal opening due to the presence of a membranous septum or to complete absence of the anal canal.

    biliary a.,   a. of the major bile ducts, causing cholestasis and jaundice.

atret'ic, atre'sic   Imperforate; relating to atresia.

a'tria   Plural of atrium.

a'trial   Relating to an atrium.

atrich'ia   [G. a- priv. + *thrix* (trich-), hair] Absence of hair, congenital or acquired.

atrio-   [L. *atrium*, q.v.] Combining form relating to an atrium.

a'triomeg'aly   [atrio- + G. *megas*, great] Enlargement of the atrium of the heart.

a'trioventric'ular (A-V)   Relating to both the atria and the ventricles of the heart.

a'trium,   pl. **a'tria** [L. entrance hall] **1.** [NA] A chamber or cavity to which are connected several chambers or passageways. **2.** A. cordis. **3.** That part of the tympanic cavity that lies immediately deep to the eardrum. **4.** In the lung, a subdivision of the alveolar duct from which alveolar sacs open.

    a. cor'dis   [NA], the upper chamber of each half of the heart.

    a. dex'trum   [NA], a. of the right side of the heart which receives the blood from the venae cavae and coronary sinus.

    a. sinis'trum   [NA], a. of the left side of the heart which receives the blood from the pulmonary veins.

atroph'ic   Denoting atrophy.

at'rophy [G. *atrophia*, fr. *a*- priv. + *trophē*, nourishment] A wasting of tissues, as from death and reabsorption of cells, diminished cellular proliferation, pressure, ischaemia, malnutrition, decreased function, or hormonal changes.

   acute yellow a. of the liver, extensive and rapid death of parenchymal cells of the liver, sometimes with fatty degeneration.

   peroneal muscular a., Charcot-Marie-Tooth disease; fasicular degeneration characterized by slowly progressive wasting of distal muscles of the extremities, usually involving the legs before the arms; autosomal dominant, autosomal recessive, and X chromosome-linked recessive types exist, with severity related to genetic type.

   Pick's a., circumscribed a. of the cerebral cortex.

   progressive muscular a., Duchenne-Aran, Aran-Duchenne, or Cruveilier's disease; a. of the cells of the anterior cornua of the spinal cord, resulting in a slow progressive wasting and paralysis of the muscles of the extremities and of the trunk.

   spinal a., *tabes* dorsalis.

at'ropine An alkaloid obtained from *Atropa belladonna*; antispasmodic, antisudorific, anticholinorgic, and mydriatic.

attack' Occurrence of some disease or episode, often with a dramatic onset.

   transient ischaemic a. (TIA), a sudden loss of neurological function with complete recovery within hours, as the result of cerebral vascular impairment.

attenua'tion [L. *at-tenuo*, pp. *-tenuatus*, to make thin or weak] **1.** Dilution; thinning. **2.** Diminution of virulence in a strain of an organism, obtained through selection of variants which occur naturally or experimentally. **3.** Reduction or weakening. **4.** Loss of energy of an ultrasonic beam as it propagates through a medium.

at'titude [Mediev. L. *aptitudo*, fr. L. *aptus*, fit] **1.** Posture; position of the body and limbs. **2.** Manner of acting. **3.** In social or clinical psychology, a relatively stable and enduring predisposition or set to behave or react in a certain way.

atyp'ical [G. *a*- priv. + *typikos*, conformed to a type] Not typical; not corresponding to the normal form or type.

audio- [L. *audio*, to hear] Combining form relating to hearing.

au'diogram [audio- + G. *gramma*, a drawing] The graphic record drawn from the results of hearing tests with the audiometer.

audiol'ogist A specialist in evaluation, habitation, and rehabilitation of those whose communication disorders centre in whole or in part in the hearing function.

audiol'ogy The study of hearing disorders through the identification and measurement of hearing function loss as well as the rehabilitation of persons with hearing impairments.

audiom'eter [audio- + G. *metron*, measure] An electrical instrument for measuring the threshold of hearing for pure tones of frequencies generally varying from 200 to 8000 Hz (recorded in terms of decibels); also records thresholds for lists of spoken words and discrimination percentage for phonetically balanced word lists.

audiom'etry Use of the audiometer.

au'ditory [L. *audio*, pp. *auditus*, to hear] Pertaining to the sense of hearing or to the organs of hearing.

au'ra, pl. **au'rae** [L. breeze, odour, gleam of light] A peculiar sensation felt by the patient immediately preceding an epileptic attack; called auditory, epigastric, vertiginous, etc., according to its seat or nature.

au'ral 1. Relating to the ear (auris). **2.** Relating to an aura.

auri- [L. *auris*, ear] Combining form denoting the ear. See also ot-, oto-.

au'ricle Auricula.

auric'ula, pl. **auric'ulae** [L. the external ear. dim. of *auris*, ear] [NA] Auricle; pinna; the projecting shell-like structure on the side of the head constituting, with the external acoustic meatus, the external ear.

auric'ular Relating to the ear, or to an auricle in any sense.

au'ris, pl. **au'res** [L.] [NA] Ear.

au'riscope [L. *auris*, ear, + *skopeō*, to view] Otoscope.

aus'cultate [L. *ausculto*, pp. *-atus*, to listen to] To perform auscultation.

ausculta'tion Listening to the sounds made by the various body structures as a diagnostic method.

auscul'tatory Relating to auscultation.

au'tism [G. *autos*, self] A tendency to morbid self-absorption at the expense of regulation by outward reality.

infantile a., severe emotional disturbance of childhood characterized by inability to form meaningful interpersonal relationships; believed by some to be a form of childhood schizophrenia.

autis'tic Pertaining to or suffering from autism.

auto-, aut- [G. *autos*, self] A prefix meaning self, same.

au'to-agglu'tinin An agglutinating autoantibody.

au'to-agglutina'tion 1. Nonspecific agglutination or clumping together of cells (*e.g.*, bacteria, erythrocytes, and the like) due to physical-chemical factors. **2.** The a. of a person's red blood cells in his own serum, as a consequence of specific autoantibody.

au'to-al'lergy An altered reactivity in which antibodies (autoantibodies) are produced against one's own tissues, causing a destructive rather than a protective effect.

au'to-an'tibody An antibody that has affinity for one or other tissue of the subject in whom the antibody was formed.

au'toclave [auto- + L. *clavis*, a key, in the sense of self-locking] **1.** An apparatus for sterilization by steam under pressure. **2.** To sterilize in an autoclave.

autoer'otism, autoerot'icism [auto- + G. *erōtikos*, relating to love] **1.** Sexual arousal or gratification using one's own body, as in masturbation. **2.** Sexual self-love, in contrast with alloerotism.

autog'enous [G. *autogenēs*, self-produced] Originating within the body, *i.e.*, endogenous; applied to vaccines prepared from bacteria obtained from the infected person.

au'tograft Autologous graft; tissue or an organ transferred by grafting into a new position in the body of the same individual.

autohaemol'ysin An autoantibody that (with complement) causes lysis of erythrocytes in the same person or animal in whose body the lysin is formed.

autoimmu'nity In immunology, the condition in which one's own tissues are subject to deleterious effects of the immunological system.

au'toimmuniza'tion Induction of autoimmunity.

autoinfec'tion 1. Reinfection by microbes or parasitic organisms on or within the body that have already passed through an infective cycle, such as a succession of boils, or a new infective cycle with production of a new generation of larvae and adults. **2.** Self-infection by direct contagion, as with parasite eggs passed in the infectious state transmitted by fingernails.

autoinfu'sion Forcing the blood from the extremities, as by the application of a bandage or pressure device, in order to raise the blood pressure and fill the vessels in the vital centres.

au'toinoc'ula'tion A secondary infection originating from a focus of infection already present in the body.

au'tointoxica'tion Self-poisoning as the result of absorption of the waste products of metabolism, decomposed matter from the intestine, or the products of dead and infected tissue as in gangrene.

autol'ogous [auto- + G. *logos*, relation] **1.** Occurring naturally and normally in a certain type of tissue or a specific structure of the body. **2.** Sometimes used to indicate a neoplasm derived from cells that occur normally in that site, *e.g.*, a squamous cell carcinoma in the oesophagus. **3.** In transplantation, referring to a graft in which the donor and recipient areas are in the same individual.

autol'ysin An antibody that (with complement) causes lysis of the cells and tissues in the body of the person (or animal) in whom the lysin is formed.

autol'ysis [auto- + G. *lysis*, dissolution] **1.** Enzymic digestion of cells (especially when dead or degenerate) by enzymes present within them (autogenous). **2.** Destruction of cells as a result of a lysin formed in those cells or others in the same organism.

autom'atism 1. The state of being independent of the will or of central innervation, as the heart's action. **2.** An act performed without intent or conscious exercise of the will, often without realization of its occurrence. **3.** A condition in which one is consciously or unconsciously, but involuntarily, compelled to the performance of certain acts.

autonom'ic [G. *autonomos*, fr. *autos*, self, + *nomos*, law] **1.** Functionally independent; not under voluntary control. **2.** Relating to the autonomic nervous system.

au'topsy [G. *autopsia*, seeing with one's own eyes] Postmortem examination; an examination of a dead body for the purpose of determining the cause of death or of studying the pathologic changes present.

autora'diograph Reproduction of the distribution and concentration of radioactivity in a tissue or other substance made by placing a photographic emulsion on the surface of, or in close proximity to, the substance.

au'toregula'tion 1. The tendency of the blood flow to an organ or part to remain at or return to the same level despite changes in the pressure in the artery which conveys blood to it. 2. In general, any biologic system equipped with inhibitory feedback systems such that a given change tends to be largely or completely counteracted.

au'toreproduc'tion The ability of a gene or virus, or nucleoprotein molecule generally, to bring about the synthesis of another molecule like itself from smaller molecules within the cell.

autoso'mal Pertaining to an autosome.

au'tosome [auto- + G. *sōma*, body] Any chromosome other than a sex chromosome, normally occurring in pairs in somatic cells and singly in gametes.

au'tosugges'tion 1. Constant dwelling upon an idea or concept, thereby inducing some change in the mental or bodily functions. 2. Reproduction in the brain of impressions previously received which become then the starting point of new acts or ideas.

au'totransfu'sion Transfusing back into the body of blood removed.

au'totransplanta'tion Performance of an autograft.

auxano-, aux-, auxo- [G. *auxanō*, to increase] Prefix denoting relation to increase.

auxe'sis [G. increase] Increase in size, especially as in hypertrophy.

avas'cular Nonvascular; without blood or lymphatic vessels.

avas'culariza'tion 1. Expulsion of blood from a part. 2. Loss of vascularity, as by scarring.

avit'amino'sis A deficiency disease state resulting from an inadequate supply of one or more vitamins in the diet.

avul'sion [L. *a-vello*, pp. *-vulsus*, to tear away] A tearing away or forcible separation.

axes Plural of axis.

ax'ial 1. Relating to an axis. 2. Relating to or situated in the central part of the body (head and trunk). 3. In dentistry, relating to or parallel with the long axis of a tooth.

axil'la, gen. and pl. **axil'lae** [L.] *Fossa axillaris.*

ax'illary Relating to the axilla.

axio- [L. *axis*] Combining form relating to an axis. See also axo-.

ax'is, pl. **ax'es** [L. axle, axis] 1. A straight line passing through a spherical body between its two poles, and about which the body may revolve. 2. The central line of the body or any of its parts. 3. [NA] The second cervical vertebra. 4. An artery that divides, immediately upon its origin, into a number of branches.

  visual a., line of vision; the straight line extending from the object seen, through the centre of the pupil, to the macula lutea of the retina.

axo- [G. *axōn*, axis] Combining form meaning axis, usually relating to an axon.

axolem'ma [axo- + G. *lemma*, husk] The delicate plasma membrane of the axon.

ax'on [G. *axōn*, axis] The single one among a nerve cell's processes that under normal conditions conducts nervous impulses away from the cell body and its remaining cell processes (dendrites). A relatively even filamentous process varying in thickness that, in contrast to dendrites, can extend far away from the parent cell body. With some exceptions, nerve cells can synaptically transmit impulses to other nerve cells or to effector cells exclusively by way of the synaptic terminals of their a.

ax'onal Pertaining to an axon.

axonotme'sis [axo- + G. *tmēsis*, a cutting] Interruption of the axons of a nerve followed by complete degeneration of the peripheral segment, without severance of the supporting structure of the nerve.

a'zoosper'mia [G. a- priv. + *zōon*, animal, + *sperma*, seed] 1. Absence of living spermatozoa in the semen. 2. Failure of spermatogenesis.

azotae'mia [azote + G. *haima*, blood] Uraemia.

azotu'ria [azote + G. *ouron*, urine] An increased elimination of urea in the urine.

azy'gos [G. a- priv. + *zygon*, a yoke] An unpaired (azygous) anatomical structure.

azy'gous [L. *azygos*] Unpaired; single.

B

Babe'sia [V. *Babés*] A genus of protozoa (family Babesiidae) characterized by multiplication in host red blood cells to form pairs and tetrads; causes babesiosis (piroplasmosis) in most types of domestic animals; several species cause malaria-like disease in splenectomized or normal people; known vectors are ixodid or argasid ticks.

ba'by An infant; a newborn child.

blue b., a child born cyanotic because of congenital cardiac or pulmonary defect causing incomplete oxygenation of the blood.

collodion b., a newborn child with lamellar ichthyosis; the skin, at birth, is bright red, shiny, translucent, and drawn tight, giving a distorted appearance (as if painted with collodion) of immobilization of the face.

bacillae'mia [bacillus + G. *haima*, blood] Presence of rod-shaped bacteria in the circulating blood.

bac'illary Rod-shaped; consisting of rods or rodlike elements.

Bacille bilié de Calmette-Guérin (BCG) [Fr.] An attenuated strain of *Mycobacterium bovis* used in the preparation of BCG vaccine.

bacil'li Plural of bacillus.

bacil'liform [L. *bacillus*, a rod, + *forma*, form] Rod-shaped.

bacil'lin An antibiotic substance produced by *Bacillus subtilis*.

bacillo'sis A general infection with bacilli.

bacillu'ria [bacillus + G. *ouron*, urine] Presence of bacilli in the urine.

Bacil'lus [L. dim of *baculus*, rod, staff] A genus of aerobic or facultatively anaerobic, sporeforming, ordinarily motile bacteria (family Bacillaceae) containing Gram-positive rods; found primarily in soil; a few species are animal pathogens; some produce antibodies.

bacil'lus, pl. **bacil'li** [L. dim. of *baculus*, a rod, staff] General term for any member of the genus *Bacillus*; formerly used to refer to any rod-shaped bacterium.

bacitra'cin An antibacterial polypeptide of known chemical structure isolated from cultures of a member of the *Bacillus subtilis* group; active against haemolytic streptococci, staphylococci, and several types of Gram-positive, aerobic, rod-shaped organisms; usually applied locally.

back'ache Nonspecific term used to describe back pain, generally below cervical level.

back'bone *Columna* vertebralis.

bacterae'mia [bacteria + G. *haima*, blood] Presence of viable bacteria in the circulating blood.

bacte'ria Plural of bacterium.

bacte'rial Relating to bacteria.

bacterici'dal Causing the death of bacteria.

bac'terid [bacteria + -id (1)] **1.** A recurrent or persistent eruption of discrete, sterile pustules of the palms and soles, thought to be an allergic response to infection at a remote site. **2.** A dissemination of a previously localized bacterial skin infection.

bacterio- [see bacterium] Combining form relating to bacteria.

bacteriolog'ic, bacteriolog'ical Relating to bacteria or to bacteriology.

bacteriol'ogist One who primarily studies or works with bacteria.

bacteriol'ogy [bacterio- + G. *logos*, study] The branch of science concerned with the study of bacteria.

bacteriol'ysin Specific antibody that combines with bacterial cells (*i.e.*, antigen) and, when adequate complement is available, causes lysis or dissolution of the cells.

bacteriol'ysis [bacterio- + G. *lysis*, dissolution] The dissolution of bacteria, as by specific antibody and complement.

bacteriolyt'ic Pertaining to lysis of bacteria; manifesting the ability to cause dissolution of bacterial cells.

bacte'riophage [bacterio- + G. *phagein*, to eat] Phage; a virus with specific affinity for bacteria, found in association with essentially all groups of bacteria; like other viruses they contain either RNA or DNA; their relationships to the host bacteria are rather specific and, as in the case of temperate b., may be genetically intimate; they are named after the bacterial species, group, or strain for which they are specific.

bacte'riostat'ic Inhibiting or retarding the growth of bacteria.

bacte'rium, pl. **bacte'ria** [Mod. L. fr. G. *baktērion*, dim. of *baktron*, a staff] A prokaryotic microorganism that differs from blue-green bacteria (blue-green algae) primarily in that the blue-green bacteria perform photosynthesis accompanied by oxygen evolution and have a photosynthetic pigment system that includes chlorophyll α- and β-carotene.

bacteriu'ria Presence of bacteria in the urine.

Bacteroid'es [G. *bacterion* + *eidos*, form] A genus of obligately anaerobic, nonsporeforming bacteria (family Bacteroidaceae, order Eubacteriales) containing Gram-negative rods; some species are pathogenic to man and other animals.

B. frag'ilis, a species that is one of the predominant organisms in the lower intestinal tracts of man and other animals; also found in specimens from appendicitis, peritonitis, rectal abscesses, pilonidal cysts, surgical wounds, and lesions of the urogenital tract.

B. melaninogen'icus, a species found in the mouth, faeces, infections of the mouth, soft tissue, respiratory tract, urogenital tract, and the intestinal tract; pathogenic, but ordinarily in association with other organisms.

bag [A.S. *baelg*] A pouch; sac; receptacle.

breathing b., a collapsible reservoir from which gases are inhaled and into which gases may be exhaled during general anaesthesia or artificial ventilation.

colostomy b., a b. worn over an artificial anus to collect faeces.

Douglas b., a large b. for the collection of expired air for several minutes to determine oxygen consumption in man under many conditions of actual work.

Politzer b., a pear-shaped rubber b. used for forcing air through the eustachian tube.

b. of waters, common term for the amniotic sac and its contained amniotic fluid.

balan'ic [G. *balanos*, acorn, glans] Relating to the glans penis or glans clitoridis.

balani'tis [G. *balanos*, acorn, glans, + *-itis*, inflammation] Inflammation of the glans penis or glans clitoridis.

balano-, balan- [G. *balanos*, acorn, glans] Combining forms relating to the glans penis.

bal'anoplasty Any reparative operation upon the glans penis.

bal'antidi'asis A disease caused by the presence of *Balantidium coli* in the large intestine; characterized by diarrhoea, dysentery, and occasionally ulceration.

Balantid'ium [G. *balantidion*, dim of *ballantion*, a bag] A genus of trichostome ciliates (family Balantidiidae) found in the digestive tract of vertebrates and invertebrates. *B. coli,* a large parasitic species; found in the caecum or large intestine, swimming actively in the lumen; usually harmless in man but may invade and ulcerate the intestinal wall, producing balantidiasis.

bald'ness Alopecia.

ballis'mus [G. *ballismos*, a jumping about] The occurrence of lively jerking or shaking movements, especially as observed in chorea.

ballis'tocar'diogram [G. *ballo*, to throw, + *kardia*, heart, + *gramma*, something written] A record of the body's recoil caused by cardiac contraction and the ejection of blood into the aorta; may be used as a basis for calculating the cardiac output in man.

ballis'tocardiog'raphy 1. The graphic recording of movements of the body imparted by ballistic forces of cardiac contraction and ejection of blood. **2.** The study and interpretation of ballistocardiograms.

balloon' An inflatable spherical or ovoid device used to retain tubes or catheters in, or provide support to, various body structures.

ballot'tement [Fr. *balloter*, to toss up] **1.** A manoeuvre in physical examination to estimate the size of an organ not near the surface, particularly when there is ascites, by a flicking motion of the hand or fingers. **2.** An infrequently used method of diagnosis of pregnancy: with the tip of the forefinger in the vagina, a sharp tap is made against the lower segment of the uterus; the fetus, if present, is moved upward and will be felt to strike against the wall of the uterus.

balm [L. *balsanum*, fr. G. *balsamon*, the balsam tree] **1.** An ointment, especially a fragrant one. **2.** A soothing or healing medication.

bancrofti'asis, bancrofto'sis Infection with *Wuchereria bancrofti*.

ban'dage 1. A piece of cloth or other material applied to a body part to make compression, absorb drainage, prevent motion, retain surgical dressings, etc. **2.** To cover a body part by application of a b.

baraesthe'sia [G. *baros*, weight, + *aisthēsis*, sensation] Pressure *sense*.

baragno'sis [G. *baros*, weight + a- priv., + *gnōsis*, a knowing] Impairment of the ability to differentiate among weights or pressures.

bar'bitone 5,5-Diethylbarbituric acid; a hypnotic and sedative.

barbit'urates Derivatives of barbituric acid that are CNS depressants; used as tranquilizers and hypnotics.

barbitu'ric acid A crystalline dibasic acid from which barbitone and other barbiturates are derived.

bar'biturism Chronic poisoning by any of the derivatives of barbituric acid.

barbotage' [Fr. *barboter*, to dabble] A method of spinal anaesthesia in which a portion of the anaesthetic solution is injected into the cerebral spinal fluid; cerebral spinal fluid is then aspirated into the syringe and a second portion of the contents of the syringe is injected; this process is repeated until the entire contents of the syringe are injected.

bariat'rics [G. *baros*, weight, + *iatreia*, medical treatment] That branch of medicine or surgery concerned with the management of obesity and allied diseases.

bar'ium [G. *barys*, heavy] A metallic, alkaline, divalent earth element; symbol Ba, atomic weight 137.36, atomic no. 56.

b. hydroxide, $Ba(OH)_2$; a caustic compound combined with calcium hydroxide in a carbon dioxide absorbent; used in anaesthetic circuits.

b. sulphate, $BaSO_4$; given orally or rectally as a suspension for x-ray visualization of the gastrointestinal tract.

baro- [G. *baros*, weight] Combining form relating to weight or pressure.

baroceptor Baroreceptor.

bar'orecep'tor Sensory nerve ending in the wall of the auricles of the heart, vena cava, aortic arch, and carotid sinus, sensitive to stretching of the wall resulting from increased pressure from within, and functioning as the elicitation point of central reflex mechanisms that tend to reduce that pressure.

bar'osinusi'tis [G. *baros*, weight, pressure + *sinusitis*] Aerosinusitis.

bar'ostat A pressure-regulating device or structure, such as the baroreceptors of the carotid sinus and aortic arch.

baroti'tis me'dia Aerotitis media.

bar'otrauma [G. *baros*, weight, + *trauma*] Injury, generally to the middle ear or paranasal sinuses, resulting from imbalance between ambient pressure and that within the affected cavity.

bar'rier 1. An obstacle or impediment. 2. In psychiatry and social psychiatry, a conflictual agent that blocks resolving behaviour.

blood-brain b., blood-cerebro-spinal fluid b., a selective mechanism opposing the passage of most large-molecular compounds from the blood to the cerebrospinal fluid and brain tissue.

placental b., the tissue intervening between fetal and maternal blood in the placenta; acts as a selective membrane regulating the passage of substances from the maternal to the fetal blood.

Bartonel'la [A. L. *Barton*] A genus of bacteria (family Bartonellaceae, order Rickettsiales) that multiply in fixed-tissue cells and in erythrocytes, and reproduce by binary fission; they are found in man and in arthropod vectors.

B. bacillifor'mis, a species found in the blood and epithelial cells of lymph nodes, spleen, and liver in Oroya fever, and in blood and eruptive elements in verruga peruana.

bartonello'sis A disease caused by *Bartonella bacilliformis* and transmitted by the bite of the sandfly, *Phlebotomus verrucarum*. It occurs in three forms: 1) Oroya fever, a generalized, acute, febrile, systemic infection, frequently fatal; 2) verruga peruana, a chronic form of the disease followed by nodular eruptions; 3) a combination (or sequence) of these.

ba'sal 1. Situated nearer the base of a pyramid-shaped organ in relation to a specific reference point. 2. In physiology, denoting the lowest level possible.

base [L. and G. *basis*] 1. Basis; the lower part or bottom; the part opposite the apex; the foundation. 2. In pharmacy, the chief ingredient of a mixture. 3. In chemistry, an electropositive element (cation) that unites with an anion to form a salt; a compound ionizing to yield hydroxyl ion. 4. Brønsted b; any molecule or ion that combines with hydrogen ion.

base pair Nucleoside or nucleotide pair; the complex of two heterocyclic nucleic acid bases, one a pyrimidine and the other a purine, brought about by hydrogen bonding; the essential element in the structure of DNA.

basi-, basio-, baso- [G. and L. *basis*, base] Combining forms meaning base, or basis.

ba'sic Relating to a base.

basic'ity 1. The valency or combining power of an acid, or the number of replaceable atoms of hydrogen in its molecule. 2. The quality of being basic.

ba'sihy'al, basihy'oid The base or body of the hyoid bone.

ba'silar Relating to the base of a pyramidal or broad structure.

basip'etal [basi- + L. *peto*, to seek] In a direction toward the base.

ba'sis [L. and G.] [NA] Base (1).

basisphe'noid Relating to the base or body of the sphenoid bone; denoting the independent centre of ossification in the embryo that forms the posterior portion of the body of the sphenoid bone.

ba'sophil, ba'sophile [baso- + G *phileo*, to love] 1. A cell with granules that stain specifically with basic dyes. 2. Basophilic.

ba'sophil'ia 1. More than the usual number of basophilic leucocytes in the circulating blood or an increase in the proportion of parenchymatous basophilic cells in an organ. 2. Basophilic erythrocytes in circulating blood, as in certain instances of leukaemia, advanced anaemia, malaria, and plumbism.

ba'sophil'ic Denoting tissue components having an affinity for basic dyes under specific pH conditions.

bath [A.S. *baeth*] 1. Immersion of the body or any of its parts in water or any other yielding or fluid medium; or application of such medium in any form to all or part of the body. 2. The apparatus used in giving a b. of any form, qualified according to the medium used, temperature of the medium, form in which the medium is applied, medicament added to the medium, and part bathed.

   colloid b., a b. prepared by adding soothing agents to the b. water.

   contrast b., a b. in which a part is immersed alternately in hot and cold water.

   douche b., local application of water in the form of a jet or stream.

   needle b., a shower in which water is projected against the body in the shape of many very fine jets.

   sitz b. [Ger. *sitzen*, to sit], immersion of only the hips and buttocks in the b.

   sponge b., a b. in which the body is washed with a wet sponge or cloth.

bathy- [G. *bathys*, deep] Combining form relating to depth.

bathyaesthe'sia [G. *bathys*, deep, + *aisthesis*, sensation] General term for all subcutaneous sensation.

bear'ing down The expulsive effort of a parturient woman in the second stage of labour.

bed In anatomy, a base or structure that supports another structure.

   capillary b., the capillaries considered collectively and their volume capacity.

   nail b., *matrix* unguis.

bed'bug *Cimex lectularius.*

bed'sore Decubitus *ulcer.*

bed-wetting Enuresis.

beha'viour 1. Any response emitted by or elicited from an organism. 2. Any mental or motor act or activity. 3. Specifically, parts of a total response pattern.

beha'vioural Pertaining to behaviour.

beha'viourism Behavioural psychology; a branch of psychology that attempts to formulate, through systematic observation and experimentation, the laws and principles which underlie the behaviour of man and animals; its major contributions have been made in the areas of conditioning and learning.

belch'ing [A.S. *baelcian*] Eructation.

belladon'na [It. *bella*, beautiful, + *donna*, lady] Deadly nightshade; *Atropa belladonna* (family Solanaceae); a perennial herb whose leaves and root contain atropine and related alkaloids which are anticholinergic; used as a powder and tincture.

bel'ly [O.E. *belig*, bag] 1. The abdomen. 2. Venter (2). 3. Popularly, the stomach or womb.

bends [fr. convulsive posture of those so afflicted] Decompression *sickness.*

benign' [thru O. Fr. fr. L. *benignus*, kind] Denoting the mild character of an illness or the nonmalignant character of a neoplasm.

ben'zene A highly toxic hydrocarbon from light coal tar oil used as the basic structure in the aromatic compounds of all chemistry and as a solvent.

ben'zocaine The ethyl ester of *p*-aminobenzoic acid; a topical anaesthetic agent.

benzodiaz'epine Parent compound for the synthesis of a number of psychoactive compounds having a common molecular configuration and similar pharmacologic activity; *e.g.*, diazepam, chlordiazepoxide.

ber'iber'i [Singhalese, extreme weakness] A specific polyneuritis resulting mainly from a deficiency of thiamine in the diet; sensory nerves are likely to be affected more than motor nerves, symptoms beginning in the feet and working upward, with the hands affected later.

berylio'sis Beryllium poisoning characterized by the occurrence of granulomatous fibrosis, especially of the lungs, from inhalation of beryllium salts.

beryl'lium A white metal element belonging to the alkaline earths; symbol Be, atomic weight 9.013, atomic no. 4.

bestial'ity Sexual relations with an animal.

betameth'asone A semisynthetic glucocorticoid with anti-inflammatory effects and toxicity similar to those of cortisol; for systemic and topical therapy, its actions are similar to those of prednisone, but more potent.

be'zoar [Pers. *padzahr*, antidote] A concretion formed in the alimentary canal of animals, and occasionally man; according to the substance forming the ball, it may be termed trichobezoar (hairball), trichophytobezoar (hair and vegetable fibre mixed), or phytobezoar (foodball).

bi- [L.] Prefix meaning twice or double, referring to double structures, dual actions, etc. See also di- and bis-.

bicam'eral [bi- + L. *camera*, chamber] Having two chambers; denoting especially an abscess divided by a more or less complete septum.

bicar'bonate HCO_3-; the ion remaining after the first dissociation of carbonic acid.

 standard b., the plasma b. concentration of a sample of whole blood that has been equilibrated at 37°C with a carbon dioxide pressure of 40 mm Hg and an oxygen pressure greater than 100 mm Hg; abnormally high or low values indicate metabolic alkalosis or acidosis, respectively.

bicel'lular Having two cells or subdivisions.

bi'ceps [bi- + L. *caput*, head] Bicipital.

bicip'ital [bi- + L. *caput*, head] Two-headed, denoting a biceps muscle.

bicon'cave Concave on two sides; denoting especially a form of lens.

bicon'vex Convex on two sides; denoting especially a form of lens.

bicor'nous, bicor'nuate, bicor'nate [bi- + L. *cornu*, horn] Two-horned; having two processes or projections.

bicus'pid [bi- + L. *cuspis*, point] Having two points, prongs, or cusps.

bi'fid [L. *bifidus*, cleft in two parts] Split or cleft; separated into two parts.

bifo'cal Having two foci.

bifur'cate, bifur'cated [bi- + L. *furca*, fork] Forked; two-pronged; having two branches.

bifurca'tion A forking; a division into two branches.

bigem'iny [bi- + L. *geminus*, twin] Twinning; pairing; especially, the occurrence of heart beats in pairs.

bilat'eral [bi- + L. *latus*, side] Relating to, or having, two sides.

bile [L. *bilis*] Gall; the yellowish brown or green fluid secreted by the liver and discharged into the duodenum where it aids in the emulsification of fats, increases peristalsis, and retards putrefaction.

Bilhar'zia [T. *Bilharz*] An early name for *Schistosoma*, the genus of trematode worms causing animal and human blood fluke disease.

bilharzi'asis Schistosomiasis.

bili- [L. *bilis*, bile] Combining form relating to bile.

bil'iary Relating to bile.

bil'iousness An imprecisely delineated congestive disturbance with anorexia, coated tongue, constipation, headache, dizziness, pasty complexion, and, rarely, slight jaundice; assumed to result from hepatic dysfunction.

biliru'bin [bili- + L. *ruber*, red] A red bile pigment found as sodium bilirubinate (soluble), or as an insoluble calcium salt in gallstones; formed from haemoglobin during normal and abnormal destruction of erythrocytes by the reticuloendothelial system.

bilirubinae'mia [bilirubin + G. *haima*, blood] Presence of bilirubin in the blood, where normally present in relatively small amounts; usually used in relation to increased concentrations observed in various pathologic conditions where there is excessive destruction of erythrocytes or interference with the mechanism of excretion in the bile.

biliru'binu'ria [bilirubin + G. *ouron*, urine] Bilirubin in the urine.

biliu'ria [bili- + G. *ouron*, urine] Presence of various bile salts, or bile, in the urine.

biliver'dine, biliver'din   A green bile pigment formed from the oxidation of bilirubin.

bilo'bate   Having two lobes.

biloc'ular, biloc'ulate   [bi- + L. *loculus*, dim. of *locus*, a place] Having two compartments or spaces.

bi'nary   [L. *binarius*, consisting of two, fr. *bini*, double] Denoting two.

binau'ral   [L. *bini*, a pair, + *auris*, ear] Relating to both ears.

bind'er   A broad bandage, especially one encircling the abdomen.

    obstetrical b.,   a garment covering the abdomen from the ribs to the trochanters, affording support after childbirth or, rarely, during childbirth.

binoc'ular   [L. *bini*, paired, + *oculus*, eye] Adapted to the use of both eyes; said of an optical instrument.

binov'ular   [L. *bini*, pair, + Mod. L. *ovulum*, dim. of L. *ovum*, egg] Relating to or derived from two ova.

binu'clear, binu'cleate   Having two nuclei.

bio-   [G. *bios*, life] Combining form denoting life.

bioas'say   Determination of the potency or concentration of a compound by its effect upon animals, isolated tissues, or microorganisms.

bi'oavailabil'ity   Physiological availability of a given amount of a drug, as distinct from its chemical potency.

biochem'ical   Relating to biochemistry, or physiological chemistry.

biochem'istry   Biological or physiological chemistry; the chemistry of living organisms and of the changes occurring therein.

biofeed'back   A training technique that enables an individual to gain some element of voluntary control over autonomic body functions; based on the learning principle that a desired response is learned when received information (feedback) indicates that a specific thought complex or action has produced the desired response.

biogen'esis   [bio- + G. *genesis*, origin] The now generally accepted view that life originates only from preexisting life and not from nonliving material.

biogenet'ic   Relating to biogenesis.

biolo'gic, biolog'ical   Relating to biology.

biol'ogy   [bio- + G. *logos*, study] The science concerned with the phenomena of life and living organisms.

    cellular b.,   cytology.

    molecular b.,   that aspect of b. concerned with biological phenomena in terms of molecular (or chemical) interactions; it differs from biochemistry in that the latter is concerned primarily with the chemical behaviour of biologically important substances and analogues thereof, and differs from general biology or parts thereof in its emphasis on chemical interactions, especially those involved in the replication of DNA, its "transcription" into RNA, and its "translation" into or expression in protein, *i.e.*, in the chemical reactions connecting genotype and phenotype.

biomechan'ics   The science of the action of forces, internal or external, on the living body.

biomed'ical   1. Pertaining to those aspects of the natural sciences, especially the biologic and physiologic sciences, that relate to or underlie medicine. 2. Biological and medical, *i.e.*, encompassing both the science(s) and the art.

biom'etry   The statistical analysis of biological data.

bion'ics   [bio- + electronics] The science of biologic functions and mechanisms as applied to electronic chemistry, such as computers, employing various aspects of physics, mathematics, and chemistry.

biophys'ics   1. The study of biological processes and materials by means of the theories and tools of physics. 2. The study of physical processes occurring in organisms.

bi'opsy   [bio- + G. *opsis*, vision] 1. The process of removing tissue from living patients for diagnostic examination. 2. A specimen so obtained.

    aspiration b.,   needle b.

    excision b.,   excision of tissue for gross and microscopic examination in such a manner that the entire lesion is removed.

    incision b.,   removal of only a part of a lesion by cutting into it.

    needle b.,   removal of the specimen for b. by aspirating it through an appropriate needle or trocar that pierces the skin, or the external surface of an organ, and into the underlying tissue to be examined.

    punch b.,   removal of a small cylindroid specimen for b. by means of a special instrument that either directly pierces the organ, or through the skin or a small incision in it.

bio'rhythm [bio- + G. *rhythmos*, rhythm] A biologically inherent cyclic variation or recurrence of an event or state, such as the sleep cycle, circadian rhythms, periodic diseases.

biostatis'tics The science of statistics applied to biological or medical data.

biosyn'thesis Formation of a chemical compound by enzymes, either in the organism (*in vivo*) or by fragments or extracts of cells (*in vitro*).

bi'otin A component of the vitamin B_2 complex occurring in or required by most organisms.

bi'otransforma'tion Conversion within an organism of molecules from one form to another; refers especially to drugs and other xenobiotics, a change often associated with change in pharmacologic activity.

bip'arous [bi- + L. *pario*, to give birth] Bearing two offspring.

bipen'nate, bipen'niform [bi- + L. *penna*, feather] Denoting a muscle with a central tendon toward which the fibres converge on either side like the barbs of a feather.

bipo'lar 1. Having two poles; denoting those nerve cells in which the branches project from two, usually opposite, points. 2. Relating to both ends or poles of a bacterial or other cell.

birth Passage of offspring from the uterus to the outside world; the act of being born.

premature b., the b. of an infant after the period of viability but before full term.

birth'mark Naevus (1).

bis- [L.] Prefix signifying two or twice. In chemical terminology, used to denote the presence of two identical but separated complex groups in one molecule. See also bi-.

bisex'ual 1. Having gonads of both sexes. 2. Denoting an individual who engages in both heterosexual and homosexual relations.

bis'muth [Ger. *Wismut*] A trivalent metallic element, chemical symbol Bi, atomic no. 83, atomic weight 209; several of its salts are used in medicine, some of which contain BiO^+, rather than Bi^{3+}, and carry the prefix sub-.

bismutho'sis Chronic bismuth poisoning.

bis'toury [Fr. *bistouri*, fr. *bisorit*, dagger] A long, narrow-bladed knife, straight or curved

on the edge, sharp or blunt pointed; used for opening abscesses, slitting sinuses and fistulas, etc.

bite [A.S. *bītan*] 1. To incise or seize with the teeth. 2. A wound or puncture of the skin made by animal or insect. See bites. 3. Jargon for terms such as interocclusal record, checkbite, maxillomandibular registration, denture space, and interarch distance.

bites [see bite] Puncture or laceration of the skin by animals or insects, with reactions as the result of mechanical injury, injection of toxic material, injection of antigenic substance capable of inducing and eliciting allergic sensitization, introduction of otherwise saprophytic flora, invasion of the tissue by the organism, or transmission of disease.

black'head Comedo.

black'out Temporary loss of consciousness due to decreased blood flow to the brain.

blad'der [A.S. *blaedre*] Vesica (1).

urinary b., *vesica* urinaria.

blad'derworm Cysticercus.

-blast [G. *blastos*, germ] Suffix indicating an immature precursor cell of the type indicated by the preceding word.

blasto- [G. *blastos*, germ] Combining form pertaining to the process of budding (and the formation of buds) by cells or tissue.

blas'tocyst [blasto- + G. *kystis*, bladder] The modified blastula stage of mammalian embryos, consisting of the inner cell mass and a thin trophoblast layer enclosing the blastocele.

blas'toderm, blastoder'ma [blasto- + G. *derma*, skin] The thin disc-shaped cell mass of a young embryo and its extraembryonic extensions over the surface of the yolk; when fully formed, all three of the primary germ layers (ectoderm, endoderm, and mesoderm) are present.

blas'togen'esis [blasto- + G. *genesis*, origin] 1. Reproduction of unicellular organisms by budding. 2. Development of an embryo during cleavage and germ layer formation. 3. Transformation of small lymphocytes of human peripheral blood in tissue culture into large, morphologically primitive blastlike cells capable of undergoing mitosis.

blasto'ma [blasto- + G. *-oma*, tumour] A neoplasm composed chiefly or entirely of immature undifferentiated cells (*i.e.*, blast forms), with little or virtually no stroma.

blas'tomere [blasto- + G. *meros*, part] One of the cells into which the egg divides after its fertilization.

Blastomy'ces dermatit'idis [blasto- + G. *mykēs*, fungus] A species of dimorphic fungus that causes blastomycosis.

blas'tomyco'sis A chronic granulomatous and suppurative disease, caused by *Blastomyces dermatitidis*, that originates as a respiratory infection and disseminates, usually with pulmonary, osseous, and cutaneous involvement predominating. Formerly called North American b.

South American b., paracoccidioidomycosis.

blas'tula [G. *blastos*, germ] An early stage of an embryo formed by the rearrangement of the blastomeres of the morula to form a hollow sphere.

bleb A large flaccid vesicle.

bleed'ing Losing blood as a result of rupture or severance of blood vessels.

dysfunctional uterine b., uterine b. due to an endocrine imbalance rather than to any organic disease.

occult b., see occult *blood*.

blenno-, blenn- [G *blennos*, mucus] Combining form relating to mucus.

blennorrha'gia [blenno- + G. *rhēgnymi*, to burst forth] Blennorrhoea.

blennorrhoe'a [blenno- + G. *rhoia*, a flow] **1.** Any mucous discharge, especially from the urethra or vagina. **2.** An obsolete term for gonorrhoea.

bleomy'cin sulphate An antineoplastic antibiotic obtained from *Streptomyces verticillus*.

blephari'tis [blepharo + G. *-itis*, inflammation] Inflammation of the eyelids.

blepharo-, blephar- [G. *blopharon*, eyelid] Combining forms meaning eyelid.

bleph'aroconjunctivi'tis Inflammation of the palpebral conjunctiva.

bleph'arophimo'sis [blepharo- + G. *phimōsis*, an obstruction] Decrease in palpebral aperture without fusion of lid margins.

bleph'aroplasty [blepharo- + G. *plassō*, to form] Surgical correction of a defect in the eyelid.

blepharople'gia [blepharo- + G. *plēgē*, stroke] Paralysis of an eyelid.

blepharopto'sis [blepharo- + G. *ptōsis*, a falling] Drooping of the upper eyelid.

bleph'arospasm Spasmodic winking, or contraction of the orbicularis palpebrarum muscle.

blind'ness Loss of the sense of sight; absolute b. connotes no light perception.

cortical b., loss of sight due to an organic lesion in the visual cortex.

day b., hemeralopia.

legal b., generally, visual acuity of less than 6/60 or 20/200 using Snellen test types, or visual field restriction to 20 degrees or less.

night b., nyctalopia.

snow b., severe photophobia secondary to ultraviolet keratoconjunctivitis.

blis'ter A fluid filled vesicle under or within the epidermis.

blood b., a b. containing blood, resulting from a minor pinch or crushing injury.

fever b., herpes simplex of the lips.

blis'tering Vesiculation (1).

bloat, bloat'ing Abdominal distension from swallowed air or intestinal gas from fermentation.

block [Fr. *bloquer*] **1.** To obstruct; to arrest passage through. **2.** A condition in which the passage of a nervous impulse is arrested, wholly or in part, temporarily or permanently. **3.** Atrioventricular b.

atrioventricular (A-V) b., impairment of the normal conduction between atria and ventricles.

nerve b., interruption of the passage of impulses through a nerve by the injection of alcohol or local anaesthetic solutions.

spinal b., (1) pathologic obstruction of the flow of cerebrospinal fluid in the spinal subarachnoid space; **(2)** inaccurate term for spinal anaesthesia.

block'ade 1. Intravenous injection of large amounts of colloidal dyes or other substances whereby the reaction of the reticuloendothelial cells to other influences is temporarily prevented. **2.** Arrest of transmission at autonomic synaptic junctions, autonomic receptor sites, or myoneural junctions by a drug.

blood [A.S. blōd] The "circulating tissue" of the body; the fluid and its suspended formed elements that are circulated through the heart, arteries, capillaries, and veins by means of which oxygen and nutritive materials are transported to tissues, and carbon dioxide and various metabolic products are removed for excretion; b. consists of plasma in which are suspended erythrocytes, leucocytes, and platelets.

occult b., b. in the faeces in amounts too small to be seen but detectable by chemical tests.

whole b., b. drawn from a selected donor under rigid aseptic precautions; contains citrate ion or heparin as an anticoagulant.

blood bank A place, usually a separate part or division of a hospital laboratory, in which blood is collected from donors, typed, and often separated into several components for transfusion to recipients.

blood count Calculation of the number of red (RBC) or white (WBC) blood cells in a cubic millimetre of blood, by means of counting the cells in an accurate volume of diluted blood; also, the determination of the percentages of various types of leucocytes, *i.e.*, a differential count, as observed in a stained film of blood.

blood group A system of genetically determined antigens or agglutinogens located on the surface of the erythrocyte, each group determined by a series of two or more genes that are allelic or at least very closely linked on a single chromosome; because of the antigen differences existing between individuals, blood groups are important with respect to blood transfusions, maternal-fetal blood group incompatibilities, and tissue and organ transplantation. See also blood type.

blood grouping The classification of blood samples by means of appropriate laboratory tests according to their agglutination reactions with respect to one or more blood groups. In general, a suspension of erythrocytes to be tested is exposed to a known specific antiserum; agglutination of the erythrocytes indicates that they possess the antigen for which the antiserum is specific, whereas absence of agglutination indicates absence of the antigen.

blood'letting Removing blood, usually from a vein; formerly used as a general remedial measure, but used now in congestive heart failure and polycythaemia.

blood'shot Locally congested, the smaller blood vessels of the part, *e.g.*, the conjunctiva, being dilated and visible.

blood'stream The flowing blood as it is encountered in the organism, as distin-

guished from blood which has been removed from the organism or sequestered in a part.

blood type The specific reaction pattern of erythrocytes of an individual to the antisera of one blood group; *e.g.*, the ABO blood group consists of four major blood types, O, A, B, and AB, depending on agglutination of erythrocytes by neither, one, the other, or both anti-A and anti-B testing sera. The blood type is the genetic phenotype of the individual for one blood group system and may vary in detail with the number of different antisera available for testing.

blood typing Blood grouping.

blood vessel A tube (artery, capillary, vein, or sinus) conveying blood.

blush A sudden and brief redness of the face and neck due to emotion.

bod'y [A.S. *bodig*] **1.** The head, neck, trunk, and extremities. **2.** The material part of man, as distinguished from the mind and spirit. **3.** The principal mass of any structure. **4.** A thing; a substance. See also corpus; soma.

ciliary b., *corpus* ciliare.

inclusion b.'s, distinctive structures frequently formed in the nucleus and/or cytoplasm in cells infected with certain filtrable viruses, observed especially in nerve, epithelial, or endothelial cells.

ketone b., acetone b., one of a group of ketones, including acetoacetic acid, its reduction product, β-hydroxybutyric acid, and its decarboxylation product, acetone; high in tissues and body fluids in ketosis.

Leishman-Donovan b., the intracytoplasmic, nonflagellated leishmanial form of certain intracellular flagellates, such as species of *Leishmania* or the intracellular form of *Trypanosoma cruz*; originally used for *Leishmania donovani* parasites in infected spleen or liver cells in kala azar.

boil [A.S. *byl*, a swelling] Furuncle.

bo'lus [L. fr. G. *bōlos*, lump, clod] **1.** A very large pill, usually of soft consistency. **2.** A masticated morsel of food ready to be swallowed.

intravenous b., a large volume of fluid given intravenously and rapidly at one time for immediate response.

bond In chemistry, the force holding two neighbouring atoms in place and resisting their separation. An **electrovalent b.** consists of the attraction between oppositely charged groups, a **covalent b.** results from the sharing of one, two, or three pairs of electrons by the bonded atoms.

bone [A.S. *bān*] A hard connective tissue consisting of cells in a matrix of ground substance and collagen fibres; the fibres are impregnated with mineral substance, chiefly calcium, phosphate and carbonate, which comprises about 67% by weight of adult bone. For anatomical definitions of bones as part of the animal skeleton, see under os.

   brittle b.'s, *osteogenesis imperfecta.*
   collar b., clavicula.
   cuboid b., os cuboideum.
   cuneiform b., os cuneiforme and os triquetrum.
   ethmoid b., os ethmoidale.
   hyoid b., os hyoideum.
   iliac b., os ilium.
   jaw b., maxilla or, especially, mandibula
   lamellar b., b. in which the tubular lamellae are formed that are characterized by having collagen fibres arranged in a parallel, spiral manner.
   parietal b., os parietale.
   sphenoid b., os sphenoidale.
   tarsal b.'s, see tarsus.
   temporal b., os temporale.
   thigh b., os femoris.
   zygomatic b., os zygomaticum.

bonelet Ossiculum.
boos'ter See under dose.
bo'rate A salt of boric acid.
bo'rax Sodium borate.
borboryg'mus, pl. **borboryg'mi** [G. *borborygmos,* rumbling in the bowels] Rumbling or gurgling noises produced by movement of gas in the alimentary canal, and audible at a distance.
Bordetel'la [J. *Bordet*] A genus of strictly aerobic bacteria (family Brucellaceae) that contain minute Gram-negative coccobacilli and are parasites and pathogens of the mammalian respiratory tract. The type species, *B. pertussis* (Bordet-Gengou bacillus), causes whooping cough.
bo'ric acid A very weak acid, used as an antiseptic dusting powder, in saturated solution as a collyrium, and with glycerin in aphthae and stomatitis.
bo'rism Symptoms caused by the ingestion of borax or any compound of boron.

bo'ron A nonmetallic trivalent element, symbol B, atomic weight 10.81, atomic no. 5; forms borates and boric acid.
Borrel'ia [A. *Borrel*] A genus of parasitic bacteria (family Treponemataceae), some of which are transmitted by the bites of arthropods. Some species cause relapsing fever.
bot'fly Robust hairy fly of the order Diptera whose larvae produce a variety of myiasis conditions in man and various domestic animals.
bot'ulism [L. *botulus,* sausage] Intoxication due to the ingestion of *Clostridium botulinum* toxin in improperly canned or preserved food; characterized by paralysis.
bou'gie [Fr. candle] A cylindrical instrument, usually somewhat flexible and yielding, used for calibrating or dilating constructed areas in tubular organs, such as the urethra or rectum; sometimes containing a medicament for local application.
bow'el [through the Fr. from L. *botulus,* sausage] The intestine.
bow'leg Genu varum.
brace An orthesis or orthopaedic appliance that supports or holds in correct position any movable part of the body and that allows motion of the part, in contrast to a splint, which prevents motion of the part.
bra'ces Colloquialism for orthodontic appliances.
bra'chial Relating to the arm.
brachio- [L. *brachium,* arm] Combining form meaning 1) arm, 2) radial.
bra'chioceph'alic Relating to both arm and head.
bra'chium, pl. **bra'chia** [L. arm, prob. akin to G. *brachiōn*] [NA] **1.** The arm, specifically the segment of the upper limb between the shoulder and the elbow. **2.** An armlike structure.
brachy- [G. *brachys,* short] Combining form meaning short.
brachydac'tyly [brachy- + G. *daktylos,* finger] Abnormal shortness of the fingers.
brach'ysyndac'tyly [brachy- + syndactyl] Abnormal shortness of fingers or toes combined with a webbing between the adjacent digits.
brachyther'apy Radiotherapy in which the source of irradiation is placed close to the surface of the body or within a body cavity.
brady- [G. *bradys,* slow] Combining form meaning slow.

brad'yarrhyth'mia [brady- + G. a-priv. + *rhythmos*, rhythm] Any disturbance of the heart's rhythm resulting in a rate under 60 beats per minute.

bradycar'dia [brady- + G. *kardia*, heart] Slowness of the heart beat, usually defined as a rate under 60 beats per minute.

bradykine'sia [brady- + G. *kinēsis*, movement] Extreme slowness in movement.

brad'yki'nin [brady- + G. *kinein*, to move] A nonapeptide normally present in blood in an inactive form and similar to trypsin in action; one of a number of the plasma kinins and a potent vasodilator, also one of the physiologic mediators of anaphylaxis released from cytotroic antibody-coated mast cells following reaction with antigen (allergen) specific for the antibody.

bradypnoe'a [brady- + G. *pnoē*, breathing] Abnormal slowness of respiration; specifically, a low respiratory frequency.

brain [A.S. *braegen*] Encephalon.

brain'case The cranium in its restricted sense, the part of the skull that encloses the brain.

brain'stem, brain stem Originally, the entire unpaired subdivision of the brain, composed of the rhombencephalon, mesencephalon, and diecephalon as distinguished from the telencephalon, the only paired subdivision. More recently, the rhombencephalon plus mesencephalon, distinguishing that complex from the prosencephalon (diencephalon plus telencephalon), exclusively to the rhombencephalon.

bran A by-product of the milling of wheat, containing approximately 20% of indigestible cellulose; a bulk cathartic, usually taken in the form of cereal or special bran products.

branch An offshoot; in anatomy, one of the primary divisions of a nerve or blood vessel. See also ramus.

breast [A.S. *breōst*] **1.** The anterior surface of the thorax. See also chest. **2.** The mamma.

    chicken b., pigeon b., *pectus* carinatum.

    funnel b., *pectus* excavatum.

breath [A.S. *braeth*] **1.** The respired air. **2.** An inspiration.

breath'ing The alternate inhalation and exhalation of air.

breech [A.S. *brēc*] The nates.

brevicol'lis [L. *brevis*, short, + *collum*, neck] Shortness of the neck.

bridge **1.** The upper part of the ridge of the nose formed by the nasal bones. **2.** One of the threads of protoplasm that appears to pass from one cell to another. **3.** Fixed partial *denture*.

    removable b., removable partial *denture*.

bridge'work Partial *denture*.

brisement' forcé' [Fr. forcible breaking] The forcible breaking or manipulation of a joint or joints, as with the adhesions in ankylosis.

broach A dental instrument for removing the pulp of a tooth or exploring the canal.

bro'mate Salt or anion of bromic acid.

bro'mated Combined or saturated with bromine or any of its compounds.

brom-, bromo- [G. *brōmos*, a stench] Prefix indicating presence of bromine in a compound.

bro'mide The anion Br-; salt of HBr.

bromidro'sis, bromhidro'sis [G. *brōmos*, a stench, + *hidrōs*, perspiration] Fetid or foul smelling perspiration.

bro'mine An element, symbol Br, atomic no. 35, atomic weight, 79.9; unites with hydrogen to form hydrobromic acid, which reacts with many metals to form bromides, some of which are used in medicine.

bro'mism, bro'minism Chronic bromide intoxication characterized by headache, mental inertia, occasionally violent delirium, muscular weakness, cardiac depression, an acneform eruption, a foul breath, anorexia, and gastric distress.

bron'chi Plural of bronchus.

bron'chial Relating to the bronchi and the bronchial tubes.

bronchiec'tasis [bronchi- + G. *ektasis*, a stretching] Chronic dilation of bronchi or bronchioles as a sequel of inflammatory disease or obstruction.

bron'chiole Bronchiolus.

bronchioli'tis Inflammation of the bronchioles, often associated with bronchopneumonia.

bronchiolo- [L. *bronchiolus*] Combining form relating to the bronchiolus.

bronchio'lus, pl. **bronchio'li** [Mod. L. dim. of *bronchus*] [NA] One of the finer subdivisions of the bronchial tubes, with no cartilage in its wall, but relatively abundant smooth muscle and elastic fibres.

bronchi'tis Inflammation of the mucous membrane of the bronchial tubes.

chronic b., b. characterized by cough, hypersecretion of mucus, and expectoration of sputum over a long period of time, associated with increased vulnerability to bronchial infection.

broncho- [G. *bronchos*, windpipe] Combining form denoting bronchus.

bron'chocele [broncho- + G. *kēlē*, hernia] Circumscribed dilation of a bronchus.

bron'chodila'tor Causing an increase in calibre of a bronchus or bronchial tube.

bron'cholith [broncho- + G. *lithos*, stone] A hard concretion in a bronchus or bronchial tube.

bron'cholithi'asis Bronchial inflammation or obstruction caused by broncholiths.

bron'chomyco'sis [broncho- + G. *mykēs*, fungus] Any fungus disease of the bronchial tubes or bronchi.

bron'chopneumo'nia Acute inflammation of the walls of the smaller bronchial tubes, with irregular areas of consolidation due to spread of the inflammation into peribronchiolar alveoli and the alveolar ducts.

bronchopul'monary Relating to the bronchial tubes and the lungs.

bron'ohoscope [broncho- + G. *skopeo*, to view] An endoscope for inspecting the interior of the tracheobronchial tree, either for diagnostic purposes (including biopsy) or for the removal of foreign bodies.

bronchos'copy Inspection of the interior of the tracheobronchial tree through a bronchoscope.

bron'chospasm Contraction of smooth muscle in the walls of the bronchi and bronchioles, causing narrowing of the lumen.

bron'ohosteno'sis Chronic stenosis or narrowing of a bronchus.

bronchotra'cheal Relating to the bronchi and trachea.

bron'chus, pl. **bron'chi** [Mod. L. fr. G. *bronchos*, windpipe] [NA] One of the primary subdivisions of the trachea that convey air to and from the lungs; the right and left main bronchi in turn form lobar, segmental, and subsegmental bronchi. In structure the intrapulmonary bronchi have a lining of pseudostratified ciliated columnar epithelium, and a lamina propria with abundant longitudinal networks of elastic fibres. There are spirally arranged bundles of smooth muscle, abundant mucoserous glands, and in the outer part of the wall irregular plates of hyaline cartilage.

brow [A.S. *brū*] **1.** The eyebrow. **2.** Frons.

brow'lift An operation to elevate the eyebrows and thereby remove excess skin folds or fullness in the upper eyelids.

Brucel'la [Sir David *Bruce*, British surgeon, 1855–1931] A genus of encapsulated, nonmotile bacteria (family Brucellaceae) containing short, rod-shaped to coccoid, Gram-negative cells; they are parasitic, invading all animal tissues and causing infection of the genital organs, the mammary gland, and the respiratory and intestinal tracts, and are pathogenic for man and various species of domestic animals. The type species is *B. melitensis*.

B. abor'tus, a species that causes abortion in cows, mares, and sheep, undulant fever in man, and a wasting disease in chickens.

B. meliten'sis, a species that causes brucellosis in man, abortion in goats, and a wasting disease in chickens; it may infect cows and hogs and be excreted in their milk; the type species of the genus *B*.

B. su'is, a species causing abortion in swine, brucellosis in man, and a wasting disease in chickens; may also infect horses, dogs, cows, monkeys, goats, and laboratory animals.

brucello'sis Undulant fever; an infectious disease caused by species of *Brucella* and characterized by fever, sweating, weakness, aches, and pains; transmitted to man by direct contact with diseased animals or through ingestion of infested meat, milk, or cheese.

Bru'gia A genus of filarial worms transmitted by mosquitoes to man, primates, felid carnivores, and a number of other mammals. *B. malayi*, is an important agent of human filariasis and elephantiasis in Southeast Asia and Indonesia.

bruise 1. An injury usually producing a haematoma without rupture of the skin. **2.** Contusion (1).

bruit [Fr.] An auscultatory sound, especially an abnormal one.

brux'ism [G. *brucho*, to grind the teeth] A clenching of the teeth, resulting in rubbing, gritting, or grinding together of the teeth, usually during sleep.

bu'bas Yaws.

bu'bo [G. *boubōn*, the groin, a swelling in the groin] Inflammatory swelling of one or more lymph nodes in the groin; the confluent mass of nodes suppurates.

bubon'ic Relating in any way to a bubo.

bubon'ocele [G. *boubōn*, groin, + *kēlē*, tumour] Inguinal hernia, especially one in which the knuckle of intestine has not yet emerged from the external abdominal ring.

buc'cal Pertaining to, adjacent to, or in the direction of the cheek.

bucco- [L. *bucca*, cheek] Combining form relating to the cheek.

buc'cola'bial 1. Relating to both cheek and lip. **2.** In dentistry, referring to that aspect of the dental arch or those surfaces of the teeth in contact with the mucosa of lip and cheek, the surfaces opposite the lingual surfaces.

buc'colin'gual Pertaining to the cheek and the tongue.

bud A structure that resembles the b. of a plant.

 taste b., one of a number of flask-shaped cell nests located in the epithelium of papillae of the tongue and also in the soft palate, epiglottis, and posterior wall of the pharynx; it consists of sustentacular, gustatory, and basal cells between which the intragemmal sensory nerve fibres terminate.

buf'fer 1. A mixture of an acid and its conjugate base (salt) that, when present in a solution, reduces any changes in pH that would otherwise occur in the solution when acid or alkali is added to it. **2.** To add a b. to a solution and thus give it the property of resisting a change in pH when it receives a limited amount of acid or alkali.

bulb [L. *bulbus*, a bulbous root] Any globular or fusiform structure.

 end b., one of the oval or rounded bodies in which the sensory nerve fibres terminate in mucous membrane.

bul'bar 1. Bulb-shaped; resembling or relating to a bulb. **2.** Relating to the rhombencephalon (pons, cerebellum, and medulla oblongata).

bulbi'tis Inflammation of the bulbous portion of the urethra.

bulbo- [L. *bulbus*, bulb] Combining form relating to a bulb or bulbus.

bulbospi'nal Relating to the medulla oblongata and spinal cord, particularly to nerve fibres interconnecting the two.

bulim'ia [G. *bous*, ox, + *limos*, hunger] A personality disorder characterized by episodic bouts of eating characterized by uncontrolled, rapid, and great amounts of ingested food followed by physical discomfort and feelings of guilt, self-disgust, and depression.

bulim'ic Relating to bulimia.

bul'la, pl. **bul'lae** [L. bubble] **1.** A large vesicle appearing as a circumscribed area of separation of the epidermis from the subepidermal structure, or as a circumscribed area of separation of epidermal cells, caused by the presence of serum, sometimes mixed with blood, or occasionally by a substance injected intra- or subepidermally. **2.** [NA] A bubble-like structure.

bul'lous Relating to, of the nature of, or marked by, bullae.

bun'dle A structure composed of a group of fibres; *e.g.*, a fasciculus.

 His b., b., of His, *truncus* atrioventricularis.

bun'ion [O.F. *buigne*, bump on the head] A localized swelling at either the medial or dorsal aspect of the first metatarsophalangeal joint, caused by an inflammatory bursa.

buphthal'mia, buphthal'mos, buphthal'mus [G. *bous*, ox, + *ophthalmos*, eye] Congenital glaucoma; an affection of infancy, marked by an increase of intraocular fluid with enlargement of the eyeball.

bur A rotary cutting instrument used in dentistry for excavating decay, shaping cavity forms, and any reduction of tooth structure. See also burr.

burn [A.S. *baernan*] A lesion caused by heat or any cauterizing agent, including friction, electricity, and electromagnetic energy. Division of burns into three degrees is recognized for geographical designation: **first degree b.,** involving only the epidermis and causing erythema and oedema without vesiculation; **second degree b.,** involving the epidermis and dermis and usually forming blisters that may be superficial or deep dermal necrosis, but with epithelial regeneration extending from the skin appendages; **third degree b.,** destruction of the entire skin; deep ones extend into subcutaneous fat, muscle, or bone and often cause much scarring.

burr A drilling tool for enlarging a trephine hole in the cranium. See also bur.

bur'sa, pl. **bur'sae** [Mediev. L., a purse] [NA] A closed sac or envelope lined with synovia and containing fluid, usually found or formed in areas subject to friction.

bursec'tomy [bursa + G. *oktomē*, oxoi sion] Surgical removal of a bursa.

bursi'tis Inflammation of a bursa; specific types of b. are named after the bursa involved.

bursot'omy [bursa + G. *tomē*, a cutting] Incision through the wall of a bursa.

but'tocks Nates.

by'pass A surgically created shunt or auxiliary flow through a diversionary channel.

cardiopulmonary b., diversion of the blood flow returning to the heart through a pump oxygenator (heart-lung machine) and then returning it to the arterial side of the circulation; used in operations upon the heart to maintain extracorporeal circulation.

coronary b., shunting of blood from the aorta to branches of the coronary arteries, to increase the flow beyond the local obstruction.

byssino'sis [G. *byssos*, flax, + *-osis*, condition] A pneumoconiosis of cotton, flax, and hemp workers, characterized by symptoms (especially wheezing) most severe at the beginning of each work week.

C

cachec'tic Relating to or suffering from cachexia.

cachet' [Fr. a seal] A seal-shaped capsule or wafer for enclosing powders of disagreeable taste.

cachex'ia [G. *kakos*, bad, + *hexis*, a habit of body] A general lack of nutrition and wasting occurring in the course of a chronic disease or emotional disturbance.

caco-, caci-, cac- [G. *kakos*, bad] Combining forms meaning bad or ill

cacogeu'sia [caco- + G. *geusis*, taste] A bad taste.

cadav'er [L. fr. *cado*, to fall] Corpse; a dead body.

cadav'erous Having the pallor and appearance of a corpse.

cae'cal **1.** Relating to the caecum. **2.** Ending blindly or in a cul-de-sac.

caecec'tomy [caeco- + G. *ektomē*, excision] Excision of the caecum.

caeco-, caec- [L. *caecum*, caecum] Combining forms denoting the caecum. See also typhlo-.

caecos'tomy [caeco- + G. *stoma*, mouth] Surgical formation of a caecal fistula.

cae'cum, pl. **cae'ca** [L. ntr. of *caecus*, blind] [NA] **1.** Blind gut; the cul-de-sac, about 6 cm in depth, lying below the terminal ileum forming the first part of the large intestine. **2.** Any similar structure ending in a cul-de-sac.

caf'feine An alkaloid obtained from the dried leaves of *Thea sinensis*, tea, or the dried seeds of *Coffea arabica*, coffee; used as a diuretic and circulatory and respiratory stimulant.

caf'feinism Chronic coffee poisoning, characterized by palpitation, dyspepsia, irritability, and insomnia.

cal'amine Zinc oxide with a small amount of ferric oxide or basic zinc carbonate suitably coloured with ferric oxide; used in dusting powders, lotions, and ointments, as a mild astringent and protective agent for skin disorders.

calca'neal, calca'nean Relating to the calcaneus or heel bone.

calca'neum [L. the heel] Calcaneus.

calca'neus, gen. and pl. **calca'nei** [L. the heel (another form of *calcaneum*)] [NA] Heel bone; the largest of the tarsal bones; it forms the heel and articulates with the cuboid anteriorly and the talus above.

cal'car [L. spur, cock's spur] **1.** [NA] A small projection from any structure; internal spurs (septa) at the level of division of arteries and confluence of veins when branches or roots form an acute angle. **2.** A dull spine or projection from a bone. **3.** A horny outgrowth from the skin.

calca'reous [L. *calcarius*, pertaining to lime, fr. *calx*, lime] Chalky; relating to or containing lime or calcium, or calcific material.

calcariu'ria [L. *calcarius*, of lime, + G. *ouron*, urine] Excretion of calcium salts in the urine.

cal'ces Plural of calx.

calcif'erol Ergocalciferol.

calcifica'tion [L. *calx*, lime, + *facio*, to make] **1.** Deposition of insoluble calcium salts. **2.** A process in which tissue or noncellular material in the body becomes hardened as the result of precipitates or larger deposits of insoluble calcium salts, normally occurring only in the formation of bone and teeth.

calcino'sis [calcium + *-osis*, condition] A condition characterized by the deposition of calcium salts in nodular foci in various tissues other than the parenchymatous viscera.

calcito'nin See thyrocalcitonin.

cal'cium [Mod. L. fr. L. *calx*, lime] A metallic dyad element; symbol Ca, atomic no. 20, atomic weight 40.09, density 1.54, melting point 810°; many of its salts have medicinal uses.

cal'culous Relating to calculi.

cal'culus, gen. and pl. **cal'culi** [L. a pebble, a calculus] Stone; a concretion formed in any part of the body, most commonly in the passages of the biliary and urinary tracts; usually composed of salts of inorganic or organic acids, or of other material such as cholesterol.

calefa'cient [L. *calefacio*, fr. *caleo*, to be warm, + *facio*, to make] Making warm or hot; causing a sense of warmth in the part to which applied.

calf, pl. **calves** [Gael. *kalpa*] Sura.

cal'ibrate 1. To graduate or standardize any measuring instrument. 2. To measure the diameter of a tube.

cal'ibrator A standard or reference material or substance used to standardize or calibrate an instrument or laboratory procedure.

calice'al Relating to a calix.

cal'ipers [a corruption of *calibre*] An instrument used for measuring diameters, as of the pelvis.

calisthen'ics [G. *kalos*, beautiful, + *sthenos*, strength] The systematic use of various exercises to preserve health and increase physical strength.

ca'lix, pl. **ca'lices** [L. fr. G. *kalyx*, the cup of a flower] [NA] A flower-shaped or funnel-shaped structure; specifically, one of the branches or recesses of the pelvis of the kidney into which the orifices of the malpighian renal pyramids project.

callo'sal Relating to the corpus callosum.

callos'ity [L. fr. *callosus*, thick skinned] A circumscribed thickening of the keratin layer of the epidermis as a result of friction or intermittent pressure.

cal'lous Relating to a callus or callosity.

cal'lus [L. hard skin] 1. Callosity. 2. The hard bonelike substance that develops between and around the ends of a fractured bone.

cal'omel Mercurous chloride; an intestinal antiseptic and laxative.

cal'or [L.] Heat, as one of the four signs of inflammation (c., rubor, tumor, dolor) enunciated by Celsus.

calor'ic [L. *calor*, heat] 1. Relating to a calorie. 2. Relating to heat.

cal'orie [L. *calor*, heat] A unit of heat content or energy; being replaced by the joule, the SI unit equal to 0.24 calorie.

large c. (C, Cal), the quantity of energy required to raise the temperature of 1 kg of water 1°C.

small c. (c, cal), the quantity of energy required to raise the temperature of 1 g of water 1°C.

calorigen'ic 1. Capable of generating heat. 2. Stimulating metabolic production of heat.

calorim'eter [L. *calor*, heat, + G. *metron*, measure] An apparatus for measuring the amount of heat liberated in a chemical reaction.

calva'ria, pl. **calva'riae** [L. a skull] [NA] Skullcap; roof of the skull, the upper domelike portion of the skull.

calx, gen. **cal'cis,** pl. **cal'ces** 1. [L. limestone] Lime (2). 2. [L. heel] Heel; the posterior rounded extremity of the foot.

Calym'matobacte'rium [G. *kalymma*, hood, veil, + *bakterion*, rod] A genus of nonmotile bacteria (family Brucellaceae) containing Gram-negative, pleomorphic rods with single or bipolar condensations of chromatin. The type species, *C. granulomatis*, causes granulomatous lesions in man, particularly in the inguinal region.

ca'lyx, pl. **ca'lyces** [G. cup of a flower] Calix.

cam'phor [mediev. L. fr. Ar. *kāfure*] A ketone distilled from the bark and wood of the Asian evergreen tree, *Cinnamomum camphora*; also prepared synthetically from oil of turpentine; used as a stimulant, carminative, expectorant, and diaphoretic.

camptocor'mia [G. *kamptos*, bent, + *kormos*, trunk of a tree] A conversion reaction or hysterical condition in which the patient is bent completely forward and is unable to straighten up.

camptome'lia [G. *kamptos*, bent, + *melos*, limb] A bending of the limbs, producing a fixed deformity.

Cam'pylobac'ter [G. *campylos*, curved, + *baktron*, staff or rod] A genus of motile bacteria containing Gram-negative, nonsporeforming, spirally curved rods with a single polar flagellum at one or both ends of the cell. The type species, *C. fetus*, contains various subspecies that can cause human infections as well as abortion in sheep and cattle.

cam'pylodac'tyly [G. *campylos*, curved, + *daktylos*, finger] Permanent flexion of one or both interphalangeal joints of one or more fingers, usually the little finger.

canal' [L. *canalis*] A duct, channel or tubular structure.

   alimentary c., digestive *tract*.

   Schlemm's c., *sinus venosus sclerae*.

   semicircular c.'s., see *canales* semicirculares ossei.

   vestibular c., *scala* vestibuli.

canaliculi'tis [L. canaliculus + G. *-itis*, inflammation] Inflammation of the lacrimal duct.

canalic'uliza'tion The formation of small canals or channels in tissue.

canalic'ulus, pl. **canalic'uli** [L. dim. fr. *canalis*, canal] [NA] A small canal or channel.

cana'lis, pl. **cana'les** [L.] [NA] A canal or channel.

   c. car'pi [NA], carpal tunnel; the space deep to the flexor retinaculum of the wrist through which the median nerve and the flexor tendons of the fingers and thumb pass.

   canales semicircula'res os'sei [NA], bony semicircular canals; the three bony tubes in the labyrinth of the ear within which the membranous semicircular ducts are located; they lie in planes at right angles to each other and are known as **canales semicirculares anterior, posterior,** and **lateralis.**

can'cellated, can'cellous [L. *cancello*, to make a lattice work] Denoting bone that has a lattice-like or spongy structure.

can'cer (CA) [L. a crab, a cancer] Any of various types of malignant neoplasms, most of which invade surrounding tissues, may metastasize to several sites, and are likely to recur after attempted removal and to cause death of the patient unless adequately treated.

can'eriform Resembling cancer.

can'croid [cancer + G. *eidos*, resemblance] **1.** Cancriform. **2.** Obsolete term for a malignant neoplasm that manifests a lesser degree of malignancy than that frequently observed with other types of carcinoma or sarcoma.

can'crum, pl. **can'cra** [Mod. L. fr. L. *cancer* (*cancr-*), cancer] A gangrenous, ulcerative, inflammatory lesion.

Can'dida [L. *candidus*, dazzling white] A genus of yeastlike fungi commonly found in nature. The gastrointestinal tract is the source of the most important species, *C. albicans*, which is ordinarily a part of the normal flora, but which becomes pathogenic when there is a disturbance in the balance of flora; resulting disease states vary from limited to generalized cutaneous or mucocutaneous infections, to severe and fatal systemic disease including endocarditis, septicaemia, and meningitis.

candidi'asis Infection with, or disease caused by, *Candida*.

ca'nine [L. *caninus*] **1.** Relating to a dog. **2.** Relating to the c. teeth. **3.** A c. (cuspid) tooth.

can'ker [L. *cancer*] An ulcerative sore, especially of the oral mucosa or lip, as in stomatitis.

can'nabis [L. fr. G. *kannabis*, hemp] Marijuana; marihuana; hashish; the dried flowering tops of the pistillate hemp plants of *Cannabis sativa* var. *indica* (family Moraceae). Preparations of c. are smoked or ingested to induce psychotomimetic effects; formerly used as a sedative and analgesic.

can'nula [L. dim. of *canna*, reed] A tube such as one inserted into a cavity by means of a trocar filling its lumen, after which the trocar is withdrawn; the c. remains as a channel for the transport of fluid.

cannula'tion, cannuliza'tion Insertion of a cannula.

can'thal Relating to a canthus.

canthec'tomy [G. *kanthos*, canthus, + *ektome*, excision] Excision of a canthus.

can'thoplasty [G. *kanthos*, canthus, + *plasso*, to form] **1.** Lengthening the palpebral fissure by cutting through the external canthus. **2.** Surgical restoration of the canthus in case of pathologic or traumatic defect.

can'thus, pl. **can'thi** [G. *kanthos*, corner of the eye] The angle at either corner of the eye.

capacita'tion [L. *capacitas*, fr. *capax*, capable of] The process occurring in the female genital tract whereby spermatozoa acquire the ability to fertilize ova, characterized by loss of the acrosome cap by spermatozoa and an increase in their respiratory metabolism and content of DNA.

capil'lary [L. *capillaris*, relating to hair] **1.** Resembling a hair; fine; minute. **2.** A capillary vessel. **3.** Relating to a blood or lymphatic c. vessel.

cap'itate [L. *caput* (*capit-*), head] Head-shaped; having a rounded extremity.

capitel'lum [L. dim. of *caput*, head] **1.** Capitulum. **2.** The small or radial head of the humerus.

capit'ium [L. *caput*, head] A bandage for the head.

capit'ular Relating to a capitulum.

capit'ulum, pl. **capit'ula** [L. dim. of *caput*, head] [NA] A small head or rounded articular extremity of a bone. See also caput.

cap'sid See virion.

cap'somer(e) A subunit of the protein coat or capsid of a virus particle.

cap'sula, pl. **cap'sulae** [L. dim. of *capsa*, a chest or box] [NA] **1.** A membranous structure, usually dense collagenous connective tissue, that envelops an organ, a joint or any other part. **2.** An anatomical structure resembling a capsule or envelope.

cap'sular Relating to any capsule.

capsule 1. Capsula. **2.** A fibrous tissue layer enveloping a tumour, especially if benign. **3.** A solid dosage form in which the drug is enclosed in a soluble container or "shell".

capsuli'tis Inflammation of the capsule of an organ or part.

   adhesive c., frozen shoulder; a condition in which there is restriction of glenohumeral and scapulothoracic motion, and pain both on motion and at rest; not caused by infection or neoplasm.

cap'sulolentic'ular Referring to the lens of the eye and its capsule.

cap'suloplasty [L. *capsula*, capsule, + G. *plassō*, to fashion] Plastic surgery of a capsule, more specifically the capsule of a joint.

capsulor'rhaphy [L. *capsula*, capsule, + *raphē*, suture] Suture of a tear in any capsule; specifically, suture of a joint capsule to prevent recurring dislocation of the articulation.

capsulot'omy [L. *capsula*, capsule, + G. *tomē*, a cutting] Incision through a capsule, especially the capsule of the lens in the extracapsular cataract operation.

cap'ut, gen. **cap'itis,** pl. **cap'ita** [L.] Head. **1.** [NA] The upper or anterior extremity of the animal body, containing the brain and the organs of sight, hearing, taste, and smell. **2.** [NA] The upper, anterior, or larger extremity, expanded or rounded, of any body, organ, or other anatomical structure. **3.** That end of a muscle which is attached to the less movable part of the skeleton.

   c. succeda'neum, an oedematous swelling formed on the presenting portion of the scalp of an infant during birth; the effusion overlies the periosteum and consists of serum.

carbenicil'lin disodium A semisynthetic form of pencillin.

carbohy'drates Saccharides; class name for the aldehydic or ketonic derivative of polyhydric alcohols, the name being derived from the fact that the most common examples of such compounds have formulas that may be written $C_n(H_2O)_n$ (*e.g.*, glucose, $C_6(H_2O)_6$; sucrose, $C_{12}(H_2O)_{11}$), although they are not true hydrates; includes compounds with relatively small molecules, such as the simple sugars (monosaccharides, disaccharides, etc.), as well as macromolecular substances (starch, glycogen, cellulose polysaccharides, etc.).

carbol'ic acid Phenol.

car'bon [L. *carbo*, coal] A nonmetallic tetravalent element, symbol C, atomic no. 6, atomic weight 12.01, with two natural isotopes, ^{12}C and ^{13}C (the former, set at 12.00000, being the standard for all molecular weights), and two artificial radioactive isotopes, ^{11}C and ^{14}C. It occurs in two pure forms, diamond and graphite; in impure form in charcoal, coke, and soot; in the atmosphere as CO_2; and in compounds found in all living tissues.

   c. dioxide, (1) CO_2; the product of the combustion of c. with an excess of air; **(2)** in concentrations not less than 99.0% by volume of CO_2, used as a respiratory stimulant.

   c. monoxide, CO; a colourless, odourless, poisonous gas formed by incomplete combustion of c.; its toxic action is due to its strong affinity for haemoglobin and cytochrome, reducing oxygen transport and blocking oxygen utilization.

   c. tetrachloride, a colourless mobile liquid having a characteristic etheral odour resembling that of chloroform.

car'bonate A salt of carbonic acid; $CO_3 =$.

carboxy- Combining form indicating addition of CO or CO_2.

carbox'yhaemoglo'bin (HbCO) A fairly stable union of carbon monoxide with haemoglobin. Formation of c. prevents the normal transfer of carbon dioxide and oxygen during the circulation of blood; thus, increasing levels of c. result in various degrees of asphyxiation, including death.

carboxyla'tion Addition of CO_2 to an organic acceptor, as in photosynthesis, to yield a —COOH group.

car'buncle [L. *carbunculus*, dim. of *carbo*, a live coal, a carbuncle] **1.** Deep-seated pyogenic infection of several contiguous hair follicles, with formation of connecting sinuses; often preceded or accompanied by fever, malaise, and prostration. **2.** Anthrax (1).

carcino-, carcin- [G. *karkinos*, crab, cancer] Combining form relating to cancer.

carcin'ogen Any cancer-producing substance.

car'cinogen'esis [carcino- + G *genesis*, generation] The origin of production of cancer, including carcinomas and other malignant neoplasms.

car'cinogen'ic Causing cancer.

carcino'ma (CA) [G. *karkinōma*, fr. *karkinos*, cancer, + *-oma*, tumour] Any of the various types of malignant neoplasm derived from epithelial tissue, occurring more frequently in the skin and large intestine in both sexes, the bronchi, stomach, and prostate gland in men, and the breast and cervix in women; c.'s are identified histologically on the basis of invasiveness and the changes that indicate anaplasia

basal cell c., a slow-growing, locally invasive, but rarely metastasizing neoplasm derived from basal cells of the epidermis or hair follicles.

giant cell c., a malignant epithelial neoplasm characterized by unusually large anaplastic cells.

c. in si'tu, a lesion observed most commonly in stratified squamous epithelium and characterized by cytologic changes of the type associated with invasive c., but with the pathologic process limited to the lining epithelium and without histologic evidence of extension to adjacent structures.

oat cell c., an anaplastic, highly malignant, and usually bronchogenic c. composed of small ovoid cells with very scanty cytoplasm.

small cell c., (1) an anaplastic c. composed of small cells; **(2)** oat cell c.

squamous cell c., a malignant neoplasm that is derived from stratified squamous epithelium, but that may also occur in sites where glandular or columnar epithelium is normally present.

car'cinomato'sis A condition resulting from widespread dissemination of carcinoma in multiple sites in various organs or tissues of the body; sometimes also used in relation to involvement of a relatively large region of the body.

car'dia [G. *kardia*, heart] The cardiac part of the stomach; the area of the stomach close to the oesophageal opening (cardiac opening) which contains the cardiac glands.

car'diac [L. *cardiacus*] Pertaining to the heart or to the oesophageal opening of the stomach.

cardial'gia [cardi- + G. *algos*, pain] **1.** Heartburn; an uncomfortable burning sensation in the stomach. **2.** Cardiodynia.

cardio-, cardi- [G. *kardia*, heart] Combining forms relating to the heart or to the oesophageal opening of the stomach.

car'dioaccel'erator That which quickens the heart beat.

car'dioac'tive Influencing the heart.

car'diocente'sis [cardio- + G. *kentesis*, puncture] Paracentesis of the heart.

car'diodyn'ia [cardio- + G. *odynē*, pain] Pain in the heart.

car'diogen'ic Of origin in the heart.

car'diogram [cardio- + G. *gramma*, a diagram] The graphic tracing made by the stylet of a cardiograph; generally, any recording derived from the heart, such prefixes as apex-, echo-, electro-, phono-, or vector-being understood.

car'diograph [cardio- + G. *graphō*, to write] An instrument for recording graphically the movements of the heart.

cardiog'raphy Use of the cardiograph.

ultrasound c., echocardiography.

car'diohepat'ic Relating to the heart and the liver.

car'dioinhib'itory Arresting or slowing the action of the heart.

cardiol'ogist Physician specializing in the diagnosis and treatment of heart disease.

cardiol'ogy [cardio- + G. *logos*, study] The medical specialty concerned with the heart and its diseases.

cardiol'ysis [cardio- + G. *lysis*, loosening] An operation for breaking up the adhesions in chronic mediastinopericarditis.

car'diomeg'aly [cardio- + G. *megas*, large] Enlargement of the heart.

cardiomus'cular Pertaining to the musculature of the heart.

car'diomyop'athy [cardio- + G. *mys*, muscle, + *pathos*, disease] Disease of the myocardium.

cardiop'athy [cardio- + G. *pathos*, disease] Any disease of the heart.

cardiople'gia [cardio- + G. *plēgē*, stroke] 1. Paralysis of the heart. 2. Elective temporary stopping of cardiac activity as by injection of chemicals, selective hypothermia, or electrical stimuli.

car'diopul'monary Relating to the heart and lungs.

car'diore'nal Relating to the heart and the kidney.

car'diospasm Oesophageal *achalasia*.

car'dioton'ic [cardio- + G. *tonos*, tension] Exerting a favourable, so-called tonic, effect upon the action of the heart.

car'diotox'ic [cardio- + G. *toxikon*, poison] Having a deleterious effect upon the action of the heart, due to poisoning of the cardiac muscle or of its conducting system.

car'diovas'cular [cardio- + L. *vasculum*, vessel] Relating to the heart and the blood vessels, or the circulation.

car'diover'sion Restoration of the heart's rhythm to normal by electrical countershock.

cardi'tis Inflammation of the heart. See myocarditis.

car'ies [L. dry rot] 1. A localized progressively destructive disease of the teeth which starts at the enamel with the apparent dissolution of the inorganic components by organic acids that are produced in immediate proximity to the tooth by the enzymic action of masses of microorganisms (in the bacterial plaque) on carbohydrates; this initial demineralization is followed by an enzymic destruction of the protein matrix with subsequent cavitation and direct bacterial invasion. 2. Obsolete term for destruction or necrosis of bone.

cari'na, pl. **cari'nae** [L. the keel of a boat] An anatomical structure forming a projecting central ridge.

car'inate Keel-shaped, relating to or resembling a carina.

cariogen'ic Producing caries; usually said of diets.

car'ious Relating to or affected with caries.

carmin'ative [L. *carmino*, pp. *-atus*, to card wool; special Mod. L. use, to expel wind] Preventing the formation or causing the expulsion of flatus.

car'otenae'mia Carotene in the blood, especially pertaining to increased quantities, which sometimes cause a pale yellow-red pigmentation of skin that may resemble icterus.

car'otene A class of yellow-red pigments (lipochromes), widely distributed in plants and animals, that include precursors of the vitamins A.

caroteno'sis cu'tis Yellow coloration of the skin caused by an increase in carotene content.

carot'id [G. *karōtides*, the carotid arteries, fr. *karoō*, to put to sleep (because compression of the c. artery results in unconsciousness)] Pertaining to any c. structure.

car'pal Relating to the carpus.

car'pus, pl. **car'pi** [Mod. L. fr. Gr. *karpos*] [NA] 1. The wrist proper, the proximal segment of the hand consisting of the carpal bones and associated soft parts. 2. The carpal bones, which articulate proximally with the radius and indirectly with the ulna, and distally with the five metacarpal bones.

car'rier 1. An individual with an asymptomatic condition that is capable of being transmitted to other individuals. 2. Any chemical capable of accepting an atom, radical, or subatomic particle from one compound, then passing it to another. 3. A substance having chemical properties closely related to or indistinguishable from those of a radioactive tracer and which engages in the process being performed or studied.

car'tilage [L. *cartilago*, gristle] A connective tissue characterized by its nonvascularity and firm consistency; consists of cells (chondrocytes), interstitial substance (matrix) of fibres, and a ground substance (chondromucoid). There are three kinds of c.: hyaline c., elastic c., and fibrocartilage.

    cricoid c., *cartilago* cricoidea.

    elastic c., c. in which the cells are surrounded by a territorial capsular matrix outside of which is an interterritorial matrix containing elastic fibre networks in addition to the collagen fibres and ground substance.

hyaline c., c. having a frosted glass appearance; in mature c. the cells are present in isogenous groups and the interstitial substance contains fine collagenous fibres obscured by the ground substance (chondromucoid).

yellow c., elastic c.

cartilag'inous Relating to or consisting of cartilage.

cartila'go, pl. **cartila'gines** [L. gristle] [NA] Cartilage.

c. cricoi'dea [NA], cricoid cartilage; the lowermost of the laryngeal cartilages, expanded into a nearly quadrilateral plate (lamina) posteriorly.

car'uncle A small fleshy protuberance, or any similar structure.

carun'cula, pl. **carun'culae** [L. a small fleshy mass, fr. *caro*, flesh] [NA] Caruncle.

caryo- [G. *karyon*, nut, kernel] See karyo-.

case [L. *casus*, an occurrence] An instance of disease with its attendant circumstances; not synonymous with "patient".

casea'tion [L. *caseus*, cheese] A form of coagulation necrosis in which the necrotic tissue resembles cheese and contains a mixture of protein and fat that is absorbed very slowly; occurs particularly in tuberculosis.

ca'sein The principal protein of cow's milk and the chief constituent of cheese; used as a constituent of some glues.

ca'seous Pertaining to or manifesting the gross and microscopic features of tissue affected by caseation.

cast 1. An object formed by the solidification of a liquid poured into an impression or mould. 2. The rigid encasement of a part, as with plaster or a plastic, for purposes of immobilization. 3. An elongated or cylindroid mould formed in a tubular structure that may be observed in histologic sections or in material such as urine or sputum; results from inspissation of fluid material secreted or excreted in the tubular structures, and named after the constituents (blood, epithelial, hyaline, etc.).

cast brace A specially designed plaster cast incorporating hinges and other brace components; used in the treatment of fractures to promote early activity and early joint motion.

cas'tor oil A fixed oil expressed from the seeds of *Ricinus communis* (family Euphorbiaceae); a purgative.

cas'trate [L. *castro*, pp. -*atus*, to deprive of generative power] To remove the testicles or the ovaries.

castra'tion [see castrate] 1. Removal of the testicles or ovaries. 2. In psychiatry, usually the fantasied loss of the penis by the female or fear of its actual loss by the male.

cata- [G. *kata*, down] Combining form meaning down. For words so beginning and not found here, see also kata .

catabol'ic Relating to catabolism.

catab'olism [G. *katabolē*, a casting down] The breaking down in the body of complex chemical compounds into simpler ones, often accompanied by the liberation of energy. *Cf.* anabolism.

catab'olite Any product of catabolism.

cat'alase A haemoprotein catalysing the decomposition of hydrogen peroxide to water and oxygen.

cat'alepsy [G. *katalēpsis*, a seizing] A morbid state in which there is a waxy rigidity of the limbs that may be placed in various positions which will be maintained for a time; there is irresponsiveness to stimuli, the pulse and respiration are slow, and the skin is pale.

catalept'ic Relating to or characteristic of catalepsy.

catal'ysis [G. *katalysis*, dissolution] The effect that a catalyst exerts upon a chemical reaction.

cat'alyst That which accelerates a chemical reaction but is not consumed or changed permanently thereby.

cataphylax'is [cata- + G. *phylaxis*, protection] A deterioration in the natural defence mechanisms by which the body resists infectious disease.

cat'aplexy [cata- + G. *plēxis*, a blow, stroke] A transient attack of extreme generalized muscular weakness, often precipitated by an emotional state such as laughing heartily.

cat'aract [L. *cataracta*, fr. G. *katarrhakēs*, a downrushing, a waterfall] A loss of transparency of the lens of the eye, or of its capsule.

catarrh' [G. *katarrheō*, to flow down] Old term for inflammation of a mucous membrane; popularly, chronic rhinitis.

catar'rhal Relating to catarrh.

catato'nia [G. *katatonos*, stretching down, depressed, fr. *kata*, down, + *tonos*, tone] A syndrome characterized by periods of physical rigidity, negativism, excitement, and stupor.

cataton'ic Relating to, or characterized by, catatonia.

cat'echolam'ines Pyrocatechols with an alkylamine side chain; *e.g.*, adrenaline, noradrenaline, dopa.

cat'gut [probably from *kit*, a small violin, through confusion with kit, a small cat] An absorbable surgical suture material made from the collagenous fibres of the submucosa of certain animals.

cathar'sis [G. purification, fr. *katharos*, pure] 1. Purgation. 2. Release or discharge of emotional tension or anxiety by psychoanalytically guided emotional reliving of past, especially repressed, events.

cathar'tic 1. Relating to catharsis. 2. An agent causing active movement of the bowels.

cath'eter [G. *katheter*, fr. *kathiemi*, to send down] A tubular instrument for the passage of fluid from or into a body cavity, especially one designed to be passed through the urethra into the bladder to drain it of retained urine.

    balloon-tip c., a tube with a balloon at its tip that can be inflated or deflated; the inflated balloon may facilitate passage of the tube through a blood vessel (propelled by the bloodstream) or to occlude the vessel.

    Swan-Ganz c., a thin (5 Fr), very flexible, flow-directed c. using a balloon to carry it through the heart to a pulmonary artery; when it is positioned in a small arterial branch, pulmonary wedge pressure is measured in front of the temporarily inflated and wedged balloon.

cath'eteriza'tion Passage of a catheter.

cathex'is [G. *kathexis*, a holding in, retention] Attachment of libido to a specific idea or object.

cat'ion [G. *kation*, going down] An ion carrying a charge of positive electricity, therefore going to the negatively charged cathode.

cation exchange The process by which a cation in a liquid phase exchanges with another cation present as the counter-ion of a negatively charged polymer, the latter being a cation exchanger.

cau'dal [Mod. L. *caudalis*] Pertaining to the tail.

cau'da, pl. **cau'dae** [L. a tail] [NA] Any tail, or tail-like structure, or tapering or elongated extremity of an organ or other part.

    c. equi'na [L. horse's tail] [NA], the bundle of spinal nerve roots running through the lower part of the subarachnoid space within the vertebral canal below the first lumbar vertebra; comprises the roots of all the spinal nerves below the first lumbar.

caul [Gaelic, *call*, a veil] The amnion forming the bag of waters, sometimes delivered unruptured with the baby; a piece of amnion capping the baby's head when born.

causal'gia [G. *kausis*, burning + *algos*, pain] Persistent severe burning sensation of the skin, usually following direct or indirect (vascular) injury of sensory fibres of a peripheral nerve, accompanied by cutaneous changes (temperature and sweating).

caus'tic [G. *kaustikos*, fr. *kaio*, to burn] Exerting an effect resembling a burn.

cau'terize To apply a cautery; to burn with an actual or potential cautery.

cau'tery [G. *kauterion*, a branding iron] An agent or device used for scarring, burning, or cutting the skin or tissues by means of heat, electric current, or caustic chemicals.

ca'va Plural of cavum. See also *vena cava*.

cav'agram Cavogram.

caverni'tis, cavernosi'tis Inflammation of the corpus cavernosum penis.

cavernos'tomy [L. *caverna*, cavern, + G. *stoma*, mouth] Surgical opening of any cavity to establish drainage.

cav'ernous Relating to a cavern or a cavity; containing many cavities.

cavita'tion Formation of a cavity, as in the lung in tuberculosis.

cav'ity [L. *cavus*, hollow] 1. A hollow space within a body structure. 2. Lay term for the loss of tooth structure due to dental caries.

    oral c., mouth; the area bounded by the lips and cheeks, teeth and gums, and isthmus of the fauces.

    tympanic c., tympanum; an air chamber in the temporal bone containing the ossicles; it is lined with mucous membrane and is continuous with the auditory tube anteriorly and the tympanic antrum and mastoid air cells posteriorly.

cav'ogram An angiogram of a vena cava.

ca'vum, pl. **ca'va** [L. ntr. of adj. *cavus*, hollow] [NA] A hollow space, hole, or cavity.

cefox'itin sodium A semisynthetic antibiotic substance structurally and pharmacologically similar to the cephalosporins; used by injection and has an antimicrobial spectrum similar to that of cephalothin.

-cele [G. *kēlē*, tumour, hernia] Suffix denoting a swelling or hernia.

cell [L. *cella*, a storeroom, a chamber] **1.** A minute structure, the living, active basis of all plant and animal organization, composed of a mass of protoplasm enclosed in a delicate membrane and containing a nucleus. **2.** A small closed or partly closed cavity.

germ c., sex c.

Hürthle c., a large, granular eosinophilic c. derived from thyroid follicular epithelium by accumulation of mitochondria, *e.g.,* in Hashimoto's disease.

Kupffer c.'s, stellate reticuloendothelial c.'s lining the hepatic sinusoids.

mast c., a connective tissue c. that contains coarse, basophilic, metachromatic granules; the c. is believed to contain heparin and histamine.

mastoid c.'s, mastoid *sinuses*.

plasma c., an ovoid c. with an eccentric nucleus having chromatin arranged radially; the cytoplasm is strongly basophilic because of abundant RNA in its endoplasmic reticulum; plasma c.'s are derived from B-lymphocytes and are active in the formation of antibodies.

Purkinje's c.'s, large nerve c.'s of the cerebellar cortex with a piriform cell body and dendrites arranged in a plane transverse to the folium.

red blood c. (RBC), erythrocyte.

Reed-Sternberg c., a large transformed lymphocyte, generally regarded as pathognomonic of Hodgkin's disease, with a pale-staining acidophilic cytoplasm and one or two large nuclei showing marginal clumping of chromatin and unusually conspicuous, deeply acidophilic nucleoli.

Schwann c.'s, c.'s of ectodermal origin that compose a continuous envelope around each nerve fibre of peripheral nerves; comparable to the oligodendroglia of the brain and spinal cord; like the latter, they may form membranous expansions that wind around axons and thus form the axon's myelin sheath.

Sertoli c.'s, elongated c.'s in the seminiferous tubules to which spermatids are attached during spermiogenesis.

sex c., a spermatozoon or an ovum.

sickle c., an abnormal crescentic erythrocyte characteristic of sickle c. anaemia, resulting from an inherited abnormality of haemoglobin (haemoglobin S) that causes decreased solubility at low oxygen tension.

white blood c. (WBC), leucocyte.

zymogenic c., a c. that secretes an enzyme; specifically a chief c. of a gastric gland or an acinar c. of the pancreas.

cel'lula, pl. **cel'lulae** [L. a small chamber, dim. of *cella*, storeroom] **1.** [NA] In gross anatomy, a small but macroscopic compartment. **2.** In histology, a cell.

cel'lular [L. *collula*, dim. of *colla*, storeroom] **1.** Relating to, derived from, or composed of cells. **2.** Having numerous compartments or interstices.

cel'lule Cellula (1).

cel'lulite Colloquial term for deposits of fat and other material believed to be trapped in pockets beneath the skin.

celluli'tis Inflammation of cellular or connective tissue.

cel'lulose A polysaccharide (polyglucose) made up of disaccharide residues which form the basis of vegetable fibre.

oxidized c., (1) cellulosic acid in the form of an absorbable gauze; used as a haemostatic in operations where ligation is not feasible because it has a pronounced affinity for haemoglobin and produces an artificial clot; **(2)** a sterile, absorbable substance prepared by the oxidation of cotton.

celo- [G. *kēlē*, hernia] Combining form meaning hernia.

cement' [see cementum] **1.** Cementum. **2.** In dentistry, a nonmetallic material used for luting, filling, permanent or temporary restorative purposes, or as an adherent sealer in attaching various dental restorations.

cemen'tum [L. *caementum*, rough quarry stone, fr. *caedo*, to cut] [NA] A layer of modified bone covering the dentine of the root and neck of a tooth which blends with the fibres of the periodontal membrane.

cen'sor [L. a judge, critic, fr. *censeo*, to value, judge] The psychic barrier which, according to psychoanalytic theory, prevents certain unconscious thoughts and wishes from coming to consciousness unless they are so cloaked or disguised as to be unrecognizable.

cen'tre [L. *centrum;* G. *kentron*] **1.** The middle point of a body; loosely, the interior of a body. **2.** A group of nerve cells governing a specific function.

  Broca's c., a small posterior part of the inferior frontal gyrus of the left hemisphere, identified as an essential component of the motor mechanisms governing articulated speech.

  ossification c., the spot where bone begins to form in a specific bone or part of a bone: **primary o. c.** is the first site of formation in the shaft of a long bone; **secondary o. c.** is a c. of formation appearing later, usually in an epiphysis.

  Wernicke's c., a large region of the parietal and temporal lobes of the left cerebral hemisphere, thought to be essential for understanding and formulating coherent, propositional speech.

cente'sis [G. *kentēsis*, puncture, fr. *kenteō*, to prick, pierce] Puncture; when used as a suffix, usually denotes paracentesis.

cen'tigrade (C) [L. *centum*, one hundred, + *gradus*, step, degree] Consisting of 100 degrees. See centigrade *scale*.

cen'tric Pertaining to a centre.

centrif'ugal [L. *centrum*, centre, + *fugio*, to flee] Denoting a direction outward (away) from an axis of rotation.

centrif'uga'tion Subjection to sedimentation, by means of the centrifuge, of solids suspended in a fluid.

cen'trifuge **1.** An apparatus by means of which particles in suspension in a fluid may be separated by centrifugal force. **2.** To subject to centrifugation.

cen'triole [G. *kentron*, a point, centre] Usually paired tubular organelles lying in the cytocentrum and having a wall having nine triple microtubules; may be multiple and numerous in cells such as the giant cells of bone marrow.

centrip'etal [L. *centrum*, centre, + *peto*, to seek] Denoting the direction of the force pulling an object toward an axis of rotation.

cen'tromere [centro- + G. *meros*, part] The nonstaining primary constriction of a chromosome which is the point of attachment of the spindle fibre, is concerned with chromosome movement during cell division, divides the chromosome into two arms, and is constant for a specific chromosome.

cen'trum, pl. **cen'tra** [L. fr. G. *kentron*] [NA] A centre of any kind, especially an anatomical centre.

cephalal'gia [cephal- + G. *algos*, pain] Headache.

cephalex'in A broad spectrum antibiotic derived from cephalosporin.

ceph'alhaemato'ma [cephal- + G. *haima*, blood, + *-ōma*, tumour] A blood cyst of the scalp in a newborn infant, due to an effusion of blood beneath the pericranium.

cephal'ic Cranial (1).

cephalo-, cephal- [G. *kephalē*, head] Combining forms denoting the head.

ceph'alocele Encephalocele.

ceph'alocente'sis [cephalo- + G. *kenetēsis*, puncture] Passage of a hollow needle or trocar and cannula into the brain to drain an abscess or the fluid of a hydrocephalus.

cephalomeg'aly [cephalo- + G. *megas*, great] Enlargement of the head.

cephalomet'rics [cephalo- + G. *metron*, measure] **1.** The scientific measurement of the bones of the cranium and face, utilizing a fixed, reproducible position for lateral radiographic exposure of skull and facial bones. **2.** A scientific study of the measurements of the head with relation to specific reference points; used for evaluation of facial growth and development, including soft tissue profile.

cephalom'etry [cephalo- + G. *metron*, measure] Any measurement of the living head.

cephalomo'tor Relating to movements of the head.

cephalo'ridine A broad spectrum antimicrobial produced from chemically modified cephalosporin.

cephalospor'in One of several antibiotic substances obtained from *Cephalosporium acremonium, C. salmosynnematum,* and other fungi. Antibiotic activity is due to the 7-aminocephalosporanic acid portion of the molecule; addition of side chains have produced semisynthetic broad spectrum antibiotics with greater antibacterial activity.

ceph'alothin A chemically modified cephalosporin; a broad spectrum antibiotic.

-ceptor [L. *capio*, pp. *captus*, to take] Suffix meaning taker or receiver.

cer'amide Generic term for a class of sphingolipid, N-acyl (fatty acid) derivatives of a long chain base or sphinoid (e.g., sphinganine or sphingosine).

cerclage' [Fr. an encircling, hooping, banding] **1.** Binding together the ends of an obliquely fractured bone or the fragments of a broken patella, brought into close apposition, by an encircling wire loop or a ring. **2.** Operation for retinal detachment in which the choroid and retinal pigment epithelium are brought in contact with the detached sensory retina by a taut encircling silicone band around the sclera. **3.** Placement of a nonabsorbable suture around an incompetent cervical os.

cerebel'lar Relating to the cerebellum.

cerebello- [L. cerebellum] Combining form relating to the cerebellum.

cerebel'lum, pl. **cerebel'la** [L. dim. of cerebrum, brain] [NA] The large posterior brain mass lying above the pons and medulla and beneath the posterior portion of the cerebrum; consists of two lateral hemispheres united by a narrow middle portion, the vermis.

cer'ebral Relating to the cerebrum.

cerebro-, cerebr-, cerebri- [L. cerebrum, brain] Combining forms relating to the cerebrum.

cer'ebroside A class of glycosphingolipid found in the myelin sheath of nerve tissue.

cer'ebrospi'nai Relating to the brain and the spinal cord.

cer'ebrovas'cular Relating to the blood supply to the brain, particularly with reference to pathologic changes.

cer'ebrum, pl. **cer'ebrums, cer'ebra** [L. brain] [NA] Originally, the largest portion of the brain, including practically all parts within the skull except the medulla, pons, and cerebellum; now, usually only the parts derived from the telencephalon and includes mainly the cerebral hemispheres (cerebral cortex and basal ganglia).

ceru'men [L. cera, wax] Earwax; the brownish yellow, waxy secretion (a modified sebum) of the ceruminous glands of the external auditory meatus.

ceru'minal, ceru'minous Relating to cerumen.

cer'vical [L. cervix (cervic-), neck] Relating to a neck, or cervix, in any sense.

cervicec'tomy [cervix + G. ektomē, excision] Excision of the cervix uteri.

cervico- [L. cervix, nook] Combining form relating to a cervix, or neck, in any sense.

cer'vix, pl. **cer'vices** [L. neck] [NA] **1.** Collum. **2.** Any necklike structure.

c. u'teri [NA], neck of the uterus or womb; the lower part of the uterus extending from the isthmus of the uterus into the vagina.

Cesto'da [G. kestos, girdle] A subclass of tapeworms (class Cestoidea), containing the typical members of this group, including the segmented tapeworms that parasitize man and domestic animals.

ces'tode, ces'toid Common name for tapeworms of the class Cestoidea or its subclasses, Cestoda and Eucestoda.

Cestoid'ea [G. kestos, girdle, + eidos, form] The tapeworms; a class of platyhelminth flatworms characterized by lack of an alimentary canal and, in typical forms, by a strobilate or segmented body with a scolex or holdfast organ at one end; adult worms are vertebrate parasites, usually found in the small intestine.

chafe [Fr. chauffer, to heat, fr. L. calefacio, to make warm] To cause irritation of the skin by friction.

chain [L. catena] **1.** In chemistry, a series of atoms held together by one or more covalent bonds. **2.** In bacteriology, a linear arrangement of living cells that have divided in one plane and remain attached to each other.

chala'sia, chala'sis [G chalaō, to loosen] Inhibition and relaxation of any previously sustained contraction of muscle, usually of a synergic group of muscles.

chala'zion, pl. **chala'zia** [G. dim. of chalaza, a sty] A chronic inflammatory granuloma in the tarsus of the eyelid, due to inflammation of a meibomian gland.

chalco'sis [G. chalkos, copper, brass] **1.** Chronic copper poisoning. **2.** A deposit of fine particles of copper in the lungs or other parts.

chalico'sis [G. chalix, gravel] A pneumonoconiosis caused by the inhalation of dust incident to the occupation of stone cutting.

cham'ber [L. camera] A compartment or enclosed space.

counting c., a special, standardized glass slide used for counting cells (especially erythrocytes and leucocytes) and other particulate material in a measured volume of fluid; such slides are frequently known as haemocytometers.

hyperbaric c., a c. employing high-pressure oxygenation.

ionization c., a c. for detecting ionization of the enclosed gas; used for determining intensity of ionizing radiation.

chan'cre [Fr. indirectly from L. *cancer*] Hard c.; the primary lesion of syphilis, a hard, nonsensitive, dull red papule or area of infiltration that begins at the site of infection after an interval of 10 to 30 days; the centre usually becomes eroded or breaks down into an ulcer that heals slowly after 4 to 6 weeks.

chan'criform Resembling chancre.

chan'croid [chancre + G. *eidos,* resemblance] Soft chancre; an infectious venereal ulcer at the site of infection by *Haemophilus ducreyi,* beginning after an incubation period of 3 to 5 days.

char'coal Carbon obtained by heating or burning organic material with restricted access of air. Activated c. is the residue from destructive distillation of various organic materials, treated to increase its adsorptive power; used in diarrhoea, as an antidote, and in purification processes in industry and research.

char'latan A quack; a fraud claiming knowledge and skills not possessed.

chart **1.** A recording, in tabular form, of clinical data relating to a case. **2.** In optics, symbols of graduated size for measuring visual acuity, or test types for examining far or near vision; *e.g.,* Snellen's test type.

cheek [A.S. *ceáce*] The side of the face forming the lateral wall of the mouth.

cheil- See cheilo-.

cheilec'tomy, chilec'tomy [cheil- + G. *ektomē,* excision] **1.** Excision of a portion of the lip. **2.** Chiseling away bony irregularities on the lips of a joint cavity that interfere with movements of the joint.

cheili'tis, chili'tis [cheil- + G. *-itis,* inflammation] Inflammation of the lips or of a lip, with redness and the production of fissures radiating from the angles of the mouth. See also cheilosis.

cheilo-, cheil- [G. cheilos, lip] Combining forms denoting relationship to the lips. See also chilo-; chil-.

chei'loplasty, chi'loplasty [cheilo- + G. *plassō,* to form] Plastic surgery of the lips.

cheilos'chisis, chilos'chisis [cheilo- + G. *schisis,* cleft] Cleft *lip.*

cheilo'sis, chilo'sis [cheil- + G. *-osis,* condition] Angular stomatitis seen in riboflavin deficiency and other B-complex deficiencies; begins with a small fissure, without much inflammation, and accumulation of dried serum, and may eventuate in deep fissures.

cheilot'omy, chilot'omy [cheilo- + G. *tomē,* incision] Incision into the lip.

cheiro- [G. *cheir,* hand] Combining forms meaning hand. See also chiro-.

chei'roplasty, chi'roplasty [cheiro- + G. *plassō,* to form] A plastic operation upon the hand.

chei'ropom'pholyx, chi'ropom'pholyx [cheiro- + G. *pompholyx,* a bubble, fr. *pomphos,* a blister] Dyshidrosis.

chei'rospasm, chi'rospasm [cheiro- + G. *spasmos,* spasm] Spasm of the muscles of the hand, as in writers' cramp.

che'late **1.** To effect chelation. **2.** Pertaining to chelation. **3.** A complex formed through chelation.

chela'tion [G. *chēlē,* claw] Complex formation involving a metal ion and two or more polar groupings of a single molecule; *e.g.,* in haem, the Fe^{2+} ion is chelated by the porphyrin ring. Chelation can be used to remove an ion from participation in biological reactions, as in the chelation of Ca^{2+} of blood by EDTA, which thus acts as an anticoagulant.

chem'exfolia'tion A chemosurgical technique designed to remove acne scars or treat chronic skin defects caused by exposure to sunlight.

chem'ist **1.** One educated in and practising the science of chemistry. **2.** One who prepares and dispenses drugs and has knowledge concerning their properties.

chem'istry [G. *chēmeia,* alchemy] The science concerned with the atomic composition of substances, with the elements and their reactions, and with the formation, decomposition and properties of molecules.

inorganic c., c. concerned with compounds not involving covalent bonds.

organic c., c. concerned with covalently linked atoms, centring around carbon compounds of this type; originally, and still including, the c. of natural (organic) products.

chemo-, chem- [G. *chēmeia*, alchemy] Combining forms relating to chemistry.

che′moprophylax′is [chemo- + prophylaxis] Prevention of disease by use of chemicals or drugs.

chem′orecep′tor   Any cell that is activated by a change in its chemical milieu and thereby originates a flow of nervous impulses.

chem′osurgery   Excision of diseased tissue after it has been fixed *in situ* by chemical means.

chemotax′is [chemo- + G. *taxis*, orderly arrangement] Attraction of living protoplasm to chemical stimuli, whereby the cells are attracted (**positive c.**) or repelled (**negative c.**) by acids, alkalies, or other bodies exhibiting chemical properties.

chem′other′apy   Treatment of disease by means of chemical substances or drugs.

cher′ubism [Hebr. *kerubh*, cherub] A familial multilocular fibro-osseous disease, with enlargement of the jaw bones in young children (producing the characteristic facies) that tends to regress in adult life.

chest [A.S. *cest*, a box] The thorax, especially the anterior aspect. See also breast.

    barrel c., a c. permanently the shape of a barrel during full inspiration, *i.e.*, with increased anteroposterior diameter and usually some degree of kyphosis, seen in cases of emphysema.

    flail c., flapping chest wall; loss of stability of thoracic cage following fracture of sternum and/or ribs.

    flat c., a c. in which the anteroposterior diameter is less than the average.

    funnel c., *pectus excavatum.*

chi′asm [G. *chiasma*, two crossing lines, fr. the letter *chi*, X] **1.** A decussation or crossing of two tracts, such as tendons or nerves. **2.** The crossing of intertwined chromosomes during prophase.

    optic c., a flattened quadrangular body in front of the tuber cinereum and infundibulum, the point of crossing or decussation of the fibres of the optic nerves.

chick′enpox   Varicella.

chig′ger   The six-legged larva of *Trombicula* species and other members of the family Trombiculidae; a bloodsucking stage of mites that includes the vectors of scrub typhus.

chig′oe   Common name for *Tunga penetrans.*

chil′blain [chill + A.S. *blegen*, a skin lesion] Erythema, itching, and burning, especially of the dorsa of the fingers and toes, and of the heels, nose, and ears on exposure to extreme cold (usually associated with high humidity).

child′birth   Parturition; the process of labour and delivery in the birth of a child. See also birth.

chill [A.S. *cele*, cold] A feeling of cold, with shivering and pallor, accompanied by an elevation of temperature in the interior of the body.

chilo-, chil- [G. *cheilos*, lip] Combining form denoting relationship to the lips. See also chello-; chell-.

chimae′ra [L. *chimoera*, fr. G. *chimaira*, a fabulous monster] **1.** One who has received a transplant of genetically and immunologically different tissue, such as bone marrow. **2.** Twins with two immunologically different types of erythrocytes. **3.** Sometimes used as a synonym for mosaic.

chin [A.S. *cin*] Mentum; the prominence formed by the anterior projection of the mandible, or lower jaw.

chiro-, chir- [G. *cheir*, hand] Combining forms denoting the hand. See also cheiro-.

chirop′odist [chiro- + G. *pous*, foot] Podiatrist.

chirop′ody   Podiatry.

chiroprac′tic [chiro- + G. *praktikos*, efficient] The science that utilizes the recuperative powers of the body and the relationship between the musculoskeletal structures and functions of the body, particularly of the spinal column and the nervous system, in the restoration and maintenance of health.

chi′ropractor   One licensed and certified to practise chiropractic.

Chlamyd′ia [G. *chlamys*, cloak] The single genus of the family Chlamydiaceae, which includes all the agents of the psittacosis-lymphogranuloma-trachoma disease groups; two species are recognized, *C. psittaci* and *C. trachomatis* (the type species).

    C. psitta′ci, a species that causes psittacosis, ornithosis, and pneumonitis, abortion, encephalomyelitis, and enteritis in various animals.

    C. tracho′matis, a species that causes trachoma, inclusion conjunctivitis, lymphogranuloma venereum, nonspecific urethritis, and proctitis; the type species of the genus *C.*

chlamyd'ial   Relating to or caused by *Chlamydia.*

chloas'ma   [G. *chloazo*, to become green] Melanoderma or melasma characterized by the occurrence of extensive brown patches of irregular shape and size on the skin of the face and elsewhere; such pigmented patches are also called the mask of pregnancy, and are associated most commonly with pregnancy, menopause, and use of oral contraceptives.

chloram'bucil   A nitrogen mustard derivative that depresses lymphocytic proliferation and maturation.

chlor-, chloro-   [G. *chloros*, green] Combining form denoting 1) green; 2) association with chlorine.

chlorac'ne   An acne-like eruption due to prolonged contact with certain chlorinated compounds (naphthalenes and diphenyls).

chlor'dane   A chlorinated hydrocarbon used as an insecticide; may be absorbed through the skin with resultant severe toxic effects.

chlo'rinated   Containing chlorine.

chlor'ine   A gaseous element; symbol Cl, atomic no. 17, atomic weight 35.46; a halogen used as a disinfectant and bleaching agent because of its oxidizing power.

chlor'oform   [chlor(ine) + form(yl)] Methylene trichloride; CHCl3; used by inhalation to produce general anaesthesia; also used as a solvent.

chloro'ma   [chloro- + G. -*oma*, tumour] Development of multiple, localized green masses of abnormal cells (in most instances, myeloblasts), especially in relation to the periosteum of the skull, spine, and ribs.

chlorophe'nol   One of several substitution products obtained by the action of chlorine on phenol; an antiseptic.

chlo'rophyll   The porphyrin derivative (phorbin) found in photosynthetic organisms as the light-absorbing, green pigments that, in living plants, convert light energy into oxidizing and reducing power, thus fixing CO_2 and evolving O_2.

chlorop'sia   [chloro- + G. *opsis*, eyesight] A condition in which all objects appear to be coloured green, as may occur in digitalis intoxication.

chlor'oquine   An antimalarial also used in the treatment of hepatic amoebiasis and for certain skin diseases.

chloro'sis   [chloro- + -*osis*, condition] A form of chronic hypochromic microcytic (iron deficiency) anaemia, characterized by a reduction in haemoglobin out of proportion to the decreased number of red blood cells; observed chiefly in females from puberty to the third decade and usually associated with deficiency in iron and protein.

chlorpro'mazine   A phenothiazine antipsychotic agent with antiemetic, antiadrenergic, and anticholinergic actions.

chlorpro'pamide   An orally effective hypoglycaemic related chemically and pharmacologically to tolbutamide.

chlorprothix'ene   An antipsychotic of the thioxanthene group; also possesses antiemetic, adrenolytic, spasmolytic, and antihistaminic actions.

chlor'tetracy'cline   A naphthacene derivative, obtained from *Streptomyces aureofaciens*, used as an antibiotic.

cho'ana,   pl. **cho'anae**   [Mod. L. fr. G. *choane*, a funnel] [NA] The posterior naris; the opening into the nasopharynx of the nasal cavity on either side.

choke   To prevent respiration by compression or obstruction of the larynx or trachea.

chokes   A manifestation of caisson disease or altitude sickness characterized by dyspnoea, coughing, and choking.

chol-   [G. *chole*, bile] Combining form denoting relationship to bile.

cholae'mia   [chole- + G. *haima*, blood] Presence of bile salts in the circulating blood.

cho'lagogue   [chol- + G. *agogos*, drawing forth] **1.** An agent that promotes the flow of bile into the intestine, especially as a result of contraction of the gallbladder. **2.** Relating to such an agent or effect.

cholangiec'tasis   [chol- + G. *angeion*, vessel, + *ektasis*, a stretching] Dilation of the bile ducts, usually a sequel to obstruction.

cholan'giogram   Radiographic image of the bile ducts obtained by cholangiography.

cholangiog'raphy   [chol- + G. *angeion*, vessel, + *grapho*, to write] Radiographic examination of the bile ducts.

cholangio'ma   [chol- + G. *angeion*, vessel, + -*oma*, tumour] A neoplasm of bile duct origin, especially within the liver; may be either benign or malignant (cholangiocarcinoma).

cholan'giopancreatog'raphy Radiographic examination of the bile ducts and pancreas.

 endoscopic retrograde c. (ERCP), a method of c. using an endoscope to inspect the pancreatic duct and common bile duct; may also involve biopsy or introduction of contrast material for radiographic examination.

cholangios'copy [chol- + G. *angeion*, vessel, + *skopeō*, to examine] Examination of bile ducts utilizing a cystoscope or fibreoptic endoscope.

cholangios'tomy [chol- + G. *angeion*, vessel, + *stoma*, mouth] Formation of a fistula into a bile duct.

cholangi'tis [chol- + G. *angeion*, vessel, + *-itis*, inflammation] Inflammation of a bile duct.

chole- [G. *cholē*, bile] Combining form relating to bile. See also cholo-.

cho'lecalcif'erol Vitamin D₃; an antirachitic, oil-soluble vitamin.

cho'lecystec'tomy [chole- + G. *kystis*, bladder, + *ektomē*, excision] Surgical removal of the gallbladder.

cholecysti'tis [chole- + G. *kystis*, bladder, + *-itis*, inflammation] Inflammation of the gallbladder.

cholecys'tocolos'tomy [chole- + G. *kystis*, bladder, + *kolon*, colon, + *stoma*, mouth] Establishment of a communication between the gallbladder and the colon.

cholecys'toduodenos'tomy [chole- + G. *kystis*, bladder, + L. *duodenum* + G. *stoma*, mouth] Establishment of a communication between the gallbladder and the duodenum.

cholecys'togastros'tomy [chole- + G. *kystis*, bladder, + *gastēr*, stomach, + *stoma*, mouth] Establishment of a communication between the gallbladder and the stomach.

cho'lecystog'raphy [chole- + G. *kystis*, bladder, + *grapho*, to write] Visualization of the gallbladder by x-rays after the administration of a radiopaque substance that is excreted by the liver and concentrated by the normal gallbladder.

cholecys'tojejunos'tomy [chole- + G. *kystis*, bladder, + jejunum, + G. *stoma*, mouth] Establishment of a communication between the gallbladder and the jejunum.

cholecystoki'nin A polypeptide hormone liberated by the upper intestinal mucosa on contact with gastric contents; stimulates the contraction of the gallbladder.

cholecys'tolithi'asis [chole- + G. *kystis*, bladder, + *lithos*, stone] Presence of one or more gallstones in the gallbladder.

cho'lecystop'athy. Disease of the gallbladder.

cho'lecystot'omy [chole- + G. *kystis*, bladder, + *tomē*, incision] Incision into the gallbladder.

choled'ochal Relating to the common bile duct.

choledocho-, cholodoch- [G. *cholēdochos*, containing bile, fr. *cholē*, bile, + *dechomai*, to receive] Combining forms relating to the common bile duct.

choled'ochodu'odenos'tomy [choledocho- + duodenum + G. *stoma*, mouth] Surgical formation of a communication between the common bile duct and the duodenum.

choled'ochoenteros'tomy [choledocho- + G. *enteron*, intestine, + *stoma*, mouth] Surgical establishment of a communication between the common bile duct and any part of the intestine.

choled'ochojejunos'tomy Anastomosis between the common bile duct and the jejunum.

choled'ocholithot'omy [choledocho- + G. *lithos*, stone, + *tomē*, incision] Incision of the common bile duct for the extraction of an impacted gallstone.

cho'ledochos'tomy [choledocho- + G. *stoma*, mouth] Establishment of a fistula into the common bile duct.

cho'ledochot'omy [choledocho- + G. *tomē*, incision] Incision into the common bile duct.

cho'lelithi'asis Presence of concretions in the gallbladder or bile ducts.

cho'lelithot'omy [chole- + G. *lithos*, stone, + *tomē*, incision] Operative removal of a gallstone.

chol'era [L. a bilious disease, fr. G. *cholē*, bile] An acute epidemic infectious disease caused by *Vibrio cholerae*, occurring chiefly in Asia, characterized by profuse watery diarrhoea, extreme loss of fluid and electrolytes, and prostration.

choler′iform Resembling cholera.

cho′lesteato′ma [chole- + steatoma] A tumour-like mass of keratinizing squamous epithelium and cholesterol in the middle ear, usually resulting from chronic otitis media, with squamous metaplasia or extension of squamous epithelium inward to line an expanding cystic cavity that may involve the mastoid and erode surrounding bone.

choles′terol The most abundant steroid in animal tissues, especially in bile and gallstones; used as an emulsifying agent.

choles′terolae′mia [cholesterol + G. *haima*, blood] Presence of enhanced quantities of cholesterol in the blood.

choles′terolo′sis 1. A condition resulting from a disturbance in metabolism of lipids, characterized by deposits of cholesterol in tissue. 2. Cholesterol crystals in the anterior chamber of the eye; it occurs in aphakia with associated retinal separation.

cho′line A substance found in most animal tissues either free or in combination as lecithin (phosphatidylcholine) or acetate (acetylcholine) or cytidine diphosphate (cytidinediphosphocholine); included in the vitamin B complex. Several of its salts are used in medicine.

choliner′gic [choline + G. *ergon*, work] 1. Relating to nerve cells or fibres that employ acetylcholine as their neurotransmitter. 2. Denoting an agent that mimics their action.

cholines′terase One of a family of enzymes capable of catalysing the hydrolysis of acylcholines and a few other compounds.

cholo- See chole-.

chon′dral [G. *chondros*, cartilage] Cartilaginous.

chon′drifica′tion [G. *chondros*, cartilage, + L. *facio*, to make] Conversion into cartilage.

chondri′tis [G. *chondros*, cartilage, + -*itis*, inflammation] Inflammation of cartilage.

chondro-, chondrio- [G. *chondrion*, grit, gristle, cartilage] Combining forms meaning, or relating to, 1) cartilage or cartilaginous, 2) granular or gritty substance.

chon′droblast [chondro- + G. *blastos*, germ] A cell of growing cartilage tissue.

chon′drocalcino′sis [chondro- + calcium + G. -*osis*, condition] Calcification of cartilage.

    articular c., a disease characterized by calcified deposits, free from urate and consisting of calcium hypophosphate crystals, in synovial fluid, articular cartilage, and adjacent soft tissue; leads to goutlike attacks of pain and swelling of the involved joints.

chondrocos′tal [chondro- + L. *costa*, rib] Relating to the costal cartilages.

chon′drocyte [chondro- + G. *kytos*, a hollow (cell)] A connective tissue cell that occupies a lacuna within the cartilage matrix.

chondrodyn′ia [chondro- + G. *odyne*, pain] Pain in cartilage.

chon′drodyspla′sia [chondro- + G. *dys*, bad, + *plasis*, a moulding] Chondrodystrophy.

chon′drodys′trophy [chondro- + G. *dys*, bad, + *trophe*, nourishment] A disturbance in the development of the cartilage primordia of the long bones, involving especially the region of the epiphyseal plates, and resulting in arrested growth of the long bones.

chondrogen′esis [chondro- + G. *genesis*, origin] The formation of cartilage.

chondro′ma [chondro- + G. -*ōma*, tumour] A benign neoplasm derived from mesodermal cells that form cartilage.

chon′dromala′cia [chondro- + G. *malakia*, softness] Abnormal softening of cartilage.

chon′dromato′sis Presence of multiple tumour-like foci of cartilage.

chon′dro-osteodys′trophy A term used for a group of disorders of bone and cartilage which includes Morquio syndrome and similar conditions.

chondrop′athy [chondro- + G. *pathos*, suffering] Any disease of cartilage.

chon′droplast [chondro- + G. *plastos*, formed] Chondroblast.

chondrosarco′ma A malignant neoplasm derived from cartilage cells, occurring most frequently in pelvic bones or near the ends of long bones.

chord- [G. *chordē*] Combining form meaning cord. See also cord-.

chor′da, pl. **chor′dae** [L., cord] 1. A tendon. 2. [NA] A tendinous or a cordlike structure.

chordee′ [Fr. corded] 1. Painful erection of the penis in gonorrhoea or Peyronie's disease, with curvature resulting from lack of distensibility of the corpus cavernosum urethrae. 2. Ventral curvature of the penis, most apparent on erection, as seen in hypospadias due to congenital shortness of the urethra.

chordi'tis [G. *chordē̄*, cord, + -*itis*, inflammation] Inflammation of a cord; usually a vocal cord.

chordot'omy Cordotomy.

chore'a [L. fr. G. *choreia*, a choral dance] **1.** Irregular, spasmodic, involuntary movements of the limbs or facial muscles. **2.** Sydenham's c.

hereditary c., Huntington's c., a chronic disorder characterized by choreic movements in the face and extremities, accompanied by a gradual loss of the mental faculties ending in dementia; autosomal dominant inheritance.

Sydenham's c., an acute toxic or infective disorder of the nervous system, usually associated with acute rheumatic fever, occurring in young persons and characterized by involuntary, irregular, jerky movement of the muscles of the face, neck, and limbs; they are intensified by voluntary effort but disappear in sleep.

chore'ic Relating to or of the nature of chorea.

chore'iform Resembling chorea.

choreo- [see chorea] Combining form relating to chorea.

chorio- [G. *chorion*, membrane] Combining form relating to any membrane, but especially that which encloses the fetus.

cho'rioadeno'ma A benign neoplasm of the chorion, especially with hydatidiform mole formation.

c. destru'ens, hydatidiform mole in which there is an unusual degree of invasion of the myometrium or its blood vessels, causing haemorrhage, necrosis, and occasionally rupture of the uterus.

cho'rioangio'ma [chorion + angioma] A benign tumour of placental blood vessels (haemangioma), usually of no clinical significance; large tumours may be associated with placental insufficiency or hydramnios.

cho'riocarcino'ma A highly malignant neoplasm derived from syncytial trophoblasts and cytotrophoblasts which forms irregular sheets and cords, which are surrounded by irregular "lakes" of blood; villi are not formed.

chorioid-, chorioido- See choroid-, choroido-.

cho'rion [G. *chorion*, membrane enclosing the fetus] The multilayered outermost fetal membrane; consisting of extraembryonic somatic mesoderm and trophoblast; on the maternal surface it possesses villi that are bathed by maternal blood; as pregnancy progresses part of the c. becomes the definitive placenta.

chorion'ic Relating to the chorion.

cho'roid [G. *choroeidēs*, a false reading for *chorioeidēs*, like a membrane] **1.** Resembling the chorion, the corium, or any membrane. **2.** Choroidea.

choroi'dea [see choroid] [NA] The middle, vascular tunic of the eye lying between the retina and the sclera.

cho'roidi'tis Inflammation of the choroid.

choroido- Combining form relating to the choroid.

chrom-, chromat-, chromato-,
chromo- [G. *chrōma*, colour] Combining forms meaning colour.

chro'maffin [chrom- + L. *affinis*, affinity] Giving a brownish-yellow reaction with chromic salts; denoting certain cells in the medulla of the adrenal glands and in paraganglia.

chro'maffino'ma A neoplasm composed of chromaffin cells derived from primitive sympathogonia, and occurring in the medullae of adrenal glands, the organs of Zuckerkandl, or the paraganglia of the thoracolumbar sympathetic chain.

chromat-, chromato- See chrom-.

chro'matin [G. *chrōma*, colour]. The genetic material of the nucleus, consisting of deoxyribonucleoprotein. During mitotic division the c. condenses and is seen as chromosomes.

sex c., Barr c. body; a small condensed mass of c. representing an inactivated X-chromosome, usually located at the periphery of the interphase nucleus just inside the nuclear membrane; the number of sex c. bodies per nucleus is one less than the number of X-chromosomes.

chro'matog'raphy [chromato- + G. *graphō*, to write] Separation of chemical substances and particles by differential movement through a two-phase system. The mixture of materials to be separated is percolated through a column or sheet of some suitable chosen absorbent. The substances least absorbed are least retarded and emerge the soonest; those more strongly absorbed emerge later.

chromatol'ysis [chromato- + G. *lysis*, dissolution] Disintegration of the granules of chromophil substance (Nissl bodies) in a nerve cell body, which may occur after exhaustion of the cell or damage to its peripheral process.

chromat'ophil, chromat'ophile Chromophil.

chromo- See chrom-.

chro'mocyte [chromo- + G. *kytos*, cell] Any pigmented cell, such as a red blood corpuscle.

chro'mophil, chro'mophile [chromo- + G. *phileō*, to love] **1.** Chromophilic. **2.** A cell or any histologic element that stains readily. **3.** Chromaffin.

chromophil'ia [chromo- + G. *phileō*, to love] The property possessed by most cells of staining readily with appropriate dyes.

chromophil'ic Staining readily; denoting certain cells and histologic structures.

chromoso'mal Pertaining to chromosomes.

chro'mosome [chromo- + G. *sōma*, body] A structure (normally 46 in man) in the cell nucleus that is the bearer of genes; it has the form of a delicate chromatin filament during interphase, contracts to form a compact cylinder segmented into two arms by the centromere during metaphase and anaphase stages of cell division, and is capable of reproducing its physical and chemical structure through successive cell divisions. In the case of microbes, the c. is prokaryotic, not being enclosed within a nuclear membrane and not being subject to a mitotic mechanism.

   sex c.'s, the pair of c.'s responsible for sex determination, designated X and Y; females have two X c.'s, whereas males have one X and one Y c.

chron'ic [G. *chronos*, time] Of long duration; denoting a disease of slow progress and long continuance.

Chrysomy'ia [G. *chrysos*, gold, + *myia*, fly] A genus of myiasis-producing fleshflies (family Calliphoridae) including the Old World screw worm, *C. bezziana.*

chrysother'apy [G. *chrysos*, gold] Treatment of disease by the administration of gold salts.

chyle [G. *chylos*, juice] A turbid, white or pale yellow fluid taken up by the lacteals from the intestine during digestion and carried by the lymphatic system via the thoracic duct into the circulation.

chylif'erous [chyl- + L. *fero*, to carry] Conveying chyle.

chylo-, -chyl [G. *chylos*, juice, chyle] Combining form relating to chyle.

chylomi'cron, pl. **chylomi'cra, chylomi'crons** [chylo- + G. *micros*, small] A microscopic particle of fat occurring in chyle, especially numerous after a meal of fat, and also in blood.

chylo'sis Formation of chyle from the food in the intestine, its absorption by the lacteals, and its mixture with the blood and conveyance to the tissues.

chylotho'rax Accumulation of milky chylous fluid in the pleural space, usually on the left.

chyme [G. *chymos*, juice] The semifluid mass of partly digested food passed from the stomach into the duodenum.

chy'mosin Renin; a proteinase structurally homologous with pepsin present as such (or as a zymogen) in the chief cells of the gastric tubules.

cic'atrix, pl. **cicatrices** [L.] Scar.

cic'atriza'tion 1. The process of scar formation. **2.** Healing of a wound otherwise than by first intention.

-cide, -cidal [L. *caedo*, to kill] Suffix denoting an agent that kills or destroys.

cil'iary [Mod. L. *ciliaris*, relating to or resembling an eyelid or eyelash] Relating to any cilia or hairlike processes; the eyelashes; certain structures of the eyeball.

cil'iated Having cilia.

cilio-, cili- [L. *cilium*, eyelid] Combining forms relating to cilia or meaning ciliary.

cil'ium, pl. **cil'ia** [L. eyelid] **1.** [NA] Eyelash; one of the stiff hairs projecting from the margin of the eyelid. **2.** A motile extension of a cell surface, *e.g.*, of certain epithelial cells, containing nine longitudinal double microtubules arranged in a peripheral ring, together with a central pair.

cimet'idine A histamine analogue and antagonist used to treat peptic ulcer and hypersecretory conditions by blocking histamine receptor sites, thus inhibiting gastric acid secretion.

Ci'mex lectula'rius [L. *cimex*, bug, L. *lectulus*, a bed] Bedbug; a biting member of the family Cimicidae that produces a characteristic pungent odour from thoracic stink glands and is a household pest.

cine-, cin- [G. *kinēō, fut. kinēsō*, to move] Combining forms denoting movement; when spelled this way, usually relating to motion pictures. See also kin-; kine-.

cin'e-angiog'raphy Motion pictures of the passage of a contrast medium through blood vessels.

cin'eradiog'raphy Radiography of an organ in motion.

cine'rea [L. fem. of *cinereus*, ashy, fr. *cinis*, ashes] The grey matter of the brain and other parts of the nervous system.

cin'gulate Relating to a cingulum.

cin'gulum, gen. **cin'guli,** pl. **cin'gula** [L. girdle, fr. *cingo*, to surround] [NA] **1.** A structure that has the form of a belt or girdle. **2.** A well marked fibre bundle passing longitudinally in the white matter of the gyrus cinguli (collateral gyrus); composed largely of fibres from the anterior thalamic nucleus to the cingulate and parahippocampal gyri, but also contains association fibres connecting these gyri with the frontal cortex, and their various subdivisions with each other.

circa'dian [L. *circa*, about, + *dies*, day] Relating to biologic variations or rhythms with a cycle of about 24 hours.

cir'cinate [L. *circinatus*, made round] Circular; ring-shaped.

cir'cle [L. *circulus*] **1.** A ring-shaped structure or group of structures. **2.** A line or process with every point equidistant from the center.

  c. of Willis, an anastomotic "circle" at the base of the brain, formed, in order from before backward, by the anterior communicating artery, the two anterior cerebral, the two internal carotid, the two posterior communicating, and the two posterior cerebral arteries.

circula'tion [L. *circulatio*] Movements in a circle, or through a circular course or one which leads back to the same point.

  extracorporeal c., c. of blood outside of the body through a heart-lung machine, artificial kidney, etc.

  systemic c., c. of blood through the arteries, capillaries, and veins of the general system, from the left ventricle to the right atrium.

cir'culatory 1. Relating to circulation. **2.** Sanguiferous.

circum- [L. around] Prefix denoting a circular movement, or a position surrounding the part indicated by the word to which it is joined. See also peri-.

circumci'sion [L. *circumcido*, to cut around] **1.** The operation of removing part or all of the prepuce. **2.** The cutting around an anatomical part.

circumduc'tion [circum- + L. *duco*, pp. *ductus*, to draw] Movement of a part in a circular direction.

cir'cumflex [circum- + L. *flexus*, to bend] Bowed; like the arc of a circle.

cirrho'sis [G. *kirrhos*, tawny, + *-osis*, condition] Fibroid or granular induration; progressive disease of the liver characterized by diffuse damage to hepatic parenchymal cells, with nodular regeneration, fibrosis, and disturbance of normal architecture; associated with failure in the function of hepatic cells and interference with blood flow in the liver, frequently resulting in jaundice, portal hypertension and ascites.

  alcoholic c., c. that frequently develops in chronic alcoholism, characterized in an early stage by enlargement of the liver due to fatty change with mild fibrosis, and later by Laënnec's c. with contraction of the liver

  biliary c., c. due to biliary obstruction, which may be a primary intrahepatic disease or secondary to obstruction of extrahepatic bile ducts.

  Laënnec's c., portal c., c. in which normal liver lobules are replaced by small regeneration nodules, sometimes containing fat, separated by a fairly regular framework of fine fibrous tissue strands (hobnail liver).

cis- [L.] **1.** Prefix meaning on this side, on the near side; opposite of trans-. **2.** In genetics, denoting the location of two or more genes on the same chromosome of a homologous pair. **3.** In organic chemistry, a form of isomerism in which similar functional groups are attached on the same side of the plane that includes two adjacent, fixed carbon atoms.

cis'tern [L. *cisterna*] Cisterna.

cister'na, gen. and pl. **cister'nae** [L. an undergound reservoir for water] **1.** [NA] Any cavity or enclosed space serving as a reservoir, especially for chyle, lymph, or cerebrospinal fluid. **2.** An ultramicroscopic space occurring between the membranes of the flattened sacs of the endoplasmic reticulum, the Golgi complex, or the two membranes of the nuclear envelope.

cis'ternog'raphy   The radiographic study of the basal cisterns of the brain after the subarachnoid introduction of an opaque or other contrast medium, or a radiopharmaceutical.

cit'rate   A salt or ester of citric acid.

cit'ric acid   The acid of citrus fruits, widely distributed in nature and a key intermediate in intermediary metabolism; its salts (citrates) are used as anticoagulants because they bind calcium ions.

Cladospor'ium   [G. *klados*, a branch, + *sporos*, seed] A genus of fungi commonly isolated in soil or plant residues. *C. carrionii* is a cause of chromomycosis in man; *C. wernekii* is the causative agent of tinea nigra.

clamp   An instrument for compression or grasping of a structure.

class   [L. *classis*, a class, division] In biologic classification, the next division below the phylum (or subphylum) and above the order.

clas'tic   [G. *klastos*, broken] Breaking up into pieces, or exhibiting a tendency so to break or divide.

claudica'tion   [L. *claudicatio*, fr. *claudico*, to limp] Limping, usually referring to intermittent c.

   intermittent c.,   Charcot's syndrome; a condition caused by ischaemia of the muscles due to sclerosis with narrowing of the arteries; characterized by attacks of lameness and pain, brought on by walking.

claus'tral   Relating to the claustrum.

claustropho'bia   [L. *claustrum*, an enclosed space, + G. *phobos*, fear] Morbid fear of being in a closed place.

claus'trum,   pl. **claus'tra** [L. barrier] One of several anatomical structures bearing a fancied resemblance to a barrier. Specifically [NA], a thin, vertically placed lamina of grey matter lying close to the outer portion (putamen) of the lenticular nucleus, from which it is separated by the external capsule.

clav'icle   Clavicula.

clavic'ula,   pl. **clavic'ulae** [L. *clavicula*, a small key] [NA] Collar bone; a doubly curved long bone that forms part of the shoulder girdle; its medial end articulates with the manubrium sterni, its lateral end with the acromion of the scapula.

clavic'ular   Relating to the clavicle.

cla'vus   [L. a nail, wart, corn] **1.** Corn; a small conical callosity caused by pressure over a bony prominence, usually on a toe. **2.** A condition resulting from healing of a granuloma of the foot in yaws, in which a core falls out, leaving an erosion.

claw'hand   Atrophy of the interosseous muscles of the hand with hyperextension of the metacarpophalangeal joints and flexion of the interphalangeal joints.

clear'ance   (C with a subscript indicating the substance removed). Removal of a substance from the blood, expressed as the volume flow of arterial blood or plasma that would contain the amount of substance removed per unit time; measured in ml/min.

clea'vage   **1.** A series of cell divisions occurring in the ovum immediately following its fertilization. **2.** The splitting of a complex molecule into two or more simpler molecules. **3.** The linear clefts in the skin, indicating the direction of the fibres in the dermis.

cleft   A fissure.

   synaptic c.,   the space between the axolemma and the postsynaptic surface. See also synapse.

climacter'ic   [G. *klimaktēr*, rung of a ladder] A period of life occurring in women, encompassing termination of the reproductive period, and characterized by endocrine, somatic, and transitory psychologic changes culminating in menopause.

cli'max   [G. *klimax*, staircase] **1.** The height of a disease; the stage of greatest severity. **2.** Orgasm.

clin'ical   **1.** Relating to the bedside of a patient or to the course of his disease. **2.** Denoting the symptoms and course of a disease, as distinguished from the laboratory findings of anatomical changes.

clini'cian   A health professional engaged in clinical practice, as distinguished from an academician.

clino-   [G. *klinō*, to slope, incline, or bend] Combining form denoting a slope or bend.

clinoceph'aly   [clino- + G. *kephalē*, head] Concavity of the upper surface of the skull, presenting a saddle-shaped appearance in profile.

clit'oridec'tomy   [clitoris + G. *ektomē*, excision] Removal of the clitoris.

clit'oris,   pl. **clito'rides** [G. *kleitoris*] [NA] A small erectile body situated at the most anterior portion of the vulva and projecting between the branched extremities of the labia minora, which form its prepuce and frenulum; homologue of the penis in the male except that it is not perforated by the urethra and does not possess a corpus spongiosum.

clit'oromeg'aly [clitoris + G. *megas*, great] An enlarged clitoris.

cli'vus, pl. **cli'vi** [L. slope] [NA] A downward sloping surface.

cloa'ca [L. sewer] In early embryos, the entodermally lined chamber into which hindgut and allantois empty.

clone [G. *klōn*, slip, cutting used for propagation] Progeny derived from a single organism or cell by asexual reproduction, all having identical characteristics.

clon'ic Of the nature of clonus, marked by alternate contraction and relaxation of muscle.

clon'icoton'ic Both clonic and tonic; said of certain forms of muscular spasm.

clo'nus [G. *klonos*, a tumult] A form of movement marked by contractions and relaxations of a muscle, occurring in rapid succession, after forcible extension or flexion of a part.

clostrid'ial Relating to any bacterium of the genus *Clostridium*.

Clostrid'ium [G. *klōstēr*, a spindle] A genus of anaerobic, sporeforming, motile bacteria (family Bacillaceae) containing Gram-positive rods. The type species is *C. butyricum*.

  C. bifermen'tans, a species found in putrid meat and gaseous gangrene, and in soil, faeces, and sewage; pathogenicity varies from strain to strain.

  C. botuli'num, a species that occurs widely in nature and is a frequent cause of food poisoning (botulism); six main types, A to F, characterized by antigenically distinct but pharmacologically similar, very potent neurotoxins.

  C. histoly'ticum, a species found in wounds, where it induces necrosis of tissue by producing a cytolytic exotoxin.

  C. no'vyi, a species consisting of three types: A, B, and C; type A causes gaseous gangrene and necrotic hepatitis.

  C. parabotuli'num, a species containing organisms formerly referred to as *C. botulinum* types A and B; produces a powerful exotoxin and is pathogenic for man and other animals.

  C. perfrin'gens, a species that is the chief causative agent of gas gangrene and may also be involved in causing enteritis, appendicitis, food poisoning, and puerperal fever.

  C. tet'ani, a species that causes tetanus; produces a potent exotoxin (neurotoxin) which is intensely toxic for man and other animals.

  C. welch'ii, *C. perfringens*.

clot 1. To coagulate. 2. A soft, nonrigid, insoluble mass formed when blood or lymph gels.

club'bing A condition affecting the fingers and toes in which the extremities of the digits are broadened and the nails are shiny and abnormally curved longitudinally.

club'foot *Talipes* equinovarus.

club'hand Talipomanus.

clu'nes [pl. of L. *clunis*, buttock] [NA] Nates.

cly'sis [G. *klysis*, a drenching by a clyster] 1. Infusion of fluid for therapeutic purposes. 2. Formerly, use of an enema or irrigation of any body space or cavity by fluids. 3. Suffix denoting injection.

CNS Central nervous *system*.

coag'ulant Causing, stimulating, or accelerating coagulation, especially with reference to blood.

coag'ulate [L. *coagulo*, pp. *-atus*, to curdle] To clot or curdle; to change from the liquid state to a solid or gel.

coagula'tion 1. Clotting; the process of changing from liquid to solid, especially of blood. 2. A clot or coagulum.

coagulop'athy A disease affecting the coagulability of the blood.

coag'ulum, pl. **coag'ula** [L. a means of coagulating, rennet] A clot or a curd, a soft insoluble mass formed when a sol is coagulated.

coarcta'tion A constriction, stricture, or stenosis.

  reversed c., aortic arch syndrome in which blood pressure in the arms is lower than in the legs.

cobal'amin A general term for compounds containing the dimethylbenzimidazolylcobamide nucleus of vitamin B_{12}.

co'balt [Ger. *kobalt*] A steel-grey metallic element, symbol Co, atomic no. 27, atomic weight 58.93; a constituent of vitamin B_{12}; some of its radioisotopes are used diagnostically and therapeutically.

cocaine' An alkaloid obtained from the leaves of *Erythroxylon coca* (family Erythroxylaceae) and other species of *Erythroxylon*, or by synthesis from ecgonine or its derivatives; has moderate vasoconstrictor activity and pronounced psychotropic effects; salts are used as a topical anaesthetic.

cocarcin'ogen A substance that works symbiotically with a carcinogen in the production of cancer.

coc'ci Plural of coccus.

Coccid'ia [Mod. L. fr. G. *kokkos*, berry] A subclass of protozoa (class Sporozoa that includes the genera *Eimeria* and *Isospora* (family Eimeriidae).

coccidio'sis Any disease due to a species of coccidia.

coccid'ium, pl. **coccid'ia** [Mod. L. dim. of G. *kokkos*, berry] Common name given to protozoan parasites of the family Eimeriidae.

coc'cus, pl. **coc'ci** [G. *kokkos*, berry] A bacterium of round, spheroidal, or ovoid form.

coccyg'eal Relating to the coccyx.

coc'cygodyn'ia, coc'cyodyn'ia [coccyx + G. *odyne*, pain] Pain in the coccygeal region.

coc'cyx, gen. **coc'cygis,** pl. **coc'cyges** [G. *kokkyx*, a cuckoo, the coccyx] *Os* coccygis.

coch'lea, pl. **coch'leae** [L. snail shell] [NA] A cone-shaped cavity in the petrous portion of the temporal bone, forming one of the divisions of the labyrinth and consisting of a spiral canal around a central core of sponge bone (modiolus).

coch'lear Relating to the cochlea.

co'deine [G. *kodeia*, head, poppy head] Methylmorphine; obtained from opium but usually made from morphine; a narcotic analgesic and antitussive; dependence may develop, but less liable to produce addiction than morphine.

co'don A sequence of three nucleotides in a strand of DNA or RNA that provides genetic code information for a specific amino acid.

coeffi'cient [L. *co-* + *efficio* (*exfacio*), to accomplish] Expression of the amount or degree of any quality possessed by a substance, or of the degree of physical or chemical change normally occurring in that substance under stated conditions.

coe'liac [G. *koilia*, belly] Relating to the abdominal cavity.

coelio- [G. *koilia*, belly] Combining form denoting relationship to the abdomen.

coeliot'omy [celio- + G. *tome*, incision] Abdominal section; transabdominal incision into the peritoneal cavity.

vaginal c., opening the peritoneal cavity through the vagina.

coe'lom, coelo'ma [G. *koiloma*, a hollow] **1.** The cavity between the splanchnic and somatic mesoderm in the embryo. **2.** The general body cavity in the adult.

coelom'ic Relating to the coelom, or body cavity.

coen'zyme A substance that enhances or is necessary for the action of enzymes; c.'s are of smaller molecular size, are dialysable and relatively heat-stable, and are usually easily dissociable from the protein portion of the enzyme.

cogni'tion [L. *cognitio*] A generic term embracing the quality of knowing, which includes perceiving, recognizing, conceiving, judging, sensing, reasoning, and imagining.

cog'nitive Pertaining to cognition.

co'hort A defined population group followed prospectively in an epidemiological study.

coi'tion [L. *co-eo*, pp. *-itus*, to come together] Coitus.

coi'tus [L.] Copulation; sexual intercourse; sexual union between male and female.

c. interrup'tus, onanism (1).

c. reserva'tus, c. in which ejaculation is delayed or suppressed.

cold A virus infection involving the upper respiratory tract; characterized by lack of fever, watery nasal discharge, and sneezing.

colec'tomy [G. *kolon*, colon, + *ektome*, excision] Excision of a segment or all of the colon.

colic [G. *kolikos*, relating to the colon] **1.** (ko'-lik) Relating to the colon. **2.** (kol'-ik) Spasmodic pains in the abdomen. **3.** Paroxysms of pain, with crying and irritability in young infants, due to a variety of causes, such as swallowing of air, emotional upset, or overfeeding.

col'icky Relating to or affected by colic.

co'liform Denoting Gram-negative, fermentative rods that inhabit the intestinal tract of man and other animals; sometimes used to refer to all enteric bacteria, or only to lactose-fermenting enteric bacteria.

coli'tis [G. *kolon*, colon, + *-itis*, inflammation] Inflammation of the colon.

ulcerative c., a chronic disease of unknown cause, characterized by ulceration of the colon and rectum, with bleeding, mucosal crypt abscesses, and inflammatory pseudopolyps; frequently causes anaemia, hypoproteinaemia, and electrolyte imbalance; less frequently complicated by perforation or carcinoma of the colon.

col'la Plural of collum.

col'lagen [G. koila, glue, + -gen, producing] The major protein of the white fibres of connective tissue, cartilage, and bone; high in glycine, alanine, proline, hydroxyproline, low in sulphur, and has no tryptophan.

collag'enous Producing or containing collagen.

collapse' [L. col-labor, pp. -lapsus, to fall together] **1.** A condition of extreme prostration, similar to hypovolaemic shock and due to the same causes. **2.** A falling together of the walls of a structure or the failure of a system.

collat'eral [L. col-] Indirect, subsidiary or accessory to the main thing; side by side. **2.** A side branch of a nerve axon or blood vessel.

colliculi'tis Inflammation of the urethra in the region of the colliculus seminalis.

collic'ulus, pl. **collic'uli** [L. mound, dim. of collis, hill] [NA] A small elevation above the surrounding parts.

   c. semina'lis [NA], **seminal c.,** an elevated portion of the urethral crest upon which open the two ejaculatory ducts and the prostatic utricle.

collima'tion [L. collineare, to direct in a straight line] The process, in radiology, of restricting and confining the x-ray beam to given area and, in nuclear medicine, of restricting the detection of emitted radiations from a given area of interest.

colliqua'tion [L. col-, together, + liquo, pp. liquatus, to cause to melt] **1.** Excessive discharge of fluid. **2.** Softening. **3.** Degeneration of tissue.

col'loid [G. kolla, glue, + eidos, appearance] **1.** Aggregates of atoms or molecules in a finely divided state (submicroscopic), dispersed in a gaseous, liquid, or solid medium, and resisting sedimentation, diffusion, and filtration, thus differing from precipitates. **2.** A homogeneous material of glue-like consistency, less fluid than mucoid or mucinoid, found in the cells and tissues in a state of c. degeneration. **3.** The stored secretion within follicles of the thyroid gland.

colloid'al Relating to a colloid.

col'lum, pl. **col'la** [L.] **1.** [NA] Neck; the body part between the shoulders or thorax and the head. **2.** A constricted or necklike portion of a structure.

col'lutory [L. colluere, to rinse] Mouthwash.

collyr'ium [G. kollyrion, poultice, eye salve] Originally, any preparation for the eye; now, an eyewash.

colo- [G. kolon, colon] Combining form relating to the colon.

colobo'ma [G. koloboma, lit., the part taken away in mutilation] Any defect, congenital, pathologic, or artificial, especially of the eye.

co'lon [G. kolon] [NA] The division of the large intestine extending from the caecum to the rectum.

   c. ascen'dens [NA], **ascending c.,** the portion of the c. between the ileocaecal orifice and the right colic flexure.

   c. descen'dens [NA], **descending c.,** the part of the c. extending from the left colic flexure to the pelvic brim.

   iliac c., that portion of the descending c. which lies in the left iliac fossa, between the crest of the left ilium and the pelvic brim.

   irritable c., a tendency to colonic hyperperistalsis, sometimes with colicky pains and diarrhoea.

   c. sigmoi'deum [NA], **sigmoid c.,** sigmoid flexure; the part of the c. describing an S-shaped curve between the pelvic brim and the third sacral segment, continuous with the rectum.

   c. transver'sum [NA], **transverse c.,** the part of the c. between the right and left colic flexures, extending transversely across the abdomen.

colon'ic Relating to the colon.

colon'oscope An elongated endoscope, usually fibre-optic.

colonos'copy [colon + G. skopeo, to view] Visual examination of the inner surface of the colon by means of a colonoscope.

col'ony [L. colonia, a colony] A discrete group of organisms, as a group of cells growing on a solid nutrient surface.

colorec'tal Relating to the colon and rectum, or to the entire large bowel.

colorim'etry A procedure for quantitative chemical analysis, based on comparison of the colour developed in a solution of the test material with that in a standard solution; the two solutions are observed simultaneously in a colorimeter, and quantitated on the basis of the absorption of light.

colos'tomy [colo- + G. *stoma*, mouth] Establishment of an artificial cutaneous opening into the colon.

colos'trum [L.] Foremilk; the first milk secreted at the termination of pregnancy, differing from the milk secreted later by containing more lactalbumin and lactoprotein, and also being rich in antibodies which confer passive immunity to the newborn.

colpi'tis [colp- + G. *-itis*, inflammation] Vaginitis.

colpo-, colp- [G. *kolpos*, any fold or hollow; specifically, the vagina] Combining forms denoting the vagina. See also vagino-, vagin-.

col'pocele [colpo- + G. *kēlē*, hernia] **1.** A hernia projecting into the vagina. **2.** Colpoptosis.

col'pocysti'tis [colpo- + G. *kystis*, bladder, + *-itis*, inflammation] Inflammation of both vagina and bladder.

colpopto'sis, colpopto'sia [colpo- + G. *ptōsis*, a falling] Prolapse of the vaginal walls.

colporrha'gia [colpo- + G. *rhēgnymi*, to burst forth] Vaginal haemorrhage.

colpor'rhaphy [colpo- + G. *rhaphē*, suture] Repair of a rupture of the vagina by freshening and suturing the edges of the tear.

colporrhex'is [colpo- + G. *rhēxis*, rupture] Tearing of the vaginal wall.

col'poscope An endoscopic instrument that magnifies cells of the vagina and cervix *in vivo* to allow direct observation and study of these tissues.

colpot'omy [colpo- + G. *tomē*, incision] Vaginotomy.

col'umn [L. *columna*] A part or structure in the form of a pillar or cylindric funiculus. See also fasciculus.

    spinal c., vertebral c., *columna* vertebralis.

colum'na, pl. **colum'nae** [L.] [NA] Column.

    c. vertebra'lis [NA], vertebral or spinal column; spine; backbone; the series of vertebrae that extend from the cranium to the coccyx, providing support and forming a flexible bony case for the spinal cord.

com- See con-.

co'ma [G. *kōma*, deep sleep] A state of profound unconsciousness from which one cannot be roused.

    diabetic c., c. that develops in severe and inadequately treated case of diabetes mellitus; results from reduced oxidative metabolism of the central nervous system that, in turn, stems from severe ketoacidosis.

co'matose In a state of coma.

com'edo, pl. **comedo'nes** [L. a glutton, fr. *com-edo*, to eat up] Blackhead; a plug of sebaceous matter, capped with a blackened mass of epithelial debris, filling the pilosebaceous orifice.

commen'sal Pertaining to or characterized by commensalism.

commen'salism [L. *con-*, with together, + *mensa*, table] A symbiotic relationship in which one organism derives benefit and the other is unharmed.

com'minuted [L. *com-minuo*, pp. *-minutus*, to make smaller, break into pieces] Broken into fragments; denoting especially a fractured bone.

commissu'ra, pl. **commissu'rae** [L. a joining together, seam] [NA] **1.** Angle or corner of the eye, lips, or labïa. **2.** A bundle of nerve fibres passing from one side to the other in the brain or spinal cord.

com'missure Commissura.

commun'icable Capable of being communicated or transmitted.

compensa'tion [L. *com-penso*, pp. *-atus*, to weigh together, counterbalance] **1.** A process in which a tendency for a change in a given direction is counteracted by another change so that the original change is not evident. **2.** An unconscious mechanism by which one tries to make up for fancied or real deficiencies.

compen'satory Relating to or characterized by compensation.

com'petence **1.** The quality of being competent or capable of performing an allotted function. **2.** Integrity; especially the normal tight closure of a cardiac valve. **3.** In psychiatry, the ability to distinguish right from wrong and to manage one's own affairs.

com'plement [L. *complementum,* that which completes] A serum protein complex, the activity of which is effected by a series of interactions resulting in enzymic cleavages and which can follow one or the other of at least two pathways. In the case of immune haemolysis, the complex comprises nine components (designated C1 through C9) which react in a definite sequence and the activation of which is effected by the antigen-antibody complex. An alternative pathway is activated by factors other than antigen-antibody complexes and involves components other than C1, C4, and C2 in the activation of C3.

com'plex [L. *complexus*, woven together] **1.** An organized constellation of feelings, thoughts, perceptions, and memories which may be in part unconscious and may strongly influence associations and attitudes. **2.** In chemistry, the relatively stable combination of two or more compounds into a larger molecule without covalent binding. **3.** A composite of chemical or immunological structures. **4.** An entity made up of three or more interrelated components. **5.** A group of individual structures known or believed to be anatomically, embryologically, or physiologically related.

inferiority c., a sense of inadequacy which is expressed in extreme shyness, diffidence, or timidity, or as a compensatory reaction in exhibitionism or aggressiveness.

Oedipus c. [*Oedipus*, G. myth. character], a developmentally distinct group of associated ideas, aims, instinctual drives, and fears generally observed in male children 3 to 6 years old; in female children, referred to as the Electra c. During this period, coinciding with the peak of the phallic phase of psychosexual development, the child's sexual interest is attached primarily to the parent of the opposite sex and is accompanied by aggressive feelings toward the parent of the same sex

compli'ance (C) 1. A measure of the ease with which a structure or substance may be deformed, usually a measure of the ease with which a hollow organ may be distended. **2.** The degree of adherence by a patient to a prescribed regimen.

complica'tion A morbid process or event occurring during a disease which is not an essential part of the disease, although it may result from it or from independent causes.

com'pos men'tis [L. possessed of one's mind] Of sound mind; sane; usually used in its opposite form, *non compos mentis*.

com'pound [thru O. Fr., fr. L. *compono*] **1.** In chemistry, a substance formed by the cova-

lent or electrostatic union of two or more elements, generally differing entirely in physical characteristics from any of its components. **2.** In pharmacy, denoting a preparation containing several ingredients.

com'press [L. *com-primo*, pp. -*pressus*, to press together] A pad of gauze or other material applied for local pressure.

compres'sion A squeezing together; exertion of pressure on a body in such a way as to tend to increase its density.

compres'sor A muscle, contraction of which causes compression of any structure.

compul'sion [L. *com- pello* pp. -*pulsus*, to drive together, compel] Uncontrollable thoughts or impulses to perform an act, often repetitively, as an unconscious mechanism to avoid unacceptable ideas and desires which, by themselves, arouse anxiety.

compul'sive Influenced by compulsion.

con- [L. *cum*, with, together] Prefix denoting with, together, in association; appears as com- before p, b, or m, and as co- before a vowel.

cona'tion [L. *conatio*, an undertaking, effort] The conscious tendency to act; in human context, usually an aspect of mental process, historically aligned with cognition and affection, but more recently used in the wider sense of impulse, desire, purposive striving

con'cave [L. *concavus*, arched or vaulted] Having a depressed or hollowed surface.

concav'ity A hollow or depression, with evenly curved sides, on any surface.

concentra'tion [L. *con-*, together, + *centrum*, centre] **1.** A preparation made by extracting a crude drug, precipitating from the solution, and drying. **2.** Increasing the strength of a fluid by evaporation. **3.** The quantity of a substance per unit volume or weight. In renal physiology, symbol U for urinary c., P for plasma c.; in respiratory physiology, symbol C for amount per unit volume in blood, F for fractional c. (mole fraction or volume per volume) in dried gas; subscripts indicate location and chemical species.

con'cept [L. *conceptum*, something understood] **1.** An abstract idea or notion. **2.** An explanatory variable or principle in a scientific system.

concep'tion [L. *conceptio;* see concept] **1.** Concept. **2.** The act of forming a general idea or notion. **3.** The act of conceiving, or

becoming pregnant; the fertilization of the oocyte (ovum) by a spermatozoon.

concep'tus The products of conception
(3); *i.e.*, embryo and membranes.

concre'tion [L. *cum*, together, + *crescere*, to grow] Aggregation or formation of
solid material.

concus'sion [L. *concussio*, fr. *con-cutio*,
pp. *-cussus*, to shake violently] **1.** A violent
shaking or jarring. **2.** An injury of a soft structure, as the brain, resulting from a blow or
violent shaking.

   brain c., a clinical syndrome, due to
   trauma of the head, characterized by immediate and transient impairment of neural function, such as alteration of consciousness, disturbance of vision and equilibrium, etc.

   spinal c., sudden transient loss of
   function of the spinal cord, caused by trauma
   but without permanent gross damage.

condi'tioning The process of acquiring,
developing, educating, establishing, learning, or training new responses in both respon-
dent and operant behaviour; refers to a
change in the frequency or form of behaviour
as a result of the influence of the environment.

con'dom A sheath or cover for the penis to
prevent conception or infection during coitus.

conduc'tion [L. *con-duco*, pp. *ductus*, to
lead, conduct] Transmission or conveyance
of certain forms of energy, such as heat,
sound, or electricity, from one point to another, without evident movement in the conducting body.

conductiv'ity Capacity for conduction.

conduc'tor **1.** A probe or sound with a
groove along which a knife is passed in slitting open a sinus or fistula; a grooved director. **2.** That which possesses conductivity.

con'dylar Relating to a condyle.

con'dyle [G. *kondylos*, knuckle of a joint]
The rounded articular surface at the extremity
of a bone.

condylec'tomy [G. *kondylos*, condyle,
+ *ektomē*, excision] Excision of a condyle.

condylo'ma [G. *kondylōma*, a knob] A
wartlike excrescence.

   c. acumina'tum, genital or venereal
   wart; a projecting warty growth on the external genitals or at the anus, consisting of fibrous overgrowths covered by thickened epithelium, due to infection by a human
   papovavirus.

cone [G. *kōnos*, cone] **1.** A figure having a
circular base with sides inclined so as to meet
at a point above. **2.** One of the photoreceptors
in the retina. See retinal c.'s.

   retinal c.'s, the photosensitive, outward-directed, cone-shaped process of a
   cone cell, one of the two types of photorecep-
   tor cell of the retina (the other being the rods),
   essential for sharp vision and for colour vision.

confabula'tion [L. *con-fabular*, pp. *-fab-
ulatus*, to talk together] Making up of tales and
recitals and a readiness to give a fluent answer to any question put; a symptom of pres-
byophrenia.

confec'tion [L. *confectio*, to prepare]
Electuary; a pharmaceutical preparation consisting of a drug mixed with a sweetener.

confine'ment [L. *confine* (ntr.), a bound-
ary] Giving birth to a child.

con'flict Tension or stress experienced by
an organism when satisfaction of a need,
drive, or motive is thwarted by the presence of
other attractive or unattractive needs, drives,
or motives.

con'fluence [L. *confluens*] A flowing or
running together; a joining.

confu'sion A mental state in which reactions to environmental stimuli are inappropriate; a state in which one is bewildered, per-
plexed, or disoriented.

congen'ital [L. *congenitus*, born with]
Existing at birth; either hereditary or due to
some influence occurring during gestation,
even up to the moment of birth.

conges'tion [L. *congestio*, a bringing
together, a heap] Presence of an abnormal
amount of fluid in the vessels or passages of a
part or organ; especially, of blood due either
to increased afflux or to obstruction of return
flow.

   hypostatic c., c. due to pooling of
   venous blood in a dependent part.

conges'tive Characterized by congestion.

conio'sis [G. *konis*, dust] Any disease or
morbid condition caused by dust.

coniza'tion Excision of a cone of tissue;
e.g., mucosa of the cervix.

conjuga'tion [L. *con-jugo*, pp. *-jugatus*, to
join together] **1.** The union of two unicellular
organisms or of the male and female gametes
of multicellular forms by which genetic material is exchanged, followed by partition. **2.**

The combination, especially in the liver, of certain toxic substances formed in the intestine, drugs, or steroid hormones with glucuronic or sulphuric acid; a means by which the biological activity of certain chemical substances can be terminated.

conjuncti'va, pl. **conjuncti'vae** [L. fem. of conjunctivus, from conjungo, pp. -junctus, to bind together] The mucous membrane covering the anterior surface of the eyeball and lining the lids.

conjunc'tivi'tis Inflammation of conjunctiva

   acute contagious c., acute epidemic c., pinkeye; an acute c. marked by intense hyperaemia and profuse mucopurulent discharge; caused by Haemophilus aegypticus.

   inclusion c., a benign follicular c. caused by Chlamydia oculogenitale.

   infantile purulent c., ophthalmia neonatorum.

consanguin'eous [L. cum, with, + sanguis, blood] Related by blood.

con'scious [L. conscius, knowing] **1.** Aware; having present knowledge or perception of oneself, one's acts and surroundings. **2.** Denoting something occurring with the perceptive attention of the individual, as a c. act or idea, as distinguished from automatic or instinctive.

conserv'ative Denoting treatment by gradual, limited, or well-established procedures, as opposed to radical.

consolida'tion [L. consolido, to make thick, condense] Solidification into a firm dense mass; applied especially to inflammatory induration of a normally aerated lung due to the presence of cellular exudate in the pulmonary alveoli.

con'stipate [L. con-stipo, pp. -atus, to press togethr] To cause a sluggishness in the action of the bowels.

constipa'tion A condition in which bowel movements are infrequent or incomplete.

constric'tion [L. con-stringo, pp. -strictus, to draw together] **1.** Binding or contraction of a part. **2.** A subjective sensation as if the body or any part were tightly bound or squeezed.

constric'tor [L. fr. constringo, to draw together] **1.** Anything that binds or squeezes a part. **2.** A muscle the action of which is to narrow a canal, as a sphincter.

con'tact [con-tingo, pp. -tactus, to touch] **1.** The touching or apposition of two bodies. **2.** A person who has been exposed to contagion.

conta'gion [L. contagio; fr. contingo, to touch closely] Transmission of disease by contact with the sick, or the disease so transmitted. The term originated long before development of modern ideas of infectious disease and has since lost much of its significance, being included under the more inclusive term "communicable disease."

conta'gious Communicable; relating to contagion; transmissible by contact with the sick.

contam'inant An impurity; that which causes contamination.

contamina'tion [L. contamino, pp. -atus, to stain, defile] **1.** Rendering harmful or unsuitable, as by the presence of radioactive substance. **2.** In chemistry or pharmacy, the presence of any extraneous material that renders a substance or preparation impure.

contra- [L.] Prefix signifying opposed, against. See also counter-.

contracep'tion Prevention of conception or impregnation.

contracep'tive [L. contra, against, + conceptive] Relating to any measure or agent designed to prevent conception or that so used.

   intrauterine c., see under device.

   "sequential" oral c., a preparation providing two types of medication; the first, containing only an oestrogen, is taken daily from the 5th to approximately the 19th day of the menstrual cycle; the second, containing an oestrogen and a semisynthetic progestational steroid, is taken daily from the 20th to the 24th days of the cycle

contract [L. con-traho, pp. -tractus, to draw together] **1.** (kon-trakt') To shorten; to become reduced in size; in the case of muscle, either to shorten or to undergo an increase in tension. **2.** To acquire by contagion or infection. **3.** (kon'trakt) An explicit, bilateral commitment by psychotherapist and patient to a defined course of action to attain the goal of the psychotherapy.

contrac'tile Having the property of contracting.

contractil'ity The ability or property of a substance, especially of muscle, of shortening, or becoming reduced in size, or developing increased tension.

contrac'tion [L. *contractio*, to draw together] **1.** A shortening or increase in tension; denoting the normal function of muscular tissue. **2.** A shrinkage or reduction in size. **3.** Heart beat, as in premature c.

contrac'ture [L. *contractura*, fr. *contraho*, to draw together] A permanent muscular contraction due to tonic spasm or fibrosis, or to loss of muscular equilibrium, the antagonists being paralysed.

Dupuytren's c., a disease of the palmar fascia resulting in thickening and c. of fibrous bands on the palmar surface of the hand and fingers.

Volkmann's c., tissue degeneration produced by ischaemia leading to a late c. involving muscles, tendons, fascia, and other soft tissues; caused by interference with blood flow.

con'traindica'tion Any special symptom or circumstance that renders the use of a remedy or the carrying out of a procedure inadvisable.

contralat'eral [L. *contra*, opposite, + *latus*, side] Relating to the opposite side, as when pain is felt or paralysis occurs on the side opposite that of the lesion.

contrecoup' [Fr. counter-blow] Denoting a fracture, as in the skull, at a point opposite that at which the blow was received.

control' [Mediev. L. *contrarotulum*, a counterroll for checking accounts, fr. L. *rotula*, dim. of *rota*, a wheel] **1.** To verify an experiment by means of another with the crucial variable omitted. **2.** A standard against which experimental observations can be compared and evaluated. **3.** Regulation of maintenance of a function, action, reflex, etc.

birth c., (1) restriction of the number of offspring by means of contraceptive measures; **(2)** projects, programs, or methods to control reproduction by either improving or diminishing fertility.

contu'sion [L. *contusio*, a bruising] **1.** Any injury caused by a blow in which the skin is not broken. **2.** Bruise (1).

co'nus, pl. **co'ni** [L. fr. G. *kōnos*, cone] [NA] Cone.

c. arterio'sus [NA], the left or anterior portion of the cavity of the right ventricle of the heart, which terminates in the pulmonary artery.

convales'cence [L. *con-valesco*, to grow strong] A period between the end of an illness, operation, or injury and the patient's recovery.

conver'gence [L. *con-vergo*, to incline together] **1.** The tending of two or more objects toward a common point. **2.** The direction of the visual lines to a near point.

negative c., slight divergence of the visual axes when c. is at rest, as when looking at the far point of normal vision or during sleep.

positive c., inward deviation of the visual axes even when c. is at rest, as in cases of convergent squint.

conver'sion [L. *con-verto*, pp. *-versus*, to turn around, to change] **1.** Change; transmutation. **2.** Transformation of an emotion into a physical manifestation, as in hysteria. **3.** In virology, lysogenic c.; the acquisition, by bacteria, of a new property associated with presence of a prophage.

con'vex [L. *convexus*, vaulted, arched, convex] Applied to a surface that is evenly curved or bulging outward, the segment of a sphere.

convex'ocon'cave Convex on one surface and concave on the oppostie surface.

convolu'tion [L. *convolutio*] **1.** A coiling or rolling of an organ by infolding upon itself. **2.** Specifically, a gyrus of the cerebral or cerebellar cortex.

convul'sion [L. *convulsio*, fr. *con-vello*, pp. *-vulsus*, to tear up] An involuntary spasm or series of jerkings of the muscles.

convul'sive Relating to convulsions; marked by or producing convulsions.

cop'per [L. *cuprum*, orig. *Cyprium*, after *Cyprus*, where mined] A metallic element, symbol Cu, atomic no. 29, atomic weight 63.55; several cupric salts are used in medicine.

copro- [G. *kopros*, dung] Combining form denoting filth or dung, usually used in referring to faeces. See also scato-, sterco-.

coprola'lia [copro- + G. *lalia*, talk] Involuntary utterance of vulgar or obscene words.

cop'rolith [copro- + G. *lithos*, stone] A hard mass consisting of inspissated faeces.

coprophil'ia [copro- + G. *philos*, fond] **1.** Attraction of microorganisms for faecal matter. **2.** In psychiatry, a morbid attraction to (with a sexual element) faecal matter.

coprosta'sis [copro- + G. *stasis*, a standing] Faecal impaction.

copula'tion [L. *copulatio*, a joining] **1.** Coitus. **2.** In protozoology, conjugation between two cells that do not fuse but separate after mutual fertilization.

cor, gen. **cor'dis** [L.] [NA] Heart.

cor'acoacro'mial Relating to the coracoid and acromial processes.

cor'acoclavic'ular Relating to the coracoid process and the clavicle.

cor'acohu'meral Relating to the coracoid process and the humerus.

cor'acoid [G. *korakōdēs*, like a crow's beak] Shaped like a crow's beak, denoting a process of the scapula.

cord- For words beginning thus, not found here, see chord-.

cord [L. *chorda*, a string] In anatomy, any long, ropelike structure.
> **spermatic c.,** *funiculus* spermaticus.
> **spinal c.,** *medulla* spinalis.
> **true vocal c.,** *plica* vocalis.
> **umbilical c.,** *funiculus* umbilicalis.

cor'dopexy [G. *chordē*, cord, + *pēxis*, fixation] Surgical fixation of a cord, as of one or both vocal cords for the relief of laryngeal stenosis.

cordot'omy [G. *chordē*, cord, + *tomē*, a cutting] **1.** Any operation on the spinal cord. **2.** Division of tracts of the spinal cord.

co'rium, pl. **co'ria** [L. *skin, hide, leather*] [NA] Dermis; a superficial, thin layer that interdigitates with the epidermis, the stratum papillare, and a deeper thick layer of dense, irregular connective tissue, the stratum reticulare; contains blood and lymphatic vessels, nerves and nerve endings, glands, and, except for glabrous skin, hair follicles.

corn [L. *cornu*, horn, hoof] Clavus.

cor'nea [L. fem. of *corneus*, horny] [NA] Transparent tissue constituting the anterior sixth of the outer wall of the eye.
> **conical c.,** keratoconus.

cor'neal Relating to the cornea.

cor'neoscle'ral Pertaining to the cornea and sclera.

cornifica'tion [L. *cornu*, horn, + *facio*, to make] Keratinization.

cor'nu, gen. **cor'nus,** pl. **cor'nua** [L. horn, hoof] A horn. **1.** [NA] Any structure resembling a horn in shape or composed of horny substance. **2.** The major subdivisions of the lateral ventricle in the cerebral hemisphere (frontal horn, occipital horn, temporal horn).

coro'na, pl. **coro'nae** [L. garland, crown] [NA] Crown; any structure, normal or pathologic, resembling or suggesting a crown or a wreath.
> **c. radia'ta** [NA], a fan-shaped fibre mass on the white matter of the cerebral cortex, composed of the widely radiating fibres of the internal capsule.

cor'onary [L. *coronarius*, fr. *corona*, a crown] **1.** Relating to or resembling a crown. **2.** Encircling; denoting various anatomical structures, as the arteries of the heart; by extension, a heart attack.

Coronavi'ridae A family of single-stranded RNA-containing viruses of medium size, some of which cause upper respiratory tract infections in man; they resemble myxoviruses except for the petal-shaped projections which give an impression of the solar corona. *Coronavirus* is the only recognized genus.

coro'navi'rus Any virus of the family Coronaviridae.

cor'oner [L. *corona*, a crown] An official whose duty it is to investigate sudden, suspicious, or violent death to determine the cause.

cor'pora Plural of corpus.

corpo'real Pertaining to the body, or to a corpus.

corpse [L. *corpus*, body] Cadaver.

cor'pulence, cor'pulency [L. *corpulentia*, magnification of *corpus*, body] Obesity.

cor'pus, gen. **cor'poris,** pl. **cor'pora** [L. body] [NA] **1.** The human body, consisting of head, neck, trunk, and limbs. **2.** Any body or mass. **3.** The main part of an organ or other anatomical structure.
> **c. al'bicans** [NA], a retrogressed c. luteum characterized by increasing cicatrization and shrinkage of the cicatricial core with a hyalinized lutein zone surrounding the central plug of scar tissue.
> **c. amygdaloi'deum** [NA], amygdala; a rounded mass of grey matter in the anterior portion of the temporal lobe of the cerebrum; its major efferent fibre connections are with the hypothalamus and mediodorsal nucleus of the thalamus; also reciprocally associated with the cortex of the temporal lobe.
> **c. callo'sum** [NA], commissure of the cerebral hemispheres; the commissural plate of nerve fibres interconnecting the cortical hemispheres, with the exception of most of the temporal lobes which are interconnected by the anterior commissure.

c. caverno'sum clitor'idis [NA], one of the two parallel columns of erectile tissue forming the body of the clitoris.

c. caverno'sum pe'nis [NA], one of two parallel columns of erectile tissue forming the dorsal part of the body of the penis.

c. cilia're [NA], ciliary body; a thickened portion of the tunica vasculosa of the eye between the choroid and the iris; consists of three parts: orbiculus ciliaris, corona ciliaris, and musculus ciliaris.

c. lu'teum, [NA], the yellow endocrine body formed in the ovary in the site of a ruptured ovarian follicle, immediately after ovulation. If pregnancy does not occur, it is called a **c. spurium,** which undergoes progressive retrogression to a c. albicans; in the event of pregnancy, the **c. verum** becomes even larger and persists to the fifth or sixth month of pregnancy before beginning to retrogress.

c. pinea'le [NA], pineal body or gland; a small, unpaired, flattened glandular structure attached to the region of the posterior and habenular commissures and lying in the depression between the two superior colliculi; despite its attachment to the brain, it appears to receive nerve fibres exclusively from the peripheral autonomic nervous system.

c. spongio'sum pe'nis [NA], the median column of erectile tissue located between the ventral to the two corpora cavernosa penis; posteriorly it expands into the bulbus penis and anteriorly it terminates as the enlarged glans penis.

c. stria'tum [NA], the caudate and lentiform nuclei considered as one structure, a striate appearance on section being caused by slender fascicles of myelinated fibres.

c. vit'reum [NA], vitreous; vitreum; a transparent jelly-like substance filling the interior of the eyeball behind the lens; composed of a delicate network enclosing in its meshes a watery fluid.

cor'puscle [L. *corpusculum,* dim. of *corpus,* body] **1.** Corpusculum. **2.** A blood cell.

 red c., erythrocyte.

 white c., any type of leucocyte.

corpus'cular Relating to a corpuscle.

corpus'culum, pl. **corpus'cula** [NA] A small mass or body.

cor'rugator [L. *cor-rugo (conr-),* pp. *-atus,* to wrinkle, fr. *ruga,* a wrinkle] A muscle that draws together the skin, causing it to wrinkle.

cor'tex, gen. **cor'ticis,** pl. **cor'tices** [L. bark] [NA] The outer portion of an organ as distinguished from the inner, or medullary, portion.

 auditory c., the region of the cerebral c. that receives auditory data from the medial geniculate body.

 c. cerebel'li [NA], **cerebellar c.,** the thin grey surface layer of the cerebellum, consisting of an outer molecular layer (including a single layer of Purkinje cells, the ganglionic layer), and an inner granular layer.

 c. cer'ebri [NA], **cerebral c.,** the layer of grey matter covering the entire surface of the cerebral hemisphere, characterized by a laminar organization of its cellular and fibrous components such that its nerve cells are stacked in defined layers varying in number from one, as in the archicortex of the hippocampus, to five or six in the larger neocortex.

 motor c., the region of the cerebral c. influencing movements of the face, neck and trunk, and arm and leg.

 c. re'nis [NA], **renal c.,** the part of the kidney containing the glomeruli and the proximal and distal convoluted tubules.

 visual c., the region of the cerebral c. occupying the entire surface of the occipital lobe and receiving the optic or visual data from the lateral geniculate body of the thalamus.

cor'tical Relating to a cortex.

cor'ticoste'roid A steroid produced by the adrenal cortex; a corticoid containing steroid.

cor'tisol Hydrocortisone.

cor'tisone [Hench's acronym for corticosterone] A steroid isolated from the adrenal cortex that exhibits no biological activity until it is converted to hydrocortisone (cortisol); acts upon carbohydrate metabolism (glucocorticoid), and influences the nutrition and growth of connective (collagenous) tissues.

corym'biform [L. *corymbus,* cluster, garland] Denoting the flower-like clustering configuration of skin lesions in granulomatous diseases.

Cor'ynebacte'rium [G. *coryne,* a club, + *bacterium,* a small rod] A genus of nonmotile, aerobic to anaerobic bacteria (family Corynebacteriaceae) containing irregularly staining Gram-positive rods. The type species, *C. diphtheriae,* the Klebs-Loeffler bacillus, causes diphtheria and produces a powerful exotoxin causing degeneration of various tissues.

cory'za [G.] Acute *rhinitis*.

cos'ta, pl. **cos'tae** [L.] **1** [NA] Rib; one of the 24 elongated curved bones forming the main portion of the bony wall of the chest. **2.** A rodlike internal supporting organelle that runs along the base of the undulating membrane of certain flagellate parasites.

cos'tal Relating to a rib.

costal'gia [L. *costa*, rib, + G. *algos*, pain] Pleurodynia.

costec'tomy [L. *costa*, rib, + G. *ektomē*, excision] Excision of a rib.

costo- [G. *costa*, rib] Combining form relating to the ribs.

cos'tochondri'tis [costo- + G. *chondros*, cartilage, + -*itis*, inflammation] Inflammation of one or more costal cartilages, characterized by pain of the anterior chest wall that may radiate.

cough **1.** A sudden explosive forcing of air through the glottis, occurring immediately on opening of the previously closed glottis, and excited by mechanical or chemical irritation of the trachea or bronchi, or by pressure from adjacent structures. **2.** To force air through the glottis by a series of expiratory efforts.

dry c., a c. not accompanied by expectoration; a non-productive c.

productive c., a c. accompanied by expectoration.

reflex c., a c. excited reflexly by irritation in some distant part, as the ear or the stomach.

whooping c., pertussis.

counter- [L. *contra*, against] Combining form meaning opposite, opposed, against. See contra-.

coun'tercondi'tioning Any of a group of specific behaviour therapy techniques in which a second conditioned response is instituted for the express purpose of counteracting or nullifying a previously conditioned or learned response.

coun'terincis'ion A second incision adjacent to a primary incision.

counterir'ritant **1.** An agent that produces counterirritation. **2.** Relating to or producing counterirritation.

coun'terirrita'tion Irritation or mild inflammation of the skin produced to relieve an inflammation of the deeper structures.

countertrac'tion Resistance, or backpull, made to extension on a limb.

coun'tertransfer'ence In psychoanalysis, the analyst's transference of his emotional needs and feelings toward the patient.

cova'lent Denoting an interatomic bond characterized by the sharing of 2, 4, or 6 electrons.

cowperi'tis Inflammation of Cowper's gland.

cox'a, pl. **cox'ae** [L] **1.** *Os* coxae. **2.** [NA] Hip or hip joint.

coxal'gia [L. *coxa*, hip, + G. *algos*, pain] Coxodynia.

Coxiel'la [H.R. *Cox*, U.S. bacteriologist, *1007] A genus of filterable parasitic bacteria (order Rickettsiales) containing small rod-shaped or coccoid, Gram-negative cells. The type species, *C. burnetii*, causes Q fever in man.

coxodyn'ia [L. *coxa*, hip, + G. *odynē*, pain] Pain in the hip joint.

coxsack'ievirus [Coxsackie, N.Y., where first isolated] A group of picornaviruses included in the genus *Enterovirus* and responsible for a variety of symptoms and infections in man. They are divided antigenically into two groups (A and B), each of which includes a number of serological types.

cra'dle A frame used to keep the bedclothes from pressing on a fractured or wounded part.

cramp **1.** A painful spasm. **2.** A professional neurosis, qualified according to the occupation of the sufferer; *e.g.*, writer's c.

heat c.'s, muscle spasm induced by hard work in intense heat, accompanied by severe pain.

intermittent c., tetany.

cra'nia Plural of cranium.

cra'nial **1.** Cephalic; relating to the cranium or head. **2.** Superior.

craniectomy [G. *kranion*, skull, + *ektomē*, excision] Excision of a portion of the skull.

cranio-, crani- [G. *kranion*, skull] Combining forms denoting relation to the cranium.

craniofa'cial Relating to both the face and the cranium.

cra'niopharyngio'ma A neoplasm, usually cystic, that develops from the nests of epithelium derived from Rathke's pouch.

cra'nioplasty [cranio- + G. *plassō*, to form] Operative repair of a defect or deformity of the skull.

cra'niopunc'ture. Surgical puncture of the skull.

cranios'chisis [cranio- + G. *schisis*, a cleavage] Congenital failure of the skull to close mid-dorsally, usually accompanied by grossly defective development of the brain.

cra'niosteno'sis [cranio- + G. *stenōsis*, a narrowing] Premature closure of cranial sutures resulting in malformation of the skull.

cra'niosynos'tosis [cranio- + synostosis] Premature ossification of the skull and obliteration of the sutures.

craniota'bes [cranio- + L. *tabes*, a wasting] A disease marked by the presence of areas of thinning and softening in the bones of the skull, usually of syphilitic or rachitic origin.

craniot'omy [cranio- + G. *tomē*, incision] Opening into the skull, either by creation of a bone flap or by trephination.

cra'nium, pl. **cra'nia** [Mediev. L. fr. G. *kranion*] [NA] Skull; the bones of the head collectively. In a more limited sense, the brain pan, the bony case containing the brain, excluding the bones of the face.

cre'atine A substance occurring in urine, generally as creatinine, and in muscle generally as phosphocreatine.

  c. kinase, an enzyme catalysing the transfer of phosphate from phosphocreatine to ADP, forming creatine and ATP; of importance in muscle contraction.

creat'inine (Cr) A component of urine and the final product of creatine catabolism.

cremaster'ic [G. *kremastēr*, a suspender] Relating to the cremaster muscle.

cre'nate, cre'nated [L. *crena*, a notch] Notched; indented; denoting the outline of a shriveled red blood cell, as observed in a hypertonic solution.

crep'itant Relating to or characterized by crepitation.

crepita'tion [L. *crepitus, q.v.*] **1.** Crackling; the quality or sound of a rale which resembles noise heard on rubbing hair between the fingers. **2.** The sensation felt on placing the hand over the seat of a fracture when the broken ends of the bone are moved, or over tissue, in which gas gangrene is present. **3.** Noise or vibration produced by rubbing bone or irregular cartilage surfaces together

as by movement of patella against femoral condyles in arthritis and other conditions.

crep'itus [L. fr. *crepo*, to rattle] **1.** Crepitation. **2.** A noisy discharge of gas from the intestine.

crest [L. *cresta*] A ridge, especially a bony ridge. See also crista.

cre'tin [Fr. *crétin*] An individual exhibiting cretinism.

cre'tinism Infantile hypothyroidism; stunting of bodily growth and of mental development that may arise from thyroid agenesis or inadequate maternal intake of iodine during gestation.

crib'riform [L. *cribrum*, a sieve, + *forma*, form] Sievelike; containing many perforations.

cri'coid [L. *cricoideus*, fr. G. *krikos*, a ring, + *eidos*, form] Ring-shaped; denoting the c. cartilage.

cri'sis, pl. **cri'ses** [G. *krisis*, separation, crisis] **1.** Sudden change, usually for the better, in the course of an acute disease, in contrast to the gradual improvement by lysis. **2.** Paroxysmal pain in an organ or circumscribed region of the body occurring in the course of tabes dorsalis.

  addisonian c., adrenal c., acute adrenocortical *insufficiency*.

  identity c., a disorientation concerning one's sense of self and role in society, often of acute onset and related to a particular and significant event in one's life.

  thyrotoxic c., thyroid c., the exacerbation of symptoms that occurs in thyrotoxicosis following shock or injury or after thyroidectomy.

cris'ta, pl. **cris'tae** [L. crest] [NA] A ridge, crest, or elevated line projecting from a level or evenly rounded surface.

cross-matching 1. A test for incompatibility between donor and recipient blood, carried out prior to transfusion to avoid potentially lethal haemolytic reactions between the donor's red blood cells and antibodies in the recipient's plasma, or the reverse; incompatibility is indicated by clumping of red blood cells and contraindicates use of the donor's blood. **2.** In allotransplantation of solid organs, a test for identification of antibody in the serum of potential allograft recipients which reacts directly with the lymphocytes or other cells of a potential allograft donor; presence of antibodies usually contraindicates the transplantation.

croup [Scots, probably from A.S. *kropan*, to cry aloud] **1.** Laryngotracheobronchitis in infants and young children caused by parainfluenza virus types 1 and 2. **2.** Any affection of the larynx in children, characterized by difficult and noisy respiration and a hoarse cough.

croup'ous Relating to croup; marked by a fibrinous exudation.

crown [L. *corona*] **1.** Corona. **2.** In dentistry, that part of a tooth that is covered with enamel or an artificial substitute for that part.

   c. of the head, the topmost part of the head.

   radiate c., corona radiata.

crown'ing 1. Preparation of the natural crown of a tooth and covering the prepared crown with a veneer of suitable dental material. **2.** That stage of childbirth when the fetal head has negotiated the pelvic outlet and the largest diameter of the head is encircled by the vulvar ring.

cru'ces Plural of crux.

cru'ciate [L. *cruciatus*] Shaped like, or resembling, a cross.

cru'ral Relating to the leg or thigh, or to any crus.

crus, gen. **cru'ris,** pl. **cru'ra** [L.] [NA] **1.** The leg, that part between the knee and the ankle. **2.** Any anatomical structure resembling a leg; in the plural, a pair of diverging bands or elongated masses.

   c. cer'ebri [NA], the massive bundle of corticofugal nerve fibres passing longitudinally over the ventral surface of the midbrain on each side of the midline.

crust [L. *crusta*] **1.** An outer layer or covering. **2.** A scab.

   milk c., seborrhoea of the scalp in an infant.

crutch [A. S. *cryce*] A device used singly or in pairs to assist in walking, when the act is impaired, by transferring weight-bearing to the upper extremity.

crux, pl. **cru'ces** [L.] Cross.

cryaesthe'sia [G. *kryos*, cold, + *aisthēsis*, sensation] **1.** Subjective sensation of cold. **2.** Sensitivity to cold.

cryalge'sia [G. *kryos*, cold, + *algos*, pain] Pain caused by cold.

cry'anaesthe'sia [G. *kryos*, cold, + *an-priv*, + *aisthēsis*, sensation] Loss of sensation of perception of cold.

cryo-, cry- [G. *kryos*, cold] Combining form relating to cold.

cry'oanaesthe'sia Localized application of cold as means of producing regional anaesthesia.

cry'oextrac'tion Removal of cataract by using a cryoprobe to extract the lens by freezing contact.

cryogen'ic [cryo- + G. *-gen*, producing] Producing, or relating to the production of, low temperatures.

cry'oprecip'itate Precipitate that forms when soluble material is cooled, especially that formed in normal blood plasma which has been subjected to cold precipitation and which is rich in factor VIII.

cry'oprobe An extremely cold instrument used in cryosurgery.

cryosur'gery An operation in which decreased temperature is used.

cryother'apy The use of cold in the treatment of disease.

crypt [L. *crypta*, fr. G. *kryptos*, hidden] A pitlike depression or tubular recess.

   tonsillar c., one of the variable number of deep recesses that extend into the palatine and pharyngeal tonsils.

crypto-, crypt- [G. *kryptoo*, hiddon, oon cealed] Combining form relating to a crypt, or meaning hidden, obscure, without apparent cause.

cryp'tococco'sis An acute, subacute, or chronic infection by *Cryptococcus neoformans*, causing a pulmonary, systemic, or meningeal mycosis.

Cryptococ'cus [crypto- + G. *kokkos*, berry] A genus of yeastlike fungi that reproduce by budding. *C. neoformans* is a species that causes cryptococcosis.

cryptogen'ic [crypto- + G. *gennesis*, origin] Of obscure, indeterminate aetiology or origin.

cryp'tomenorrhoe'a [crypto- + G. *mēn*, month, + *rhoia*, flow] Occurrence each month of the general symptoms of the menses without any flow of blood, as in cases of imperforate hymen.

cryptor'chism, cryptor'chidism Failure of descent of a testis into the scrotum.

cryp'tosporidio'sis Infection with members of the genus *Cryptosporidium*, characterized by chronic protracted diarrhoea.

Cryp′tosporid′ium A genus of parasitic coccidian sporozoans (family Cryptosporiidae, suborder Eimeriina) that infect epithelial cells of the gastrointestinal tract in vertebrates and flourish under conditions of intense immunosuppression in man.

crys′tal [G. *krystallos*, clear ice, crystal] A solid of regular shape and, for a given compound, characteristic angles, formed when an element or compound solidifies.

crys′talline 1. Clear; transparent. **2.** Relating to a crystal or crystals.

cu′bitus, pl. **cu′biti** [L. elbow] [NA] **1.** Elbow (1). **2.** Ulna.

 c. val′gus, deviation of the extended forearm to the outer (radial) side of the axis of the limb.

 c. va′rus, deviation of the extended forearm to the inward (ulnar) side of the axis of the limb.

cuff A bandlike structure encircling a part.

 musculotendinous c., rotator c. of the shoulder, the upper half of the capsule of the shoulder joint reinforced by the tendons of insertion of the supraspinatus, infraspinatus, teres minor, and subscapularis muscles.

cul-de-sac′, pl. **culs-de-sac′** [Fr. bottom of a sack] A blind pouch or tubular cavity closed at one end.

 Douglas c., *excavatio* rectouterina.

cul′docente′sis [cul-de-sac + G. *kentesis*, puncture] Aspiration of fluid from the cul-de-sac (rectouterine excavation) by puncture of the vaginal vault near the midline between the uterosacral ligaments.

cul′doplasty [cul-de-sac + G. *plasso*, to fashion] A surgical procedure to remedy relaxation of the posterior fornix of the vagina.

culdos′copy [cul-de-sac + G. *skopeō*, to view] Introduction of an endoscope through the posterior vaginal wall to view the rectovaginal pouch and pelvic viscera.

Cu′lex [L. gnat] A genus of mosquitoes (family Culicidae) including over 2000 species that are worldwide in distribution and vectors for a number of diseases of man and of domestic and wild animals.

cul′ture [L. *cultura*, tillage, fr. *colo*, pp. *cultus*, to till] **1.** The propagation of microorganisms on or in media of various kinds. **2.** A mass of microorganisms on or in a medium.

cu′mulative Tending to accumulate or pile up, as with certain drugs that may have a c. effect.

cu′neate, cune′iform [L. *cuneus*, wedge] Wedge-shaped.

cura′re [S. Am.] An extract of various plants, especially *Strychnos toxifera*, *S. castelnaei*, *S. crevauxii*, and *Chondodendron tomentosum*, that produces nondepolarizing paralysis of skeletal muscle by blocking transmission at the myoneuronal junction; used clinically (*e.g.*, as *d*- tubocurarine) to provide muscle relaxation during operations.

cu′rative Tending to heal or cure.

cure [L. *curo*, to care for] **1.** To heal; to make well. **2.** A restoration to health. **3.** A special method or course of treatment.

curet′ Curette.

curettage′ A scraping, usually of the interior of a cavity or tract, for the removal of new growths or other abnormal tissues, or to obtain material for tissue diagnosis.

curette′ [Fr.] **1.** An instrument in the form of a loop, ring, or scoop with sharpened edges used for curettage. **2.** To use a c.

cur′vature [L. *curvatura*, fr. *curvo*, pp. *-atus*, to bend, curve] A bending or flexure.

 spinal c., see kyphosis; lordosis; scoliosis.

cush′ingoid Resembling the signs and symptoms of Cushing's syndrome.

cusp [L. *cuspis*, point] **1.** In dentistry, a conical elevation arising on the surface of a tooth from an independent calcification centre. **2.** A leaflet of one of the heart's valves.

cuta′neous [L. *cutis*, skin] Relating to the skin.

cut′down Dissection of a vein for insertion of a cannula or needle for the administration of intravenous fluids or medication.

cu′ticle [L. *cuticula*, dim. of *cutis*, skin] **1.** An outer thin layer, usually horny. **2.** The layer, sometimes chitinous in invertebrates, which occurs on the surface of epithelial cells. **3.** Epidermis.

cu′tireac′tion [L. *cutis*, skin, + reaction] Cutaneous reaction; inflammatory reaction in the case of a skin test in a sensitive (allergic) subject.

cu′tis [L.] [NA] Skin; the membranous protective covering of the body, consisting of epidermis and corium (dermis).

 c. anseri′na, contraction of the arrectores pilorum muscles produced by cold, fear, or other stimulus, causing the orifices of hair follicles to become prominent.

c. hyperelas'tica, Ehlers-Danlos *syndrome*.

c. lax'a, a congenital condition characterized by an excessive amount of skin hanging in folds; vascular anomalies may be present; inheritance is either dominant or recessive, the latter sometimes in association with pulmonary emphysema.

cy'anide A compound containing the radical —CN or ion (CN)—; some c. compounds are extremely poisonous.

cyano-, cyan- [G. *kyanos*, a dark blue mineral] **1.** Combining form meaning blue. **2.** Chemical prefix frequently used in naming compounds that contain the cyanide group, CN, as part of the molecule.

cy'anocobal'amin Vitamin B_{12}; a complex of cyanide and cobalamin; a haematopoietic agent apparently identical with the anti-anaemia factor of liver.

cyano'sis [G. dark blue colour, fr. *kyanos*, blue substance] A dark bluish or purplish coloration of the skin and mucous membrane due to deficient oxygenation of the blood, evident when reduced haemoglobin in the blood exceeds 5 g per 100 ml.

cyanot'ic Relating to or marked by cyanosis.

cy'cle [G. *kyklos*, circle] **1.** A recurrent series of events. **2.** A recurring period of time.

menstrual c., the period in which an ovum matures, is ovulated, and enters the uterine lumen via the fallopian tubes; ovarian hormonal secretions effect endometrial changes such that, if fertilization occurs, nidation will be possible; In the absence of fertilization, ovarian secretions wane, the endometrium sloughs, and menstruation begins; day 1 of the c. is that day on which menstrual flow begins.

cyclec'tomy [cyclo- + G. *ektomē*, excision] Excision of a portion of the ciliary body.

cy'clic 1. Occurring periodically. **2.** In chemistry, continuous, without end.

cycli'tis [G. *kyklos*, circle (ciliary body), + -*itis*, inflammation] Inflammation of the ciliary body.

cyclo-, cycl- [G. *kyklos*, circle] **1.** Combining form relating to a circle or cycle, or denoting association with the ciliary body. **2.** Chemical combining form indicating a continuous molecule, without end, or formation of such a structure between two parts of a molecule.

cy'clodial'ysis [cyclo- + G. *dialysis*, separation] Establishment of a communication between the anterior chamber and the suprachoroidal space in order to reduce intraocular pressure in glaucoma.

cy'clodiather'my Diathermy applied to the ciliary region in glaucoma.

cyclople'gia [cyclo- + G. *plēgē*, stroke] Paralysis of accommodation; loss of power in the ciliary muscle of the eye.

cyclo'sis [G. fr. *kykloō*, to move around] Movement of the protoplasm and contained plastids within the protozoan cell.

cyclospo'rin A An immunosupressant produced by the fungus *Tolypocladium inflatum;* used to inhibit organ transplant rejection.

cyclothy'mic [cyclo- + G. *thymos*, rage] Denoting a disorder marked by swings of mood, from elation to depression, within normal limits.

cye'sis [G. *kyēsis*] Pregnancy.

oylindru'ria Presence of renal casts in the urine.

cyst [G. *kystis*, bladder] **1.** A bladder. **2.** An abnormal sac containing gas, fluid, or a semi-solid material, with a membranous lining.

dermoid c., a tumour consisting of displaced ectodermal structures along lines of embryonic fusion, the wall being formed of epithelium-lined connective tissue, including skin appendages, and containing keratin, sebum, and hair; a common benign cystic teratoma of the ovary.

hydatid c., a c. formed by the larval stage of *Echinococcus granulosus;* may be unilocular or osseous.

meibomian c., chalazion.

ovarian c., a cystic tumour of the ovary, usually retricted to benign c.'s.

sebaceous c., pilar c., wen; a common c. of the skin and subcutis containing sebum and keratin which is lined by pale-staining stratified epithelial cells derived from the pilosebaceous follicle.

cyst'adeno'ma A histologically benign neoplasm derived from glandular epithelium, in which cystic accumulations of retained secretions are formed.

cystad'enocarcino'ma A malignant neoplasm derived from glandular epithelium, in which cystic accumulations of retained secretions are formed; develops frequently in the ovaries, where pseudomucinous and serous types are recognized.

cystal'gia [cyst- + G. *algos*, pain] Pain in the urinary bladder.

cystathi'onine An intermediate in the conversion of methionine to cysteine.

cys'tathi'oninu'ria A heritable disorder characterized by inability to metabolize cystathionine normally, with development of elevated concentrations of the amino acid in blood, tissue, and urine; mental retardation is an associated condition.

cystec'tomy [cyst- + G. *ektomē*, excision] **1.** Excision of the gallbladder or of the urinary bladder. **2.** Removal of a cyst.

cys'teine (Cys) An α-amino acid found in most proteins; especially abundant in keratin.

cysti- See cysto-.

cys'tic **1.** Relating to the urinary bladder or gallbladder. **2.** Relating to a cyst. **3.** Containing cysts.

cys'ticerco'sis Disease caused by encystment of cysticercus larvae in subcutaneous, muscle, or central nervous system tissues; results from the hatching of the eggs of *Taenia solium* in the intestines or by accidental ingestion of eggs from human faeces.

cysticer'cus, pl. **cysticer'ci** [G. *kystis*, bladder, + *kerkos*, tail] Bladderworm; the larval form of certain *Taenia* species.

cys'tine An oxidation product of cysteine; sometimes occurs as a deposit in the urine, or forming a vesical calculus.

cystino'sis The most common of a group of disease with characteristic renal tubular dysfunction disorders, termed collectively Fanconi's *syndrome*; a recessive hereditary disease of early childhood characterized by deposits of cystine crystals throughout the body; abnormality in cystine metabolism; associated with a marked generalized aminoaciduria, glycosuria, polyuria, chronic acidosis, hypophosphataemia with vitamin D-resistant rickets, and often with hypokalaemia.

cystinu'ria [cystine + G. *ouron*, urine] Excessive urinary excretion of cystine, along with lysine, arginine, and ornithine, as a result of a defect in renal tubular reabsorption.

cysti'tis [cyst- + G. *-itis*, inflammation] Inflammation of the urinary bladder.

cysto-, cysti-, cyst- [G. *kystis*, bladder] Combining forms relating to the bladder; the cystic duct; a cyst.

cys'tocele [cysto- + G. *kēlē*, hernia] Herniation of the bladder.

cystog'raphy [cysto- + G. *graphō*, to write] Radiography of the bladder following injection of a radiopaque substance.

cys'tolith [cisto- + G. *lithos*, stone] A urinary calculus formed or lodged in the bladder.

cystom'eter [cysto- + G. *metron*, measure] A device for studying bladder function by measuring capacity, sensation, intravesical pressure, and residual urine.

cystom'etry, cys'tometrog'raphy Measurement of bladder function, as by a cystometer.

cys'topexy [cysto- + G. *pēxis*, fixation] Surgical attachment of the gallbladder or of the urinary bladder to the abdominal wall or to other supporting structures.

cys'toscope [cysto- + G. *skopeō*, to examine] A lighted tubular endoscope for examining the interior of the bladder.

cystos'copy Inspection of the interior of the bladder by means of a cystoscope.

cystos'tomy [cysto- + G. *stoma*, mouth] Formation of an opening into the urinary bladder or gallbladder.

cys'totome **1.** An instrument for incising the urinary bladder or gallbladder. **2.** A surgical instrument used for incising the capsule of a cataractous lens.

cystot'omy [cysto- + G. *tomē*, incision] Incision into urinary bladder or gallbladder.

suprapubic c., opening into the bladder through an incision above the symphysis pubis.

cys'tourethrog'raphy Radiography of the bladder and urethra after visualization by means of a radiopaque substance.

cystoure'throscope An instrument combining the uses of a cystoscope and a urethroscope, whereby both the bladder and urethra can be visually inspected.

cy'tidine (C, Cyd) A major component of ribonucleic acids.

cyto-, cyt- [G. *kytos*, a hollow (cell)] Combining forms meaning cell; as a suffix, -cyte.

cy'tochrome [cyto- + G. *chrōma*, colour] A class of haemoprotein whose principal biological function is electron and/or hydrogen transport by virtue of a reversible valency change of the haem iron; classified in four groups. (*a, b, c, d*) according to spectrochemical characteristics.

cy'todiagno'sis Diagnosis of a pathologic process by means of microscopic study of cells.

cytolog'ic Relating to cytology.

cytol'ogy [cyto- + G. *logos*, study] Cellular biology; the study of the anatomy, physiology, pathology, and chemistry of the cell.

   exfoliative c., the examination, for diagnostic purposes, of cells denuded from a lesion and recovered from the sediment of the exudate, secretions, or washings from the tissue.

cytol'ysin An antibody that, in association with complement, effects partial or complete destruction of an animal cell.

cytol'ysis [cyto- + G. *lysis*, loosening] Dissolution of a cell.

cytomeg'alovi'rus A group of species-specific herpetoviruses infecting man and other animals and causing enlargement of cells of various organs and development of characteristic inclusions in the cytoplasm or nucleus.

cytopathology The medical science and subspecialty concerned with studies and diagnoses of health and disease by microscopic examination and evaluation of cellular specimens.

cy'toplasm [cyto- + G. *plasma*, thing formed] The substance of a cell exclusive of the nucleus; contains various organelles and inclusions within a colloidal protoplasm.

cy'tosine (Cyt) A pyrimidine found in nucleic acids.

cytotox'ic Detrimental or destructive to cells; pertaining to the effect of noncytophilic antibody on specific antigen, frequently, but not always, mediating the action of complement.

cytotox'in [cyto- + G. *toxikon*, poison] A specific substance, usually with reference to antibody, that inhibits or prevents the functions of cells, or causes destruction of cells, or both.

D

d- Prefix indicating a chemical compound to be dextrorotatory.

dac'ryagogue [dacry- + G. *agōgos*, drawing forth] An agent that stimulates the lacrimal gland to secretion, promoting the flow of tears.

dacryo-, dacry- [G. *dakryon*, tear] Combining forms relating to tears, or to the lacrimal sac or duct.

dac'ryoadeni'tis [dacryo- + G. *adēn*, gland, + *-itis*, inflammation] Inflammation of a lacrimal gland.

dac'ryocyst [dacryo- + G. *kystis*, sac] *Saccus lacrimalis.*

dac'ryocysti'tis [dacryocyst + G. *-itis*, inflammation] Inflammation of the lacrimal sac.

dac'ryocys'torhinos'tomy [dacryocyst + G. *rhis(rhin-)*, nose, + *stoma*, mouth] Surgical anastomosis between the lacrimal sac and the nasal mucosa through an opening in the lacrimal bone.

dac'ryocystot'omy [dacryocyst + G. *tomē*, incision] Incision of the lacrimal sac.

dac'ryolith [dacryo- + G. *lithos*, stone] Lacrimal calculus; a concretion in the lacrimal apparatus.

dacryo'ma [dacryo- + G. *-ōma*, tumour] **1.** A cyst formed by the accumulation of tears in an obstructed lacrimal duct. **2.** A tumour of the lacrimal apparatus.

dac'tyl [G. *daktylos*] Digit.

dactyli'tis Inflammation of one or more fingers.

dactylo-, dactyl- [G. *daktylos*, finger] Combining forms relating to the fingers, and sometimes to the toes.

dam [A.S. *fordemman*, to stop up] Any barrier to the flow of fluid; especially, in surgery and dentistry, a sheet of thin rubber arranged so as to shut off the part operated upon from the access of fluid.

dan'der Scales from skin, hair, or feathers; may cause an allergic reaction in sensitive persons.

dan'druff The presence, in varying amounts, of scales in the scalp hair, due to the normal branny exfoliation of the epidermis.

de- [L. *de*, from, away] Prefix, often privative or negative, denoting away from, cessation.

deaf [A.S. *déaf*] Unable to hear; hearing indistinctly; hard of hearing.

deaf'ferenta'tion [L. *de*, from, + afferent] A loss of the sensory nerve fibres from a portion of the body.

deaf'ness General term for loss of the ability to hear, without designation of the degree of loss or the cause.

conductive d., hearing impairment caused by interference with sound or vibratory energy in the external canal, middle ear, or ossicles.

cortical d., d. resulting from a lesion of the cerebral cortex.

sensorineural d., hearing loss due to lesions or dysfunction of the cochlea or retrocochlear nerve tracts and centres, as opposed to conductive d.

death [A.S. *dēath*] Cessation of life. In multicellular organisms, a gradual process at the cellular level, with tissues varying in their ability to withstand deprivation of oxygen; in higher organisms, a cessation of integrated tissue and organ functions; in man, manifested by the loss of heart beat, by the absence of spontaneous breathing, and by cerebral d.

cerebral d., brain d., in the presence of cardiac activity, the permanent loss of cerebral function, manifested clinically by absence of purposive responsiveness to external stimuli, absence of cephalic reflexes, apnoea, and an isoelectric electroencephalogram for at least 30 minutes in the absence of hypothermia and poisoning by central nervous system depressants.

cot d., sudden infant death *syndrome.*

debil'itating [L. *debilitas,* fr. *debilis,* weak] Causing weakness.

débridement' [Fr. unbridle] Excision of devitalized tissue and foreign matter from a wound.

debt [L. *debitum,* debt] That which is owed; a liability to be rendered.

oxygen d., the extra oxygen, taken in by the body during recovery from exercise, beyond the resting needs of the body; sometimes used as if synonymous with oxygen deficit.

decal'cifica'tion [L. *de-,* away, + *calx(calc-),* lime, + *facio,* to make] **1.** Removal of lime salts from bones and teeth, either *in vitro* or as a result of a pathologic process. **2.** Precipitation of calcium from blood as by oxalate or fluoride, or the conversion of blood calcium to an un-ionized form as by citrate, thus preventing or delaying coagulation.

decapsula'tion Incision and removal of a capsule or enveloping membrane, as of the kidney.

decay' [L. *de,* down, + *cado,* to fall] **1.** Destruction of an organic substance by slow combustion or gradual oxidation. **2.** Putrefaction. **3.** To deteriorate; to undergo slow combustion or putrefaction. **4.** In dentistry, caries. **5.** In psychology, loss of information which was registered by the senses and processed into the short term memory system. **6.** Loss of radioactivity with time.

decer'ebrate **1.** To cause decerebration. **2.** Denoting an animal so prepared, or a patient whose brain has suffered an injury which results in neurologic function comparable to a decerebrate animal.

decerebra'tion Removal of the brain above the lower border of the corpora quadrigemina or a complete section of the brain at about this level or somewhat below, or destroying the function of the cerebrum by tying the common carotid arteries and the basilar artery at about the middle of the pons.

dec'ibel (db, dB) [L. *decimus,* tenth, + bel] One-tenth of a bel; unit for expressing the relative loudness of sound on a logarithmic scale.

decid'ua [L. *deciduus,* falling off] *Membrana* decidua.

deciduo'ma An intrauterine mass of decidual tissue, probably the result of hyperplasia of decidual cells retained in the uterus. It is doubtful that d. is a true neoplasm.

decid'uous [L. *deciduus,* falling off] **1.** Not permanent; denoting that which eventually falls off. **2.** (abbreviated D in dental formulas) In dentistry, often used to designate the first or primary dentition.

de'compensa'tion **1.** A failure of compensation in heart disease. **2.** The appearance or exacerbation of a mental disorder due to failure of defence mechanisms.

decomposi'tion Decay; disintegration; lysis.

decompres'sion [L. *de-,* from, down, + *com-primo,* pp. *-pressus,* to press together, fr. *premo,* to press] Removal of pressure.

cerebral d., removal of a piece of the cranium, usually in the subtemporal region, with incision of the dura, to relieve intracranial pressure.

nerve d., release of pressure on a nerve trunk by the surgical excision of constricting bands or widening of the bony canal.

spinal d., removal of pressure upon the spinal cord as by a tumour, cyst, haematoma, or bone.

deconges'tant, deconges'tive Having the property of reducing congestion.

de'contamina'tion Removal or neutralization of toxic substances, radioactive materials, etc.

decortica'tion [L. decortico, pp. -atus, to deprive of bark] **1.** Removal of the cortex, or external layer, beneath the capsule from any organ or structure. **2.** Surgical removal of the residual clot and/or newly organized scar tissue that form after a haemothorax or neglected empyema.

decrudes'cence [L. de, from, + crudesco, to become worse] Abatement of the symptoms of disease.

decu'bitus [L. decumbo, to lie down] **1.** The position of the patient in bed, as dorsal d., lateral d. **2.** A decubitus ulcer.

decus'sate [L. decusso, pp. -atus, to make in the form of an X] **1.** To cross. **2.** Crossed like the arms of an X.

decussa'tio, pl. **de'cussatio'nes** [L. (see decussate)] [NA] **1.** In general, any crossing over or intersection of parts. **2.** Intercrossing of two homonymous fibre bundles as each crosses over to the opposite side of the brain in the course of its ascent or descent through the brainstem or spinal cord.

decussa'tion Decussatio.

defaeca'tion [L. defaeco, pp. -atus, to remove the dregs] The discharge of faeces from the rectum.

de'fect An imperfection or malformation.

ventricular septal d., a congenital d. in the septum between the cardiac ventricles, usually resulting from failure of the spiral septum to close the interventricular foramen.

defence' [L. defendo, to ward off] Methods used to control anxiety.

def'erent [L. deferens, pres. p. of defero, to carry away] Carrying away.

deferves'cence [L. de-fervesco, to cease boiling] Falling of an elevated temperature; abatement of fever.

de'fibrilla'tion Arrest of fibrillation of the cardiac muscle (atrial or ventricular) with restoration of the normal rhythm.

defib'rillator That which arrests fibrillation of the ventricular muscle and restores the normal heart beat.

defi'ciency [L. deficio, to fail, fr. facio, to do] A lacking; something wanting.

immunological, immune, or **immunity d.,** immunodeficiency.

def'icit [L. deficio, to fail] The result of temporarily consuming something faster than it is being replenished.

oxygen d., the difference between oxygen uptake of the body during early stages of exercise and during a similar duration in a steady state of exercise; sometimes considered as the formation of the oxygen debt.

deform'ity A deviation from the normal shape or size, resulting in disfigurement.

Arnold–Chiari d., elongation of the cerebellar tonsils and drawing of the cerebellum into the fourth ventricle, together with smallness of the medulla and pons and internal hydrocephalus; frequently associated with spina bifida.

lobster-claw d., a hand or foot, with the medial digits missing or fused so that it suggests the shape of a lobster claw; usually autosomal dominant inheritance.

degenera'tion [L. degeneratio] **1.** Deterioration; a declining to a lower level of mental, physical, or moral qualities. **2.** A retrogressive pathologic change in cells or tissues, in consequence of which the functions may be impaired or destroyed.

hepatolenticular d., a disorder of copper metabolism characterized by cirrhosis, d. in the basal ganglia of the brain, and deposition of green pigment in the periphery of the cornea; autosomal recessive inheritance.

degen'erative Relating to degeneration.

degluti'tion [L. de-glutio, to swallow] The act of swallowing.

dehis'cence [L. dehiscere, to split apart or open] A bursting open, splitting, or gaping along natural or sutured lines.

dehydra'tion [L. de, from + G. hydōr (hydr-), water] **1.** Deprivation of water. **2.** Reduction of water content. **3.** Exsiccation (2). **4.** Desiccation.

dehydro- Prefix used in the names of those chemical compounds that differ from other and more familiar compounds in the absence of two hydrogen atoms.

dehy'drogena'tion **1.** Removal of a pair of hydrogen atoms from a compound, by the action of enzymes (dehydrogenases) or other catalysts. **2.** Removal of hydrogen from the lungs by breathing oxygen in a semiclosed or nonbreathing system for several minutes prior to the induction of inhalation anaesthesia.

déjà vu [Fr. already seen] See under phenomenon.

dejec'tion [L. *dejectio,* fr. *de-jicio,* pp. *-jectus,* to cast down] **1.** Depression (3). **2.** Discharge of excrementitious matter. **3.** The matter so discharged.

delete'rious [G. *dēlētērios,* fr. *dēleomai,* to injure] Injurious; noxious; harmful.

delir'ium [L. fr. *deliro,* to be crazy] A condition of extreme mental, and usually motor, excitement marked by defective perception, impaired memory, and a rapid succession of confused and unconnected ideas, often with illusions and hallucinations.

  d. tre'mens, a form of acute insanity due to alcoholic withdrawal and marked by sweating, tremor, atonic dyspepsia, restlessness, anxiety, precordial distress, mental confusion, and hallucinations.

deliv'ery Passage of the child and the fetal membranes through the genital canal into the external world.

  forceps d., assisted birth of the child by an instrument designed to grasp the head of the child; **high f. d.** occurs before engagement has taken place; **low f. d.** occurs when the fetal head is clearly visible, the skull has reached the perineal floor, and the sagittal suture is in the anteroposterior diameter of the pelvis; **midforceps d.** before the criteria of low forceps d. have been met, but after engagement has taken place.

del'toid [G. *deltoeidēs,* shaped like the letter *delta*] **1.** Resembling the Greek letter delta (Δ); triangular. **2.** *Musculus* deltoideus.

delu'sion [L. *de-ludo,* pp. *-lusus,* to deceive] A false belief or wrong judgment held with conviction despite incontrovertible evidence to the contrary.

  d. of grandeur, a d. in which one believes himself possessed of great wealth, intellect, importance, power, etc.

  d. of negation, nihilistic d., a depressive d. in which one imagines that the world and all that relates to it have ceased to exist.

  d. of persecution, a false notion that one is being persecuted; characteristic symptom of paranoid schizophrenia.

delu'sional Relating to a delusion or delusions.

demen'tia [L. fr. *de-* priv. + *mens,* mind] A general mental deterioration due to organic or psychological factors.

  d. prae'cox, [L. precocious], any one of the group of psychotic disorders known as the schizophrenias; formerly used to describe schizophrenia as a single entity.

  presenile d., d. preseni'lis, (1) d. developing before old age; **(2)** Alzheimer's *disease.*

  senile d., an organic brain syndrome associated with aging and marked by progressive mental deterioration, loss of recent memory, lability of affect, difficulty with novel experience, self-centredness, and childish behaviour.

demi- [Fr. fr. L. *dimidius,* half] Prefix denoting half, lesser. See also hemi-, semi-.

demin'eraliza'tion A loss or decrease of the mineral constituents of the body or individual tissues, especially of bone.

De'modex [G. *dēmos,* tallow, + *dēx,* a woodworm] A genus of minute follicular parasitic mites (family Demodicidae) that invade the skin and are usually found in the sebaceous glands and hair follicles of man and animals; seldom pathogenic.

demog'raphy [G. *demos,* people, + *graphō,* to write] The statistical study of groups of people, their environment, and their geographic distribution.

demul'cent [L. *de-mulceo,* pp. *-mulctus,* to stroke lightly, to soften] Soothing; relieving irritation, especially of mucous surfaces.

demy'elina'tion,

demy'eliniza'tion Destruction or loss of myelin from the medullary sheath of Schwann or of myelin associated with oligodendroglia.

den'driform [G. *dendron,* tree, + L. *forma,* form] Tree-shaped, or branching.

den'drite [G. *dendritēs,* relating to a tree] One of the two types of branching protoplasmic processes of the nerve cell (the other being the axon).

dendrit'ic **1.** Dendriform. **2.** Relating to the dendrites of nerve cells.

den'dron [G. a tree] Dendrite.

dener'vate To cut off the nerve supply of a part by incision, excision, or local anaesthesia.

den'gue [Sp. a corruption of "dandy" fever] A disease of tropical and subtropical regions occurring epidemically, transmitted by an *Aëdes* mosquito, and caused by dengue virus. Four grades of severity are recognized: *I*, fever and constitutional symptoms; *II*, grade I plus spontaneous bleeding of skin, gums, or gastrointestinal tract; *III*, grade II plus agitation and circulatory failure; *IV*, profound shock.

deni'al Negation; unconscious defence mechanism used to allay anxiety by denying the existence of important conflicts or troublesome impulses.

denida'tion [L. *de*, from, + *nidus*, nest] Exfoliation of the superficial portion of the mucous membrane of the uterus.

dens, pl **den'tes** [L.] [NA] **1.** Tooth. **2.** A toothlike process projecting upward from the body of the axis around which the atlas rotates.

d. cani'nus, pl. **den'tes cani'ni** [NA], canine, cuspid, or eye tooth; a tooth having a crown of thick conical shape and a long conical root; there are two canine tooth in each jaw, adjacent to the distal surface of the lateral incisors, in both deciduous and permanent dentition.

d. decid'uus, pl. **den'tes decidu'ui** [NA], baby, primary, or deciduous tooth; deciduous or primary dentition; a tooth of the first set of teeth, 20 in all, that erupts between the mean ages of 6 and 28 months of life.

d. incisi'vus, pl. **den'tes incisi'vi** [NA], incisor tooth; a tooth with a chisel shaped crown and a single conical root; there are four in the anterior part of each jaw, in both deciduous and permanent dentitions.

d. mola'ris, pl. **den'tes mola'res** [NA], molar tooth; a tooth having a crown with four or five cusps on the grinding surface, a bifid root in the lower jaw, and three conical roots in the upper jaw; in permanent dentition, there are three on either side behind the premolars; in deciduous dentition, there are two on either side behind the canines.

d. per'manens, pl. **den'tes permane'tes** [NA], permanent tooth; secondary dentition; one of the 32 teeth whose eruptions begin from the 5th to the 7th year, and last until

the 17th to the 23rd year, when the last of the wisdom teeth appears.

d. premola'ris, pl. **den'tes premola'res** [NA], premolar or bicuspid tooth; a tooth usually having two cusps on the grinding surface and a flattened root; there are two on either side between the canine and the molars.

d. seroti'nus [NA], wisdom tooth; the third molar tooth on each side in each jaw that erupt from the 17th to the 23rd year.

dent-, denti-, dento- [L. *dens*, tooth] Combining forms relating to the teeth.

den'tal [L. *dens*, tooth] Relating to the teeth.

dental'gia [L. *dens*, tooth, + G. *algos*, pain] Toothache.

den'tate [L. *dentatus*, toothed] Notched; toothed; cogged.

den'tinal Relating to dentine.

den'tine [L. *dens*, tooth] The ivory substance forming the mass of a tooth.

hereditary opalescent d., dentinogenesis imperfecta.

den'tinogen'esis [dentine + G. *genesis*, production] The process of dentine formation in the development of teeth.

d. imperfec'ta, a defect of dentine formation characterized by translucent or opalescent colour of teeth, easy fracturing of enamel, wearing of occlusal surfaces, and staining of exposed dentine; autosomal dominant inheritance.

den'tist A licensed practitioner of dentistry.

den'tistry The healing science and art concerned with the prevention, diagnosis, and treatment of deformities, diseases, and traumatic injuries of the teeth and orofacial complex.

denti'tion [L. *dentitio*, to teethe] The natural teeth, considered collectively, in the dental arch.

den'toalve'olar Denoting that portion of the alveolar bone immediately about the teeth; also the functional unity of teeth and alveolar bone.

den'ture An artificial substitute for missing natural teeth and adjacent tissues.

complete d., full d., a dental prosthesis that is a substitute for the lost natural dentition and associated structures of the maxillae or mandible.

fixed partial d., bridge; a restoration of one or more missing teeth permanently attached to natural teeth or roots which furnish the primary support to the appliance.

partial d., bridgework; a dental prosthesis that restores one or more, but less than all, of the natural teeth and/or associated parts and is supported by the teeth and/or the mucosa; may be removable or fixed.

11-deoxycor'tisone An adrenocortical steroid, with weak biologic activity, and biosynthetic precursor of cortisol.

deoxygena'tion Removing or depriving of oxygen.

deoxyri'bonucle'ic acid (DNA). Nucleic acid containing deoxyribose as the sugar component and found principally in the chromatin and chromosomes of animal and vegetable cells, usually loosely bound to protein; considered to be the autoreproducing component of chromosomes and of many viruses, and the repository of hereditary characteristics.

complementary DNA (cDNA), DNA that is complementary to messenger RNA.

depen'dence [L. *dependeo,* to hang from] The quality or condition of lacking independence by relying upon, being influenced by, or being subservient to a person or object reflecting a particular need.

deper'sonaliza'tion A state in which a person loses the feeling of his own identity in relation to others in his family or peer group, or loses the feeling of his own reality.

depigmenta'tion Loss of pigment; it may be partial or complete.

depil'atory 1. Epilatory (1). **2.** An agent that causes the falling out of hair.

depres'sant [L. *de-primo,* pp. *-pressus,* to press down] Reducing functional tone or activity.

depres'sion 1. A sinking below the surrounding level. **2.** A hollow or sunken area. **3.** A sinking of spirits so as to constitute a clinically discernible condition.

depres'somo'tor Retarding motor activity.

depres'sor 1. A muscle that flattens or lowers a part. **2.** Anything that depresses or retards functional activity. **3.** An instrument or device used to push certain structures out of the way during an operation or examination. **4.** An agent producing decreased blood pressure.

depriva'tion Absence, loss, or withholding of something needed.

emotional d., lack of adequate and appropriate interpersonal or environmental experiences, or both, usually in the early developmental years.

sensory d., diminution or absence of usual external stimuli or perceptual opportunities, commonly resulting in psychological distress and aberrant functioning.

de'reism [L. *de,* away, + *res,* thing] Mental activity in fantasy, in contrast to reality.

derm-, derma-, dermat-, dermato-, dermo- [G. *derma,* skin] Combining forms signifying skin.

dermabra'sion Operative removal of disfigured skin using sand paper, wire brushes, or other abrasive materials.

Der'macen'tor [derm- + G. *kentōr,* a goader] A characteristically marked genus of hard ticks (family Ixodidae).

D. anderso'ni, the Rocky Mountain spotted-fever, or wood tick; a species that is the vector of spotted fever in the Rocky Mountain regions of the U.S., and also transmits tularaemia and causes tick paralysis.

D. variabi'lis, the American dog or wood tick, a species that transmits tularaemia and is a principal vector of spotted fever in the central and eastern U.S.

der'mal Relating to the skin.

dermati'tis, pl. **dermatit'ides** [derm- + G. *-itis,* inflammation] Inflammation of the skin.

actinic d., eruption of sensitivity produced by exposure to sunlight, usually of specific electromagnetic energy.

contact d., a delayed type of induced sensitivity (allergy) of the skin with varying degrees of erythema, oedema, and vesiculation, resulting from cutaneous contact with a specific allergen.

exfoliative d., Wilson's disease; generalized exfoliation with scaling of the skin and usually with erythema (erythroderma).

d. herpetifor'mis, a chronic disease of the skin marked by a severe, extensive, itching eruption of vesicles and papules which occur in groups.

napkin d., colloquially referred to as napkin rash; d. of thighs and buttocks supposedly due to ammonia produced in decomposing urine in infants' napkins.

seborrhoeic d., d. seborrhoe'ica, a scaly macular eruption that occurs primarily on the face, scalp, interscapular area, pubic area, and about the anus; the lesions are covered with a slightly adherent oily scale.

dermato- See derm-.

der'matoglyph'ics [dermato- + glyphē, carved work] **1.** Configurations of the characteristic ridge patterns of the volar surfaces of the skin; the distal segment of each digit has three types of configurations: whorl, loop, and arch. See also fingerprint. **2.** The science or study of these configurations or patterns.

der'matograph'ism [dermato- + G. graphō, to write] A form of urticaria in which wealing occurs in the site and in the configuration of stroking.

der'matol'ogy [dermato- + G. logos, study] The medical specialty concerned with the study of the skin and the relationship of cutaneous lesions to systemic disease.

der'matome [dermato- + tomē, a cutting] **1.** An instrument for cutting thin slices of skin for grafting, or excising small lesions. **2.** The area of skin supplied by cutaneous branches from a single spinal nerve.

der'matomyco'sis Dermatophytosis.

Dermatophagoi'des pteronys-si'nus [dermato- + G. phagein, to eat] A common species of cosmopolitan sarcoptiform mites found in house dust and a common contributory cause of atopic asthma.

dermat'ophyte [dermato- + G. phyton, plant] A fungus that causes infections of the skin, hair, and/or nails.

der'matophyto'sis Infection of the hair, skin, or nails caused by a dermatophyte; characterized by erythema, small papular vesicles, fissures, and scaling.

der'matosclero'sis [dermato- + G. sclerō, to harden] Scleroderma.

dermato'sis, pl. **dermato'ses** [dermato- + G. -osis, condition] Any cutaneous lesion or group of lesions, or eruptions of any type.

radiation d., skin changes caused by ionizing radiation, particularly erythema in the acute stage and chronic changes in the epidermis and dermis resembling actinic keratosis.

seborrhoeic d., seborrhoeic dermatitis.

der'mis [G. derma, skin] [NA] Corium.

dermo- See derm-.

der'moid [dermo- + G. eidos, resemblance] Dermoid cyst.

des- See de-.

descent' [L. descensus] In obstetrics, the passage of the presenting part of the fetus into and through the birth canal.

desen'sitiza'tion **1.** Reduction or abolition of allergic sensitivity or reactions to the specific antigen (allergen). **2.** The act of removing an emotional complex.

des'iccant [L. de-sicco, pp. -siccatus, to dry up] Drying; causing or promoting dryness.

des'iccate To dry thoroughly, to render free from moisture.

desicca'tion Dehydration; the process of being desiccated.

desmo-, desm- [G. desmos, a band] Combining forms meaning fibrous connection or ligament.

desmop'athy [desmo- + G. pathos, suffering] A disease of ligaments.

desquama'tion [L. desquamo, pp. -atus, to scale off] The shedding of the epidermis in scales or shreds, or of the outer layer of any surface.

detach'ment **1.** A voluntary or involuntary separation from normal associations or environment. **2.** Separation of a structure from its support.

retinal d., d. of retina, loss of apposition between the sensory retina and the retinal pigment epithelium.

dete'riora'tion [L. deterior, worse] The process or condition of becoming worse.

detoxica'tion, detox'ifica'tion **1.** Recovery from toxic effects. **2.** Removal of toxic properties. **3.** Metabolic conversion of pharmacologically active principles to pharmacologically less active principles.

detri'tion [L. de tero, pp. tritus, to rub off] A wearing away by use or friction.

detri'tus [L. (see detrition)] Matter resulting from or remaining after decomposition or disintegration of a substance.

detru'sor [L. detrudo, to drive away] A muscle that has the action of expelling a substance.

detumes'cence [L. de, from, + tumesco, to swell up] Subsidence of a swelling.

devas'culariza'tion [L. de, away, + vasculus, small vessel, + G. izo, to cause] Occlusion of all or most of the blood vessels to any part or organ.

devel'opment The act or process of natural progression from a previous, lower, or embryonic stage to a later, more complex, or adult stage.

psychosexual d., maturation and development of the psychic phase of sexuality from birth to adult life through the oral, anal, phallic, latency, and genital phases.

de'viance [see deviation] Departure from an accepted norm, role, or rule.

devia'tion [L. *devio*, to turn from the straight path] **1.** Deflection; a turning away or aside from the normal point or course. **2.** An abnormality. **3.** In psychiatry, deviance.

conjugate d. of the eyes, (1) the turning of eyes equally and simultaneously in the same direction, as occurs normally; **(2)** a condition in which both eyes are pathologically turned to the same side as a result of either paralysis or muscular spasm.

device' A contrivance, usually mechanical, designed to perform a specific function.

contraceptive d., a d. used to prevent pregnancy; *e.g.,* occlusive diaphragm, condom, intrauterine d.

intrauterine d.'s (IUD), intrauterine contraceptive d.'s (IUCD), plastic or metal of various shapes inserted into the uterus to exert a contraceptive effect.

devi'talized Devoid of life; dead, as a tooth in which the pulp has been destroyed.

dex'ter (D) [L. f. *dextra*, neut. *dextrum*] [NA] Right.

dextral'ity Right-handedness; preference for the right hand in performing manual tasks.

dex'tran Any of several water-soluble, high molecular weight glucose polymers produced by the action of *Leuconostoc mesenteroides* on sucrose; used in isotonic sodium chloride solution for the treatment of shock, in distilled water for the relief of the oedema of nephrosis, and as plasma substitutes or expanders.

dextro-, dextr- [L. *dexter*, right] **1.** Prefix meaning right, or toward or on the right side. **2.** Chemical prefix meaning dextrorotatory. See also *d-*.

dextrocar'dia [dextro- + G. *kardia*, heart] Displacement of the heart to the right, usually as one of two kinds: 1) dextroposition, in which the heart is simply displaced to the right; 2) cardiac heterotaxia, in which there is complete transposition of the right and left chambers, the heart thus presenting a mirror picture of the normal.

dextroro'tatory (d-) Denoting certain crystals or solutions capable of giving a clockwise twist to the plane of plane-polarized light.

dex'trose Glucose.

dextrover'sion [dextro- + L. *verto*, pp. *versus*, to turn] **1.** Version (a turning) toward the right. **2.** In ophthalmology, rotation of both eyes to the right.

di- [G. *dis*, two] Prefix denoting two, twice. See also bi-, bis-.

dia- [G. *dia*, through] Prefix meaning through, throughout, completely.

diabe'tes [G. *diabētēs*, a compass, a siphon] Either d. insipidus or d. mellitus, diseases having in common the symptom polyuria; when used without qualification, refers to d. mellitus.

bronze d., a type of d. associated with haemochromatosis, with iron deposits in the skin, liver, and other viscera, and often with severe liver damage and glycosuria.

d. insip'idus, the chronic excretion of very large amounts of pale urine of low specific gravity, accompanied by extreme thirst; ordinarily results from inadequate output of pituitary antidiuretic hormone.

juvenile d., severe d. mellitus, usually of abrupt onset during the first two decades of life.

maturity-onset d., an often mild form of d. mellitus, of gradual onset in obese individuals over the age of 35.

d. melli'tus [L. sweetened with honey], a metabolic disorder in which carbohydrate utilization is reduced and that of lipid and protein enhanced; caused by deficiency of insulin and is characterized, in more severe cases, by glycosuria, water and electrolyte loss, ketoacidosis, and coma; chronic complications include neuropathy, retinopathy, nephropathy, and generalized degenerative changes in large and small blood vessels.

diabet'ic Relating to or suffering from diabetes.

diabetogen'ic Causing diabetes.

di'agnose [G. *diagignōskō*, to distinguish] To make a diagnosis.

diagno'sis [G. *diagnōsis*, a deciding] Determination of the nature of a disease.

clinical d., d. made from a study of the signs and symptoms of a disease.

differential d., determination of which of two or more diseases with similar symptoms is the one from which the patient is suffering.

laboratory d., d. made by a chemical, microscopic, bacteriologic, or biopsy study of secretions, discharges, blood, or tissue.

diagnos'tic Relating to or aiding in diagnosis.

dial'ysate That part of the mixture that passes through the dialysing membrane.

di'alyser A device used in dialysis; a haemodialyser.

dial'ysis [G. a separation] Separation of crystalloid from colloid substances (or smaller molecules from larger ones) in a solution by interposing a semipermeable membrane between the solution and water; the crystalloid (smaller) substances pass through the membrane into the water on the other side, the colloids do not

diapede'sis [G. *dia*, through, + *pēdēsis*, a leaping] The passage of blood, or any of its formed elements, through the intact walls of blood vessels.

diaphore'sis [G. *diaphorēsis*] Perspiration (1).

diaphoret'ic Relating to or promoting perspiration.

di'aphragm [G. *diaphragma*, a partition wall] **1.** A thin partition separating adjacent regions. **2.** Midriff; the musculomembranous partition between the abdominal and thoracic cavities. **3.** A flexible metal ring covered with a dome-shaped sheet of elastic material used in the vagina to prevent pregnancy.

di'aphragmat'ic Relating to the diaphragm.

di'aphragmat'ocele [diaphragm + G. *kēlē*, hernia] Diaphragmatic *hernia.*

diaphys'eal, diaphys'ial Relating to the diaphysis.

diaphysec'tomy [diaphysis + G. *ektomē*, excision] Partial or complete removal of the shaft of a long bone.

diaph'ysis, pl. **diaph'yses** [G. a growing between] [NA] The shaft of a long bone, as distinguished from the epiphyses, or extremities, and apophyses, or outgrowths.

diarrhoe'a [G. *diarrhoia,* fr. *dia,* through, + *rhoia,* a flow, flux] An abnormally frequent discharge of fluid faecal matter from the bowel.

summer d., d. of infants in hot weather, usually an acute gastroenteritis due to the presence of a microorganism of the *Shigella* or *Salmonella* groups.

traveler's d., d. of sudden onset occurring sporadically in travelers in all parts of the world, usually during the first week of a trip, and most commonly caused by *Escherichia coli.*

diarrhoe'al, diarrhoe'ic Relating to diarrhoea.

diarthro'sis, pl. **diarthro'ses** [G. articulation] *Articulatio* synovialis.

diaste'ma, pl. **diaste'mata** [G. *diastēma*, an interval] **1.** A fissure or abnormal opening in any part, especially if congenital. **2.** [NA] A space between two adjacent teeth in the same dental arch.

dias'tole [G. *diastolē*, dilation] Dilation of the heart cavities, during which they fill with blood; d. alternates rhythmically with systole or contraction of the heart musculature.

diastol'ic Relating to diastole.

di'athermy [G. *dia*, through, + *thermē*, heat] Local elevation of temperature within the tissues, produced by high frequency current, ultrasonic waves, or microwave radiation.

diath'esis [G. arrangement, condition] A constitutional or inborn predisposition to a disease, group of diseases, or anomaly.

diathet'ic Relating to a diathesis.

diaz'epam A skeletal muscle relaxant, sedative, and antianxiety agent; also used as an anticonvulsant.

di'azines A group of synthetic tuberculostatic drugs.

dichromat'ic **1.** Having or exhibiting two colours. **2.** Relating to dichromatism (2).

dichro'matism [G. *di-*, two, + *chrōma*, colour] **1.** State of being dichromatic (1). **2.** The abnormality of colour vision in which only two of the three retinal cone pigments are present.

di'cophane (DDT) An insecticide that was once very effective, but insect populations rapidly developed tolerance for it; general usage is now widely discouraged because of the toxicity that results from the environmental persistence of this agent.

dicou'marol An anticoagulant agent that inhibits the formation of prothrombin in the liver.

didac'tic [G. *didaktikos*, fr. *didaskō*, to teach] Instructive; denoting medical teaching by lectures or textbooks as distinguished from clinical demonstration with patients.

didym-, didymo- [G. *didymos*, twin] Combining form denoting relationship to the didymus, testis.

didymi'tis [G. *didymoi*, the testes, + -*itis*, inflammation] Orchitis.

-didymus, [G. *didymos*, twin] Termination denoting a conjoined twin, the first element of the word designating the part or parts of the twins which have remained *unfused;* the more common usage is to designate the parts *fused* by use of the suffix -pagus. See also -dymus.

diel'drin A chlorinated hydrocarbon used as an insecticide; may cause toxic effects through skin contact, inhalation, or food contamination.

dienceph'alon, pl. **dienceph'ala** [G. *dia*, through, + *enkephalos*, brain] [NA] That part of the prosencephalon that is composed of the thalamus, the subthalamus, and the hypothalamus.

Dientamoe'ba frag'ilis A species of small amoeba parasitic in the large intestine and capable of sometimes causing low grade inflammation with mucous diarrhoea and gastrointestinal disturbance.

di'et [G. *diaita*, a way of life; a diet] **1.** Food and drink in general. **2.** A prescribed course of eating and drinking, in which the amount and kind of food, as well as the times at which it is to be taken, are regulated for therapeutic purposes. **3.** Reduction of caloric intake so as to lose weight. **4.** To follow any prescribed or specific d.

   bland d., a regular d. omitting foods that irritate the gastrointestinal tract.

   elimination d., a d. designed to detect what foodstuffs cause allergic manifestations by separate and succesive withdrawl of foods from the d. until that which causes the symptoms is discovered.

   high calorie d., a d. containing upward of 4000 calories per day.

   low calorie d., a d. of 1200 calories or less per day.

dietet'ic 1. Relating to diet. **2.** Descriptive of food that, naturally or through processing, has a low caloric content.

dietet'ics The branch of therapeutics concerned with food and drink in relation to health and disease.

dieth'yl e'ther A pungent volatile liquid the vapour of which produces inhalation anaesthesia.

dif'ferentia'tion 1. The acquiring or the possession of character or function different from that of the original type. **2.** Differential *diagnosis*.

diffrac'tion [L. *dif-fringo*, pp. -*fractus*, to break in pieces] Deflection of the rays of light from a straight line in passing by the edge of an opaque body.

diffuse' [L. *dif-fundo*, pp. -*fusus*, to pour in different directions] Spread about, not circumscribed or limited.

digest' [L. *digero*, pp. -*gestus*, to force apart, divide, dissolve] **1.** To soften by moisture and heat. **2.** To hydrolyse or break up into simpler chemical compounds by means of hydrolysing enzymes or chemical action; denoting the action of the secretions of the alimentary tract upon the food.

diges'tion [L. *digestio*, see digest] The process whereby ingested food is converted into material suitable for assimilation for synthesis of tissues or liberation of energy.

dig'it [L. *digitus*] A finger or toe.

   clubbed d.'s, A bulbous enlargement of the terminal phalanges produced by clubbing.

digital'in A standardized mixture of glycosides obtained from digitalis and used as a cardiotonic.

digital'is [L. *digitalis*, relating to the fingers (in allusion to the finger-like flowers)] Foxglove, a genus of perennial flowering plants (family Schrophulariaceae). *D. lanata* and *D. purpurea* are the main sources of cardioactive steroid glycosides used in the treatment of certain heart diseases, especially heart failure.

digitaliza'tion Administration of digitalis by a dosage schedule until sufficient amounts are present in the body to produce the desired therapeutic effects.

digox'in A cardioactive steroid glycoside obtained from Digitalis lanata.

dihydroco'deine A narcotic analgesic derivative of codeine, about one-sixth as potent as morphine.

dila'tion Dilation.

dil'atator Dilator.

dila'tion [L. *dilato*, pp. *dilatatus*, to spread out, dilate] **1.** Physiologic, pathologic, or artificial enlargement of a cavity, canal, blood vessel, or opening. **2.** The act of such enlargement.

dilation and curettage' (D & C) Dilation of the cervix and curettement of the endometrium.

dilation and evacua'tion (D & E) Dilation of the cervix and removal of the early products of conception.

di'lator 1. An instrument or substance for enlarging a cavity, canal, blood vessel, or opening. **2.** A muscle that opens an orifice or dilates the lumen of a structure; the opening or dilating component of a pylorus.

dil'uent 1. Diluting; making weaker or more watery. **2.** That which dilutes the strength of a solution or mixture.

dilu'tion [L. *di-luo*, pp. *-lutus*, to wash away, dilute] **1.** The act of reducing the concentration of a mixture or solution. **2.** A weakened (diluted) solution.

dimercap'rol A chelating agent, developed as an antidote for lewisite and other arsenical poisons; also used as an antidote for antimony, bismuth, chromium, mercury, gold, and nickel poisoning.

dimeth'yltryp'tamine (DMT) A psychotomimetic agent present in several South American snuffs and in the leaves of *Prestonia amazonica* (family Apocynaceae); produces effects similar to those of LSD, but with more rapid onset, greater likelihood of a panic reaction, and a shorter duration.

dinoflag'ellate [G. *dinos*, whirling, + L. *flagellum*, a whip] A plantlike flagellate of the subclass Phytomastigophorea, some species of which produce a potent neurotoxin that may cause severe food intoxication following ingestion of parasitized shellfish.

diop'tre (D) [G. *dioptra*, a leveling instrument] The unit of refracting power of lenses, denoting the reciprocal of the focal length expressed in metres.

diox'in Popular abbreviation for dibenzodioxin, a contaminant in the herbicide, 2,4,5-T; its potential toxicity and carcinogenicity are controversial.

Dipet'alone'ma [G. *di-*, two, + *petalon*, leaf, + *nema*, thread] A large genus of nematode filariae (including the genus *Acanthocheilonema*) transmitted by species of *Culicoides;* it produces microfilariae in blood or tissue fluids, and adults in deep connective tissue, membranes, or visceral surfaces.

D. per'stans, the persistant "filaria" species characterized by unsheathed microfilariae without periodicity in the circulating blood and by adult forms in the peritoneal, pleural, or pericardial cavities.

D. streptocer'ca, a species characterized by unsheathed microfilariae without periodicity in the circulating blood and by adult forms in the dermis and subcutaneous tissues.

dipha'sic [G. *di-*, two, + *phasis*, appearance] Occurring in or referring to two phases or stages.

diphthe'ria [G. *diphthera*, leather] A specific infectious disease due to *Corynebacterium diphtheriae* and its toxin, marked by inflammation, with formation of a fibrinous exudate, of the mucous membrane of the throat, the nose, and sometimes the tracheobronchial tree; the toxin produces degeneration in peripheral nerves, heart muscle, and other tissues.

diphthe'rial, diphtherit'ic Relating to diphtheria, or the membrane characteristic of this disease.

diph'theroid [diphtheria + G. *eidos*, resemblance] **1.** A local infection suggesting diphtheria, caused by a microorganism other than *Corynebacterium diphtheriae*. 2. Any of the species resembling *Corynebacterium diphtheriae*.

diphyl'lobothri'asis Infection with *Diphyllobothrium latum*, caused by ingestion of raw or inadequately cooked fish infected with the larva; leucocytosis and eosinophilia may occur.

Diphyllobothr'ium [G. *di-*, two, + *phyllon*, leaf, + *bothrion*, little ditch] A large genus of tapeworms (order Pseudophyllidea). *D. latum*, the broad tapeworm, is a species that causes diphyllobothriasis.

diple'gia [G. *di-*, two, + *plēgē*, a stroke] Paralysis of corresponding parts on both sides of the body.

diplo- [G. *diplous*, double] Combining form meaning double or twofold.

diplobacil'lus Two rod-shaped bacterial cells linked end to end.

Diplococ'cus [diplo- + G. *kokkos*, berry] *Streptoccuccus*.

diplococ'cus, pl. **diplococ'ci** [diplo- + G. *kokkos*, berry] **1.** Spherical or ovoid bacterial cells joined together in pairs. **2.** Common name of any member of the bacterial genus *Diplococcus*.

diploë [G. *diploē*, fem. of *diplous*, double] [NA] The central layer of spongy bone between the two layers of compact bone, outer and inner plates, or tables, of the flat cranial bones.

dip'loid [diplo- + G. *eidos* resemblance] Containing twice the normal gametic number of chromosomes, one member of each chromosome pair derived from the father and one from the mother; the normal chromosome complement (46) of somatic cells in man.

diplop'agus [diplo- + G. *pagos*, something fixed] General term for conjoined twins, each with fairly complete bodies, although one or more internal organs may be in common.

diplo'pia [diplo- + G. *ōps*, eye] Double vision; the condition in which a single object is perceived as two objects.

dipse'sis [G. *dipsein*, to thirst] Abnormal or excessive thirst, or a craving for certain unusual forms of drink.

dipsoma'nia [G. *dipsa*, thirst, + *mania*, madness] A recurring compulsion to drink alcoholic beverages to excess.

Dip'tera [G. *di-*, two, + *pteron*, wing] An important order of insects (the two-wing flies and gnats), including many important disease vectors such as the mosquito, tsetse fly, sandfly, and biting midge.

dis- [L. inseparable particle denoting separation, taking apart, sundering in two] Prefix having the same force as the original Latin preposition.

disabil'ity Medicolegal term signifying loss of function and earning power.

disac'charide Condensation product of two monosaccharides by elimination of water, usually between an alcoholic OH and a hemiacetal OH.

dis'articula'tion [L. *dis-*, apart, + *articulus*, joint] Amputation of a limb through a joint, without cutting of bone.

disc [L. *discus*; G. *diskos*, a quoit, disc] **1.** Discus. **2.** Lamella (2).

herniated d., protruded d., ruptured d., protrusion of a degenerated or fragmented intervertebral d. into the intervertebral foramen, compressing the nerve root.

intervertebral d., *discus* intervertebralis.

optic d., *discus* nervi optici.

discec'tomy [G. *diskos*, disc, + *ektomē*, excision] Excision, in part or whole, of an intervertebral disc.

dis'charge 1. That which is emitted or evacuated, as an excretion or a secretion. **2.** The activation or firing of a neurone.

dis'ci Plural of discus.

disc'iform Disc-shaped.

discis'sion [L. *di-scindo*, pp. *-scissus*, to tear asunder] **1.** Incision or cutting through a part. **2.** Specifically, needling, splitting the capsule, and breaking up the substance of the crystalline lens with a knife needle, in cases of soft cataract.

disci'tis Nonbacterial inflammation of an intervertebral disc or disc space.

disco-, disc- [G. *diskos*, disc] Combining forms indicating relation to, or similarity to, a disc.

discog'raphy [disco- + G. *graphō*, to write] Radiographic visualization of intervertebral disc space by injection of contrast media.

discop'athy [disco- + G. *pathos*, disease] Disease of a disc, particularly of the intervertebral disc.

traumatic d., an injury characterized by fissuration, laceration and/or fragmentation of the disc or surrounding ligaments, with or without displacement of fragments against spinal cord, nerve roots, or ligaments.

discot'omy [disco- + G. *tomē*, incision] Discectomy.

discrete' [L. *dis-cerno*, pp. *-cretus*, to separate] Separate; distinct; not joined to or incorporated with another; especially denoting certain lesions of the skin.

dis'cus, pl. **dis'ci** [L. fr. G. *diskos*, a quoit, disc] [NA] Disc; any approximately flat circular surface.

d. intervertebra'lis [NA], intervertebral disc or cartilage; a disc interposed between the bodies of adjacent vertebrae; composed of an outer fibrous part (anulus fibrosus) that surrounds a central gelatinous mass (nucleus pulposus).

d. ner'vi op'tici [NA], blind spot; optic disc; an oval area of the ocular fundus, devoid of light receptors, where retinal ganglion cell axons converge to form the optic nerve.

disease' [Eng. *dis-* priv. + *ease*] **1.** Illness; sickness; an interruption, cessation, or disorder of body functions, systems, or organs. **2.** A pathologic entity characterized usually by at least two of these criteria: a recognized aetiologic agent(s), an identifiable group of signs and symptoms, or consistent anatomical alterations. See also syndrome and subentries.

Addison's d., chronic adrenocortical insufficiency.

Albers-Schönberg d., osteopetrosis.

Albright's d., polyostotic fibrous dysplasia with irregular brown patches of cutaneous pigmentation and endocrine dysfunction, especially precocious puberty, in girls

Alzheimer's d., organic dementia occurring usually in persons under 50 years of age, associated with Alzheimer's sclerosis, neurofibrillary degeneration, and senile plaques.

aortoiliac occlusive d., obstruction of the abdominal aorta and its main branches by atherosclerosis.

Aran-Duchenne d., progressive muscular atrophy.

autoimmune d., a d. resulting from an immune reaction produced by an individual's leucocytes or antibodies acting on the subject's own tissues or extracellular proteins.

Bechterew's d., spondylitis deformans.

Boeck's d., sarcoidosis.

Bright's d., nonsuppurative nephritis with albuminuria and oedema, corresponding stages of glomerulonephritis; sometimes used in general reference to unspecified kidney d.

Brill-Symmers d., nodular lymphoma.

Brill-Zinsser d., Brill's d., recrudescent typhus; an endogenous infection associated with the "carrier state" in persons who previously had epidemic typhus fever.

Buerger's d., thromboangiitis obliterans.

Busse-Buschke d., cryptococcosis.

Caffey's d., infantile cortical hyperostosis.

cais'son d., [Fr. caisson, a water-tight box or cylinder containing air under high pressure, used in sinking structural pilings underwater] decompression sickness.

Calvé-Perthes d., Legg-Calvé-Perthes d.

Canavan's d., spongy degeneration.

cat-scratch d., cat-scratch fever; benign inoculation lymphoreticulosis, an ulceroglandular d. that frequently follows the scratch or bite of a cat, producing regional lymphadenitis, indolent reaction, and benign low grade infection.

Chagas d., Chagas-Cruz d., South American trypanosomiasis.

Charcot's d., amyotrophic lateral sclerosis.

Charcot-Marie-Tooth d., peroneal muscular atrophy.

Chiari's d., Chiari's syndrome.

Christensen-Krabbe d., poliodystrophia cerebri progressiva infantilis.

Christian's d., (1) Hand-Schüller-Christian d.; **(2)** nodular nonsuppurative panniculitis.

Christmas d., [surname of child with the d.], haemophilia B.

chronic obstructive pulmonary d., general term used for those diseases in which forced expiratory flow is slowed, especially when no aetiologic or other more specific term can be applied.

Coats d., exudative retinitis.

Cockayne's d., Cockayne's syndrome.

coeliac d., A disease characterized by sensitivity to gluten and atrophy of the mucosa of the upper small intestine; mainifestations include diarrhoea, malabsorption, steatorrhoea, and nutritional and vitamin deficiencies.

collagen, collagen-vascular d.'s, a group of non-mendelian, although sometimes familial, generalized d.'s affecting connective tissue and frequently characterized by fibrinoid necrosis or vasculitis, included in this group are lupus erythematosus, progressive systemic sclerosis rheumatoid arthritis, rheumatic fever, polyarteritis nodosa, and dermatomyositis. See also connective tissue d.

communicable d., contagious d., any d. that is transmissible by infection or contagion directly or through the agency of a vector.

Concato's d., polyserositis.

connective-tissue d., a group of generalized d.'s affecting connective tissue, especially d.'s not inherited as mendelian characteristics; rheumatic fever and rheumatoid arthritis were first proposed as such d.'s, and other so-called collagen d.'s have been added.

Cori's d., type 3 *glycogenosis*.

Creutzfeldt-Jakob d., spastic pseudosclerosis with corticostriatal-spinal degeneration, a form of spongiform encephalopathy caused by a slow virus and characterized by dementia, myoclonus, ataxia, and other neurologic manifestations; progresses rapidly to coma and death.

Crigler-Najjar d., Crigler-Najjar *syndrome*.

Crohn's d., regional *enteritis*.

Crouzon's d., craniofacial *dysostosis*.

Cruveilhier's d., progressive muscular *atrophy*.

Cushing's d., Cushing's syndrome associated with a pituitary basophil adenoma.

cystine storage d., cystinosis.

cytomegalic inclusion d., the presence of inclusion bodies within the cytoplasm and nuclei of enlarged cells of various organs or newborn infants dying with jaundice, hepatomegaly, splenomegaly, purpura, thrombocytopenia, and fever; also occurs, at all ages, as a complication of other d.'s in which immune mechanisms are severely depressed.

deficiency d., any d. resulting from lack of calories, proteins, essential amino acids, fatty acids, vitamins, or trace minerals.

degenerative joint d., osteoarthritis.

Duchenne's d., (1) pseudohypertrophic muscular *dystrophy;* **(2)** progressive bulbar *paralysis*.

Erb's d., progressive bulbar *paralysis*.

fibrocystic d. of the breast, a benign d. common in women of the third, fourth, and fifth decades, characterized by formation, in one or both breasts, of small cysts containing fluid, associated with stromal fibrosis and variable degrees of intraductal epithelial hyperplasia and sclerosing adenosis.

Freiberg's d., epiphyseal ischaemic (aseptic) necrosis of second metatarsal head.

Friedreich's d., *myoclonus* multiplex.

Gaucher's d., glycocerebroside accumulation in macrophages due to a genetic deficiency of glucocerebrosidase; marked by hepatosplenomegaly, lymphadenopathy, and bone destruction by characteristic cells containing cytoplasmic tubules; autosomal recessive inheritance.

Gilles de la Tourette's d., Gilles de la Tourette's syndrome; motor incoordination with echolalia and coprolalia; a form of tic.

glycogen storage d., glycogenosis.

Goldflam d., *myasthenia* gravis.

graft versus host d., a type of incompatibility reaction of transplanted cells against those host tissues that possess an antigen not possessed by the donor.

Graves d., toxic goitre characterized by diffuse hyperplasia of the thyroid gland; a form of hyperthyroidism.

H d., Hartnup d.

hand-foot-and-mouth d., an exanthematous eruption of the fingers, toes, palms, and soles, accompanied by often painful vesicles and ulceration of the buccal mucous membrane and the tongue and by slight fever; caused by a Coxsackie virus.

Hand-Schüller-Christian d., generalized lipid histiocytosis of bones, especially the skull, with bone destruction by accumulation of cells containing cholesterol esters, and eosinophil leucocytes.

Hansen's d., leprosy (2).

Hartnup d., H d.; a congenital metabolic disorder consisting of aminoaciduria due to a defect in renal tubular absorption of neonatal α-amino acids and urinary excretion of tryptophan derivatives; characterized by a pellagra-like, light-sensitive skin rash with temporaray cerebellar ataxia; autosomal recessive inheritance.

Hashimoto's d., Diffuse infiltration of the thyroid gland with lymphocytes, resulting in diffuse goitre and progressive destruction of the parenchyma and hypothyroidism.

Heine-Medin d., acute anterior *poliomyelitis*.

Hirschsprung's d., congenital *megacolon*.

Hodgkin's d., a d. marked by chronic enlargement of the lymph nodes, enlargement of the spleen and often of the liver, by anaemia and fever, and by transformed lymphocytes (Reed-Sternberg cells) associated with inflammatory infiltration of lymphocytes and eosinophilic leucocytes and fibrosis; classified into lymphocytic predominant and nodular sclerosing types, mixed cellularity type, and lymphocytic depletion type.

Hurler's d., Hurler's *syndrome*.

Hutchinson-Gilford d., progeria.

hyaline membrane d. respiratory distress syndrome of the newborn; a d. seen especially in premature neonates with respiratory distress, characterized post mortem by atelectasis and an eosinophilic membrane lining alveolar ducts and associated with reduced amounts of lung surfactant.

infectious d., a d. resulting from the presence and activity of a microbial agent.

Kimmelstiel-Wilson d., A nodular hyaline deposit in tufts of the glomeruli of the kidneys associated with diabetes, albuminuria, hypertension, and oedema of the nephrotic type.

Legg-Calvé-Perthes, Legg-Perthes, or **Legg's d.,** epiphyseal aseptic necrosis of the upper end of the femur.

Legionnaires' d., [American *Legion* convention, 1976, at which many delegates were so affected], an acute infectious d., caused by *Legionella pneumophila*, with prodromal influenza-like symptoms and a rapidly rising high fever, followed by severe pneumonia and production of usually nonpurulent sputum, mental confusion, hepatic fatty changes, and renal tubular degeneration.

Lyme d. [*Lyme*, Connecticut, where first recognized], an inflammatory disorder caused by the spirochaete *Borrelia burgdorferi* and transmitted by ixodid ticks, typically occurring during the summer months; the characterizing lesion, erythema chronicum migrans, usually is preceded or accompanied by fever, malaise, fatigue, headache, and stiff neck; neurologic or cardiac manifestations, or arthritis (Lyme arthritis) may occur weeks to months later.

maple syrup urine d. a disorder caused by deficient oxidative decarboxylation of α-keto acid metabolites of leucine, isoleucine, and valine which are present in blood and urine in elevated concentrations, the urine having an odour similar to that of maple syrup; mental and physical retardation are associated; autosomal recessive inheritance.

marble bone d., osteopetrosis.

Marburg virus d., human infection by Marburg virus, causing fever, diarrhoea, a maculopapular rash, and disseminated intravascular coagulation with high mortality.

Marie-Strümpell d., ankylosing *spondylitis*.

Ménière's d., an affection characterized clinically by vertigo, nausea, vomiting, tinnitus, and progressive deafness.

Milroy's d., the congenital type of hereditary lymphoedema.

Minamata d. [*Minamata* Bay, Japan], a neurological disorder resulting from poisoning by organic mercury compounds and characterized by peripheral paraesthesis, dysarthria, ataxia, and loss of peripheral vision.

Morvan's d., syringomyelia.

motor neurone d., general term including progressive muscular atrophy (infantile, juvenile, and adult), amyotrophic lateral sclerosis, progressive bulbar paralysis, and primary lateral sclerosis; frequently familial.

Niemann-Pick d., Lipid histiocytosis with accumulation of phospholipid (sphingomyelin) in histiocytes in the liver, spleen, lymph nodes and bone marrow; cerebral involvement may occur at a late stage, with red macular spots less common than in Tay-Sachs d.; autosomal recessive inheritance.

notifiable d., a d. that, by statutory requirements, must be reported to public health authorities at diagnosis because of its importance to human or animal health

Oppenheim's d., amyotonia congenita.

organic d., a d. in which there is anatomical change in some tissue or organ.

Osgood-Schlatter d., Epiphyseal aseptic necrosis of the tibial tubercle.

Paget's d., (1) osteitis deformans; a generalized skeletal disease, frequently familial, of older persons in which bone resorption and formation are both increased, leading to thickening and softening of bones, and bending of weight-bearing bones; **(2)** a d. of elderly women, characterized by an infiltrated, somewhat eczematous lesion surrounding and involving the nipple and areola, and associated with subjacent intraductal cancer of the breast and infiltration of the lower epidermis by malignant cells; **(3)** cancer of the vulva arising from apocrine sweat glands.

Parkinson's d., parkinsonism (1).

Pel-Ebstein d., Hodgkin's d. with periodic pyrexia.

pelvic inflammatory d. (PID), acute or chronic inflammation in the pelvic cavity, particularly, suppurative lesions of the female genital tract.

Perthes d., Legg-Calvé-Perthes d.

Peyronie's d., a d. of unknown cause in which there are plaques or strands of dense fibrous tissue surrounding the corpus cavernosum of the penis, causing deformity and painful erection.

Pick's d., (1) [F. Pick], a form of multiple serositis (or polyserositis) characterized by chronic congestive hepatomegaly, persistent or recurrent ascites, sometimes recurrent pleural effusion, peritonitis, and pleuritis, occurring in a patient with previous (or concurrent) hyalinizing pericarditis; **(2)** [A. Pick], Pick's *atrophy*.

pink d., acrodynia (1).

polycystic d. of kidneys, polycystic *kidney*.

Pott's d., tuberculous *spondylitis*.

pulseless d., a progressive obliterative arteritis of the vessels arising from the arch of the aorta.

Raynaud's d., idiopathic paroxysmal bilateral cyanosis of the digits, due to arterial and arteriolar contraction, caused by cold or emotion.

Recklinghausen's d., neurofibromatosis.

Recklinghausen's d. of bone, *osteitis* fibrosa cystica.

Reiter's d., Reiter's *syndrome* .

rheumatic heart d., d. of the heart resulting from rheumatic fever, chiefly manifested by abnormalities of the valves.

Ritter's d., (1) toxic epidermal *necrolysis;* **(2)** *icterus* neonatorum.

Scheuermann's d., epiphyseal aseptic necrosis of vertebral bodies.

Schlatter-Osgood d., Osgood-Schlatter d.

Schönlein's d., Henoch-Schönlein *purpura*.

Schüller's d., Hand-Schüller-Christian d.

Still's d., juvenile rheumatoid *arthritis*.

Stokes-Adams d., Adams-Stokes *syndrome*.

storage d., accumulation of a specific substance within tissues, generally because of congenital deficiency of an enzyme necessary for further metabolism of the substance.

Sturge-Weber d., Sturge-Weber *syndrome*.

Takahara's d., acatalasaemia.

Takayasu's d., pulseless d.

Tay-Sachs d., infantile type of cerebral *sphingolipidosis*.

venereal d., a contagious d. acquired during sexual intercourse; e.g., syphilis, gonorrhoea, chancroid.

Vincent's d., necrotizing ulcerative *gingivitis*.

von Recklinghausen's d., neurofibromatosis.

von Willebrand's d., pseudohaemophilia; a haemorrhagic diathesis characterized by tendency to bleed primarily from mucous membranes, prolonged bleeding time, normal platelet count, normal clot retraction, partial and variable deficiency of factor VIII, and possibly a morphologic defect of platelets; autosomal dominant inheritance with reduced penetrance and variable expressivity.

Weil's d., leptospirosis caused by a leptospire and characterized clinically by fever, jaundice, muscular pains, conjunctival congestion, and albuminuria.

Wernicke's d., Wernicke's *syndrome*.

Wilson's d., (1) [S. A. K. Wilson], hepatolenticular *degeneration;* **(2)** [Sir W. J. E. Wilson], exfoliative *dermatitis*.

disengage'ment [Fr.] Emergence of the fetal head from the vulva during childbirth, or ascent of the presenting part from the pelvis after the inlet has been negotiated.

disimpac'tion Withdrawal of impaction in a fractured bone.

disinfect' To destroy pathogenic microorganisms in or on any substance or to inhibit their growth and vital activity.

disinfec'tant Destroying organisms of putrefaction or disease, or inhibiting their activity.

disloca'tion [L. *dislocatio*, fr. *dis-*, apart, + *locatio*, a placing] Displacement of an organ or any part; specifically a disturbance or disarrangement of the normal relation of the bones entering into the formation of a joint.

dismem'ber To amputate an arm or leg.

disor'der A disturbance of function, structure, or both.

affective d.'s, a class of mental d.'s characterized by a disturbance in mood.

bipolar d., an affective d. characterized by the occurrence of manic episodes or manic episodes alternating with depressive episodes.

personality d., general term for a group of behavioural d.'s, each characterized by usually lifelong, ingrained, maladaptive patterns of deviant behaviour, life style, and social adjustment that are different in quality from psychotic and neurotic symptoms; former designations for these personality d.'s were psychopath and sociopath.

post-traumatic stress d., a form of neuropsychologic d., classified as an anxiety d. and characterized by the development of symptoms subsequent to a psychologically traumatic event outside the range of usual human experience.

disorienta'tion Loss of the sense of familiarity with one's surroundings; loss of one's bearings.

displace'ment 1. Removal from the normal location or position. 2. Transfer of impulses from one expression to another, as from fighting to talking.

dissect' [L. dis-seco, pp. -sectus, to cut asunder] 1. To cut apart or separate the tissues of the body for study. 2. In an operation, to separate the different structures along natural lines by dividing the connective tissue framework.

dissem'inated [L. dis-semino, pp. -atus, to scatter seed] Widely scattered throughout an organ, tissue, or the body.

dissocia'tion [L. dis-socio, pp. -atus, to disjoin, separate] 1. The change of a complex into a more simple chemical compound by any lytic reaction or by ionization. 2. An unconscious process by which a group of mental processes is separated from the rest of the thinking processes, resulting in an independent functioning of these processes and a loss of the usual relationships.

dis'tal [L. distalis] 1. Situated away from the centre of the body, or from the point of origin; applied to the extremity or distant part of a limb or organ. 2. In dentistry, away from the median sagittal plane of the face, following the curvature of the dental arch.

disten'sion [L. dis-tendere, to stretch apart] The act or state of being distended or stretched.

distomi'asis Presence in any of the organs or tissues of a fluke formerly known as Distoma or Distomum; in general, infection by any parasitic trematode or fluke.

distribu'tion [L. dis-tribuo, pp. -tributus, to distribute] 1. Passage of the branches of arteries or nerves to the tissues and organs. 2. The area in which the branches of an artery or a nerve terminate, or the area supplied by such artery or nerve.

disulf'iram An antioxidant that interferes with the normal metabolic degradation of alcohol in the body, resulting in increased acetaldehyde concentrations in blood and tissues; used in the treatment of chronic alcoholism. When a small quantity of alcohol is consumed an unpleasant reaction results.

diuret'ic Promoting the excretion of urine.

diur'nal [L. diurnus, of the day] 1. Pertaining to the daylight hours; opposite of nocturnal. 2. Repeating once each 24 hours, as a d. rhythm.

divertic'ula Plural of diverticulum.

diverticulec'tomy Excision of a diverticulum.

diverticuli'tis Inflammation of a diverticulum, especially of the small pockets in the wall of the colon which fill with stagnant faecal material and become inflamed.

diverticulo'sis Presence of a number of diverticula of the intestine.

divertic'ulum, pl. **divertic'ula** [L. deverticulum (or di-), a by-road] [NA] A pouch or sac opening from a tubular or saccular organ, such as the gut or bladder.

divul'sion [L. di-vello, pp. -vulvus, to pull apart] 1. Removal of a part by tearing. 2. Forcible dilation of the walls of a cavity or canal.

dizygot'ic [G. di-, two, + zygotos, yoked together] Relating to twins derived from two separate zygotes.

diz'ziness [A. S. dyzig, foolish] Imprecise term commonly used to describe various peculiar subjective symptoms such as faintness, giddiness, light-headedness, or unsteadiness. See also vertigo.

DNA Deoxyribonucleic acid.

dolicho- [G. dolichos, long] Combining form meaning long.

dolichocephal'ic [dolicho- + G. kephale, head] Having a disproportionately long head.

dolichopel'lic, dolichopel'vic [dolicho- + G. pellis, bowl (pelvis)] Having a disproportionately long pelvis.

dom'inance The state of being dominant.

d. of genes, an expression of the apparent physiologic relationship existing between two or more genes that may occupy the same chromosome locus (alleles); *e.g.*, if a heterozygous individual presents only the hereditary characteristic determined by one gene, while the effect of the other gene is not apparent, the former is said to be dominant and the latter is said to be recessive. D. relationships may in some cases be modified by environmental factors and in a series of multiple alleles, complex d. relationships may exist.

dom'inant [L. pres. p. of *dominor*, pp. -*atus*, to rule] **1.** Ruling or controlling. **2.** In genetics, denoting an allele possessed by one of the parents of a hybrid which is expressed in the latter to the exclusion of a contrasting allele (the recessive) from the other parent.

do'nor [L. *dono*, pp. *donatus*, to donate, to give] **1.** An individual from whom blood, tissue, or an organ is taken for transplantation. **2.** A compound that will transfer an atom or a radical to an acceptor. **3.** An atom that readily yields electrons to an acceptor.

universal d., in blood grouping, a person belonging to group O; *i.e.*, one whose erythrocytes do not contain either agglutinogen A or B and are, therefore, not agglutinated by plasma containing either of the ordinary isoagglutinins, alpha or beta.

do'pa (Dopa, DOPA) An intermediate in the catabolism of phenylalanine and tyrosine, and in the biosynthesis of noradrenaline, adrenaline, and melanin. The L form (laevodopa) is biologically active.

do'pamine An intermediate in tyrosine metabolism and the precursor of noradrenaline and adrenaline present in the central nervous system and localized in the basal ganglia (caudate and lentiform nuclei).

dor'sal [Mediev. L. *dorsalis*, fr. *dorsum*, back] **1.** Pertaining to the back or any dorsum. **2.** In human anatomy, synonymous with posterior (2). **3.** In veterinary anatomy, pertaining to the back or upper surface of an animal; often used to indicate the position of one structure relative to another. **4.** Old term meaning thoracic, in a limited sense; *e.g.*, dorsal vertebrae.

dorsal'gia [L. *dorsum*, back, + G. *algos*, pain] Pain in the upper back.

dorsiflex'ion Turning of the foot or the toes upward.

dor'sum, gen. **dor'si,** pl. **dor'sa** [L. back] [NA] **1.** The back of the body. **2.** The upper or posterior surface, or the back, of any part.

do'sage 1. The giving of medicine or other therapeutic agent in prescribed amounts. **2.** The determination of the proper dose of a remedy; often incorrectly used for *dose*.

dose [G. *dosis, a giving,* fr. +IL *didōmi,* fut. *dōsō,* to give] The quantity of a drug or other remedy to be taken or applied within a given period.

dosim'etry [G. *dosis,* dose, + *metron,* measure] The accurate determination of dosage.

douche [Fr. fr. *doucher,* to pour] **1.** A current of water, gas, or vapour directed against the surface or projected into a cavity. **2.** An instrument for giving a d. **3.** To apply a d.

draconti'asis [G. *drakōn* (*drakont*-), dragon] Infection with *Dracunculus medinensis.*

Dracun'culus [L. dim. of *draco,* serpent] A genus of nematodes (superfamily Dracunculoidea) that have some resemblances to true filarial worms. *D. medinensis* is a species of skin-infecting, yard-long parasites, the females of which migrate along fascial planes to subcutaneous tissues, where chronic ulcers are formed in the skin.

drain [A. S. *drehnian,* to draw off] **1.** To draw off fluid from a cavity as it forms. **2.** A device, usually in the shape of a tube or wick, for removing fluid as it collects in a cavity, wound, or infected area.

dres'sing Material applied, or its application, to a wound for protection, absorbance, drainage, etc.

drip 1. To flow a drop at a time. **2.** A flowing in drops.

intravenous d., continuous introduction of solutions intravenously, a drop at a time.

postnasal d., the sensation of excessive mucoid or mucopurulent discharge from the posterior nares.

drive A basic compelling urge; in psychology, classified as innate (*e.g.,* hunger), learned (*e.g.,* hoarding) and appetitive (*e.g.,* hunger, thirst, sex), or aversive (*e.g.,* fear, pain, grief).

drop'sical Relating to or suffering from dropsy.

drop'sy [G. *hydrōps*] An old term for oedema.

drug 1. A therapeutic agent; any substance, other than food, used in the prevention, diagnosis, alleviation, treatment, or cure of disease. **2.** To give or take a d., usually implying an overly large quantity. **3.** To narcotize.

drug interac'tions The pharmacological result, either desirable or undesirable, of drugs interacting with themselves or other drugs, with endogenous physiologic chemical agents; with components of the diet, and with chemicals used in diagnostic tests or the results of such tests.

duct [L. *duco*, pp. *ductus*, to lead] A tubular structure giving exit to the secretion of a gland, or conducting any fluid. See also canal.

   bile d., biliary d., any of the d.'s conveying bile between the liver and the intestine, including the hepatic, cystic, and common bile d.'s.

duc'tal Relating to a duct.

duct'less Having no duct; denoting certain glands having only an internal secretion.

duc'tus, pl. **duc'tus** [L. a leading, fr. *duco*, pp. *ductus*, to lead] [NA] Duct.

   d. arterio'sus [NA], arterial canal or duct; a fetal vessel connecting the left pulmonary artery with the descending aorta; after birth, it normally becomes changed into a fibrous cord, the ligamentum arteriosum; occasional failure to close postnatally causes a cardiovascular handicap (patent d. arteriosus) that can be surgically corrected.

   d. def'erens [NA], vas deferens; the secretory duct of the testicle, running from the epididymis, of which it is the continuation, to the prostatic urethra where it terminates as the ejaculatory duct.

duode'nal Relating to the duodenum.

duodeno- [L. *duodenum*] Combining form relating to the duodenum.

duode'noenteros'tomy [duodeno- + G. *enteron*, intestine, + *stoma*, mouth] Establishment of communication between the duodenum and another part of the intestinal tract.

duode'nojejunos'tomy [duodeno- + jejunum, + G. *stoma*, mouth] The operative formation of an artificial communication between the duodenum and the jejunum.

duodenos'tomy [duodeno- + G. *stoma*, mouth] Establishment of a fistula into the duodenum.

duode'num, gen. **duode'ni,** pl. **duode'na** [Mediev. L. fr. L. *duodeni*, twelve] [NA] The first division of the small intestine, about 25 cm or 12 fingerbreadths (hence the name) in length, extending from the pylorus to the junction with the jejunum at the level of the first or second lumbar vertebra on the left side.

du'ral Relating to the dura mater.

du'ra ma'ter [L. hard mother] A tough, fibrous membrane forming the outer envelope of the brain and the spinal cord.

dwarf [A.S. *dweorh*] A markedly undersized person.

dwarf'ism The condition of being markedly undersized.

   mesomelic d., d. with shortness of the forearms and lower legs.

   pituitary d., a rare form of d. caused by the absence of a functional anterior pituitary gland.

-dymus [g. -*dymos*, fold] **1.** Suffix combined with number roots; *e.g.*, didymus, tridymus. **2.** An occasionally used shortened form for -didymus.

dynam'ics [G. *dynamis*, force] **1.** The science of motion in response to forces. **2.** In psychiatry, the determination of how behaviour patterns and emotional reactions develop. **3.** In the behavioural sciences, any of the numerous intrapersonal and interpersonal influences or phenomena associated with personality development and interpersonal processes.

dynamo- [G *dynamis*, force] Combining form relating to force or energy.

dynamom'eter [dynamo- + G. *metron*, measure] An instrument for measuring the degree of muscular power.

dys- [G] Prefix meaning bad or difficult. Cf dis-.

dysaesthe'sia [G. *dysaisthesia*, fr. *dys-*, hard, difficult, + *aisthēsis*, sensation] **1.** Impairment of sensation short of anaesthesia. **2.** A condition in which a disagreeable sensation is produced by ordinary stimuli.

dysar'thria [dys- + G. *arthroō*, to articulate] Disturbance of articulation due to emotional stress or to paralysis, incoordination, or spasticity of muscles.

dysarthro'sis [dys- + G. *arthrōsis*, joint] **1.** Dysarthria. **2.** Malformation of a joint. **3.** A false joint.

dysautono'mia [dys- + G. *autonomia*, self-government] Abnormal functioning of the autonomic nervous system.

dysbar'ism [dys- + G. *baros*, weight] The symptom complex resulting from exposure to decreased or changing barometric pressure, including all physiologic effects resulting from such changes with the exception of hypoxia, and including the effects of rapid decompression.

dyschei'ria, dyschi'ria [dys- + G. *cheir*, hand] A disorder of sensibility in which, although there is no apparent loss of sensation, the patient is unable to tell which side of the body has been touched (acheiria), or refers it to the wrong side (allocheiria), or to both sides (syncheiria).

dysche'zia [dys- + G. *chezō*, to defaecate] Difficulty in defaecation.

dyschon'drogen'esis [dys- + G. *chondros*, cartilage, + *genesis*, production] Abnormal development of cartilage.

dyschon'dropla'sia [dys- + G. *chondros*, cartilage, + *plasis*, a forming] Enchondromatosis.

dyschon'drosteo'sis [dys- + G. *chondros*, cartilage, + *osteon*, bone, + *-osis*, condition] A bone dysplasia characterized by bowing of the radius, dorsal dislocation of the distal ulna and proximal carpal bones, and mesomelic dwarfism; autosomal dominant inheritance.

dyschromatop'sia [dys- + G. *chrōma*, colour, + *opsis*, vision] Dichromatism (2).

dyscra'sia [G. bad temperament] **1.** A morbid general state. **2.** An old term to indicate disease.

    blood d., a diseased state of the blood; usually refers to abnormal cellular elements of permanent character.

dys'entery [G. *dysenteria*, fr. *dys-*, bad, + *entera*, bowels] A disease marked by frequent watery stools, often with blood and mucus, abdominal pain, tenesmus, fever, and dehydration.

    amoebic d., diarrhoea resulting from ulcerative inflammation of the colon, caused chiefly by *Entamoeba hystolytica*.

    bacillary d., d. caused by infection with *Shigella dysenteriae*, *Shigella flexneri*, or other organisms.

dysfibrin'ogenae'mia A familial disorder of qualitatively abnormal fibrinogens; various types are classified according to the major defect, thrombin time, effect on clotting, and symptoms such as bleeding and thrombosis.

dysfunc'tion Difficult or abnormal function.

    minimal brain d., a mild degree of impaired cerebration which may be manifested by dyslexia, dysgraphia, hyperactivity, and/or mental retardation.

dysgam'maglob'ulinae'mia An immunoglobulin abnormality, especially a disturbance of the percentage distribution of γ-globulins.

dysgen'esis [dys- + G. *genesis*, generation] Defective embryonic development.

dysgermino'ma [dys- + L. *germen*, a bud or sprout, + G. *-oma*, tumour] A rare malignant neoplasm of the ovary, a counterpart of seminoma of the testis, composed of undifferentiated gonadal germinal cells.

dysgeu'sia [dys- + G. *geusis*, taste] Impairment or perversion of the gustatory sense.

dyshidro'sis [dys- + G. *hidrōs*, sweat] A vesicular or vesicopustular eruption that occurs primarily on the hands and feet; the lesions spread peripherally but have a tendency to central clearing.

dyskerato'sis [dys- + G. *keras*, horn, + *-osis*, condition] **1.** Appearance of premature keratinization in individual cells that have not reached the keratinizing surface layer. **2.** Epidermalization of the conjunctival and corneal epithelium.

dyskine'sia [dys- + G. *kinēsis*, movement] Difficulty in performing voluntary movements.

    tardive oral d., involuntary movement of the lips or jaw and other dystonic gestures; an extrapyramidal effect of certain psychotropic drug treatments.

dysla'lia [dys- + G. *lalia*, talking] Disorder of articulation due to structural abnormalities of the articulatory organs or impaired hearing.

dyslex'ia [dys- + G. *lexis*, word, phrase] A level of reading ability markedly below that expected on the basis of the individual's level of over-all intelligence or ability in skills.

dysmatur'ity Syndrome of an infant born with relative absence of subcutaneous fat, wrinkling of the skin, prominent fingernails and toenails, and meconium staining of the dysmelia / dystrophy — page 105

dysmelia [dys- + G. *melos*, limb] A congenital abnormality characterized by missing or foreshortened extremities, sometimes with associated spinal abnormalities.

dysmenorrhoea [dys- + G. *mēn*, month, + *rhoia*, a flow] Difficult and painful menstruation.

dysmorphism [G. *dysmorphia*, badness of form] Abnormality of shape.

dysostosis [dys- + G. *osteon*, bone, + *-osis*, condition] Defective bone formation.

craniofacial d., Crouzon's disease; cranial stenosis with widening of the skull and high forehead, ocular hypertelorism, exophthalmos, beaked nose, and hypoplasia of the maxilla; usually autosomal dominant inheritance.

dyspareunia [dys- + G. *pareunos*, lying beside, fr. *para*, beside, + *eunē*, a bed] The occurrence of pain during sexual intercourse.

dyspepsia [dys- + G. *pepsis*, digestion] Gastric indigestion; impaired digestion or "upset stomach" due to some disorder of the stomach.

dyspeptic Relating to or suffering from dyspepsia.

dysphagia, dysphagy [dys- + G. *phagein*, to eat] Difficulty in swallowing.

dysphasia [dys- + G. *phasis*, speaking] Lack of coordination in speech, and failure to arrange words in an understandable way; due to cortical lesion.

dysphonia [dys- + G. *phōnē*, voice] Difficulty or pain in speaking.

dysphoria [G. extreme discomfort, fr. *dys-*, difficult, bad, + *phora*, a bearing] A feeling of unpleasantness or discomfort.

dysplasia [dys- + G. *plasis*, a moulding] Abnormal tissue development.

dysplastic Pertaining to or marked by dysplasia.

dyspnoea [G. *dyspnoia*, fr. *dys-*, bad, + *pnoē*, breathing] Shortness of breath, a subjective difficulty or distress in breathing.

paroxysmal nocturnal d., acute d. appearing suddenly at night, usually waking the patient after an hour or two of sleep; caused by pulmonary congestion and oedema which result from left-sided heart failure.

dyspnoeic Relating to or suffering from dyspnoea.

dyspraxia [dys- + G. *praxis*, a doing] Impaired or painful functioning in any organ.

dysraphism, dysraphia [dys- + g. *raphē*, suture] Defective fusion of a raphe, especially of the neural folds.

dysrhythmia [dys- + G. *rhythmos*, rhythm] Defective rhythm.

cardiac d., any abnormality in the rate, regularity, or sequence of cardiac activation.

electroencephalographic d., a diffusely irregular brain wave tracing.

dysspermatism, dysspermia [dys- + G. *sperma*, seed] Occurrence of pain or discomfort in the discharge of seminal fluid.

dysstasia [dys- + G. *stasis*, standing] Difficulty in standing.

dysstatic Characterized by dysstasia.

dyssynergia [dys- + G. *syn*, with, + *ergon*, work] Ataxia.

d. cerebellaris myoclonica, an affection with symptoms similar to those of d. cerebellaris progressiva, with the addition of myoclonus and epilepsy.

d. cerebellaris progressiva, Hunt's *syndrome* (1).

dyssystole A defective cardiac systole.

dystaxia [dys- + G. *taxis*, order] A mild degree of ataxia.

dysthymia [dys- + G. *thymos*, mind, emotion] Any disorder of mood.

dystocia [G. *dystokia*, fr. dys-, difficult, + *tokos*, childbirth] Difficult childbirth.

dystonia [dys- + G. *tonos*, tension] Abnormal tonicity in any of the tissues.

dystonic Pertaining to dystonia.

dystopia [dys- + G. *topos*, place] Malposition, faulty or abnormal position of a part or of the body.

dystopic Pertaining to, or characterized by, dystopia. See also ectopic.

dystrophia [L. fr. G. dys-, bad, + *trophē*, nourishment] Dystrophy.

d. adiposogenitalis, a disorder characterized primarily by obesity and genital hypoplasia; when caused by an adenohypophyseal tumour it is called Frölich's syndrome; may also be caused by hypothalamic lesions in areas regulating appetite and gonadal development.

dystrophic Relating to dystrophy.

dystrophy [dys- + G. *trophē*, nourishment] Defective nutrition.

adiposogenital d., *dystrophia adiposogenitalis.*

childhood muscular d., pseudohypertrophic muscular d.

Duchenne's d., pseudohypertrophic muscular d.

facioscapulohumeral muscular d., Landouzy-Déjérine d., a relatively benign type of d. commencing in childhood and characterized by wasting and weakness, mainly of the muscles of the face, shoulder girdle, and arms; autosomal dominant inheritance.

muscular d., inborn abnormality of muscle associated with dysfunction and ultimately with deterioration.

pseudohypertrophic muscular d., a type of muscular d. occurring in males in childhood; characterized by muscular weakness in the pelvic girdle that spreads with relative rapidity to the musculature of the pectoral girdle, trunk, and extremities, muscular pseudohypertrophy, and contractures of muscle and tendon; X-linked recessive inheritance.

dysu'ria [dys- + G. *ouron,* urine] Difficulty or pain in urination.

dysu'ric Relating to or suffering from dysuria.

dysver'sion [dys- + L. *verto,* to turn] A turning in any direction, less than inversion; particularly d. of the optic nerve head (situs inversus of the optic disc).

E

ear [A.S. *eáre*] The organ of hearing: composed of the **external e.,** which includes the auricle and the external acoustic, or auditory, meatus; the **middle e.,** or the tympanic cavity with its ossicles; and the **internal** or **inner e.,** or labyrinth, which includes the semicircular canals, vestibule, and cochlea.

ear'ache Otalgia; pain in the ear.

ear'drum *Membrana* tympani.

eburna'tion [L. *eburneus,* of ivory] A change in exposed subchondral bone in degenerative joint disease in which it is converted into a dense, smooth substance like ivory.

ec- Prefix fr. G. preposition meaning out of, away from.

eccen'tric [G. *ek,* out, + *kentron,* centre] **1.** Abnormal or peculiar in ideas, actions, or speech. **2.** Proceeding from a centre. **3.** Peripheral.

eccen'trochondropla'sia [G. *ek,* out + *kentron,* centre, + *chondros,* cartilage, + *plasis,* a moulding] Abnormal epiphyseal development from eccentric centres of ossification.

ecchondro'ma [G. *ek,* from, + *chondros,* cartilage, + *-oma,* tumour] **1.** A cartilaginous neoplasm arising as an overgrowth from normally situated cartilage, as a mass protruding from the articular surface of a bone. **2.** An enchondroma that has burst through the shaft of a bone and become pedunculated.

ecchondro'sis Ecchondroma.

ecchymo'ma [G. *ek,* out, + *chymos,* juice, + *-oma,* tumour] A slight haematoma following a bruise.

ec'chymosed Characterized by or affected with ecchymosis.

ecchymo'sis, pl. **ecchymo'ses** [G. *ekchymōsis,* ecchymosis, fr. *ek,* out, + *chymos,* juice] A purplish patch caused by extravasation of blood into the skin, differing from petechiae only in size.

ecchymot'ic Relating to an ecchymosis.

ec'crine [G. *ek-krino,* to secrete] **1.** Exocrine (1). **2.** Denoting the flow of sweat.

ec'crisis [G. separation] **1.** The removal of waste products. **2.** Any waste product; excrement.

eccrit'ic Promoting the expulsion of waste matters.

eccye'sis [G. *ek,* out, + *kyēsis,* pregnancy] Ectopic *pregnancy.*

ecdem'ic [G. *ekdēmos,* foreign, from home] Denoting a disease brought into a region from without, not epidemic or endemic.

echino-, echin- [G. *echinos,* hedgehog, sea urchin] Combining forms meaning prickly or spiny.

echi'nococco'sis Infection with *Echinococcus;* larval infection is hydatid *disease.*

Echinococ'cus [echino- + G. *kokkos,* a berry] A genus of very small taeniid tapeworms. Adults are found in various carnivores but not in man; larvae, in the form of hydatid cysts, are found in the liver and other organs of ruminants, rodents, and, under certain epidemiological circumstances, man.

echoacou'sia [echo + G. *akouō,* to hear] A subjective disturbance of hearing in which a sound heard appears to be repeated.

echoaortog'raphy [echo + aortography] Application of ultrasound techniques to the diagnosis and study of the aorta, particularly the abdominal aorta.

echocar'diogram The ultrasonic record obtained by echocardiography.

echocardiog'raphy [echo + cardiography] Ultrasound cardiography. Use of ultrasound in the diagnosis of cardiovascular lesions and recording of the size, motion, and composition of various cardiac structures.

ech'oencephalog'raphy [echo + encephalography] Use of reflected ultrasound in the diagnosis of intracranial processes.

ech'ogram [echo + G gramma, a diagram] Ultrasonic display of reflection techniques appropriate for any field of application, but applied especially to the heart.

echog'raphy [echo + G. graphō, to write] Ultrasonography.

echola'lia [echo + G. lalia, a form of speech] Involuntary repetition of a word or sentence just spoken by another person.

echomim'ia [echo + G. mimēsis, imitation] Echopathy.

echop'athy [echo + G. pathos, suffering] A mental disorder in which the words or actions of another are imitated and repeated by the patient.

echophra'sia [echo + phrasis, speech] Echolalia.

echoprax'ia [echo + G. praxis, action] The involuntary imitation of movements made by another.

ech'ovirus ECHO virus.

eclamp'sia [G. eklampsis, a shining forth] Occurrence of one or more convulsions, not attributable to other cerebral conditions such as epilepsy or cerebral haemorrhage, in a patient with pre-eclampsia.

   puerperal e., convulsions and coma associated with hypertension, oedema, or proteinuria occurring in a woman following delivery.

eclamp'sism A state in which general signs point to the early occurrence of puerperal eclampsia, but convulsions do not take place.

eclamp'tic. Relating to eclampsia.

eclamptogen'ic Causing eclampsia.

ecmne'sia [G. ek, out, + mnēsis, relating to memory] Loss of memory for recent events.

eco- [G. oikos, house, household, habitation] Combining form denoting relationship to environment.

ecol'ogy [eco- + G. logos, study] The branch of biology concerned with the total complex of interrelationships among living organisms, encompassing the relations of organisms to each other, to the environment, and to the entire energy balance within a given ecosystem.

ecphy'ma [G. a pimply eruption] A warty growth or protuberance.

écraseur' [Fr. écraser, to crush] A snare, especially one of great strength for cutting through the base or pedicle of a tumour.

ect-. See ecto-.

ec'tad [G. ektos, outside, + L. ad, to] Outward.

ec'tal [G. ektos, outside] Outer; external.

-ectasia, -ectasis [G. ektasis, a stretching] Combining form in suffix position used to denote dilation or expansion.

ecta'sia, ec'tasis [G. ektasis, a stretching.] Dilation of a tubular structure.

ectat'ic Relating to or marked by ectasis.

ecthy'ma [G. a pustule] A pyogenic infection of the skin due to staphylococci or streptococci and characterized by adherent crusts beneath which ulceration occurs.

ecto-, ect- [G. ektos, outside] Combining forms denoting outer, on the outside. See also exo-.

ec'toblast [ecto + G. blastos, germ] Ectoderm.

ectocar'dia [ecto- + G. kardia, heart] Congenital displacement of the heart.

ec'toderm [ecto- + G. derma, skin] The outer layer of cells in the embryo, after the establishing of the primary germ layers.

ectoder'mal, ectoder'mic Relating to the ectoderm.

ec'todermo'sis A disorder of any organ or tissue developed from the ectoderm.

ectoen'zyme An enzyme that is excreted externally.

ectog'enous [ecto- + G. -gen, producing] Exogenous.

ec'tomorph [ecto- + G. morphē, form] A constitutional body type or build in which tissues that originated from the ectoderm prevail; from the morphological standpoint, the limbs predominate over the trunk.

-ectomy [G. *ektomē*, excision] Combining form used as a suffix to denote removal of any anatomical structure. See also -tomy.

ectopar'asite A parasite that lives on the surface of the host body.

ec'tophyte [ecto- + G. *phyton*, plant] A plant parasite of the skin.

ecto'pia [G. *ektopos*, out of place, fr. *ektos*, outside, + *topos*, place] Congenital displacement of any organ or part of the body.

    e. cor'dis, congenital condition in which the heart is exposed on the chest wall because of maldevelopment of the sternum and pericardium.

    e. len'tis, displacement of the lens of the eye.

ectop'ic [see ectopia] **1.** Out of place; said of an organ that is not in its proper position, or of a pregnancy occurring elsewhere than in the cavity of the uterus. **2.** In cardiography, denoting a heart beat that has its origin in a focus other than the sinoatrial node.

ec'topy Ectopia.

ectos'teal [ecto- + G. *osteon* bone] Relating to the external surface of a bone.

ectos'tosis [ecto- + G. *osteon*, bone, + *-osis*, condition] Ossification in cartilage beneath the perichondrium, or the formation of bone beneath the periosteum.

ectozo'on [ecto- + G. *zōon*, animal] An animal parasite living on the surface of the body.

ectro- [G. *ektrōsis*, miscarriage] Combining form denoting congenital absence of a part.

ectrodac'tyly, ec'trodactyl'ia, ectrodac'tylism [ectro- + G. *dactylos*, finger] Congenital absence of one or more fingers or toes.

ectrogen'ic. Relating to ectrogeny.

ectrog'eny [ectro- + G. *-gen*, producing] Congenital absence of any part.

ectrome'lia [ectro- + G. *melos*, limb] Congenital absence of one or more limbs.

ectromel'ic. Pertaining to, or characterized by, ectromelia.

ectro'pion [G. *ek*, out, + *tropē*, a turning] A rolling outward of the margin of a part.

ec'trosyndac'tyly [ectro- + G. *syn*, together, + *dactylos*, finger] A congenital deformity marked by the absence of one or more digits and the fusion of others.

ec'zema [G. fr. *ekzeō*, to boil over] Generic term for acute or chronic inflammatory conditions of the skin, typically erythematous, oedematous, papular, vesicular, and crusting; followed often by lichenification and scaling, occasionally by duskiness of the erythema, and infrequently hyperpigmentation; often accompanied by sensations of itching and burning.

eczem'atoid Resembling eczema in appearance.

eczem'atous Marked by or resembling eczema.

eden'tate [L. *edentatus*] Toothless.

eden'tulous [L. *edentulus*, toothless] Toothless; without teeth.

effect' [L. *ef-ficio*, pp. *effectus*, to accomplish] The result or consequence of an action.

    additive e., an e. wherein two substances or actions used in combination produce a total e. the same as the sum of the individual e.'s.

    cumulative e., the condition in which repeated administration of a drug may produce e.'s that are more pronounced than those produced by the first dose.

effec'tor [L. producer] A peripheral tissue that receives nerve impulses and reacts by contraction (muscle) or secretion (gland).

effemina'tion [L. *ef-femino*, pp. *-atus*, to make feminine, fr. *ex*, out, + *femina*, woman] Acquisition of feminine characteristics, either physiologically by women, or pathologically by individuals of either sex.

ef'ferent [L. *efferens*, fr. *effero*, to bring out] Conducting outward from a given organ or part thereof.

effloresce' [L. *ef-floresco*, to blossom] To become powdery by losing the water of crystallization on exposure to a dry atmosphere.

efflu'vium, pl. **efflu'via** [L. a flowing out] **1.** A shedding, especially of hair. **2.** Obsolete term for an exhalation, especially one of bad odour or injurious influence.

effu'sion [L. *effusio*, a pouring out] **1.** The escape of fluid from the blood vessels or lymphatics into the tissues or a cavity. **2.** The fluid so escaped.

egest' [L. *e-gero*, pp. *-gestus,* to carry out, discharge] To discharge unabsorbed food residues from the digestive tract.

eges'ta Matter that is egested.

egg [A.S. *aeg*] The female sexual cell or gamete; after fertilization and fusion of the pronuclei it is a zygote. See also oocyte, ovum.

e'go [L. I] In psychoanalysis, one of the three components of the psychic apparatus in the freudian structural framework, the other two being the id and superego. Although the e. has some conscious components, many of its functions are learned and automatic. It occupies a position between the primal instincts (pleasure principle) and the demands of the outer world (reality principle), and mediates between the person and external reality, and is also responsible for certain defensive functions to protect the person against the demands of the id and superego.

ego-dyston'ic [ego + G. *dys*, bad, + *tonos*, tension] Repugnant to or at variance with the aims of the ego.

egoma'nia [ego + G. *mania*, frenzy] Extreme self-appeciation or self-content.

ego-synton'ic [ego + G. *syn*, together, + *tonos*, tension] Acceptable to the aims of the ego.

eidoptom'etry [G. *eidos*, form, + *optikos*, referring to vision, + *metron*, measure] The measurement of the acuteness of form vision.

Eime'ria [Theodor *Eimer*] The largest, most economically important, and most widespread genus of the coccidial protozoa (family Eimeriidae, class Sporozoa); highly pathogenic, especially in young domesticated mammals and birds.

ejac'ulate. **1.** To expel suddenly, as semen. **2.** Semen expelled in ejaculation.

ejacula'tio [L.] Ejaculation.

    e. prae'cox, premature *ejaculation*.

ejacula'tion [L. *ejaculatio*] Emission of seminal fluid.

    premature e., during sexual intercourse, too rapid achievement of climax and e. in the male relative to his own or his partner's wishes.

ejac'ulatory. Relating to an ejaculation.

ejec'ta [L. ntr. pl. of *ejectus*, pp. of *ejicio*, to throw out] Ejection (2).

ejec'tion [L. *ejectio*, from *ejicio*, to cast out] **1.** The act of driving or throwing out by physical force from within. **2.** That which is ejected.

elas'tance A measure of the tendency of a hollow viscus to recoil toward its original dimensions upon removal of a distending or compressing force, the recoil pressure resulting from a unit distension or compression of the viscus; the reciprocal of compliance.

elas'tic [G. *elastreō*, epic form of *elaunō*, drive, push] Having the property of returning to the original shape after being distorted.

elastic'ity The quality or condition of being elastic.

elas'tofibro'ma A nonencapsulated slow-growing mass of poorly cellular, collagenous, fibrous tissue and elastic tissue; occurs usually in subscapular adipose tissue of elderly persons.

elastorrhex'is [G. *rhēxis*, rupture] Fragmentation of elastic tissue in which the normal wavy strands appear shredded and clumped.

elasto'sis **1.** Degenerative change in elastic tissue. **2.** Degeneration of collagen fibres, with altered staining properties resembling elastic tissue.

el'bow [A.S. *elnboga*] **1.** The joint between the arm and the forearm. **2.** An angular body resembling a flexed e.

    tennis e., pain in or near the lateral epicondyle of the humerus, and lateral epicondylitis, as a result of unusual strain (not necessarily from playing tennis).

electro- [G. *ēlektron*, amber (on which static electricity can be generated by friction)] Prefix denoting electric or electricity.

elec'troanalge'sia Analgesia induced by the passage of an electric current.

elec'troanaesthe'sia Anaesthesia produced by an electric current.

elec'trobiol'ogy The science concerned with electrical phenomena in living organisms.

electrocar'diogram **(ECG, EKG)** [electro- + G. *kardia*, heart, + *gramma*, a drawing] The graphic record of the heart's action currents obtained with the electrocardiograph.

elec'trocar'diograph An instrument for recording the potential of the electrical currents that traverse the heart and initiate its contraction.

elec'trocardiograph'ic Relating to an electrocardiograph.

elec'trocardiog'raphy **1.** A method of recording electrical currents traversing the heart muscle just previous to each heart beat. **2.** The study and interpretation of electrocardiograms.

elec'trocauteriza'tion Cauterization by an electrocautery.

electrocau'tery 1. An instrument for directing a high frequency current through a local area of tissue. 2. A metal cauterizing instrument heated by electricity.

electrochem'ical Relating to chemical reactions effected by means of electricity and the mechanisms involved.

elec'trocoagula'tion Coagulation produced by an electrocautery.

elec'trocontractil'ity. The power of contraction of muscular tissue in response to an electrical stimulus.

elec'troconvul'sive Denoting a convulsive response to an electrical stimulus. See electroshock *therapy*.

electrocor'ticogram The record obained by electrocorticography.

elec'trocorticog'raphy The technique of surveying the electrical activity of the cerebral cortex.

elec'trode [electro- + G. *hodos*, way] 1. One of the two extremities of an electric circuit; one of the two poles of an electric battery or of the end of the conductors connected thereto. 2. An electrical terminal specialized for a particular electrochemical reaction.

electroder'mal [electro- + G. *derma*, skin] Pertaining to electric properties of the skin, usually referring to altered resistance.

elec'trodesicca'tion [electro- + L. *desicco*, to dry up] Destruction of lesions or sealing off of blood vessels by monopolar high frequency electric current.

elec'trodiagno'sis Determination of the nature of a disease through observation of changes in electrical irritability.

electrodial'ysis The removal in an electric field of ions from larger molecules and particles.

elec'troenceph'alogram (EEG) The record obtained by means of the electroencephalograph.

elec'troenceph'alograph [electro- + G. *encephalon*, brain, + *graphō*, to write] An apparatus for recording the electric potentials of the brain derived from electrodes attached to the scalp.

elec'troencephalog'raphy Registration the electrical potentials recorded by an electroencephalograph.

elec'trogram 1. Any record made by an electrical event. 2. In electrophysiology, a recording taken directly from the surface by unipolar or bipolar leads.

elec'trohaemos'tasis [electro- + G. *haima*, blood, + *stasis*, halt] Arrest of haemorrhage by means of the electrocautery.

electroky'mogram (EKY) The graphic record produced by the electrokymograph.

electroky'mograph An apparatus for recording, from changes in the x-ray silhouette, the movements of the heart and great vessels.

electrokymog'raphy [electro- + G. *kyma*, wave, + *graphō*, to write] 1. The registration of the movements of the heart and great vessels by means of the electrokymograph. 2. The science and technique of interpreting electrokymograms.

electrol'ysis [electro- + G. *lysis*, dissolution] 1. Decomposition of a salt or other chemical compound by means of an electric current. 2. Destruction of certain body tissues by means of galvanic electricity.

elec'trolyte [electro- + G. *lytos*, soluble] Any compound that, in solution, conducts a current in electricity and is decomposed by it; an ionizable substance in solution.

electrolyt'ic Referring to or caused by electrolysis.

electromy'ogram (EMG) The graphic representation produced by an electromyograph.

electromy'ograph An instrument used in electromyography.

electromyog'raphy [electro- + G. *mys*, muscle, + *graphō*, to write] A method of recording the electrical currents generated in an active muscle.

elec'tron One of the negatively charged subatomic particles that, distributed about the positive nucleus, constitute the atom.

elec'tronarco'sis Production of insensibility to pain by the use of electrical current.

elec'tronystagmog'raphy (ENG) [electro- + nystagmus + G. *graphō*, to write] A method of nystagmography in which skin electrodes are placed at outer canthi to register horizontal nystagmus or above and below each eye for vertical nystagmus.

elec'trophore'sis [electro- + G. *phorēsis*, a carrying] The movement of particles in an electric field toward one or other electric pole, anode, or cathode.

elec'trophoret'ic Relating to electrophoresis.

electroret'inogram (ERG) [electro- + retina + G. *gramma*, something written] A record of the retinal action currents produced in the retina by an adequate light stimulus.

elec'troretinog'raphy The recording and study of the retinal action currents.

elec'troshock See electroshock *therapy*.

electrosur'gery Division of tissues by high frequency current applied locally with an instrument or needle.

elec'trotherapeu'tics, electrother'apy Use of electricity in the treatment of disease.

electroto'nus [electro- + G. *tonos*, tension] Changes in excitability and conductivity in a nerve or muscle cell caused by the passage of a constant electric current.

elec'tuary [G. *eleikton*, a medicine that melts in the mouth, fr. *eleichō*, to lick up] Confection.

el'ement [L. *elementum*, a rudiment, beginning] **1.** A substance composed of atoms of only one kind, *i.e.*, of identical atomic number, that therefore cannot be decomposed into two or more substances, and that can lose its chemical property only by union with some other e. **2.** An indivisible structure or entity

    trace e.'s., e.'s present in minute amounts in the body; many are essential in metabolism or for the manufacture of essential compounds.

el'ephanti'asis [G. fr. *elephas*, elephant] Hypertrophy and fibrosis of the skin and subcutaneous and lymphoid tissue due to longstanding obstructed circulation in the blood or lymphatic vessels, chiefly by the presence of the filarial worms *Wuchereria bancrofti* or *Brugia malayi*.

el'evator [L. fr. *e-levo*, pp. *-atus*, to lift up] **1.** An instrument for prying up a sunken part, as the depressed fragment of bone in fracture of the skull, or for elevating tissues. **2.** An instrument used to luxate and remove teeth and roots that cannot be engaged by the beaks of a forceps, or to loosen teeth and roots prior to forceps application.

elimina'tion [L. *elimino*, pp. *-atus*, to turn out of doors] Expulsion; removal of waste material from the body.

elix'ir [Med. L. fr. Ar. *al-iksir*, the philosopher's stone] A clear, sweetened, hydroalcoholic liquid intended for oral use; used either

as vehicles or for the therapeutic effect of the active medicinal agents.

el'uant Eluent.

el'uate [see elution] The material washed out of paper or out of a column of adsorbent in chromatography.

el'uent [see elution] A liquid used in the process of elution.

elu'tion [L. *e-luo*, pp. *lutus*, to wash out] **1.** Separation, by washing, of one solid from another. **2.** Removal, by means of a suitable solvent, of one material from another that is insoluble in that solvent.

em- See en-.

emacia'tion [L. *e-macio*, pp. *-atus*, to make thin] Wasting; becoming abnormally thin from extreme loss of flesh.

emana'tion [L. *-e-mano*, pp. *-atus*, to flow out] Any substance that flows out or is emitted from a source or origin.

emascula'tion [L. *emasculo*, pp. *atuo*, to castrate] Castration of the male by removal of the testis and/or penis.

embalm' [L. *in*, in, + *balsamum*, balsam] To treat a dead body with balsams or antiseptics to preserve it from decay.

embolec'tomy [G. *embolos*, a plug (embolus), + *ektome*, excision] Removal of an embolus.

embol'ic Relating to an embolus or to embolism.

em'bolism [G. *embolisma*, a piece or patch] Obstruction or occlusion of a vessel by a transported clot or vegetation, a mass of bacteria, or other foreign material (embolus).

    air e., presence of bubbles of air in the vascular system, which may obstruct blood flow; due to entry of air into the venous circulation following trauma or operations.

    fat e., occurrence of fat globules in the circulation following fractures of a long bone, in burns, in parturition, and in association with fatty degeneration of the liver.

    pulmonary e., e. of pulmonary arteries, most frequently by detached fragments of thrombus from a leg or pelvic vein.

    pyaemic e., infective e., plugging of an artery by an embolus detached from a suppurating thrombus.

emboliza'tion Therapeutic introduction of various substances into the circulation to occlude vessels, either to arrest or prevent haemorrhaging or to defunctionalize a structure or organ.

em'bolus, pl. **em'boli** [G. *embolos*, a plug, wedge or stopper] A plug, composed of a detached clot or vegetation, mass of bacteria, or other foreign body, occluding a blood vessel (embolism).

embryec'tomy [embryo- + G. *ektomē*, excision] Operative removal of the product of conception, especially in ectopic pregnancy.

embryo-, embry- [G. *embryon*, embryo] Combining forms relating to the embryo.

em'bryo [G. *embryon*] **1.** An organism in the early stages of development. **2.** In man, the developing organism from conception until approximately the end of the second month; developmental stages from this time to birth are commonly designated as fetal. **3.** A primordial plant within a seed.

embryocar'dia [embryo- + G. *kardia*, heart] A condition in which the cadence of the heart sounds resembles that of the fetus, the first and second sounds becoming alike and evenly spaced; a sign of serious myocardial disease.

embryogen'esis [embryo- + G. *genesis*, production] That phase of prenatal development involved in the establishing of the characteristic configuration of the embryonic body, usually regarded as extending from the end of the 2nd week, when the embryonic disc is formed, to the end of the 8th week, after which the conceptus is usually spoken of as a fetus.

embryogen'ic, embryogenet'ic Producing an embryo; relating to the formation of an embryo.

embryog'eny The origin and growth of the embryo.

embryol'ogy [embryo- + G. *logos*, study] The science of the origin and development of the organism from the fertilization of the ovum to the period of extrauterine or extraovular life.

embryo'ma Embryonal *tumour*.

   e. of the kidney, Wilms' *tumour*.

em'bryonal, embryon'ic Of, pertaining to, or in the condition of an embryo.

em'bryoniza'tion Reversion of a cell or a tissue to an embryonic form.

embryot'omy [embryo- + G. *tomē*, cutting] Any operation on the fetus to make possible its removal when delivery is impossible by natural means.

emed'ullate [L. *e-*, from, + *medulla*, marrow] To extract any marrow or pith.

em'esis [G. fr. *emeō*, to vomit] Vomiting. Also used as a combining form in suffix position.

emet'ic [G. *emetikos*, producing vomiting] Relating to or causing vomiting.

em'etocathar'tic Both emetic and cathartic, causing vomiting and purging.

emic'tion Urination.

emigra'tion [L. *e-migro*, pp. *-atus*, to emigrate] Passage of white blood cells through the endothelium and wall of small blood vessels.

em'inence [L. *eminentia*, prominence] A circumscribed prominence or elevation.

emis'sion [L. *emissio*; fr. *e-mitto*, to send out] A discharge; referring usually to a seminal discharge occurring during sleep (nocturnal e.).

emmenagog'ic Relating to or acting as an emmenagogue.

emmen'agogue [G. *emmēnos*, monthly, + *agōgos*, leading] An agent that induces or increases menstrual flow.

emmen'ia [G. *emmēnos*, monthly] Menses.

emmen'ic Menstrual.

emmetro'pia [G. *emmetros*, according to measure, + *ōps*, eye] The state of refraction of the eye in which parallel rays, when the eye is at rest, are focused exactly on the retina.

emol'lient [L. *emolliens*, pres. p. of *e-mollio*, to soften] Soothing to skin or mucous membrane.

emo'tion [L. *e-moveo*, pp. *-motus*, to move out, agitate] A strong feeling, aroused mental state, or intense state of drive or unrest directed toward a definite object and evidenced in both behaviour and in psychologic changes.

empath'ic Relating to or marked by empathy.

em'pathy [G. *en(em)*, in, + *pathos*, feeling] **1.** The intellectual and occasionally emotional identification with another person's mental and emotional states, as distinguished from sympathy. **2.** The anthropomorphization or humanizing of objects and feeling oneself as in and part of them.

emphyse'ma [G. inflation of stomach] **1.** The presence of air in the interstices of the connective tissue of a part. **2.** Pulmonary e.; a condition of the lung characterized by increase beyond the normal in the size of air spaces distal to the terminal bronchiole (those parts containing alveoli), with destructive changes in their walls and reduction in their number. Two structural varieties are described: panlobular e. and centrilobular e.

subcutaneous e., the presence of air or gas in the subcutaneous tissues.

surgical e., subcutaneous e. from air trapped in the tissues by an operation or injury.

emphyse'matous Relating to or affected with emphysema.

empir'ic, empir'ical [G. *empeirikos;* fr. *empeiria,* experience] Founded on practical experience but not proved scientifically, in contrast to rational.

emprosthot'onos [G. *emprosthen,* forward, + *tonos,* tension] A tetanic contraction of the flexor muscles, curving the back with concavity forward.

empye'ma [G. *empyēma,* suppuration] Pus in a body cavity; when used without qualification, refers to pyothorax.

empye'sis [G. suppuration] A pustular eruption.

emul'gent [L. *e-mulgeo,* pp. *-mulsus,* to milk or drain out] Denoting a straining, extracting, or purifying process.

emul'sifier An agent used to make an emulsion of a fixed oil.

emul'sion [Mod. L. fr. *e-mulgeo,* pp. *-mulsus,* to milk or drain out] A system containing two immiscible liquids in which one is dispersed, in the form of very small globules, throughout the other. That in the form of globules is called the internal phase; the second liquid is called the external phase.

en- Prefix fr. G. preposition meaning in; appears as em- before b, p, or m.

enam'el The hard, glistening substance covering the exposed portion of the tooth. It is composed of an inorganic portion (about 96%) made up of hydroxyapatite with small amounts of carbonate, magnesium, fluoride, and an organic matrix of glycoprotein and a keratin-like protein.

enamelo'ma A developmental anomaly in which there is a small nodule of enamel below the cementoenamel junction, usually at the bifurcation of molar teeth.

enan'them, enan'thema [G. *en,* in, + *anthēma,* bloom, eruption] A mucous membrane eruption, especially one occur-

ring in connection with one of the exanthemas.

en'anthem'atous Relating to an enanthem.

enanthe'sis [G. *en,* in, + *anthēsis,* full bloom] The skin eruption of a general disease, such as scarlatina or typhoid fever.

encapsula'tion [L. *in* + capsula, dim of *capsa,* box] Enclosure in a capsule or sheath.

enceph'aloscle ro'sis [encephalo- + G. *sklerōsis,* hardening] A sclerosis, or hardening, of the brain.

encephalal'gia [encephalo- + G. *algos,* pain] Headache.

enceph'al'ic Relating to the brain, or to the structures within the cranium.

encephalit'ic Relating to encephalitis.

encephali'tis, pl. **encephalit'ides** [G. *enkephalos,* brain, + *-itis,* inflammation] Inflammation of the brain.

encephalo-, encephal- [G. *enkephalos,* brain] Combining forms indicating the brain or some relationship thereto.

enceph'alocele [encephalo- + G. *kēlē,* hernia] A congenital gap in the skull, usually with herniation of brain substance.

enceph'alogram [encephalo- + G. *gramma,* a drawing] The record obtained by encephalography.

encephalog'raphy [encephalo- + G. *graphō,* to write] Radiographic imaging of the brain.

encephalo'ma. Herniation of brain substance.

enceph'alomala'cia [encephalo- + G. *malakia,* softness] Infarction of brain tissue, usually caused by vascular insufficiency.

enceph'alomeningi'tis [encephalo- + G. *mēninx,* membrane, + *-itis,* inflammation] Meningoencephalitis.

encephalom'eter [encephalo- + G. *metron,* measure] An apparatus for indicating on the skull the location of the cortical centres.

enceph'alomyeli'tis [encephalo- + G. *myelon,* marrow, + *-itis,* inflammation] An acute inflammation of the brain and spinal cord.

enceph'alon, pl. **enceph'ala** [G. *enkephalos,* brain, fr. *en,* in, + *kephalē,* head] [NA] Brain; that portion of the cerebrospinal axis contained within the cranium, comprised of the prosencephalon, mesencephalon, and rhombencephalon.

encephalop'athy [encephalo- + G. *pathos*, suffering] Any disease of the brain.

lead e., a rapidly developing e. caused by the ingestion of lead compounds and seen particularly in early childhood; clinical manifestations are convulsions, delirium, hallucinations, and other cerebral symptoms due to chronic lead poisoning.

traumatic e., disturbance of structure of cerebral nerve cells, glia, or intracranial vessels resulting from injury.

Wernicke's e., Wernicke's *syndrome*.

enceph'alopyo'sis [encephalo- + G. *pyōsis*, suppuration] Purulent inflammation of the brain.

enceph'alorrha'gia [encephalo- + G. *rhēgnymi*, to burst forth] Cerebral *haemorrhage*.

encephalo'sis Any organic disease of the brain.

encephalot'omy [encephalo- + G. *tomē*, incision] Dissection or incision of the brain.

enchondro'ma [Mod. L. fr. G. *en*, in, + *chondros*, cartilage, + *-oma*, tumour] A benign cartilaginous growth starting within the medullary cavity of a bone originally formed from cartilage.

enchon'dromato'sis Nonfamilial hamartomatous proliferation of cartilage in the metaphyses of several bones, most commonly of the hands and feet, causing distorted growth in length or pathological fractures.

enchondro'matous Relating to or having the elements of enchondroma.

en'clave [Fr. fr. L. *clavis*, key] An enclosure; a detached mass of tissue enclosed in tissue of another kind.

enclit'ic [G. *enkilitikos*, leaning on] Inclined; denoting especially the relation of the planes of the fetal head to those of the pelvis of the mother.

encopre'sis [G. *enkopros*, full of manure] Involuntary passage of faeces.

encys'ted [G. *kystis*, bladder] Encapsulated by a membranous bag.

endangii'tis [endo- + G. *angeion*, vessel, + *-itis*, inflammation] Inflammation of the intima of a blood vessel.

endaorti'tis Inflammation of the intima of the aorta.

endarterec'tomy [endo- + artery + G. *ektomē*, excision] Excision of diseased endothelial lining of an artery and occluding atheromatous deposits, so as to leave a smooth lining.

endarteri'tis [endo- + arteritis] Inflammation of the intima of an artery.

end'brain. Telencephalon.

endem'ic [G. *endēmos*, native, fr. *en*, in, + *dēmos*, the people] **1.** Present in a community or among a group of people; said of a disease prevailing continually in a region. **2.** Enzootic.

endo-, end- [G. *endon*, within] Prefix indicating within, inner, absorbing, containing. See also ento-.

en'doangii'tis Endangiitis.

en'doappendici'tis Simple catarrhal inflammation, limited to the mucosal surface of the vermiform appendix.

en'doarteri'tis Endarteritis.

en'docardi'tis Inflammation of the endocardium.

bacterial e., e. caused by the direct invasion of bacteria and leading to deformity of the valve leaflets; **acute b. e.** is caused by pyogenic organisms such as haemolytic streptococci or staphylococci; **subacute b. e.** is usually due to *Streptococcus viridans* or *S. faecalis*.

endocar'dium, pl. **endocar'dia** [endo- + G. *kardia*, heart] [NA] The innermost tunic of the heart, which includes endothelium and subendothelial connective tissue.

endocer'vical 1. Within any cervix, specifically within the cervix uteri. **2.** Relating to the endocervix.

en'docervici'tis Inflammation of the mucous membrane of the cervix uteri.

endocer'vix The mucous membrane of the cervical canal.

endocoli'tis Simple inflammation of the colon.

endocra'nial 1. Within the cranium. **2.** Relating to the endocranium.

endocra'nium The lining membrane of the cranium, or dura mater of the brain.

en'docrine [endo- + G. *krinō*, to separate] Secreting internally, most commonly into the systemic circulation; of or pertaining to such secretion or to a gland that furnishes such a secretion.

en'docrinol'ogist. One specializing in endocrinology.

en'docrinol'ogy [endocrine + G. *logos*, study] The science concerned with internal secretions and their physiologic and pathologic relations.

en'docrino'ma A tumour with endocrine tissue that retains the function of the parent organ, usually to an excessive degree.

en'docrinop'athy A disorder in the function of an endocrine gland and the consequences thereof.

endocysti'tis [endo- + G. kystis, bladder, + -itis, inflammation] Inflammation of the mucous membrane of the bladder.

endocyto'sis [endo- + kytos, cell, + -osis, condition] The process, including pinocytosis and phagocytosis, whereby materials are taken into a cell by the invagination of the plasma membrane, which it breaks off as a boundary membrane of the part engulfed.

en'doderm [endo- + G. derma, skin] The innermost of the three primary germ layers of the embryo, giving rise to the epithelial lining of the primitive gut tract, its glands, and the epithelial component of structures arising as outgrowths from the gut.

endodon'tia Endodontics.

endodon'tics [endo- + G. odous, tooth] A field of dentistry concerned with the prevention, diagnosis, and treatment of diseases and traumatic injuries in the dental pulp and periapical tissues.

endodon'tist One who specializes in endodontics.

en'dodontol'ogy. Endodontics.

en'doenteri'tis [endo- + G. enteron, intestine, + -itis, inflammation] Inflammation of the intestinal mucous membrane.

endog'enous [endo- + G. -gen. production] Originating or produced within the organism or one of its parts.

en'dointoxica'tion Poisoning by an endogenous toxin.

en'dolymph [endo- + L. lympha, a clear fluid] The fluid contained within the membranous labyrinth of the inner ear.

endome'tria Plural of endometrium.

endome'trial Relating to or composed of endometrium.

en'dometrio'sis Ectopic occurrence of endometrial tissue, frequently forming cysts containing altered blood.

endometri'tis Inflammation of the endometrium.

endome'trium, pl. **endome'tria** [endo- + G. + metra, uterus] [NA] The mucous membrane comprising the inner layer of the uterine wall.

en'domorph [endo- + G. morphē, form] A constitutional body type or build in which tissues that orginated in the endoderm prevail; from a morphological standpoint, the trunk predominates over the limbs.

endomor'phic Relating to, or having the characteristics of, an endomorph.

en'domy'ocardi'tis Inflammation of both endocardium and myocardium.

endoneuri'tis Inflammation of the endoneurium.

endoneu'rium [endo- + G. neuron, nerve] The delicate connective tissue enveloping individual nerve fibres within a peripheral nerve.

endopar'asite A parasite living within the body of its host.

en'dopericardi'tis [endo- + G. peri, around, + kardia, heart, + -itis, inflammation] Simultaneous inflammation of the endocardium and pericardium.

en'doperitoni'tis Superficial inflammation of the peritoneum.

endophlebi'tis [endo- + G. phleps (phleb-), vein, + -itis, inflammation] Inflammation of the intima of a vein.

en'dophyte [endo- + G. phyton, plant] A plant parasite living inside another organism.

en'doplasm In certain cells, especially motile ones and protozoa, the inner or medullary part of the cytoplasm.

en'dorphin One of a family of opioid like polypeptides originally isolated from the brain but now found in many parts of the body; in the brain, it binds to the same receptors that bind exogenous opiates.

en'doscope [endo- + G. skopeō, to examine] An instrument for the examination of the interior of a canal or hollow viscus.

endos'copy [see endoscope] Examination of the interior of a canal or hollow viscus by means of an endoscope.

endoskel'eton The internal bony framework of the body; the skeleton in its usual context.

endosmo'sis Osmosis in a direction toward the interior of a cell or a cavity.

endos'teal Relating to the endosteum.

endostei'tis, endosti'tis Inflammation of the endosteum or of the medullary cavity of a bone.

endosteo'ma [endo- + G. osteon, bone, + -ōma, tumour] A benign neoplasm of bone tissue in the medullary cavity of a bone.

endos'teum [endo- + G. *osteon*, bone] [NA] A thin membrane lining the inner surface of bone in the central medullary cavity.

en'dotendin'eum [endo- + L. *tendon*, tendon] The fine connective tissue surrounding secondary fascicles of a tendon.

endothe'lial Relating to the endothelium.

en'dothelio'ma A generic term for a group of neoplasms derived from the endothelial tissue of blood vessels of lymphatic channels.

endothe'lium, pl. **endothe'lia** [endo- + G. *thēlē*, nipple] A layer of flat squamous cells lining especially blood and lymphatic vessels and the heart.

en'dothrix [endo- + G. *thrix*, hair] A trichophyton (notably *Trichophyton violaceum* and *T. tonsurans*) whose spores and, occasionally, mycelia characteristically invade the interior of the hair shaft.

en'dotoxico'sis Poisoning by an endotoxin.

endotox'in 1. A bacterial toxin not freely liberated into the surrounding medium. **2.** The complex phospholipid-polysaccharide macromolecules which form an integral part of the cell wall of a variety of relatively avirulent as well as virulent strains of Gram-negative bacteria; they are released only when the of the cell wall is disturbed, are relatively heat-stable, are less potent than most exotoxins, are less specific, and do not form toxoids.

endotra'cheal Within the trachea.

en'dovasculi'tis Endangiitis.

end-piece The terminal part of the tail of a spermatozoon consisting of the axoneme and the flagellar membrane.

end'plate, end-plate The ending of a motor nerve fibre in relating to a skeletal muscle fibre.

end-ti'dal At the end of a normal expiration.

en'ema [G.] A substance introduced into the rectum to evacuate the bowel, or to administer drugs or nutrients.

barium e., contrast e., administration of barium as a radiopaque medium, for radiographic study of the lower intestinal tract.

enerva'tion [L. *enervo*, pp. *-atus*, to enervate] Failure of nerve force; weakening.

engage'ment In obstetrics, the mechanism by which the biparietal diameter of the fetal head enters the plane of the inlet.

engorged' [O. Fr. fr. Mediev. L. *gorgia*, throat, narrow passage, fr. L. *gurges*, a whirlpool] Congested, distended with fluid.

en'gram [G. *en*, in, + *gramma*, mark] A hypothetical physical habit or memory trace made on the protoplasm of an organism by the repetition of stimuli.

enkeph'alin A pentapeptide, found in many parts of the brain, which binds to specific receptor sites, some of which may be pain-related opiate receptors.

enophthal'mos [G. *en*, in, + *ophthalmos*, eye] Recession of the eyeball within the orbit.

enosto'sis [G. *en*, in, + *osteon*, bone, + *-osis*, condition] A mass of proliferating bone tissue within a bone.

en'siform [L. *ensis*, sword, + *forma*, appearance] Xiphoid.

ent- See ento-.

en'tad [G. *entos*, within, + L. *ad*, to] Toward the interior.

Entamoe'ba [G. *entos*, within + *emoibē*, change] A genus of amoeba parasitic in the caecum and large bowel of man and other primates and many domestic and wild mammals and birds. *E. histolytica*, the only distinct pathogen of the genus, causes tropical or amoebic dysentery, and hepatic amoebiasis.

ent'amoebi'asis Infection with *Entamoeba histolytica*.

en'teral Within or by way of the intestine, as distinguished from parenteral.

enteral'gia [entero- + G. *algos*, pain] Severe abdominal pain accompanying spasm of the bowel.

enterec'tasis [entero- + G. *ektasis*, a stretching] Dilation of the bowel.

enterec'tomy [entero- + G. *ektomē*, excision] Resection of a segment of the intestine.

enter'ic [G. *enterikos*, from *entera*, bowels] Relating to the intestine.

enteri'tis [entero- + *-itis*, inflammation] Inflammation of the intestine, especially of the small intestine.

regional e., granulomatous e., Crohn's disease; granulomatous segmented e. of unknown cause, involving the terminal ileum and less frequently other parts of the gastrointestinal tract, characterized by patchy deep ulcers that may cause fistulas, and narrowing and thickening of the bowel by fibrosis and lymphocytic infiltration, with non-caseating tuberculoid granulomas which may also be found in regional lymph nodes.

entero-, enter- [G. *enteron*, intestine] Combining form relating to the intestines.

en'terobi'asis Infection with *Enterobius vermicularis*, the human pinworm.

Entero'bius [entero- + G. *bios*, life] A genus of nematode worms that includes the pinworms (*E. vermicularis*) of man and primates.

en'terocele [entero- + G. *kēlē*, hernia] 1. A hernial protrusion through a defect in the rectovaginal or vasicovaginal pouch. 2. An intestinal hernia.

en'terocente'sis [entero- + G. *kentēsis*, puncture] Puncture of the gut with a hollow needle (cannula or trocar) to withdraw substances.

en'terococ'cus, pl. **en'terococ'ci** [entero- + G. *kokkos*, a berry] A streptococcus that inhabits the intestinal tract.

enterocoli'tis [entero- + G. *kolon*, colon, + -*itis*, inflammation] Inflammation of varying extent of the mucous membrane of both small and large intestines.

en'terocolos'tomy [entero- + G. *kōlon*, colon, + *stoma*, mouth] Establishment of an artificial opening between the small intestine and the colon.

en'terogastri'tis [entero- + G. *gastēr*, belly, + -*itis*, inflammation] Gastroenteritis.

en'terohepati'tis [entero- + G. *hēpar* (*hēpat-*), liver, + -*itis*, inflammation] Inflammation of both the intestine and the liver.

enterohy'drocele Hydrocele in which the sac contains also a loop of intestine.

en'terokine'sis [entero- + G. *kinēsin*, movement] Muscular contraction of the alimentary canal, as in peristalsis.

en'terokinet'ic Relating to, or producing, enterokinesis.

en'terolith [entero- + G. *lithos*, stone] An intestinal calculus formed of layers surrounding a nucleus of some hard indigestible substance swallowed.

en'terolithi'asis Presence of calculi in the intestine.

enterol'ogy [entero- + G. *logos*, study] The branch of medical science concerned with the intestinal tract.

en'teropare'sis [entero- + G. *paresis*, slackening, relaxation] A state of diminished or arrested peristalsis with flaccidity of the intestinal walls.

en'teropath'ogen'ic Pathogenic for the alimentary canal.

enterop'athy [entero- + G. *pathos*, suffering] A disorder of the intestine.

en'teropexy [entero- + G. *pēxis*, fixation] Fixation of a segment of the intestine to the abdominal wall.

en'teroplasty [entero- + G. *plassō*, to mould] Reconstructive operation on the intestine.

enterople'gia [entero- + G. *plēgē*, stroke] See ileus.

en'terorrha'gia [entero- + G. *rhēgnymi*, to burst forth] Bleeding within the intestinal tract.

enteror'rhaphy [entero- + G. *rhaphē*, suture] Suture of the intestine.

en'terorrhex'is [entero- + G. *rhēxis*, rupture] Rupture of the gut or bowel.

en'terosep'sis [entero- + G. *sēpsis*, putrefaction] Sepsis occurring in or derived from the alimentary canal.

en'terospasm [entero- + G. *spasmos*, spasm] Increased, irregular, and painful peristalsis.

en'terosta'sis [entero- + G. *stasis*, a standing] Intestinal stasis; a retardation or arrest of the passage of the intestinal contents.

en'terostax'is [entero- + G. *staxis*, a dripping] Oozing of blood from the mucous membrane of the intestine.

en'terosteno'sis [entero- + G. *stenōsis*, narrowing] Narrowing of the lumen of the intestine.

enteros'tomy [entero- + G. *stoma*, mouth] An artificial anus or fistula into the intestine through the abdominal wall.

enterot'omy Incision into the intestine.

enterotox'in A cytotoxin specific for the cells of the mucous membrane of the intestine.

Enterovi'rus A proposed genus of viruses (family Picornaviridae) that includes poliovirus types 1 to 3, coxsackievirus A and B, echoviruses, and the enteroviruses.

enterozo'ic Relating to an enterozoon.

enterozo'on [entero- + G. *zōon*, animal] An animal parasite in the intestine.

en'thesis [G. an insertion, fr. *en*, in, + *thesis*, a placing] Insertion of synthetic or other nonvital material to replace lost tissue.

enthet'ic 1. Relating to enthesis. **2.** Exogenous.

ento-, ent- [G. *entos*, within] Prefixes meaning inner, or within. See also endo-.

en'toblast [ento- + G. *blastos*, germ] Endoblast.

en'toderm [ento- + G. *derma*, skin] Endoderm.

entomol'ogy [G. *entomon*, insect, + *logos*, study] The science concerned with insects, especially as affecting man.

entop'ic [G. *en*, within, + *topos*, place] Placed within; occurring or situated in the normal place.

entop'tic [ento- + G. *optikos*, relating to vision] Within the eyeball.

entozo'on, pl. **entozo'a** [ento- + G. *zōon*, animal] An animal parasite inhabiting any of the internal organs or tissues.

entro'pion [G. *en*, in, + *tropē*, a turning] Inversion or turning inward of a part.

   e. u'veae, inversion of the pupillary margin.

enu'cleate To perform enucleation.

enuclea'tion [L. *enucleo*, to remove the kernel, fr. *e*, out, + *nucleus*, nut, kernel] **1.** The entire removal of a tumour or structure (such as the eyeball), without rupture, as one shells out the kernel of a nut. **2.** The removal or destruction of the nucleus of a cell.

enure'sis [G. *en-oureō*, to urinate in] Bedwetting; involuntary passage of urine, usually occurring at night or during sleep.

en'velope In anatomy, a structure that encloses or covers.

envenoma'tion Injection of a poisonous material by sting, spine, bite, or other venom apparatus.

enzoot'ic [G. *en*, in, + *zōon*, animal] Denoting a disease of animals which is indigenous to a certain locality, more precisely, the temporal pattern of occurrence of a disease in a population of animals with only minor changes in its incidence with time.

enzygot'ic [G. *eis(en)*, one, + zygote] Derived from a single fertilized ovum, denoting twins so derived.

en'zyme [G. *en*, in, + *zymē*, leaven] A protein, secreted by cells, that acts as a catalyst to induce chemical changes in other substances, itself remaining apparently unchanged by the process. E.'s, with the exception of those discovered long ago (*e.g.*, pepsin, emulsin), are generally named by adding -*ase* to the name of the substrate on which the e. acts (*e.g.*, glucosidase) or the substance activated (*e.g.*, hydrogenase) and/or the type of reaction (*e.g.*, oxidoreductase, transferase, hydrolase, lyase, isomerase, ligase or synthetase—these being the six main groups).

enzy'mic, enzymat'ic Relating to an enzyme.

e'osin [G. *ēōs*, dawn] Any of a group of acid dyes used as cytoplasmic stains and counterstains in histology and especially in the staining of blood cells.

eosin'ophil, eosin'ophile [eosin + G. *philos*, fond] Eosinophilic *leucocyte*.

eosinophil'ia Eosinophilic *leucocytosis*.

   tropical e., e. associated with cough and asthma, caused by occult filarial infection without evidence of microfilaraemia, occurring most frequently in India and southeast Asia.

eosinophil'ic Staining readily with eosin dyes; denoting such cell or tissue elements.

epax'ial [G. *epi*, upon, + L. *axis*, axis] Above or behind any axis, such as the spinal axis or the axis of a limb.

epen'dyma [G. *ependyma*, an upper garment] [NA] The cellular membrane lining the central canal of the spinal cord and the brain ventricles.

epen'dymal Relating to the ependyma.

ependymi'tis Inflammation of the ependyma.

ependymo'ma A glioma derived from relatively undifferentiated ependymal cells; the neoplastic cells tend to be arranged radially about blood vessels, to which they are attached by means of fibrillary processes.

ephe'bic [G. *ephēbikos*, relating to youth, fr. *hēbē*, youth] Relating to the period of puberty or to adolescence.

eph'edrine An alkaloid from the leaves of *Ephedra equisetina*, *E. sinica*, and other species, or produced synthetically; an adrenergic (sympathomimetic) agent with actions similar to those of adrenaline.

ephe'lis, pl. **ephe'lides** [G.] Freckle.

epi- G. preposition, used as a prefix, meaning upon, following, or subsequent to.

ep'iblast [epi- + G. *blastos*, germ] A potential ectoderm.

epibul'bar Upon the eyeball.

epican'thus [epi- + G. kanthos, canthus] A fold of skin extending from the root of the nose to the medial termination of the eyebrow, overlapping the medial angle of the eye; normal in fetal life and in various Oriental peoples.

epicar'dia [epi- + cardia] The portion of the oesophagus from where it passes through the diaphragm to the stomach.

epicar'dial Relating to the epicardia.

epicon'dyle [epi- + G. kondylos, a knuckle] A projection from a long bone near the articular extremity above or upon the condyle.

ep'icondyli'tis Infection or inflammation of an epicondyle.

epicra'nium [epi- + G. kranion, skull] The muscle, aponeurosis, and skin covering the cranium.

epicri'sis A secondary crisis, a crisis terminating a recrudescence of morbid symptoms following a primary crisis.

epicrit'ic [G. epikritikos, adjudicatory] Denoting that component of the somatic sensory modality by which one is enabled to discriminate the finer degrees of touch and temperature stimuli, and to localize them on the body surface.

epicysti'tis [epi- + G. kystis, bladder, + -itis, inflammation] Inflammation of the cellular tissue around the bladder.

epidem'ic [epi- + G. dēmos, the people] 1. A disease attacking many in a community simultaneously; distinguished from endemic, since the disease is not continuously present but has been introduced from outside. 2. A temporary increase in number of cases of an endemic disease.

epidemio'ity The state of prevailing disease in epidemic form.

epidemiol'ogy [G. epidēmios, epidemic, | logos, study] 1. The study of the prevalence and spread of disease in a community. 2. The field of medicine concerned with determination of specific causes of occurrences of health problems or diseases in a locality.

epider'mal, epider'mic Relating to the epidermis.

epider'mis, pl. **epider'mides** [G. epidermis, the outer skin] [NA] The outer epithelial portion of the skin (cutis).

epidermi'tis Inflammation of the epidermis or superficial layers of the skin.

epider'modyspla'sia [epidermis + G. dys-, bad, + plasis, a moulding] Faulty growth or development of the epidermis.

e. verrucifor'mis, numerous flat warts on the hands and feet, sometimes familial, in which intranuclear viral particles with the appearance of infectious wart virus have been demonstrated.

epider'moid [epidermis + G. eidos, appearance] 1. Resembling epidermis. 2. A cholesteatoma or other cystic tumour arising from aberrant epidermic cells.

epidermol'ysis [epidermis + G. lysis, loosening] A condition in which the epidermis is loosely attached to the corium, readily exfoliating or forming blisters.

Epidermoph'yton [epidermis + G phyton, plant] A genus of fungi distinguished from Trichophyton in that it never invades the hair follicles. E. floccosum, is a common cause of tinea pedis.

epidid'ymal Relating to the epididymis.

ep'ididymec'tomy [epididymis + G. ektomē, excision] Operative removal of the epididymis.

epidid'ymis, pl. **epidid'ymides** [Mod. L. fr G. epididymis, fr. epi, on, + didymos, twin, in pl. testes] [NA] An elongated structure connected to the posterior surface of the testis; the main component is the ductus epididymidis which in the tail and the beginning of the ductus deferens is a reservoir for spermatozoa.

epididymi'tis Inflammation of the epididymio.

epididymot'omy [epididymis + G. tomē, a cutting] Incision into the epididymis.

epidu'ral Upon (or outside) the dura mater.

epidurog'raphy Radiographic visualization of the epidural space following the regional instillation of a radiopaque contrast medium.

epigastral'gia [epigastrium + G. algos, pain] Pain in the epigastric region.

epigas'tric Relating to the epigastrium.

epigas'trium [G. epigastrion] [NA] Epigastric region; the topographical area of the abdomen located between the costal margins and the subcostal plane.

epigas'trocele [epigastrium + G. kēlē, hernia] A hernia in the epigastric region.

epigen'esis [epi- + G. genesis, creation] Development of offspring as a result of the union of the ovum and sperm.

ep'igenet'ic Relating to epigenesis.

epiglot'tic Relating to the epiglottis.

ep'iglottidec'tomy [epiglottis + G. *ektomē*, excision] Excision of the epiglottis.

ep'iglottidi'tis Epiglottitis.

epiglot'tis [G. *epiglōttis*, fr. *epi*, on, + *glōttis*, the mouth of the windpipe] [NA] A plate shaped of elastic cartilage at the root of the tongue that serves as a diverter valve over the superior aperture of the larynx during the act of swallowing.

epiglotti'tis Inflammation of the epiglottis.

ep'ilate [L. *e*, out, + *pilus*, a hair] To extract a hair; to remove the hair from a part by forcible extraction, electrolysis, or loosening at the root by chemical means.

epila'tion Depilation; the act or result of removing hair.

epil'atory 1. Depilatory (1); having the property of removing hair; relating to epilation. **2.** Depilatory (2).

ep'ilepsy [G. *epilēpsia*, seizure] A chronic disorder characterized by paroxysmal attacks of brain dysfunction due to excessive neuronal discharge, and usually associated with some alteration of consciousness; attacks may remain confined to elementary or complex impairment of behaviour or may progress to a generalized convulsion.

    focal e., cortical e., an epileptic attack beginning with an isolated disturbance of cerebral function such as a twitching of a limb, a somatosensory or special sense phenomenon, or a disturbance of higher mental function.

    generalized e., grand mal e., grand mal; a seizure characterized by loss of consciousness and tonic spasm of the musculature, usually followed by repetitive generalized clonic jerking.

    petit mal e., absence.

    psychomotor e., temporal lobe e. attacks characterized clinically by impairment of consciousness and amnesia for the episode, often associated with semipurposeful movements of the arms or legs and sometimes with psychic disturbances such as hallucinations.

    tonic e., a convulsive attack in which the body is rigid.

epilep'tic Relating to or suffering from epilepsy.

epilep'tiform Epileptoid.

ep'ileptogen'ic, epileptog'enous Causing epilepsy.

epilep'toid [G. *epilēpsia*, seizure, epilepsy, + *eidos*, resemblance] Resembling epilepsy; denoting certain convulsions, especially of functional nature.

epimandib'ular [epi- + L. *mandibulum*, mandible] Upon the lower jaw.

ep'imenorrhoe'a Too frequent menstruation.

ep'imere [epi- + G. *meros*, part] The dorsal part of the myotome.

epimorpho'sis [epi- + G. *morphē*, shape] Regeneration of a part of an organism by growth at the cut surface.

epineph'rine The term preferred in the U.S. for adrenaline.

epineu'ral On a neural arch of a vertebra.

epineu'rium [epi- + G. *neuron*, nerve] The connective tissue encapsulating a nerve trunk and binding together the fascicles; contains the blood vessels and lymphatics supplying the nerves.

ep'iphenom'enon An unusual and unassociated symptom appearing during the course of a disease.

epiph'ora [G. a sudden flow] Tearing; an overflow of tears upon the cheek, due to imperfect drainage by the tear-conducting passages.

epiphys'eal, epiphys'ial Relating to an epiphysis.

epiph'ysis, pl. **epiph'yses** [G. an excrescence, fr. *epi*, upon, + *physis*, growth] [NA] A part of a long bone developed from a center of ossification distinct from that of the shaft and separated at first from the latter by a layer of cartilage.

epiphysi'tis Inflammation of an epiphysis.

epiplo- [G. *epiploon*, omentum] Combining form relating to the omentum. See also omento-.

epiplo'ic Omental.

episcle'ra [epi- + sclera] The connective tissue between the sclera and the conjunctiva.

episcle'ral 1. Upon the sclera. **2.** Relating to the episclera.

episcleri'tis (ep'i-u-skle-ri'tis). Inflammation of the episcleral or subconjunctival connective tissue. See also scleritis.

episio- [G. *episeion*, pudenda] Combining form relating to the vulva. See also vulvo-.

epi′sioplasty [episio- + G. *plasso*, to form] Repair of a defect of the vulva.

episior′rhaphy [episio- + G. *rhaphe*, a stitching] Repair of a lacerated vulva or an episiotomy.

episiosteno′sis [episio- + G. *stenosis*, narrowing] Narrowing of the vulvar orifice.

episiot′omy [episio- + G. *tome*, incision] Surgical incision of the vulva to prevent laceration at the time of delivery or to facilitate vaginal surgery.

epispad′ias [epi- + G. *spadon*, a rent] A malformation in which the urethra opens on the dorsum of the penis.

epistax′is [G. fr. *epistazo*, to bleed at the nose] Nosebleed; profuse bleeding from the nose.

epithe′lial Relating to or consisting of epithelium.

epithe′lializa′tion Formation of epithelium over a denuded surface.

epithe′lioid [epithelium + G. *eidos*, resemblance] Resembling or having some of the characteristics of epithelium.

ep′ithelio′ma [epithelium + G. *-oma*, tumor] **1.** An epithelial neoplasm or harmartoma of the skin, especially of skin appendage orgin. **2.** A carcinoma of the skin derived from squamous, basal, or adnexal cells.

epithe′lium, pl. **epithe′lia** [G. *epi*, upon, + *thele*, nipple; originally, the thin skin covering the nipples and the papillary layer of the border of lips] [NA] The purely cellular, avascular layer covering all the free surfaces, cutaneous, mucous, and serous, including the glands and other structures derived therefrom.

epizo′ic Living as a parasite on the skin surface.

epizo′on, pl. **epizo′a** [epi- + G. *zoon*, animal] An animal parasite living on the body surface.

ep′onym [G. *eponymos*, named after] The name of a disease, structure, operation, or procedure, supposedly derived from the name of the person who first discovered or described it.

eponym′ic 1. Relating to an eponym. **2.** An eponym.

ep′ulis [G. *epoulis*, gumboil] Persisting inflammatory hyperplasia of the gingiva, a nonspecific growth on the gingiva that may be present at birth as a benign tumour resembling a granular cell myoblastoma.

ep′uloid A nodule or mass (in the gingival tissue) that resembles an epulis.

epulo′sis [G. *epoulosis*, a scarring over] Cicatrization (1).

epulot′ic 1. Cicatricial. **2.** Cicatrizant.

erec′tile Capable of erection.

erec′tion [L. *erectio*, fr. *erigo*, pp. *erectus*, to set up] The condition of erectile tissue when filled with blood, becoming hard and unyielding; denoting especially this state of the penis.

erec′tor [Mod. L.] That which raises or makes erect, denoting specifically certain muscles having such action.

er′ethism [G. *erethismos*, irritation] An abnormal state of excitement or irritation, either general or local.

erethis′mic, erethis′tic, erethit′ic Marked by or causing erethism.

erga′sia [G. work] **1.** Any form of activity, especially mental. **2.** The total of functions and reactions of an individual.

ergo- [G. *ergon*, work] Combining form relating to work.

er′gocalcif′erol Vitamin D₂; calciferol; activated ergosterol, the vitamin D of plant origin which arises from ultraviolet irradiation of ergosterol.

er′gograph [ergo- + G. *grapho*, to write] An instrument for recording the amount of work done by muscular contractions, or the amplitude of contraction.

ergograph′ic Relating to the ergograph and the record made by it.

ergom′eter [ergo- + G. *metron*, measure] Dynamometer.

ergonom′ics [ergo- + G. *nomos*, law] A branch of ecology dealing with human factors in the design and operations of machines and the physical environment.

ergos′terol The most important of the provitamins D₂; ultraviolet irradiation converts e. to lumisterol, tachysterol, and vitamin D₂.

er′got Rye smut; the resistant, over-wintering stage of the fungus *Claviceps purpura*, a pathogen of rye grass that transforms the seed of rye into a compact spur-like mass of fungal pseudotissue containing five or more optically isomeric pairs of alkaloids; the laevorotory isomers induce uterine contractions, control bleeding, and alleviate certain localized vascular disorders (migraine headaches).

ergot'amine An alkaloid from ergot that is a potent stimulant of smooth muscle, particularly of the blood vessels and the uterus, and produces adrenergic blockade (chiefly of the alpha receptors).

er'gotism Poisoning by a toxic substance contained in the sclerotia of the fungus, *Claviceps purpurea*, growing on rye grass; symptoms are necrosis of the extremities due to contraction of the peripheral vascular bed.

erog'enous Capable of producing sexual excitement when stimulated.

ero'sion [L. *erosio*, fr. *erodere*, to gnaw away] **1.** A wearing away or a state of being worn away, as by friction or pressure. **2.** A shallow ulcer; in the stomach and intestine, an ulcer limited to the mucosa, with no penetration of the muscularis mucosa. **3.** The wearing away of a tooth by chemical or abrasive action.

ero'sive Having the property of eroding or wearing away.

erot'ic [G. *erōtikos*, relating to love, fr. *erōs*, love] Relating to sexual passion; lustful; having the quality to arouse sexual drive.

erot'ism, erot'icism A condition of sexual excitement.

erotogen'ic [G. *erōs*, love, + *-gen*, production] Causing sexual excitement.

erotoma'nia [G. *erōs*, love, + *mania*, frenzy] Excessive or morbid inclination to erotic thoughts and behaviour.

eructa'tion [L. *eructo*, pp. *-atus*, to belch] Belching; the raising of gas or of a small quantity of acid fluid from the stomach.

erup'tion [L. *e-rumpo*, pp. *-ruptus*, to break out] **1.** A breaking out, especially the appearance of lesions on the skin. **2.** A rapidly developing dermatosis of the skin or mucous membranes, especially when appearing as a local manifestation of a general disease; characterized, according to the nature of the lesion, as macular, papular, vesicular, pustular, bullous, nodular, erythematous, etc. **3.** Passage of a tooth through the alveolar process and perforation of the gums.

  drug e., any e. caused by the ingestion, injection, inhalation, or insertion of a drug, most often the result of allergic sensitization; reactions to drugs applied to the skin are generally designated as a contact dermatitis.

erup'tive Characterized by eruption.

erysip'elas [G. from *erythros*, red, + *pella*, skin] A specific, acute, inflammatory disease caused by a haemolytic streptococcus and characterized by an eruption, limited to the skin and sharply defined, usually accompanied by severe constitutional symptoms.

er'ysipel'atous Relating to erysipelas.

erysip'eloid [G. *erysipelas* + *eidos*, resemblance] A specific, usually self-limiting cellulitis of the hand, caused by *Erysipelothrix rhusiopathiae*; appears as a dusky erythema at the site of a wound sustained in handling fish or fowl.

Erysip'elothrix [*erysipelas* + G. *thrix*, hair] A genus of bacteria (family Corynebacteriaceae) that are parasitic on mammals, birds, and fish. The type species, *E. rhusiopathiae*, causes swine erysipelas, human erysipeloid, and mouse septicaemia, and commonly infects fish handlers.

erythe'ma [G. *erythēma*, flush] Inflammatory redness of the skin.

  e. multifor'me, an acute eruption of macules, papules, or subdermal vesicles presenting a multiform appearance, the characteristic lesion being the target or iris lesion over the dorsal aspect of the hands and forearms; its origin may be allergic, seasonal, or from drug sensitivity; the eruption may be recurrent or may run a severe course with fatal termination (Stevens-Johnson syndrome).

  e. nodo'sum, a dermatosis marked by the sudden formation of painful nodes on the extensor surfaces of the lower extremities, with lesions that are self-limiting, but that tend to recur; associated with arthralgia and fever or may be evidence of drug sensitivity, sarcoidosis, or infections.

erythe'matous Relating to or marked by erythema.

erythe'matovesic'ular Denoting a condition characterized by oedema, erythema, and vesiculation, as in allergic contact dermatitis.

erythrae'mia [erythro- + G. *haima*, blood] Polycythaemia vera: a chronic form of polycythaemia of unknown cause; characterized by bone marrow hyperplasia, an increase in blood volume as well as in the number of red cells, redness or cyanosis of the skin, and splenomegaly.

erythral'gia [erythro- + G. *algos*, pain] Painful redness of the skin. See also erythromelalgia.

erythras'ma [G. *erythraino̅*, to redden] An eruption of reddish brown patches, in the axillae and groins especially, due to the presence of *Corynebacterium minutissimum*.

er'ythrism [G *erythros*, red] Redness of the hair with a ruddy, freckled complexion.

erythris'tic Relating to or marked by erythrism.

erythro-, erythr- [G. *erythros*, red] Combining forms meaning red or denoting relationship to redness.

eryth'roblast [erythro- + G. *blastos*, germ] Originally, a term denoting all forms of human red blood cells containing a nucleus, both pathologic (*i.e.*, megaloblastic) and normal (*i.e.*, normoblastic). Now, the nucleated precursor from which a reticulocyte develops into an erythrocyte.

eryth'roblastae'mia [erythroblast + G. *haima*, blood] Presence of nucleated red cells in the peripheral blood.

eryth'roblastope'nia [erythroblast + G. *penia*, poverty] A primary deficiency of erythroblasts in bone marrow, seen in aplastic anaemia.

eryth'roblasto'sis [erythroblast + *osis*, condition] Presence in considerable number of erythroblasts in the blood.

  e. feta'lis, fetal e., haemolytic disease of newborn; haemolytic anaemia that, in most instances, results from development in the mother of anti-Rh antibody in response to the Rh factor in the (Rh-positive) fetal blood; characterized by many erythroblasts in the circulation, and often generalized oedema (hydrops fetalis) and enlargement of the liver and spleen.

erythroc'lasis [erythro- + G. *klasis*, a breaking] Fragmentation of the red blood cells.

erythroclas'tic Pertaining to erythroclasis; destructive to red blood cells.

eryth'rocyano'sis [erythro- + G. *kyanos*, blue, + -*osis*, condition] A condition seen particularly in girls and women in which exposure of the limbs to cold causes them to become swollen and dusky red.

eryth'rocyte [erythro- + G. *kytos*, cell] Red blood cell or corpuscle: a mature red blood cell.

erythrocythae'mia [erythro- + G. *kytos*, cell, + *haima*, blood] Polycythaemia.

erythrocyto'sis Polycythaemia, especially that which occurs in response to some known stimulus.

ery'throdegen'erative. Pertaining to or characterized by degeneration of the red blood cells.

erythroder'ma [erythro- + G. *derma*, skin] A nonspecific designation for intense and usually widespread reddening of the skin, often preceding, or associated with exfoliation.

erythrodon'tia [erythro- + G. *odous*, tooth] Reddish discoloration of the teeth, as may occur in porphyria.

erythroede'ma [erythro- + G. *oidēma*, swelling] Acrodynia (1).

erythrogen'ic [erythro- + -*gen*, producing] **1.** Producing red, as causing an eruption or a red colour sensation. **2.** Pertaining to the formation of red blood cells.

eryth'rokinet'ics [erythro- + G. *kinēsis*, movement] A consideration of the kinetics of erythrocytes from their generation to destruction; erythrokinetic studies are sometimes made in cases of anaemia to evaluate the balance between erythrocyte production and destruction.

eryth'roleukae'mia Simultaneous neoplastic proliferation of erythroblastic and leucoblastic tissues.

eryth'romelal'gia [erythro- + G. *melos*, limb, + *algos*, pain] Paroxysmal throbbing and burning pain in the skin, affecting one or both legs and feet, sometimes one or both hands, accompanied by a dusky mottled redness of the parts; associated with polycythaemia vera, thrombocythaemia; gout, neurological disease, or heavy-metal poisoning.

erythromy'cin An antibiotic agent obtained from cultures of a strain of *Streptomyces erythraeus;* Gram-positive bacteria are in general more susceptible to its action than are Gram-negative bacteria.

eryth'roneocyto'sis [erythrocyte + G. *neos*, new, + *kytos*, cell, + -*osis*, condition] Presence in the peripheral circulation of regenerative forms of red blood cells.

erythrope'nia [erythrocyte + G. *penia*, poverty] Deficiency in the number of red blood cells.

eryth'ropoie'sis [erythrocyte + G. *poiēsis*, a making] Formation of red blood cells.

eryth'ropoiet'ic Pertaining to or characterized by erythropoiesis.

erythropoi'etin A sialic acid-containing protein that enhances erythropoiesis by stimulating formation of proerythroblasts and release of reticulocytes from bone marrow; secreted by the kidney and possibly by other tissues, and can be detected in human plasma and urine.

erythrop'sia [erythro- + G. $\bar{o}ps$, eye] A condition in which all objects appear to be tinged with red.

erythru'ria [erythro- + G. $ouron$, urine] Passage of red urine.

es'char [G. $eschara$, a fireplace, a scab caused by burning] A thick, coagulated crust or slough which develops following a thermal burn or chemical or physical cauterization of the skin.

escharot'ic [G. $eschar\bar{o}tikos$] Caustic or corrosive.

escharot'omy [eschar + G. $tom\bar{e}$, incision] A surgical incision in a burn eschar to lessen constriction.

Escherich'ia A genus of aerobic, facultatively anaerobic bacteria found in faeces; occasionally they are pathogenic to man, causing enteritis, peritonitis, cystitis, etc. The type species, *E. coli*, occurs normally in the intestines of man and other vertebrates, is widely distributed in nature and is a frequent cause of infections of the urogenital tract and of diarrhoea in infants.

-esis [G. suffix -*esis*, condition or process] Suffix meaning condition, action, or process.

esopho'ria [G. $es\bar{o}$, inward, + $phora$, a carrying] A tendency of the eyes to deviate inward.

esotro'pia [G. $es\bar{o}$, inward, + $trop\bar{e}$, turn] Crossed eyes; convergent strabismus; strabismus in which the visual axes converge; may be paralytic or concomitant, monocular or alternating, accommodative or nonaccommodative.

espun'dia [Sp. fr. L. *spongia*, sponge] A type of American leishmaniasis caused by *Leishmania braziliensis* that affects the mucous membranes, particularly in the nasal and oral region, resulting in grossly destructive changes.

essen'tial 1. Necessary, indispensable (*e.g.*, e. amino acids). 2. Characteristic of. 3. Determining. 4. Idiopathic, inherent.

es'ter An organic compound formed by the elimination of H_2O between the —OH of an acid group and the —OH of an alcohol group.

ester'ifica'tion The process of forming an ester.

eth'anol Alcohol (2).

eth'ene Ethylene.

e'ther [G. $aith\bar{e}r$, the pure upper air] 1. Any organic compound in which two carbon atoms are independently linked to a common oxygen atom, thus containing the group —C—O—C—. 2. Loosely used to refer to diethyl e. or an anaesthetic e., although a large number of e.'s have anaesthetic properties.

ethe'real [g. $aitherios$, etherial, fr. $aith\bar{e}r$, the upper air] Relating to or containing ether.

eth'ical Relating to ethics; in conformity with the rules governing personal and professional conduct.

eth'ics [G. $ethikos$, arising from custom, fr. $ethos$, custom] The science of morality; the principles of proper professional conduct concerning the rights and duties of the health care professional, his patients, and his colleagues.

ethmo- [G. $\bar{e}thmos$, sieve] Combining form meaning ethmoid; relating to the ethmoid bone.

eth'moid [G. $\bar{e}thmos$, sieve, + $eidos$, resemblance] 1. Resembling a sieve. 2. The e. bone, os ethmoidale.

ethmoidec'tomy [ethmo- + G. $ektom\bar{e}$, excision] Removal of all or part of the mucosal lining and bony partitions between the ethmoid sinuses.

ethmoidi'tis Inflammation of the ethmoid sinuses.

ethnocen'trism [G. $ethnos$, race, tribe, + $kentron$, centre of a circle, + ism] The tendency to evaluate other groups according to the values and standards of one's own ethnic group, especially with the conviction that one's own ethnic group is superior to the other groups.

eth'ylene An explosive constituent of ordinary illuminating gas; an inhalation anaesthetic, now infrequently used, slightly more potent than nitrous oxide.

eth'ylenedi'aminetet'raace'tic acid (EDTA) A chelating agent used to remove multivalent cations from solution as chelates. As the sodium salt, it is used as a water softener, to stabilize drugs rapidly decomposed in the presence of traces of metal ions, and as an anticoagulant; as the sodium calcium salt, used to remove radium, lead, strontium, plutonium, and cadmium from the skeleton.

etiola'tion [Fr. *étioler*, to blanch] **1.** Paleness or pallor resulting from deprivation of light. **2.** The process of blanching or making pale by withholding light.

eu- G. particle used as a prefix, meaning good, well.

Eubacte'rium A genus of anaerobic, nonsporeforming, nonmotile bacteria occurring in the intestinal tract; they attack carbohydrates and may be pathogenic. The type species is *E. foedans*.

euca'ryote Eukaryote.

eu'caryot'ic Eukaryotic.

eugen'ic Relating to eugenics.

eugen'ics [G. *eugeneia*, nobility of birth] Practices and policies that tend to better the innate qualities of man and to develop them to the highest degree.

euglob'ulin That fraction of the serum globulin less soluble in $(NO_4)_2SO_4$ solution than the pseudoglobulin fraction.

euglycae'mia [eu- + G. *glykys*, sweet, + *haima*, blood]. Normal blood glucose concentration.

eu'karyot'ic Eukaryotic; pertaining to a eukaryote.

eukar'yote [eu- + G. *karyou*, kernel, nut] An organism whose cells contain a limiting membrane around the nuclear material and which undergoes mitosis.

eu'nuch [G. *eunouchos*, fr. *eunē*, bed, + *echein*, to have, because used as a chamberlain] One whose testes have been removed or have never developed.

eu'nuchoid [G. *eunouchos*, eunuch, + *eidos*, resembling] Partially resembling, or having the general characteristics of, a eunuch.

eu'nuchoidism Male hypogonadism; a state in which testes are present but fail to function.

eupho'ria [eu- + G. *pherō*, to bear] A feeling of well-being, commonly exaggerated and not necessarily well founded.

eu'ploid Relating to euploidy.

euploi'dy [eu- + G. *-ploos*, -fold] The state of a cell whose number of chromosomes is an exact multiple of the haploid number normal for the species.

eusta'chian Described by or attributed to Eustachio.

euthana'sia [eu- + G. *thanatos*, death] **1.** A quiet, painless death. **2.** The intentional putting to death by artificial means of persons with incurable or painful disease.

evac'uant Promoting evacuation.

evacua'tion [L. *e-vacuo*, pp. *-vacuatus*, to empty out] **1.** Removal of waste material, especially from the bowels. **2.** Stool (2).

evac'uator An instrument for removal of material from a body cavity.

evagina'tion [L. *e*, out, + *vagina*, sheath] The protrusion of some part or organ from its normal position.

evanes'cent [L. *e*, out, + *vanescere*, to vanish] Of short duration.

evap'ora'tion [L. *e*, out, + *vaporare*, to emit vapour] Volatilization. **1.** A change from liquid to vapour form. **2.** Loss of volume of a liquid by conversion into vapour.

eventra'tion [L. *e*, out, + *venter*, belly] **1.** Protrusion of omentum and/or intestine through an opening in the abdominal wall. **2.** Removal of the contents of the abdominal cavity.

ever'sion [L. *e-everto*, pp. *-versus*, to overturn] A turning outward, as of the eyelid.

evert' [L. *e-verto*, to overturn] To turn outward.

eviscera'tion [L. *eviscero*, pp. *-atus*, to disembowel] **1.** Exenteration. **2.** Removal of the contents of the eyeball, leaving the sclera and sometimes the cornea. **3.** Disembowelling. **4.** Protrusion of the abdominal viscera, *e.g.*, through a defect created by wound dehiscence.

evolu'tion [L. *e-volvo*, pp. *-volutus*, to roll out] A continuing process of change from one state, condition, or form to another.

 biologic e., the doctrine that all forms of life have been derived by gradual changes from simpler forms or from a single cell.

evul'sion [L. *evulsio*, fr. *e-vello*, pp. *-vulsus*, to pluck out] A forcible pulling out or extraction.

ex- [L. and G. out of] Prefix denoting out of, from, away from.

exac'erba'tion [L. *ex-acerbo*, pp. *-auts*, to exacerbate] An increase in the severity of a disease or any of its signs or symptoms.

examina'tion Any investigation or inspection made for the purpose of diagnosis, usually qualified by the method used; *e.g.,* cytologic, physical.

exan'them [G. *exanthēma,* efflorescence; an eruption] Exanthema.

exanthe'ma [G.] A skin eruption occurring as a symptom of an acute viral or coccal disease.

   e. subi'tum, a viral disease of infants and young children, marked by sudden onset with fever lasting several days (sometimes with convulsions) and followed by a fine macular (sometimes maculopapular) rash.

exanthem'atous Relating to an exanthema.

excava'tio [L. fr. *ex-cavo,* pp. *-cavatus,* to hollow out, *ex,* out, + *cavus,* hollow] [NA] Excavation (1).

   e. rectouteri'na [NA], rectouterine pouch; Douglas pouch; a pocket formed by the deflection of the peritoneum from the rectum to the uterus.

excava'tion **1.** A natural cavity, pouch, or recess. **2.** A cavity formed artificially or as the result of a pathologic process.

ex'cavator An instrument like a sharp spoon or curette, used in scraping out pathologic tissue.

excemento'sis Outgrowth of cementum or root surface of a tooth.

excen'tric Eccentric (2, 3).

excip'ient [L. *excipiens;* pres. p. of *excipio,* to take out] A more or less inert substance added in a prescription as a diluent or vehicle or to give form or consistency when the remedy is given in pill form.

excise' Exsect; to cut out.

exci'sion [L. *excidere,* to cut out] **1.** Operative removal of a portion of a structure or organ. **2.** In molecular biology, a recombination event in which a genetic element is removed.

exci'table **1.** Capable of quick response to a stimulus; having potentiality for emotional arousal. **2.** In neurophysiology, referring to a tissue, cell, or membrane capable of undergoing excitation in response to an adequate stimulus.

excita'tion **1.** The act of increasing the rapidity or intensity of the physical or mental processes. See also stimulation. **2.** In neurophysiology, the complete, all-or-none response of a nerve or muscle to an adequate stimulus, ordinarily including propagation of

e. along the membranes of the cell or cells involved.

excite'ment An emotional state characterized by its potential for impulsive or poorly controlled activity.

excoria'tion [L. *excorio,* to skin, strip] A scratch mark; a linear break in the skin surface, usually covered with blood or serous crusts.

ex'crement [L. *ex-cerno,* pp. *-cretus,* to separate] Waste matter or any excretion cast out of the body; *e.g.,* faeces.

excres'cence [L. *ex-cresco,* pp. *-cretus,* to grow forth] Any outgrowth from the surface.

excre'ta [L. neut. pl. of *excretus,* pp. of *excerno,* to separate] Excretion (2).

excre'tion [see excrement] **1.** The process whereby the undigested residue of food and the waste products of metabolism are eliminated. **2.** The product of a tissue or organ that is waste material to be passed out of the body.

ex'cretory Relating to excretion.

exencephal'ic Relating to exencephaly.

exenceph'aly [G. *ex,* out, + *enkephalos,* brain] A condition in which the skull is defective, the brain being exposed or extruding.

exentera'tion [G. *ex,* out, + *enteron,* bowel] Removal of internal organs and tissues, usually radical removal of the contents of a body cavity.

exenteri'tis [G. *exō,* on the outside, + enteritis] Inflammation of the peritoneal covering of the intestine.

ex'ercise **1.** *Active:* bodily exertion for the sake of restoring the organs and functions to a healthy state or keeping them healthy. **2.** *Passive:* motion of limbs without effort by the individual.

exer'esis [G. *exairesis,* a taking out] Excision, or surgical removal of any part or organ; also used as combining form in suffix position.

exfolia'tion [L. *exfolatio,* fr. *ex,* out, + *folium,* leaf] **1.** Detachment and shedding of superficial cells of an epithelium or from any tissue surface. **2.** Scaling or desquamation of the horny layer of epidermis. **3.** Loss of deciduous teeth following physiological loss of root structure. **4.** Extrusion of permanent teeth as a result of disease or loss of their antagonists.

exfo'liative [Mod. L. *exfoliativus*] Marked by exfoliation, desquamation, or profuse scaling.

exhala'tion [L. *ex-halo*, pp. *-halatus*, to breathe out] **1.** Expiration; breathing out. **2.** The giving forth of gas or vapour. **3.** Any exhaled or emitted gas or vapour.

exhale' **1.** To breathe out. **2.** To emit a gas or vapour or odour.

exhaus'tion [L. *ex-haurio*, pp. *-haustus*, to draw out, empty] **1.** Extreme fatigue; inability to respond to stimuli. **2.** Removal of contents; using up of a supply of anything. **3.** Extraction of the active constituents of a drug by treating with water, alcohol, or other solvent.

heat e., a form of reaction to heat, marked by prostration, weakness, and collapse, resulting from unrecognized or unavoidable dehydration.

exhibi'tionist One who has a morbid compulsion to expose the genitals to a person of the opposite sex.

exhuma'tion [L. *ex*, out of + *humus*, earth] Disinterment.

exo- [G. *exō*, outside] Prefix meaning exterior, external, or outward. See also ecto-.

ex'ocrine [exo- + G. *krinō*, to separate] **1.** Denoting glandular secretion that is delivered to a surface. **2.** Pertaining to a gland that secretes outwardly through excretory ducts.

exodon'tia [exo- + G. *odous*, tooth] The branch of dental practice concerned with the extraction of teeth.

exodon'tist One who specializes in the extraction of teeth.

exog'enous [exo- + G. *-gen*, production] Originating or produced outside of the organism.

exom'phalos [G. *ex*, out, + *omphalos*, umbilicus] **1.** Protrusion of the umbilicus **2.** Umbilical *hernia*. **3.** Omphalocele.

exophthal'mic Relating to exophthalmos, marked by prominence of the eyeball.

exophthal'mos [G. *ex*, out, + *ophthalmos*, eye] Protrusion of the eyeballs.

exoskel'eton **1.** All hard parts, such as hair, teeth, nails, feathers, dermal plates, scales, etc., developed from the ectoderm or mesoderm in vertebrates. **2.** The outer chitinous envelope of an insect, or the chitinous or calcareous covering of certain Crustacea and other invertebrates.

exosto'sis, pl. **exosto'ses** [exo- + G. *osteon*, bone, + *-osis*, condition] A cartilage-capped bony projection arising from any bone that develops from cartilage.

ex'other'mic [exo- + G. + *thermē*, heat] **1.** Denoting a chemical reaction attended by the development of heat. **2.** Relating to the external warmth of the body.

exotox'ic **1.** Relating to an exotoxin. **2.** Relating to the introduction of an exogenous poison or toxin.

exotox'in An antigenic, injurious substance elaborated within the cells of certain Gram-positive bacteria and released into the environment where it is rapidly active in small amounts.

exotro'pia [exo- + G *tropē*, turn] Divergent strabismus; wall-eye; that type of strabismus in which the visual axes diverge; may be paralytic or concomitant, monocular or alternating; constant or intermittent.

expec'torant [L. *ex*, out, + *pectus*, chest] Promoting secretion from the mucous membrane of the air passages or facilitating its expulsion.

expec'torate To spit; to eject saliva, mucus, or other fluid from the mouth.

expectora'tion **1.** Mucus and other fluids formed in the air passages and the mouth, and expelled by coughing. **2.** Spitting; the expelling from the mouth of saliva, mucus, and other material.

expira'tion [L. *expiro* or *ex-spiro*, pp. *-atus*, to breathe out] Exhalation (1).

expi'ratory Relating to expiration.

explora'tion [L. *ex-ploro*, pp. *-ploratus*, to explore] An active examination, usually involving endoscopy or a surgical procedure, to ascertain conditions present as an aid in diagnosis.

explor'atory Relating to or with a view to exploration.

explo'rer A sharp, pointed probe used to investigate tooth surfaces in order to detect caries or other defects.

express' [L. *ex-premo*, pp. *-pressus*, to press out] To press or squeeze out.

expres'sion **1.** Squeezing out; expelling by pressure. **2.** Mobility of the features giving a particular emotional significance to the face. **3.** Any act determined by the nature of an individual.

expul'sive [L. *ex-pello*, pp. *-pulsus*, to drive out] Tending to expel.

exsan'guinate [L. *ex*, out, + *sanguis* (*-guin*), blood] **1.** To deprive of blood; to make bloodless. **2.** Exsanguine.

exsanguina'tion Depriving of blood; making exsanguine.

exsan'guine Deprived of blood.

exsect' [L. *ex-seco*, pp. *-sectus*, to cut out] Excise.

exsec'tion Excision.

exsicca'tion 1. Desiccation. 2. Dehydration; removal of water of crystallization.

exsorp'tion [G. *ex*, out, + *sorbēre*, to suck] Movement of substances from the blood into the lumen of the gut.

ex'strophy [G. *ex*, out, + *strophē*, a turning] A congenital turning out or eversion of a hollow organ.

extend' [L. *ex-tendo*, pp. *-tensus*, to stretch out] To straighten a limb, to diminish or extinguish the angle formed by flexion; to place the distal segment of a limb in such a position that its axis is continuous with that of the proximal segment.

exten'sion [L. *extensio*, to stretch out] 1. The act of bringing the distal portion of a joint in continuity (though only parallel) with the long axis of the proximal portion. 2. A pulling or dragging force exerted on a limb in a distal direction.

  Buck's e., an apparatus for applying skin traction on the leg through contact between the skin and adhesive tape connected to a suspended weight.

  skeletal e., skeletal *traction.*

exten'sor [L. one who stretches] [NA] A muscle the contraction of which tends to straighten a limb; the antagonist of a flexor.

exte'riorize 1. To direct a patient's interest, thoughts, or feelings into a channel leading outside himself, to some definite aim or object. 2. To expose an organ temporarily for observation, or permanently for purposes of physiologic experiment.

exter'nal [L. *externus*] Exterior; on the outside or farther from the centre.

extirpa'tion [L. *extirpo*, pp. *-atus*, to root out] The removal of an organ, in part or completely, or of a diseased tissue.

extor'sion [L. *extorsio*, fr. *ex-torqueo*, pp. *-tortus*, to twist out] 1. Outward rotation of a limb or of an organ. 2. Positive declination; rotation of the eye temporally around its anteroposterior axis.

extra- Prefix fr. L. preposition meaning without, outside of.

extracel'lular Outside a cell.

ex'tracorpo'real Outside of, or unrelated to, the body or any anatomical "corpus."

extract 1. (ek'strakt) A concentrated preparation of a drug obtained by removing the active constituents of the drug with suitable solvents, evaporating all or nearly all of the solvent, and adjusting the residual mass or powder to the prescribed standard. 2. (ek-strakt') To remove part of a mixture with a solvent.

extrac'tion [L. *ex-traho*, pp. *-tractus*, to draw out] 1. Removal by withdrawing or pulling out, as a tooth from its alveolus, or a baby from the genital canal in assisted delivery. 2. The active portion of a drug; the making of an extract.

extrac'tor An instrument for use in drawing or pulling out any natural part or a foreign body.

ex'tra-embryon'ic Outside the embryonic body; *e.g.*, pertaining to structures concerned with the embryo's protection and nutrition, and discarded at birth without being incorporated into the embryo.

extrasen'sory Ouside or beyond the ordinary senses; not limited to the senses; *e.g.*, clairvoyance or thought transference.

ex'trasys'tole An ectopic, usually premature, contraction of the heart; such beats arise from the atrium, the A-V node, or the ventricle and interrupt the dominant, usually sinus, rhythm; they are in some way dependent on the preceding beat and are therefore "forced" beats.

extrav'asate [L. *extra*, out of, + *vas*, vessel] 1. To exude from or pass out of a vessel into the tissues, said of blood, lymph, or urine. 2. The substance thus exuded.

extrav'asa'tion 1. The act of extravasating. 2. Extravasate (2).

ex'traver'sion Extroversion.

extrem'itas [L. from *extremus*, last, outermost] [NA] Extremity (1).

extrem'ity [L. *extremitas*] 1. An end of an elongated or pointed structure. 2. An arm or a leg.

extrin'sic [L. *extrinsecus*, from without] Originating outside of the part where found or upon which it acts; denoting especially a muscle.

extrover'sion [fr. L. *extra*, outside, + *verto*, pp. *versus*, to turn] 1. A turning outward. 2. A trait involving social intercourse.

ex'trovert A gregarious person whose chief interests lie outside himself, and who is involved in the affairs of others.

extru'sion 1. A thrusting or forcing out of a normal position. 2. The overeruption or migration of a tooth beyond its normal occlusal position.

extuba'tion [L. *ex*, out, + *tuba*, tube] Removal of a tube from an organ, structure, or orifice; specifically, the removal of the tube after intubation of the larynx or trachea.

exu'berant [L. *exubero*, to abound, be abundant] Denoting excessive proliferation or growth, as of a tissue or granulation.

ex'udate [L. *ex*, out, + *sudare*, to sweat] Any fluid that has exuded out of a tissue or its capillaries, specifically because of injury or inflammation.

exuda'tion 1. The act or process of exuding. 2. Exudate.

exu'dative Relating to the process of exudation or to an exudate.

exude' [L. *ex*, out, + *sudare*, to sweat] To ooze or pass gradually out of a body structure or tissue; specifically, restricted to a fluid or semisolid that so passes and may become encrusted or infected, because of injury or inflammation.

eye [A.S. *ēage*] Oculus; the organ of vision.
  black e., ecchymosis of the lids and their surroundings.
  crossed e.'s, esotropia.

eye bank A place where corneas of eyes removed immediately after death are preserved for subsequent keratoplasty.

eye'brow Supercilium (1).

eye'glasses Spectacles.

eye'lash Cilium (1).

eye'lid Palpebra.

eye'strain Asthenopia.

eye'wash A soothing solution for bathing or medicating the eye.

F

face The front portion of the head, from forehead to chin.
  moon f., the round, usually red face, with large jowls, seen in Cushing's disease or in hyperadrenocorticalism.

face-lift See rhytidectomy.

fac'et [Fr. *facette*] 1. A small smooth area on a bone or other firm structure. 2. A worn spot on a tooth, produced by chewing or grinding.

fa'cial Relating to the face.

-facient [L. *facio*, to make] Suffix meaning that which brings about.

fa'cies, pl. **facies** [L.] 1. [NA] Face. 2. [NA] Surface. 3. Expression (2).
  adenoid f., the open-mouthed and often stupid appearance in children with adenoid hypertrophy, associated with a pinched nose and narrow nares.
  myasthenic f., the facial expression in myasthenia gravis: drooping of the eyelids and corners of the mouth, and weakness of the muscles of the face.
  Parkinson's f., the expressionless or masklike f. characteristic of parkinsonism (1).

facio- [L. *facies*, face] Combining form relating to the face.

facti'tious [L. *factitius*, made by art] Artificial; self-induced; not natural; produced either unintentionally (accidentally) or deliberately (consciously or unconsciously).

fac'tor [L. maker, causer, fr. *facio*, to make] 1. One of the contributing causes in any action. 2. One of the components which by multiplication makes up a number or expression. 3. Gene. 4. Vitamin or other essential element.
  f. I, fibrinogen.
  f. II, (1) prothrombin; **(2)** lipoic acid.
  f. III, tissue thromboplastin.
  f. IV, calcium ions.
  f. V, proaccelerin; a blood clotting f. deficiency of which leads to a rare haemorrhagic tendency known as parahaemophilia or hypoproaccelerinaemia, with autosomal recessive inheritance; heterozygous individuals are recognized by reduced levels of f. V but have no bleeding tendency.
  f. VII, proconvertin; serum accelerator; a blood clotting f. known to be involved in: 1) congenital deficiency of f. VII, with purpura and bleeding from mucous membranes, autosomal recessive inheritance; 2) the acquired deficiency of f. VII in association with a deficiency of vitamin K, the neonatal period, and administration of prothrombinopenic drugs; and 3) acquired excess of f. VII in some patients with thromboembolism. F. VII accelerates the conversion of prothrombin to thrombin, in the presence of tissue thromboplastin, calcium, and f. V.

f. VIII, antihaemophilic f.; proconvertin; a blood clotting f. deficiency of which is associated with classic haemophilia A, an X-linked recessive haemorrhagic tendency that occurs almost exclusively in males; clotting time is prolonged, less thromboplastin is formed, and the conversion of prothrombin is diminished.

f. IX, a blood clotting f. deficiency of which causes haemophilia B or Christmas disease, which resembles haemophilia A and is an X-linked recessive defect that leads to a severe haemorrhagic disorder. F. IX is required for the formation of intrinsic blood thromboplastin and affects the amount formed (rather than the rate).

f. X, prothrombinase.

f. XI, A component of the contact system absorbed from plasma and serum by glass and similar surfaces. Deficiency of f. XI results in a haemorrhagic tendency and is caused by an autosomal recessive gene.

f. XII, a blood clotting f. deficiency of which results in prolongation of the clotting time of venous blood, rarely in a haemorrhagic tendency, and is caused by an autosomal recessive gene.

f. XIII, in the clotting of blood, thrombin catalyses the conversion of this f. into its active form, fibrinase, which cross-links subunits of the fibrin clot to form insoluble fibrin.

clotting f., coagulation f., various plasma components involved in the clotting process, including, notably, fibrinogen (f. I), prothrombin (f. II), thromboplastin (f. III), and calcium ion (f. IV).

releasing f. (RF), a substance of hypothalamic origin capable of accelerating the rate of secretion of a given hormone by the anterior pituitary gland.

fac′ultative Able to live under more than one specific set of environmental conditions; with an alternative pathway.

fae′cal Relating to faeces.

fae′calith [faeces, + G. *lithos,* stone] Coprolith.

faecalu′ria [faeces, + G. *ouron,* urine] Commingling of faeces with urine passed from the urethra in persons with a fistula connecting the intestinal tract and bladder.

fae′ces [L., pl. of *faex (faec-),* dregs] The matter discharged from the bowel during defaecation.

fail′ure Inability to function or perform satisfactorily.

congestive heart f., heart f. (1).

heart f., (1) cardiac or myocardial insufficiency; mechanical inadequacy of the heart to maintain the circulation of blood, with congestion and edema developing in the tissues; **(2)** the resulting clinical syndrome consisting of shortness of breath, pitting oedema, enlarged tender liver, engorged neck veins, and pulmonary rales.

faint 1. Extremely weak; threatened with syncope. **2.** An attack of syncope.

fal′ciform [L. *falx,* sickle, + *forma,* form] Crescentic or sickle-shaped.

fallo′pian Described by or attributed to Fallopius.

falx, pl. **fal′ces** [L. sickle] [NA] A sickle-shaped structure.

f. cer′ebri [NA], the scythe-shaped fold of dura mater in the longitudinal fissure between the two cerebral hemispheres.

famil′ial [L. *familia,* family] Affecting several members of the same family, usually within a single sibship.

fam′ily [L. *familia*] **1.** A group of blood relatives; strictly, the parents and their children. **2.** In biologic classification, a division between order and tribe or genus.

fan′tasy [G. *phantasia,* idea, image] Imagery that is more or less coherent, as in dreams and daydreams, yet unrestricted by reality.

far′sight′edness Hyperopia.

fas′cia, pl. **fas′ciae** [L. a band or fillet] [NA] A sheet of fibrous tissue that envelops the body beneath the skin; also encloses muscles and muscle groups, and separates their several layers or groups.

fas′cial Relating to any fascia.

fas′cicle Fasciculus.

fascic′ular, fascic′ulate, fascic′ulated Relating to a fasciculus; arranged in the form of a bundle or collection of rods.

fascic′ula′tion 1. An arrangement in the form of fasciculi. **2.** Involuntary contractions, or twitchings, of groups (fasciculi) of muscle fibres, a coarser form of muscular contraction than fibrillation.

fascic′ulus, gen. and pl. **fascic′uli** [L. dim. of *facis,* bundle] [NA] A band or bundle of fibres, usually of muscle or nerve fibres.

fascii′tis 1. Inflammation in fascia. **2.** Reactive proliferation of fibroblasts in fascia.

fascio- [L. *fascia*, a band or fillet] Combining form denoting a fascia.

Fascio'la [L. dim of *fascia*, a band] A genus of large digenetic liver flukes (family Fasciolidae, class Trematoda) of mammals. *F. hepatica*, the common liver fluke inhabiting the bile ducts of sheep and cattle, is rarely reported from man, where it may cause considerable biliary damage.

fascio'la, pl. **fascio'lae** [L. dim of *fascia*, band, fillet] A small band or group of fibres.

fas'cioli'asis Infection with a species of Fasciola.

fasciot'omy [fascio- + G. *tome̅*, incision] Incision through a fascia.

fastig'ium [L. top, as of a gable; a pointed extremity] **1.** Summit of the roof of the fourth ventricle of the brain. **2.** The acme or period of full development of a disease.

fat [A.S. *faet*] **1.** Adipose *tissue*. **2.** Obese; corpulent. **3.** A greasy, soft-solid material, found in animal tissues and many plants, composed of a mixture of glycerol esters; together with oils these make up that class of foodstuffs known as simple lipids.

fa'tal [L. *fatalis*, of or belonging to fate] **1.** Inevitable. **2.** Pertaining to or causing death; denoting especially inevitability or inescapability of death.

fatigue' [Fr. fr. L. *fatigo*, to tire] **1.** That state following a period of mental or bodily activity characterized by a lessened capacity for work and reduced efficiency of accomplishment when from any cause energy expenditure outstrips restorative processes. **2.** Sensation of boredom and lassitude due to absence of stimulation, monotony, or lack of interest in one's surroundings.

fat-pad An accumulation of somewhat encapsulated adipose tissue.

fat'ty acid Any acid derived from fats by hydrolysis; any long-chain monobasic organic acid.

fau'ces [L. the throat] [NA] The space between the cavity of the mouth and the pharynx.

fau'cial Relating to the fauces.

fauci'tis Inflammation of the fauces.

fave'olus, pl. **fave'oli** [Mod. L. dim of *favus*, honeycomb] A small pit or depression.

fa'vid An allergic reaction in the skin observed in favus.

fa'vism [Ital. *favismo*, from *fava*, bean] An acute condition following the ingestion of certain species of beans, e.g., *Vicia faba*, or inhalation of the pollen of its flower; characterized by fever, headache, abdominal pain, severe anaemia, prostration, and coma, and occurs in certain individuals with genetic erythrocytic deficiency of glucose 6-phosphate dehydrogenase.

fa'vus [L. honeycomb] A severe type of chronic ringworm of the scalp and nails caused by three dissimilar dermatophytes, *Trichophyton schönleinii*, *T. violaceum*, and *Microsporum gypseum*.

fear [A.S. *faer*] Apprehension; dread; alarm. F has an identifiable stimulus, and thus is differentiated from anxiety which has no easily identifiable stimulus.

febrifa'cient [L. *febris*, fever, + *facio*, to make] Causing fever.

feb'rifuge [L. *febris*, fever, + *fugo*, to put to flight] Antipyretic; reducing fever.

feb'rile Feverish; relating to fever.

fecunda'tion [L. *fecundo*, pp. -*atus*, to make fruitful, fertilize] The act of rendering fertile.

fecun'dity Pronounced fertility; capability of repeated fertilization.

feed'back **1.** In a given system, the return, as input, of some of the output, as a regulatory mechanism. **2.** An explanation for the learning of motor skills. sensory stimuli set up by muscle contractions modulate the activity of the motor system.

fella'tio [L.] The sexual act of taking a penis into the mouth.

fel'on [M.E. *feloun*, malignant] Whitlow; a purulent infection or abscess involving the bulbous distal end of a finger.

fe'male In zoology, denoting the sex that bears the young or the sexual cell which develops into a new organism.

   genetic f., (1) An individual with a normal female karyotype, including two X chromosomes; **(2)** an individual whose cell nuclei contain Barr sex chromatin bodies, which are normally present in f.'s and absent in males.

feminiza'tion The acquisition of female characteristics by the male.

fem'oral Relating to the femur or thigh.

fem'orotib'ial Relating to the femur and the tibia.

fe'mur, pl. **fem'ora,** gen. **fem'oris** [L. thigh] **1.** [NA] The thigh. **2.** *Os femoris*.

fenes'tra, pl. **fenes'trae** [L.] Window. **1.** [NA] An anatomical aperture, often closed by a membrane. **2.** A specialized opening, as in an instrument.

   f. vestib'uli [NA], **f. of the vestibule,** an oval opening on the medial wall of the tympanic cavity leading into the vestibule, closed in life by the foot of the stapes.

fen'estrated Having fenestrae or window-like openings.

fen'estra'tion The presence or making of openings or fenestrae in a part.

fermenta'tion [L. *fermento*, pp. *-atus*, to ferment] **1.** A chemical change induced in a complex organic compound by the action of an enzyme, whereby the substance is split into more simple compounds. **2.** In bacteriology, the anaerobic dissimilation of substrates with the production of energy and reduced compounds.

ferment'ative Causing or having the ability to cause fermentation.

ferri- [L. *ferrum*, iron] Prefix designating the presence in a compound of a ferric ion.

fer'ric Relating to iron, especially denoting a salt containing iron in its higher (triad) valency, Fe^{3+}.

fer'ritin An iron protein complex containing up to 23% iron, formed by the union of ferric iron with apoferritin; found in the intestinal mucosa, spleen, liver.

ferro- [L. *ferrum*, iron] Prefix designating the presence of metallic iron or of the divalent ion Fe^{2+}.

fer'ropro'teins Proteins containing iron in a prosthetic group, *e.g.*, haem, cytochrome.

fer'tile [L. *fertilis*; *fero*, to bear] **1.** Fecund; fruitful; capable of conceiving and bearing young. **2.** Impregnated; fertilized.

fertil'ity. The state of being fertile; specifically, the ability to produce young.

fer'tiliza'tion The process that begins with the penetration of the secondary oocyte by the spermatozoon and is completed with the fusion of the male and female pronuclei.

fes'ter [L. *fistula*] **1.** To ulcerate. **2.** An ulcer. **3.** To form pus or putrefy.

fes'tinant [L. *festino*, to hasten] Rapid; quick; hastening; accelerating.

festina'tion [L. *festino*, to hasten] The peculiar acceleration of gait noted in parkinsonism and some other nervous affections.

fe'tal Relating to a fetus.

fe'tid [L. *foetidus*] Foul-smelling.

fet'ish [Fr. *fétiche*, fr. L. *factitius*, made by art, artificial] An inanimate object or nonsex-

ual body part that is regarded as endowed with magic or erotic qualities.

fet'ishism The act of worshipping or using for sexual arousal and gratification that which is regarded as a fetish.

fetog'raphy [L. *fetus* + G. +*IL graphō*, to write] Radiography of the fetus *in utero*.

fetom'etry [L. *fetus* + G. +*IL metron*, measure] Estimation of the size of the fetus, especially of its head, prior to delivery.

fe'toplacen'tal Relating to the fetus and its placenta.

fetopro'tein A fetal protein found in adults; α-f. (AFP) increases in maternal blood during pregnancy and, when detected by amniocentesis, is an important indicator of open neural tube defects; β-f., although a fetal liver protein, has been detected in adult patients with liver disease; γ-f., occurs in various neoplasms.

fe'tor [L. an offensive smell, fr. *feteo*, to stink] A very offensive odour.

fe'toscope A fibre-optic endoscope used in fetoscopy.

fetos'copy Use of a fibre-optic endoscope to view the fetus and placenta, and for collection of fetal blood.

fe'tus, pl. **fe'tuses** [L. offspring] The unborn young of a viviparous animal after it has taken form in the uterus; in man, it represents the product of conception from the end of the eighth week to the moment of birth.

fe'ver [A.S. *fefer*] **1.** Pyrexia; a bodily temperature above the normal of 98.6°F (37°C). **2.** A disease in which there is an elevation of the body temperature above the normal.

   cat-scratch f., cat-scratch *disease.*

   enteric f., (1) typhoid f.; **(2)** the group of typhoid and paratyphoid A and B f.'s.

   hay f., a form of atopy characterized by an acute irritative inflammation of the mucous membranes of the eyes and upper respiratory passages accompanied by itching and profuse watery secretion, followed occasionally by bronchitis and asthma; recurs annually at the same or nearly the same time of the year as an allergic reaction to the pollen of trees, grasses, weeds, flowers, etc.

   haemorrhagic f., a syndrome that occurs in perhaps 20 to 40% of infections by arboviruses of the haemorrhagic f. group; clinical manifestations are generally indistinguishable from those of the undifferentiated type f.'s caused by other arboviruses or by viruses of other taxonomic groups. The syndrome is associated with high f., scattered petechiae, gastrointestinal tract and other organ bleeding, hypotension, and shock; kidney damage may be severe, especially in epidemic haemorrhagic f., and neurologic signs may appear, especially in the case of the Argentinian-Bolivian types. Aetiologic agents are distributed among several taxonomic groups: alphaviruses, flaviviruses, bunyaviruses, and arenaviruses; some types are tick-borne, others mosquito-borne, and some seem to be zoonoses.

Oroya f., a specific, acute, febrile, endemic disease of the Peruvian Andes, caused by *Bartonella bacilliformis* and marked by high fever, rheumatic pains, progressive, severe anaemia, and albuminuria.

paratyphoid f., an acute infectious disease with symptoms and lesions resembling those of typhoid f., though milder in character; associated with the presence of the paratyphoid bacillus, of which at least three varieties (types A, B, and C) have been described.

puerperal f., postpartum sepsis with a rise in f. after the first 24 hours following delivery, but before the 11th postpartum day.

relapsing f., recurrent f., an acute infectious disease caused by any one of a number of strains of *Borrelia*, transmitted by lice or ticks and marked by a number of febrile attacks lasting about six days and separated from each other by apyretic intervals of about the same length; the microorganism is found in the blood during the febrile periods but not during the intervals, the disappearance being associated with specific antibodies and previously evoked antibodies.

rheumatic f., f. occurring during recovery from infection, usually of the throat, with group A streptococci and is variably associated with acute migratory polyarthritis, Sydenham's chorea, subcutaneous nodules over bony prominences, myocarditis with formation of Aschoff bodies, which may cause acute cardiac failure, and endocarditis which is frequently followed by scarring of valves, causing stenosis or incompetence.

Rocky Mountain spotted f., an acute infectious disease characterized by frontal and occipital headache, intense lumbar pain, malaise, a moderately high continuous f., and a rash on wrists and ankles later

spreading to all parts of the body; it occurs in the spring of the year, primarily in the southeast U.S. and the Rocky Mountain region, and is caused by *Rickettsia rickettsi*, transmitted by two or more tick species of the genus *Dermacentor*.

scarlet f., scarlatina.

swamp f., malaria.

typhoid f., an acute infectious disease caused by *Salmonella typhi* and characterized by a continued f., physical and mental depression, an eruption of rose-coloured spots on the chest and abdomen, tympanites, often diarrhoea, sometimes intestinal haemorrhage or perforation of the bowel.

undulant f., [referring to the wavy appearance of the long temperature curve], brucellosis.

yellow f., a tropical mosquito-borne viral hepatitis, due to yellow f. virus, with an urban form transmitted by *Aedes aegypti*, and a rural, jungle, or sylvatic form from tree-dwelling mammals by various mosquitoes of the *Haemagogus* species complex; characterized clinically by fever, slow pulse, albuminuria, jaundice, congestion of the face, and haemorrhages, especially haematemesis.

fibr- See fibro-.

fibrae'mia [fibrin + G. *haima*, blood] Presence of formed fibrin in the blood, causing thrombosis or embolism.

fi'bre [L. *fibra*] A slender thread or filament. In anatomy, refers to 1) extracellular filamentous structures such as collagenic or elastic connective tissue f.'s; 2) the nerve cell axon with its glial envelope; 3) certain elongated, threadlike cells such as muscle cells and the epithelial cells composing the major part of the eye lens.

myelinated f., an axon enveloped by a myelin sheath formed by oligodendroglia cells (in brain and spinal cord) or Schwann cells (in peripheral nerves).

unmyelinated f.'s, nerve f.'s (axons) lacking a fatty sheath but in common with others enveloped by a sheath of Schwann cells.

fibre-op'tic Pertaining to fibre-optics.

fibre-op'tics An optical system whereby light or an image is conveyed by a compact, coherent bundle of fine flexible glass or plastic fibres.

fi'brescope An optical instrument that transmits images by fibre-optics.

fi'bril [Mod. L. *fibrilla*] A minute fibre.

fi'brilla, pl. **fi'brillae** [Mod. L. dim. of L. *fibra*, a fibre] Fibril.

fi'brillar, fi'brillary 1. Filar (1); relating to a fibril. **2.** Denoting the fine rapid contractions or twitchings of fibres or of small groups of fibres in skeletal or cardiac muscle.

fi'brillate 1. To make or to become fibrillar. **2.** Fibrillated. **3.** To be in a state of fibrillation (3).

fi'brillated Composed of fibrils.

fibrilla'tion 1. The condition of being fibrillated. **2.** Formation of fibrils. **3.** Exceedingly rapid contractions or twitching of muscular fibrils, but not of the muscle as a whole. **4.** Vermicular twitching, usually slow, of individual muscular fibres, commonly occurs in atria or ventricles of the heart as well as in recently denervated skeletal muscle fibres.

   atrial f., auricular f., f. in which the normal rhythmical contractions of the cardiac atria are replaced by rapid irregular twitchings of the muscular wall; the ventricles respond irregularly to the dysrhythmic bombardment from the atria.

   ventricular f., fine, rapid, fibrillary movements of the ventricular muscle that replace the normal contraction.

fi'brin [L. *fibra*, fibre] An elastic filamentous protein derived from fibrinogen by the action of thrombin, which releases fibrinopeptides A and B from fibrinogen, in coagulation of the blood.

fi'brinae'mia Fibraemia.

fibrino- [L. *fibra*, fibre] Combining form relating to fibrin.

fi'brinocel'lular Composed of fibrin and cells, as in certain types of exudates resulting from acute inflammation.

fibrin'ogen Factor I; a globulin of the blood plasma that is converted into fibrin by the action of thrombin in the presence of ionized calcium; produces coagulation of the blood.

fi'brinogen'ic, fibrinog'enous Pertaining to fibrinogen; producing fibrin.

fi'brinol'ysin Plasmin.

fibrinol'ysis [fibrino- + G. *lysis*, dissolution] The hydrolysis of fibrin.

fi'brinous Pertaining to or composed of fibrin.

fibro-, fibr- [L. *fibra*, fibre] Combining forms denoting fibre.

fi'broadeno'ma A benign neoplasm derived from glandular epithelium, in which there is a conspicuous stroma of proliferating fibroblasts and connective tissue elements.

fi'broblast A stellate or spindle-shaped cell with cytoplasmic processes present in connective tissue, capable of forming collagen fibres.

fi'broblas'tic. Relating to fibroblasts.

fi'brocar'tilage. A variety of cartilage that contains visible collagenic fibres.

fi'brocartilag'inous Relating to or composed of fibrocartilage.

fi'brochondri'tis Inflammation of a fibrocartilage.

fi'brocyst Any cystic lesion that is circumscribed by or situated within a conspicuous amount of fibrous connective tissue.

fi'brocys'tic Pertaining to or characterized by the presence of fibrocysts.

fi'brodyspla'sia Abnormal development of fibrous connective tissue.

fi'broelas'tic Composed of collagen and elastic fibres.

fi'broid [fibro- + G. *eidos*, resemblance] **1.** Resembling or composed of fibres or fibrous tissue. **2.** Old term for certain types of leiomyoma, especially those occurring in the uterus.

fibro'ma [fibro- + G. *-oma*, tumour] A benign neoplasm derived from fibrous connective tissue.

fi'bromato'sis 1. The occurrence of multiple fibromas, with a relatively large distribution. **2.** Abnormal hyperplasia of fibrous tissue.

fi'bromus'cular Both fibrous and muscular; relating to both fibrous and muscular tissues.

fibromyo'ma A leiomyoma that contains a relatively abundant amount of fibrous tissue.

fi'bromyosi'tis [fibro- + G. *mys*, muscle, + *-itis*, inflammation] Chronic inflammation of a muscle with an overgrowth, or hyperplasia, of the connective tissue.

fibropla'sia [fibro- + G. *plasis*, a moulding] Production of fibrous tissue, usually implying an abnormal increase of non-neoplastic fibrous tissue.

   retrolental f., abnormal replacement of the sensory retina by fibrous tissue and blood vessels, occurring mainly in premature infants placed in a high oxygen environment.

fibroplas'tic [fibro- + G. *plastos*, formed] Producing fibrous tissue.

fi′brosarco′ma A malignant neoplasm derived from fibrous connective tissue and characterized by immature proliferating fibroblasts or undifferentiated anaplastic spindle cells.

fibro′sis Formation of fibrous tissue as a reparative or reactive process.

 cystic f. (of the pancreas), a congenital metabolic disorder, inherited as a recessive trait, in which exocrine glands secrete excessively viscid mucus, causing obstruction of passageways (including pancreatic and bile ducts, intestines, and bronchi); the sodium and chloride content of sweat is increased.

fi′brosi′tis [fibro- + G. -*itis*, inflammation] **1.** Inflammation of fibrous tissue. **2.** A term used to denote aching, soreness, or stiffness in the absence of objective abnormalities.

fi′brous Composed of or containing fibroblasts, and also the fibrils and fibres of connective tissue formed by such cells.

fib′ula [L. *fibula* (contr. fr. *figibula*), that which fastens, a clasp, buckle, fr. *figo*, to fix, fasten] [NA] Calf bone; the lateral and smaller of the two bones of the leg; articulating with the tibia above and the tibia and talus below.

fib′ular [L. *fibularis*] Relating to the fibula.

field [A.S. *feld*] A definite area of plane surface, considered in relation to some specific object.

 visual f. (F), the area simultaneously visible to one eye without movement; usually measured by means of an arc (perimeter) located 330 mm from the eye.

fila [L.] Plural of filum.

fil′ament [L. *filamentum*, fr. *filum*, a thread] A fibril, fine fibre, or threadlike structure.

filamen′tous. 1. Threadlike in structure. **2.** Composed of filaments or threadlike structures.

fi′lar [L. *filum*, a thread] **1.** Fibrillar. **2.** Filamentous.

Fila′ria Former genus of nematodes now classified in several genera and species of the family Onchocercidae.

fila′ria, pl. **fila′riae** [L. *filum*, a thread] Common name for nematodes of the family Onchocercidae, which live as adults in the blood, tissue fluids, tissues, or body cavities of many vertebrates.

fila′rial Pertaining to a filaria (or filariae), including the microfilaria stage.

filari′asis The presence of filariae in the tissues of the body or in blood or tissue fluids (microfilaraemia or microfilariasis); death of the adult worms leads to granulomatous inflammation and permanent fibrosis causing obstruction of the lymphatic channels from dense hyalinized scars in the subcutaneous tissues; the most serious consequence is elephantiasis or pachyderma.

filar′icide [filaria + L. *caedo*, to kill] An agent that kills filariae.

filar′iform 1. Resembling filariae or other types of small nematode worms. **2.** Thin or hairlike.

fil′ial [L. *filialis*, fr. *filius*, son, *filia*, daughter] Denoting the relationship of offspring to parents.

fil′let [Fr. *filet*, a band] **1.** Lemniscus. **2.** A skein or loop of cord or tape used for making traction on a part of the fetus.

fil′ling Lay term for a dental restoration.

fi′lopres′sure [L. *filum*, thread] Temporary pressure on a blood vessel by a ligature, which is removed when the flow of blood has ceased.

fil′ter [Mediev. L. *filtro*, pp. -*atus*, to strain through felt] **1.** To pass a fluid through a porous substance that arrests suspended solid particles. **2.** A porous substance through which a fluid is passed in order to separate it from contained particulate matter. **3.** A translucent screen, used in both diagnostic and therapeutic radiology, that permits the passage of certain rays and inhibits the passage of others which have a lower and less desirable energy. **4.** A device used in spectrophotometric analysis to isolate a segment of the spectrum.

fil′trable, fil′terable Capable of passing through a filter; frequently applied to smaller viruses and some bacteria.

fil′trate [see filter] Liquid that has passed through a filter.

filtra′tion Percolation (1); the process of passing a liquid through a filter.

fi′lum, pl. **fi′la** [L. thread] [NA] A structure of filamentous or threadlike appearance.

fim′bria, pl. **fim′briae** [L. fringe] **1.** [NA] Any fringelike structure. **2.** Pilus (2).

fim′briate, fim′briated Having fimbriae.

fin′ger [A.S.] *Digitus manus*; one of the digits of the hand.

webbed f.'s, two or more f.'s united by a common sheath of skin.

fin'gerprint 1. An impression of the inked bulb of the distal phalanx of a finger, showing the configuration of the ridges, used as a means of identification. **2.** Any analytical method capable of making fine distinctions between similar compounds.

first aid Immediate assistance given in the case of injury or sudden illness by a bystander before the arrival of a health care professional.

fis'sion [L. *fissio*, a cleaving] **1.** The act of splitting, *e.g.*, amitotic division of a cell or its nucleus. **2.** Splitting of the nucleus of an atom.

fissu'ra, pl. **fissu'rae** [L. fr. *findo*, to cleave] [NA] **1.** A deep fissure, cleft, or slit. **2.** In neuroanatomy, a particularly deep sulcus of the surface of the brain or spinal cord.

fis'sure [L. *fissura*] **1.** A deep furrow, cleft, or slit. **2.** In dentistry, a developmental break or fault in the enamel of a tooth.

fis'tula, pl. **fis'tulae** or **fis'tulas** [L. a pipe, tube] An abnormal passage from a hollow organ to the surface, or from one organ to another.

anal f., a f. opening at or near the anus, usually opening into the rectum above the internal sphincter.

blind f., incomplete f., a f. that ends in a cul-de-sac, being open at one extremity only.

intestinal f., faecal f., stercoral f., a tract leading from the lumen of the bowel to the exterior.

fistulec'tomy [fistula + G. *ektomē*, excision] Excision of a fistula.

fistulot'omy [fistula + G. *tomē*, incision] Incision or surgical enlargement of a fistula.

fit [A.S. *fitt*] An acute attack or the sudden appearance of some symptom, such as coughing or a convulsion.

fixa'tion [L. *figo*, pp. *fixus*, to fix, fasten] **1.** The condition of being stabilized, firmly attached, or set. **2.** Fixing; in histology, rapid killing of tissue elements and their preservation and hardening, to retain as nearly as possible the same relations they had in the living body. **3.** In chemistry, conversion of a gas into solid or liquid form by chemical reactions either with or without the help of living tissue. **4.** In psychoanalysis, the quality of being firmly attached or fixed to a particular person or object, such as a close and paralyz-

ing attachment. **5.** In physiological optics, the coordinated positioning and accommodation of both eyes that results in bringing or maintaining a sharp image of a stationary or moving object on the fovea of each eye.

fix'ative 1. Serving to fix, bind, or make firm or stable. **2.** A substance used for the preservation of gross and histologic specimens of tissue, or individual cells, usually by denaturing and precipitating or cross-linking the protein constituents.

flac'cid [L. *flaccidus*] Relaxed; flabby; without tone.

flagel'lar Relating to a flagellum or to the extremity of a protozoan.

flag'ellate 1. Possessing one or more flagella. **2.** Common name for a member of the class Mastigophora.

flag'ellated Possession one or more flagella.

flagella'tion [L. *flagellatus*, fr. *flagellāre*, to whip or scourge] Whipping either one's self or another as a means of arousing or heightening sexual feeling.

flagel'lum, pl. **flagel'la** [L. dim. of *flagrum*, a whip] A whiplike locomotory organelle consisting of nine double peripheral microtubules and two single central microtubules; it arises from a deeply staining basal granule, often connected to the nucleus by a fibre, the rhizoplast.

flank Latus.

flap 1. A mass or tongue of tissue for transplantation, vascularized by a pedicle or stem; specifically, a pedicle f. **2.** An uncontrolled movement, as of the hands.

flare A diffuse redness of the skin extending beyond the local reaction to the application of an irritant; due to a vasomotor reaction.

flat'foot *Talipes* planus.

flat'ulence [Mod. L. *flatulentus*, fr. L. *flatus*, a blowing] Presence of an excessive amount of gas in the stomach and intestines.

fla'tus [L. a blowing] Gas or air in the gastrointestinal tract which may be expelled through the anus.

flat'worm A member of the phylum Platyhelminthes, including the free-living Turbellaria and parasitic tapeworms and flukes.

Fla'vivirus A genus of viruses (family Togaviridae) formerly classified as group B arboviruses.

Fla'vobacte'rium [L. *flavus*, yellow] A genus of bacteria (family Achromobacteraceae) that characteristically produce yellow, orange, red, or yellow-brown pigments; found in soil and fresh and salt water; some species are pathogenic. The type species is *F. aquatile*.

flea An insect of the order Siphonaptera, marked by lateral compression, sucking mouthparts, extraordinary jumping powers, and ectoparasitic adult life in the hair and feathers of warm-blooded animals. Important f.'s include *Ctenocephalides* (*C. felis*, cat f., or *C. canis*, dog f.), *Pulex irritans*, (human f.), *Tunga penetrans* (chigger, chigoe, or sand f.), *Echidonophaga gallinacea* (sticktight f.), *Xenopsylla* (rat f.), and *Ceratophyllus*.

flesh [A.S. *flaesc*] **1.** The meat of animals used for food. **2.** Muscular *tissue*.

proud f., exuberant granulations in the granulation tissue on the surface of a wound.

flesh'flies Members of the order Diptera, whose larvae (maggots) develop in putrifying or living tissues.

flex [L. *flecto*, pp. *flexus*, to bend] To bend; to move a joint in such a direction as to approximate the two parts which it connects.

flexibil'itas ce'rea [L. waxy flexibility] The peculiar rigidity of catalepsy which may be overcome by slight external force, but which returns at once, holding the limb firmly in the new position.

flex'ion [L. *flecto*, pp. *flectus*, to bend] **1.** The act of flexing or bending. **2.** The condition of being flexed or bent.

flex'or [NA] A muscle the action of which is to flex a joint.

flexu'ra, pl. **flexu'rae** [L. a bending] [NA] A bend, as in an organ or structure.

flex'ure [L. *flexura*] Flexura.

sigmoid f., *colon* sigmoideum.

float'ing 1. Free or unattached. **2.** Out of the normal position; unduly movable; wandering; denoting an occasional abnormal condition of certain organs.

floccilla'tion [Mod. L. *flocculus*] An aimless plucking at the bedclothes, as if one were picking off threads or tufts of cotton, occurring in the delirium of a fever.

floc'cular Relating to a flocculus of any sort; specifically to the flocculus of the cerebellum.

floc'culate To become flocculent.

floc'culent 1. Resembling tufts of cotton or wool; denoting a fluid, such as the urine, containing numerous shreds or fluffy particles of grey-white or white mucus or other material. **2.** In bacteriology, denoting a fluid culture in which there are numerous colonies either floating in the fluid medium or loosely deposited at the bottom.

flo'ra [L. *Flora*, goddess of flowers, fr. *flos* (*flor-*), a flower] **1.** Plant life, usually of a certain locality or district. **2.** The various bacterial and other microscopic forms of life inhabiting an individual.

flor'id [L. *floridus*, flowery] Of a bright red colour; denoting certain cutaneous lesions.

flow [A.S. *flōwan*] The movement of a fluid or gas; specifically, the volume of fluid or gas passing a given point per unit of time. In respiratory physiology, the symbol for gas flow is V-. and for blood flow is Q-., followed by subscripts denoting location and chemical species. **4.** In rheology, a permanent deformation of a body which proceeds with time.

flow'ers A mineral substance in a powdery state after sublimation.

flow'meter A device for measuring velocity or volume of flow of liquids or gases.

fluc'tuate [L. *fluctuo*, pp. -*atus*, to flow in waves] **1.** To move in waves. **2.** To vary, to change from time to time, as in referring to any quantity or quality.

flu'id [L. *fluridus*, fr. *fluo*, to flow] **1.** Flowing; liquid; gaseous. **2.** A nonsolid substance, either liquid or gas.

amniotic f., a liquid within the amnion that surrounds the fetus and protects it from injury.

cerebrospinal f. (CSF), f. secreted by the choroid plexuses of the ventricles of the brain, filling the ventricles and the subarachnoid cavities of the brain and spinal cord.

extracellular f., (1) the interstitial f. and the plasma, constituting about 20% of the weight of the body; **(2)** sometimes used to mean all f. outside of cells, usually excluding transcellular f.

interstitial f., the f. in spaces between the tissue cells; constituting about 16% of the weight of the body.

seminal f., semen (1).

synovial f., synovia.

flu'idex'tract Pharmacopoeial liquid preparation of vegetable drugs, containing alcohol as a solvent, preservative, or both, and so made that each millilitre contains the therapeutic constitutents of 1 g of the standard drug that it represents.

fluke [A.S. *flōc*, flatfish] Common name for members of the class Trematoda (phylum Platyhelminthes). All f.'s of mammals (subclass Digenea) are internal parasites in the adult stage and are characterized by complex digenetic life cycles involving a snail initial host, in which larval multiplication occurs, and the release of swimming larvae (cercariae) which directly penetrate the skin of the final host, encyst on vegetation, or encyst in or on another intermediate host.

fluor-, fluoro- Prefixes denoting fluorine.

fluores'cence The emission of a longer wavelength radiation by a substance as a consequence of absorption of energy from a shorter wavelength radiation, continuing only as long as the stimulus is present.

fluorida'tion Addition of fluorides to the drinking water, usually 1 p.p.m., to reduce incidence of dental decay.

flu'oride A compound of fluorine with a metal, a nonmetal, or an organic radical; the anion of fluorine.

flu'oriza'tion Therapeutic use of fluorides to reduce the incidence of dental decay, as by topical application of fluoride agents to the teeth.

flu'orine A gaseous chemical element, symbol F, atomic no. 9, atomic weight 19.00.

fluoro- See fluor-.

fluorog'raphy Photofluorography.

flu'oroscope [fluorescence + G. *skopeō*, to examine] An apparatus for rendering visible the shadows of the x-rays which, after passing through the body examined, are projected on a fluorescent screen.

fluoros'copy Examination of the tissues and deep structures of the body by x-ray, using the fluoroscope.

fluoro'sis A condition caused by an excessive intake of fluorides in drinking water, characterized mainly by mottling of the enamel of the teeth, although the skeletal bones are also affected.

flush 1. To wash out with a full stream of fluid. **2.** A transient erythema due to heat, exertion, stress, or disease. **3.** Flat, or even with another surface.

flux [L. *fluxus*, a flow] **1.** The discharge of a fluid material in large amount from a cavity or surface of the body. **2.** Material thus discharged from the bowels.

fly [A.S. *fleóge*] A two-winged insect in the order Diptera. Typical flies of the housefly type and similar forms are in the family Muscidae.

fo'cal Relating to a focus.

fo'cus, pl. **fo'ci** [L. a hearth] **1.** The point at which the light rays meet after passing through a convex lens. **2.** The centre, or the starting point, of a disease process.

fo'late A salt or ester of folic acid.

fold 1 A ridge or margin apparently formed by the doubling back of a lamina. See also plica. **2.** In the embryo, a transient elevation or reduplication of tissue in the form of a lamina.

fo'lic acid The growth factor for *Lactobacillus casei*, and a member of the vitamin B complex necessary for the normal production of red blood cells; present in peptide linkages in liver, green vegetables, and yeast.

folie' [Fr. folly] Old term for madness or insanity.

　f. à deux (á-dü′) [Fr. *deux*, two] double insanity; identical or similar mental disorders affecting two individuals, usually members of the same family living together.

fo'lium, pl. **folia** [L. a leaf] [NA] A broad, thin, leaflike structure, as of the cerebellar cortex.

fol'licle [L. *folliculus*, a small sac] **1.** Folliculus. **2.** Ovarian f.

　graafian f., vesicular ovarian f.

　hair f., *folliculus* pili.

　ovarian f., one of the spheroidal cell aggregations in the ovary containing an ovum.

　vesicular ovarian f., a f. in which the oocyte attains its full size and is surrounded by the (zona pellucida) at the periphery of the fluid-filled antrum; the follicular cells proliferate and form the membrana granulosa; the theca of the f. develops into internal and external layers.

follic'ular Relating to a follicle or follicles.

follic'uli Plural of folliculus.

follic'uli'tis An inflammatory reaction in hair follicles.

folliculo'sis Presence of lymph follicles in abnormally great numbers.

follic'ulus, pl. **follic'uli** [L. a small sac] [NA] **1.** A more or less spherical mass of cells usually containing a cavity. **2.** A crypt or minute cul-de-sac or lacuna, such as the depression in the skin, from which the hair emerges.

f. pi'li [NA], hair follicle; a deep narrow pit formed by invagination of the epidermis and corium; it contains the root of the hair and the ducts of the sebaceous glands open into it.

fomenta'tion [L. fomento, pp. -atus, to foment] **1.** A warm application; a poultice. **2.** Application of warmth and moisture in the treatment of disease.

fo'mes, pl. **fomi'tes** [L. tinder, fr. foveo, to keep warm] A substance, such as clothing, capable of absorbing and transmitting the contagium of disease; usually used in the plural.

fontanel', fontanelle' [Fr. dim. of fontaine, fountain, spring] Fonticulus.

fontic'ulus, pl. **fontic'uli** [L. dim. of fons (font-), fountain, spring] [NA] One of several membranous intervals at the angles of the cranial bones in the infant; the midline anterior and posterior fontanels, and the paired sphenoidal and mastoid fontanels.

foot [A.S. fōt] The lower, pedal, podalic, extremity of the leg.

athlete's f., tinea pedis.

club f., talipes equinovarus.

flat f., talipes planus.

immersion f., trench f., a condition resulting from prolonged exposure to damp and cold; the extremity is initially cold and anaesthetic, but on rewarming becomes hyperaemic, paraesthetic, and hyperhidrotic.

foot-drop Paralysis or weakness of the dorsiflexor muscles of the foot and ankle, as a consequence of which the foot falls and the toes drag on the ground in walking.

fora'men, pl. **foram'ina** [L. an aperture, fr. foro, to pierce] [NA] An aperture or perforation through a bone or a membranous structure.

f. mag'num [NA], the large opening in the basal part of the occipital bone through which the spinal cord becomes continuous with the medulla oblongata.

f. interventricula're [NA], **interventricular f.,** the short, often slitlike passage that, on both the left and right side, connects the third ventricle (in the diencephalon) with the lateral ventricle (in the cerebral hemisphere).

f. ova'le, oval f., (1) [NA], in the fetal heart, the oval opening in the septum secundum; the persistent part of septum primum acts as a valve for this interatrial communication during fetal life and postnatally becomes fused to septum secundum to close it; **(2)** [NA], a large oval opening in the greater wing of the sphenoid bone, transmitting the mandibular nerve and a small meningeal artery; **(3)** valvular incompetence of the f. ovale of the heart; a condition contrasting with probe patency of the f. ovale in that the valvula foraminis ovalis has abnormal perforations in it or is of insufficient size to afford adequate valvular action at the f. ovale prenatally, or effect a complete closure postnatally.

forced feeding Giving nourishment through a nasal tube passed into the stomach of someone unable or unwilling to eat.

for'ceps [L. a pair of tongs] **1.** An instrument for seizing a structure, and making compression or traction. **2.** [NA] Bands of white fibres (f. major and f. minor) composing the radiation of the corpus callosum to the cerebrum.

bone f., strong f. used for seizing or removing fragments of bone.

dental f., extracting f., f. used to luxate teeth and remove them from the alveolus.

obstetrical f., f. used for grasping and making traction on or rotation of the fetal head; they are introduced separately into the genital canal, permitting the fetal head to be grasped firmly but with minimal compression and then are articulated after being placed in correct position.

fore'brain Prosencephalon.

fore'head Frons.

fore'milk Colostrum.

foren'sic [L. forensis, of a forum] Pertaining to, or used in, legal proceedings.

fore'skin Preputium.

fore'waters Bulging membranes filled with amniotic fluid presenting in front of the fetal head.

-form [L. -formis] Suffix denoting in the form or shape of; equivalent to -oid.

formal'dehyde [form(ic) + aldehyde] A pungent gas used as an antiseptic, disinfectant, and histologic fixative.

formica'tion [L. formica, ant] A form of paraesthesia in which there is a sensation as of ants running over the skin.

for'mula, pl. **for'mulas, for'mulae** [L. dim. of forma, form] **1.** A recipe or prescription containing directions for the compounding of a medicinal preparation. **2.** In chemistry, a symbol or collection of symbols expressing the number of atoms of the element or elements forming one molecule of a substance, together with, *e.g.*, information concerning the arrangement of the atoms within the molecule, their electronic structure, their charge, the nature of the bonds within the molecule. **3.** An expression by symbols and numbers of the normal order or arrangement of parts or structures.

for'mulary A collection of formulas for the compounding of medicinal preparations.

for'nicate **1.** [L. *fornicatus*, arched, fr. *fornix*, vault, arch] Vaulted or arched; resembling a fornix. **2.** [see fornication] To commit fornication.

fornica'tion [L. *fornicatio*, an arched or vaulted basement (brothel)] Sexual intercourse, especially between unmarried partners.

for'nix, gen. **for'nicis,** pl. **for'nices** [L. arch, vault] **1.** [NA] An arch-shaped structure; often the arch-shaped roof (or roof portion) of an anatomical space. **2.** [NA] The compact white fibre bundle by which the hippocampus of each cerebral hemisphere projects to the contralateral hippocampus and to the septum, anterior nucleus of the thalamus, and mamillary body.

fos'sa, gen. and pl. **fos'sae** [L. a trench or ditch] [NA] A depression, usually longitudinal in shape, in the surface of a part.

f. axilla'ris [NA], **axillary f.,** axilla; armpit; the space below the shoulder joint, bounded by the pectoralis major, the latissimus dorsi, the serratus anterior, and the humerus; contains the axillary artery and vein, the infraclavicular part of the brachial plexus, lymph nodes and vessels, and areolar tissue.

fos'sula, pl. **fos'sulae** [L. dim. of *fossa*, ditch] [NA] A small fossa.

foulage' [Fr. impression] Kneading and pressure of the muscles, constituting a form of massage.

fourchette' [Fr. dim. of *fourché*, fr. L. *furca*, fork] Frenulum labiorum pudendi.

fo'vea, pl. **fo'veae** [L. a pit] [NA] A cup-shaped depression or pit.

f. centra'lis ret'inae [NA], **central f.,** a depression in the centre of the macula retinae where only cones are present and blood vessels are lacking.

fovea'tion [L. *fovea*, a pit] Pitted scar formation as in smallpox, chickenpox, or vaccina.

fove'ola, pl. **fove'olae** [Mod. L. dim. of L. *fovea*, pit] [NA] A minute fovea or pit.

fractiona'tion **1.** To separate components of a mixture. **2.** Protraction of a total therapeutic radiation dose over a period of time, ordinarily days or weeks, in order to minimize untoward radiation effects on normal contiguous tissue.

frac'ture [L. *fractura*, a break] **1.** To break. **2.** A break, especially the breaking of a bone or cartilage.

avulsion f., a f. that occurs when a joint capsule, ligament, or muscle insertion of origin is pulled from the bone as a result of a sprain dislocation or strong contracture of the muscle against resistance; as the soft tissue is pulled away from the bone, a fragment or fragments of the bone may come away with it.

closed f., one in which skin is intact at site of f.

Colles f., a f. of the lower end of the radius with displacement of the distal fragment dorsally; volar displacement of the distal fragment in the same location is sometimes called a reversed Colles f., or Smith's f.

comminuted f., a f. in which the bone is broken into pieces.

compound f., open f.

green-stick f., the bending of a bone with incomplete f. involving the convex side of the curve only.

hairline f., a f. without separation of the fragments, the line of break being fine, as seen sometimes in the skull.

longitudinal f., a f. involving the bone in the line of its axis.

simple f., closed f.

open f., compound f.; f. in which the skin is perforated and there is an open wound down to the f.

stellate f., a f. in which the lines of break radiate from a central point.

transverse f., a f. the line of which forms a right angle with the axis of the bone.

fragil'ity [L. *fragilitas*] Brittleness; liability to break, burst, or disintegrate.

f. of the blood, increased susceptibility of the red blood cells to break down when the proportion of the saline content of the fluid is altered.

framboe'sia [Fr. *framboise*, raspberry] Yaws.

frame A structure made of parts fitted together.

Balkan f., Balkan splint; an overhead pole or f., supported on uprights attached to the bedposts or to a separate stand, from which a splinted limb is slung.

Bradford f., an oblong rectangular f. made of pipe, over which are stretched transversely two strips of canvas; permits trunk and lower extremities to move as a unit.

Stryker f., a f. that holds the patient and permits turning in various planes without individual motion of parts.

Francisel'la A genus of nonmotile, non-sporeforming, aerobic bacteria that contain small, Gram-negative cocci and rods. The type species, *F. tularensis* (*Pasteurella tularensis*), causes tularaemia in man.

frank Unmistakable; manifest; clinically evident.

freck'le [O. Eng. *freken*] A yellowish or brownish macule developing on the exposed parts of the skin, especially in persons of light complexion, due to an increase in melanin from exposure to the sun.

Hutchinson's f., melanotic f., *lentigo* maligna.

frem'itus [L. a dull roaring sound] A vibration imparted to the hand resting on the chest or other part of the body.

rhonchal f., f. produced by vibrations from the passage of air in the bronchial tubes partially obstructed by mucous secretion.

vocal f., the vibration in the chest wall, felt on palpation, produced by the spoken voice.

frenot'omy [frenum + G. *tomē*, a cutting] Division of any frenum, especially of the frenulum linguae.

fren'ulum, pl. **fren'ula** [Mod. L. dim. of L. *frenum,* bridle] [NA] A small frenum.

f. lin'guae [NA], f. of the tongue; a fold of mucous membrane extending from the floor of the mouth to the midline of the undersurface of the tongue.

f. labio'rum puden'di [NA], the fold connecting the two labia minora posteriorly.

fre'num, pl. **fre'na, fre'nums** [L. a bridle, curb] **1.** A narrow reflection or fold of mucous membrane passing from a more fixed to a movable part, serving to check undue movement of the part. **2.** An anatomical structure resembling such a fold.

freu'dian Relating to or described by Freud.

freudian slip A mistake which presumably suggests some underlying motive, often sexual or aggressive in nature.

frig'id [L. *frigidus*, cold] **1.** Cold. **2.** Temperamentally, especially sexually, cold or irresponsive.

frons, gen. **fron'tis** [L.] [NA], Forehead; brow; the part of the face between the eyebrows and the hairy scalp.

fron'tal 1. In front; relating to the anterior part of a body. **2.** Frontalis.

fronta'lis [L.] [NA] Referring to the frontal (coronal) plane or to the frontal bone or forehead.

fron'toma'lar Frontozygomatic.

frontomax'illary Relating to the frontal and the maxillary bones.

frontona'sal Relating to the frontal and the nasal bones.

fron'to-occip'ital Relating to the frontal and the occipital bones, or to the forehead and the occiput.

frontopari'etal Relating to the frontal and the parietal bones.

frontotem'poral Relating to the frontal and the temporal bones.

fron'tozygomat'ic Relating to the frontal and zygomatic bones.

frost'bite Local tissue destruction resulting from exposure to extreme cold or contact with extremely cold objects; in mild cases, it results in erythema and slight pain; in severe cases, it can be painless or paraesthetic and result in blistering, deep-seated destruction, and gangrene.

frottage' [F., a rubbing] **1.** The rubbing movement in massage. **2.** Production of sexual excitement by rubbing against someone

fruc'tose (Fru) In D form, physiologically the most important of the ketohexoses, and one of the two products of sucrose hydrolysis; metabolized or converted to glycogen in the absence of insulin.

fructosu'ria [G. *ouron*, urine] Excretion of fructose in the urine.

essential f., a benign, asymptomatic metabolic abnormality due to deficiency of fructokinase in which fructose appears in the blood and urine, but is simply excreted unchanged; autosomal recessive inheritance.

-fuge [L. *fuga*, flight] Suffix meaning flight, denoting the place from which flight takes place or that which is put to flight.

fugue [Fr. fr. L. *fuga*, flight] A period in the past for which one alleges almost complete amnesia, accompanied by life elsewhere with different conduct; afterward, earlier events are remembered but those of the f. period are alleged to be forgotten.

ful'gurant [L. *fulgur*, flashing lightning] Sharp and piercing.

ful'gurating 1. Fulgurant. 2. Relating to fulguration.

fulgura'tion [L. *fulgur*, lightning stroke] Destruction of tissue by means of a high-frequency electric current.

ful'minant [L. *fulmino*, pp. -*atus*, to hurl lightning] Occurring suddenly, with lightning-like rapidity, and with great intensity or severity; applied to certain pains, such as those of tabes dorsalis.

ful'minating Running a speedy course, with rapid worsening.

fu'migant [see fumigate] Any vaporous substance used as a disinfectant or pesticide.

fu'migate [L. *fumigo*, pp. -*atus*, to fumigate] To expose to the action of smoke or of fumes of any kind as a means of disinfection.

fu'ming [L. *fumus*, smoke] Giving forth a visible vapour, a property of concentrated nitric, sulphuric, and hydrochloric acids.

func'tion [L. *functio*, fr. *fungor*, pp., *functus*, to perform] 1. The special action or physiologic property of an organ or body part. 2. To perform its special work or office, said of an organ or other body part. 3. The general properties of any substance, depending on its chemical character and relation to other substances, according to which it may be grouped among acids, bases, alcohols, esters, etc. 4. A particular reactive grouping in a molecule; *e.g.*, a functional group, is the —OH group of an alcohol.

func'tional 1. Relating to a function. 2. Nonorganic, not caused by a structural defect.

fun'diform [L. *funda*, a sling, + *forma*, shape] Looped; sling-shaped.

fun'doplica'tion [fundus + L. *plico*, to fold] Suture of the fundus of the stomach around the oesophagus to prevent reflux in repair of hiatal hernia.

fun'dus, pl. **fun'di** [L. bottom] [NA] The bottom or lowest part of a sac or hollow organ; that part farthest removed from the opening or exit.

f. oc'uli, f. of the eye; the portion of the interior of the eyeball around the posterior pole, visible through the ophthalmoscope.

f. u'teri [NA], **f. of the uterus,** the upper rounded extremity of the uterus above the openings of the uterine (fallopian) tubes.

fun'gal Fungous.

fun'gate To grow exuberantly like a fungus or spongy growth.

Fun'gi [L. *fungus*, a mushroom] A division of plantlike organisms growing in irregular masses, without roots, stems, or leaves, and devoid of chlorophyll or other pigments capable of photosynthesis; they reproduce sexually or asexually (spore formation), and may obtain nutrition as parasites or as saprophytes.

fun'gicide An agent that has a destructive killing action upon fungi.

fun'giform Shaped like a fungus or mushroom; applied to any structure with a broad, often branched, free portion and a narrower base.

Fungi Imperfec'ti A class of fungi in which sexual reproduction is not known or in which one of the mating types has not yet been discovered.

fun'goid Resembling a fungus; denoting an exuberant morbid growth on the surface of the body.

fun'gous Relating to a fungus.

fun'gus, pl. **fun'gi** [L. *fungus*, a mushroom] General term used to encompass the diverse morphological forms of yeasts and moulds; originally classified as primitive plants without chlorophyll, the fungi are being placed increasingly in the kingdom Protoetista, along with the algae (all but the blue-green algae), protozoa, and slime moulds. Relatively few fungi are pathogenic for man, whereas most plant diseases are caused by fungi.

funic'ular Relating to a funiculus.

funiculi'tis [funiculus + G. -*itis*, inflammation] 1. Inflammation of a funiculus, especially of the spermatic cord. 2. Inflammation of that portion of a spinal nerve that lies within the intervertebral canal.

funic'ulopexy [funiculus + G. *pēxis*, a fixing] Suturing of the spermatic cord to the surrounding tissue in the correction of an undescended testicle.

funic'ulus, pl. **funic'uli** [L. dim. of *funis*, cord] [NA] A small, cordlike structure composed of several to many longitudinally oriented fibres, vessels, ducts, or combinations thereof.

f. spermat'icus [NA], spermatic or testicular cord; the cord formed by the ductus deterens and its associated structures extending from the deep inguinal ring through the inguinal canal into the scrotum.

f. umbilica'lis [NA], umbilical cord; the definitive connecting stalk between the embryo or fetus and the placenta.

fu'nis [L. a rope, cord] **1.** *Funiculus* umbilicalis. **2.** A cordlike structure.

furca'tion [L. *furca*, fork] **1.** A forking, or a forklike part or branch. **2.** In dental histology, the region of a multirooted tooth at which the roots divide.

furfura'ceous [L. *furfuraceus*, fr. *furfur*, bran] Branny, or composed of small scales; denoting a form of desquamation.

fu'ror epilep'ticus Attacks of anger to which epileptics are occasionally subject, occurring without apparent provocation and without disturbance of consciousness.

fu'runcle [L. *furunculus*, a petty thief] Boil; a localized pyogenic infection originating in a hair follicle.

furun'cular Relating to a furuncle.

furunculo'sis A condition marked by the presence of furuncles.

furun'culus, pl. **furun'culi** [L. a petty thief, a boil, dim. of *fur*, a thief] Furuncle.

fus'cin [L. *fuscus*, dusky] The melanin-like pigment of the retinal pigment epithelium.

fu'siform [L. *fusus*, a spindle, + *forma*, form] Spindle-shaped; tapering at both ends.

fu'sion [L. *fusio*, a pouring, fr. *fundo*, pp. *fusus*, to pour] **1.** Liquefaction, as by melting by heat. **2.** Union, as by joining together. **3.** The blending of slightly different images from each eye into a single perception. **4.** The growth together, as one, of two or more teeth, in consequence of the abnormal union of their formative organs.

Fusobacte'rium [L. *fusus*, a spindle, + bacterium] A genus of bacteria (family Bacteroidaceae) that produce butyric acid as a major metabolic product and are found in cavities of man and other animals; some species are pathogenic. The type species is *F. nucleatum.*

fu'sospirochae'tal Referring to the associated fusiform and spirochaetal orga-

nisms such as those found in the lesions of Vincent's angina.

G

gag 1. To retch; to cause to retch or heave. **2.** To prevent from talking. **3.** An instrument adjusted between the teeth to keep the mouth from closing during operations in the mouth or throat.

gait Manner of walking.

galac'tagogue [galact- + G. *agōgos*, leading] An agent that promotes the secretion and flow of milk.

galacto-, galact- [G. *gala*, milk] Combining forms indicating milk.

galac'tocele [galacto- + G. *kele*, tumour] A retention cyst caused by occlusion of a lactiferous duct.

gal'actorrhoe'a [galacto- + G. *rhoia*, a flow] A continued discharge of milk from the breasts in the intervals of nursing or after weaning.

galac'tosae'mia [galactose + G. *haima*, blood] An inborn error of galactose metabolism characterized by nutritional failure, hepatosplenomegaly with cirrhosis, cataracts, mental retardation, galactosuria, aminoaciduria, and albuminuria; autosomal recessive inheritance.

galac'tose (Gal) A hexose found (in D form) as a constituent of lactose, cerebrosides, mucoproteins, etc.

galac'tother'apy 1. Treatment of disease by means of an exclusive or nearly exclusive milk diet. **2.** Medicinal treatment of a nursing infant by giving to the mother a drug that is excreted in part by the milk.

gall [A.S. *gealla*] Bile.

gall'bladder Vesica fellea.

gal'lium-67 (^{67}Ga) A cyclotron-produced radionuclide with a physical half-life of 78 hr and major gamma ray emmisions of 93, 184, and 296 kiloelectron volts; used in the citrate form as a tumour- and inflammation-localizing radiotracer.

gallium-68 (^{68}Ga) A positron emitter with a physical half-life of 1.13 hr; used in brain scanning.

gal'lop Gallop rhythm; a triple cadence to the heart sounds at rates of 100 beats per minute or more due to an abnormal third or fourth heart sound being heard in addition to the first and second sounds; usually indicative of a serious disease.

gall'stone A concretion in the gallbladder or a bile duct, composed chiefly of cholesterol crystals and occasionally mixed with calcium.

gam'ete [G. *gametēs*, husband; *gametē*, wife] **1.** One of two cells undergoing karyogamy or true conjugation. **2.** In heredity, any germ cell, whether ovum, spermatozoon, or pollen cell.

gameto- [see gamete] Combining form relating to a gamete.

game'tocyte [gameto- + G. *kytos*, cell] A cell capable of dividing to produce gametes; *e.g.,* a spermatocyte or oocyte.

gam'etogen'esis [gameto- + G. *genesis,* production] Formation and development of gametes.

gammop'athy A primary disturbance in immunoglobulin (γ-globulin) synthesis.

gamogen'esis [G. *gamos,* marriage, + *genesis,* production] Sexual reproduction.

gan'glion, pl. **gan'glia, gan'glions** [G. a swelling or knot] **1.** [NA] Originally, any group of nerve cell bodies in the central or peripheral nervous system; currently, an aggregation of nerve cell bodies located in the peripheral nervous system. **2.** A cyst containing mucopolysaccharide-rich fluid within fibrous tissue or, occasionally, muscle or a semilunar cartilage; usually attached to a tendon sheath in the hand, wrist, or foot.

  basal ganglia, originally, all of the large masses of grey matter at the base of the cerebral hemisphere; currently, the corpus striatum (caudate and lentiform nuclei) and cell groups associated with the corpus striatum.

  dorsal root g., g. spinale.

  gasse'rian g., g. trigeminale.

  g. spina'le [NA], **spinal g.,** the g. of the posterior root of each spinal segmental nerve, containing the cell bodies of the pseudounipolar pimary sensory neurones whose peripheral axon branch becomes part of the mixed segmental nerve, whereas the central axon branch enters the spinal cord as a component of the sensory posterior root.

  g. trigemina'le [NA], **trigeminal g.,** the large flattened sensory g. of the trigeminal nerve lying in close relation to the cavernous sinus along the medial part of the middle cranial fossa.

ganglionec'tomy [ganglion + G. *ektomē,* excision] Excision of a ganglion.

ganglioni'tis Inflammation of a lymphatic or of a nerve ganglion.

gan'glioside A substance chemically similar to cerebrosides but containing one or more sialic acid residues; found principally in nerve tissue and spleen.

gan'gliosidos'is Any disease characterized, in part, by the abnormal accumulation within the nervous system of specific gangliosides.

gan'grene [G. *gangraina,* an eating sore] Necrosis due to obstruction, loss, or diminution of blood supply; may be localized to a small area or involve an entire extremity or organ, and may be wet or dry.

  dry g., g. in which the involved part is dry and shriveled.

  gas g., g. occurring in a wound infected with various anaerobic, sporeforming bacteria, especially *Clostridium perfringens,* and *C. oedematiens;* crepitation of the surrounding tissues is due to gas liberated by bacterial fermentation and constitutional septic symptoms.

  moist g., g. in which the necrosed part is moist and soft.

  wet g., ischaemic necrosis of an extremity with bacterial infection, producing cellulitis adjacent to the necrotic areas.

gan'grenous Relating to or affected with gangrene.

gar'gle [thru Old Fr. fr. L. *gurgulio,* gullet, windpipe] **1.** To rinse the fauces with fluid in the mouth through which expired breath is forced to produce a bubbling effect while the head is held far back. **2.** A medicated fluid used for gargling; a throat wash.

gar'goylism [gargoyle, fr. L. *gurgulio,* gullet] The gargoyle-like facies and related characteristics of Hurler's syndrome (**autosomal recessive type g.**) and Hunter's syndrome (**X-linked recessive type g.**).

gas **1.** A thin fluid, like air, capable of indefinite expansion but convertible by compression and cold into a liquid and, eventually, solid. **2.** To subject to the action of a g.

  blood g.'s, a clinical expression for the determination of the partial pressures of oxygen and carbon dioxide in blood.

  laughing g. [so called because its inhalation sometimes excites a hilarious delirium preceding insensibility], nitrous oxide.

mustard g., a poisonous vesicating gas introduced in World War I; the progenitor of the so-called nitrogen mustards.

noble g.'s, inert g.'s; zero group in the periodic series: helium, neon, argon, krypton, xenon, and radon.

tear g., a g., such as acetone, benzene bromide, and xylol, that causes irritation of the conjunctiva and profuse lacrimation.

gas'eous Of the nature of gas.

gastral'gia [gastr- + G. *algos*, pain] A stomach ache.

gastrec'tomy [gastr- + G. *ektomē*, excision] Excision of a part or all of the stomach.

gas'tric Relating to the stomach.

gastrino'ma A gastrin-secreting tumour associated with the Zollinger-Ellison syndrome.

gas'trins Hormones secreted in the pyloric-antral mucosa of the mammalian stomach that stimulate secretion of HCl by the parietal cells of the gastric glands.

gastri'tis [gastr- + G. -*itis*, inflammation] Inflammation, especially mucosal, of the stomach.

gastro-, gastr- [G. *gastēr*, stomach] Combining forms denoting the stomach.

gas'trocar'diac Relating to both the stomach and the heart.

gastrocne'mius [G. *gastroknēmia*, calf of the leg] *Musculus* gastrocnemius.

gastroco'lic Relating to the stomach and the colon.

gas'trocolos'tomy [gastro- + G. *kōlon*, colon, + *stoma*, mouth] Establishment of a communication between stomach and colon.

gas'troduode'nal Relating to the stomach and duodenum.

gas'trodu'odenos'copy [gastro- + duodenum, + G. *skopeō*, to view] Visualization of the interior of the stomach and duodenum by a gastroscope.

gas'troenteri'tis [gastro- + G. *enteron*, intestine, + -*itis*, inflammation] Inflammation of the mucous membrane of both stomach and intestine.

gas'troenterol'ogy [gastro- + G. *enteron*, intestine, + *logos*, study] The medical specialty concerned with the function and disorders of the stomach and intestines.

gas'troenterop'athy [gastro- + G. *enteron*, intestine, + *pathos*, suffering] Any disorder of the alimentary canal.

gas'trointes'tinal (GI). Relating to the stomach and intestines.

gas'trostolavage' Lavage of the stomach through a gastric fistula.

gas'tro-oesophage'al [gastro- + G. *oisophagos*, gullet (oesophagus)] Relating to both stomach and oesophagus.

gas'troparal'ysis Paralysis of the muscular coat of the stomach.

gas'troplasty [gastro- + G. *plassō*, to form] Operative repair of a defect in the stomach or lower oesophagus.

gastros'chisis [gastro- + G. *schisis*, a fissure] a congenital muscular defect in the abdominal wall, not at the umbilical ring, usually with protrusion of the viscera.

gas'troscope [gastro- + G. *skopeō*, to examine] An endoscope for inspecting the inner surface of the stomach.

gastros'copy Inspection of the inner surface of the stomach through an endoscope.

gas'trospasm Spasmodic contraction of the walls of the stomach.

gastros'tomy [gastro- + G. *stoma*, mouth] Establishment of a new opening into the stomach.

gastrot'omy [gastro- + G. *tomē*, incision] Incision into the stomach.

gas'trula [Mod. L. dim. of G. *gastēr*, belly] The embryo in the stage of development following the blastula.

gastrula'tion Tranformation of the blastula into the gastrula; development and invagination of the embryonic germ layers.

gauze A bleached cotton cloth of plain weave, used for dressings, bandages, and absorbent sponges.

gavage' [Fr. *gaver*, to gorge fowls] **1.** Forced feeding by stomach tube. **2.** Therapeutic use of a high-potency diet.

gel [Mod. L. *gelatum*] **1.** A jelly or the solid or semisolid phase of a colloidal solution. **2.** To form a g. or jelly; to convert a sol into a g.

gel'atin [L. *gelo*, pp. *gelatus*, to freeze, congeal] A derived protein formed from the collagen of tissues by boiling in water.

gelo'sis [L. *gelo*, to freeze, congeal, + G. -*osis*, condition] An extremely firm mass in tissue (especially in a muscle) with a consistency resembling that of frozen tissue.

gen-, -gen [G. *genos*, birth] **1.** Combining form meaning "producing" or "coming to be." **2.** In chemistry, use as a suffix indicates "precursor of."

gen′der The anatomical sex of an individual.

gene [G. *genos*, birth] The functional unit of heredity that occupies a specific place or locus on a chromosome, is capable of reproducing itself exactly at each cell division, and is capable of directing formation of an enzyme or other protein.

    autosomal g., a g. located on any chromosome other than a sex chromosome (X or Y).

    histocompatibility g.'s, g.'s that control HLA antigens.

    recessive g., see *dominance* of g.'s.

    sex-linked g., a g. located on a sex chromosome, in usual usage the X chromosome.

gen′era Plural of genus.

gen′erator [*generatus*, pp. *generare*, to beget, produce] An apparatus for conversion of chemical, mechanical, atomic, or other forms of energy into electricity.

    pulse g., in an electronic pacemaker, a device that produces an electrical discharge at regular intervals, which may be modified by a sensory circuit which can reset the timebase for subsequent discharge on the basis of other electrical activity, such as that produced by spontaneous cardiac beating.

gener′ic [L. *genus* (*gener-*), birth] **1.** Relating to or denoting a genus. **2.** General. **3.** Characteristic or distinctive.

generic name 1. In chemistry, a noun that indicates the class or type of a single compound; "class" is more appropriate and more often used. **2.** Misnomer for nonproprietary name. **3.** In the biologic sciences, the first part of the scientific name (Latin binary combination or binomial) of an organism.

gen′esis [G.] An origin or beginning process. Also used as combining form in suffix position.

genet′ic Relating to (1) genetics, and (2) ontogenesis.

genetic code Genetic information carried by the specific DNA molecule of the chromosomes; specifically, the system whereby particular combinations of three adjacent nucleotides in a DNA molecule control the insertion of particular amino acids in equivalent places in a protein molecule.

genet′ics [G. *genesis*, origin or production] The branch of science concerned with heredity.

    clinical g., the means of diagnosis, prognosis, management, and prevention of genetic disease.

    medical g., study of the aetiology, pathogenesis, and natural history of diseases that are at least partially genetic in origin.

-genic Suffix denoting producing or forming, produced or formed by.

genic′ular Commonly used to mean genual.

genic′ulate [L. *geniculo*, pp. *-atus*, to bend the knee, fr. *genu*, knee] **1.** Bent like a knee. **2.** Referring to the geniculum of the facial nerve, denoting the ganglion there.

genic′ulum, pl. **genic′ula** [L. dim. of *genu*, knee] **1.** [NA] A small genu or angular kneelike structure. **2.** A knotlike structure.

geni′oplasty [G. *geneion*, chin, cheek, + *plassō*, to form] Mentoplasty.

gen′ital 1. Relating to reproduction, or generation. **2.** Relating to the organs of reproduction (genitalia). **3.** Relating to or characterized by genitality.

genita′lia [L. neut. pl. of *genitalis*, genital] Genital *organs*.

genital′ity In psychoanalysis, a term referring to the genital components of sexuality (penis and vagina), as opposed to orality and anality.

genitou′rinary (GU) Urogenital; relating to the organs of reproduction and urination.

ge′nome [gene + chromosome] **1.** A complete set of chromosomes derived from one parent, the haploid number of a gamete. **2.** The total gene complement of a set of chromosomes found in higher life forms, or the functionally similar but simpler linear arrangements found in bacteria and viruses.

ge′notype [G. *genos*, birth, descent, + *typos*, type] The genetic constitution of an individual; may be used with respect to gene combination at one specified locus or with respect to any specified combination of loci.

gentami′cin A broad spectrum antibiotic complex, obtained from *Micromonospora purpurea* and *M. echinospora;* inhibits the growth of both Gram-positive and Gram-negative bacteria.

ge′nu, gen. **ge′nus,** pl. **gen′ua** [L.] [NA] **1.** The knee. **2.** Any structure of angular shape resembling a flexed knee.

g. recurva'tum, a condition of hyperextension of the knee, the lower extremity making a curve with concavity forward.

g. val'gum, knock-knee; a deformity marked by abduction of the leg in relation to the thigh.

g. va'rum, bowleg; an outward bowing of the legs.

gen'ual [L. *genu*, knee] Relating to the knee.

ge'nus, pl. **gen'era** [L. birth, descent] In natural history classification, the division between the family, or tribe, and the species; a group of species alike in the broad features of their organization but different in detail.

geo- [G. *gē*, earth] Combining form relating to the earth, or to soil.

geopha'gia, geoph'agism, geoph'agy [geo- + G. *phagein*, to eat] The practice of eating dirt or clay; variously referred to as earth-eating; dirt-eating.

geriat'rics [G. *gēras*, old age, + *iatrikos*, healing] The branch of medicine concerned with the diseases and problems of the elderly.

germ [L. *germen*, sprout, bud, germ] **1.** A microbe; a microorganism. **2.** A primordium; the earliest trace of a structure within an embryo.

germici'dal Germicide (1).

ger'micide [germ + L. *caedo*, to kill] **1.** Destructive to germs or microbes. **2.** An agent with this action.

germino'ma A neoplasm of germinal tissue that normally differentiates to form sperm cells or ova.

gero-, geront-, geronto- [G. *gerōn*, old man] Combining forms denoting old age. See also presby-.

geroder'ma [gero- + G. *derma*, skin] **1.** The atrophic skin of the aged. **2.** Any condition in which the skin is thinned and wrinkled, resembling the integument of old age.

gerontol'ogy [geronto- + G. *logos*, study] Scientific study of the process and problems of aging.

gestalt' [Ger. shape] A system of phenomena so integrated as to constitute a functional unit with properties not derivable from its parts.

gestalt'ism [see gestalt] The theory in psychology that the objects of mind come as complete forms or configurations which cannot be split into parts; *e.g.*, a square is perceived as such rather than as four discrete lines.

gesta'tion [L. *gestatio*, from *gesto*, pp. *gestatus*, to bear] Pregnancy in viviparous animals.

Giar'dia [Alfred *Giard*, French biologist, 1846–1908] A genus of parasitic flagellates that parasitize the small intestine of mammals, including most domestic animals and man. *G. lamblia*, the common species in man, is usually asymptomatic except in heavy infections, when it may interfere with absorption of fats and produce flatulence, steatorrhoea, and acute discomfort.

giardi'asis Infection with *Giardia lamblia*.

gib'bous [L. *gibbosus*] Humped; humpbacked.

gib'bus [L. a hump] Extreme kyphosis, hump, or hunch; a deformity of spine in which there is a sharply angulated segment, the apex of the angle being posterior.

gigan'tism [G. *gigas*, giant] Abnormal size, or overgrowth, of the entire body or of any of its parts.

gin'giva, gen. and pl. **ging'ivae** [L.] [NA] Gum; the dense fibrous tissue; covered by mucous membrane, that envelops the alveolar processes of the upper and lower jaws and surrounds the necks of the teeth.

gin'gival Relating to the gums.

Gingival Index (GI). An index of periodontal disease based upon the severity and location of the lesion.

Gingival-Periodontal Index (GPI). An index of gingivitis, gingival irritation, and advanced periodontal disease.

gingivec'tomy [gingiva + G. *ektomē*, excision] Gum resection; surgical resection of unsupported gingival tissue.

gingivi'tis [gingiva + G. -*itis*, inflammation] Inflammation of the gingival tissue.

necrotizing ulcerative g. (NUG), Vincent's disease; trench mouth; an acute, sometimes recurrent lesion of the gingivae characterized by ulceration and necrosis of the gingival margin and destruction of the interdental papillae; commonly associated with fusiform bacilli and spirochaetes.

gingivo- [L. *gingiva*] Combining form relating to the gingivae.

gin'givoglossi'tis Inflammation of both the tongue and gingival tissues.

gin'givoplas'ty Surgical reshaping and recontouring of the gingival tissue to attain aesthetic, physiologic, and functional form.

gin'givostomato'sis [gingivo- + G. *stoma*, mouth, + *-osis*, condition] Any disease of both the gingiva and portions of the oral mucosa.

gin'glymus [G. *ginglymos*] [NA] Hinge joint; a uniaxial joint in which a broad, transversely cylindrical convexity on one bone fits into a corresponding concavity on the other, allowing motion in one plane only, as in the elbow.

gir'dle [A.S. *gyrdel*] A belt; a zone. See also cingulum (1).

glabel'la [L. *glabellus*, hairless, smooth] **1.** [NA] A smooth prominence, most marked in the male, on the frontal bone above the root of the nose. **2.** The most forward projecting point of the forehead in the midline at the level of the supraorbital ridges.

gla'brous, gla'brate [L. *glaber*, smooth] Smooth or hairless; denoting areas of the body where hair does not normally grow.

gland [L. *glans*, acorn] A secreting organ.

  adrenal g., *glandula suprarenalis.*

  Bartholin's g., *glandula vestibularis major.*

  Cowper's g., *glandula bulbourethralis.*

  ductless g.'s, *glandulae sine ductibus.*

  endocrine g.'s, *glandulae sine ductibus.*

  exocrine g., a g. from which secretions reach a free surface of the body by ducts.

  holocrine g., a g. whose secretion consists of disintegrated cells of the g. itself.

  lymph g., lymph *node.*

  mammary g., *glandula mammaria.*

  meibomian g.'s, *glandulae tarsales.*

  parathyroid g., *glandula parathyroidea.*

  parotid g., *glandula parotidea.*

  pineal g., *corpus pineale.*

  pituitary g., *hypophysis.*

  prostate g., *prostata.*

  salivary g.'s, *glandula parotidea, sublingualis,* and *submandibularis.*

  sebaceous g.'s, *glandulae sebaceae.*

  thyroid g., *glandula thyroidea.*

glan'dula, pl. **glan'dulae** [L. gland, dim. of *glans*, acorn] [NA] A glandule or small gland.

  g. bulbourethra'lis [NA], Cowper's gland; one of two small compound racemose glands side by side along the membranous urethra just above the bulb of the corpus spongiosum; they produce a mucoid secretion and discharge through a small duct into the spongy portion of the urethra.

  g. mamma'ria [NA], mammary gland; the compound alveolar gland that forms the breast; consists of lobes separated by adipose tissue and fibrous septa, each lobe consisting of many lobules.

  g. parathyroi'dea [NA], parathyroid gland; one of two small paired endocrine glands (superior and inferior) embedded in the connective tissue capsule on the posterior surface of the thyroid gland; concerned with the metabolism of calcium and phosphorus.

  g. parotid'ea [NA], parotid gland; the largest of the salivary glands; a compound acinous gland situated below and in front of the ear, on either side, extending from the angle of the jaw to the zygomatic arch and backward to the sternocleidomastoid muscle; it discharges through the parotid duct.

  glan'dulae seba'ceae [NA], sebaceous glands; numerous holocrine glands in the corium that usually open into the hair follicles and secrete sebum.

  glan'dulae sine duc'tibus [NA], ductless or endocrine glands; glands that have no ducts, their secretions being absorbed directly into the blood.

  g. suprarena'lis [NA], suprarenal or adrenal gland, a flattened, roughly triangular body upon the upper end of each kidney; a ductless gland furnishing adrenaline and noradrenaline from the medulla and steroid hormones from the cortex.

  glan'dulae tarsa'les [NA], meibomian glands; sebaceous glands embedded in the tarsal plate of each eyelid, discharging at the edge of the lid near the posterior border.

  g. thyroi'dea [NA], thyroid gland; a horseshoe-shaped ductless gland in front and to the sides of the upper part of the trachea; it is supplied by branches from the external carotid and subclavian arteries, and its nerves are derived from the middle cervical and cervicothoracic ganglia of the sympathetic system.

  g. vestibula'ris ma'jor [NA], Bartholin's gland; one of two mucoid-secreting tubuloalveolar glands on either side of the lower part the vagina; equivalent of the bulbourethral glands in the male.

glan'dular, glan'dulous Relating to a gland.

glans, pl. **glan'des** [L. acorn] [NA] A conical acorn-shaped structure.

  g. clitor'idis [NA], a small mass of erectile tissue capping the body of the clitoris.

  g. pe'nis [NA], the conical expansion of the corpus spongiosum that forms the head of the penis.

glas'ses 1. Spectacles. **2.** Lenses for correcting refractive errors in the eyes.

glauco'ma [G. glaukōma, opacity of the crystalline lens] A disease of the eye characterized by increased intraocular pressure due to restricted outflow of the aqueous humour through the aqueous veins and Schlemm's canal, excavation and degeneration of the optic disc, and nerve fibre bundle damage producing arcuate defects in the field of vision.

  congenital g., buphthalmos.

glauco'matous Relating to glaucoma.

gleet A slight chronic discharge of thin mucus from the urethra, following gonorrhoea.

gle'noid [G. glēnoeidēs, fr. glēnē, socket of joint, + eidos, appearance] Resembling a socket; denoting the articular depression of the scapula entering into the formation of the shoulder joint.

gli'a [G. glue] Neuroglia.

gli'acyte [G. glia, glue, + kytos, cell] A neuroglia cell. See neuroglia.

gli'al Pertaining to glia or neuroglia.

glio- [G. glia, glue] Combining form meaning glue or gluelike, relating specifically to the neuroglia.

gli'oblasto'ma [glio- + G. blastos, germ, sprout, + -oma, tumour] A glioma, consisting chiefly of undifferentiated anaplastic cells frequently arranged radially about an irregular focus of necrosis, that grows rapidly and invades extensively, occurring most frequently in the cerebrum of adults.

glio'ma [glio- + G. -oma, tumour] Any neoplasm derived from one of the various types of cells that form the interstitial tissue of the brain, spinal cord, pineal gland, posterior pituitary gland, and retina.

gliomato'sis Neoplastic growth of neuroglial cells in the brain or spinal cord, especially with reference to a relatively large neoplasm or to multiple foci.

glio'matous Pertaining to or characterized by a glioma.

glio'sis Occurrence of overgrowth or tumours of the neuroglia.

glo'bin The protein of haemoglobin.

glob'ule [L. globulus, dim. of globus, a ball] **1.** A small spherical body of any kind. **2.** A fat droplet in milk.

glob'ulin [L. globulus, globule] A family of proteins precipitated from plasma (or serum) by half-saturation with ammonium sulphate and which may be further fractionated by separation methods into many subgroups, the main groups being α-, β-, and γ-g.; these differ with respect to associated lipids or carbohydrates and in their content of many physiologically important factors.

globulinu'ria Excretion of globulin in the urine, usually, if not always, in association with serum albumin.

glo'bus, pl. **glo'bi** [L.] [NA] A round body; sphere; ball.

  g. pal'lidus [NA], the inner and lighter grey portion of the lentiform or lenticular nucleus.

glomer'ular Relating to or affecting a glomerulus or the glomeruli.

glomeruli'tis Inflammation of a glomerulus, specifically of the renal glomeruli, as in glomerulonephritis.

glomer'ulonephri'tis [glomerulus + G. nephros, kidney, + -itis, inflammation] Glomerular nephritis; renal disease characterized by bilateral inflammatory changes in glomeruli that are not the result of infection of the kidneys.

glomerulop'athy [glomerulus + G. pathos, suffering] Glomerular disease of any type.

glomer'uloscloro'sis [glomerulus + G. sklerōsis, hardness] Hyaline deposits or scarring within the renal glomeruli, a degenerative process occurring in association with renal arteriosclerosis or diabetes.

glomer'ulus, pl. **glomer'uli** [Mod. L. dim. of L. glomus, a ball of yarn] [NA] **1.** A plexus of capillaries. **2.** A tuft formed of capillary loops at the beginning of each uriniferous tubule in the kidney; this tuft with its capsule (Bowman's capsule) constitutes the corpusculum renis (malpighian body). **3.** The twisted secretory portion of a sweat gland. **4.** A cluster of dendritic ramifications and axon terminals in often complex synaptic relationship with each other, surrounded by a glial sheath.

glo'mus [L. *glomus* (*glomer-*), pl. *glomera*, a ball] **1.** [NA] A small globular body. **2.** A richly innervated, highly organized arteriolovenular anastomosis forming a tiny nodular focus in the nailbed, pads of the fingers and toes, ears, hands, and feet and many other organs of the body; functions as a shunt or bypass regulation mechanism in the flow of blood, temperature, and conservation of heat in the part as well as in the indirect control of the blood pressure and other functions of the circulatory system.

glos'sal Lingual (1).

glossal'gia [gloss- + G. *algos*, pain] Glossodynia.

glossec'tomy [gloss- + G. *ektomē*, excision] Excision or amputation of the tongue.

Glossi'na [G. *glōssa*, tongue] A genus of bloodsucking Diptera (tsetse flies) confined to Africa that serve as vectors of the pathogenic trypanosomes that cause various forms of African sleeping sickness.

glossi'tis [gloss- + G. -*itis*, inflammation] Inflammation of the tongue.

glosso-, gloss- [G. *glōssa*, tongue] Combining forms relating to the tongue.

glos'socele [glosso- + G. *kēlē*, tumour, hernia] Protrusion of the tongue from the mouth, owing to its excessive size.

glossodyn'ia [glosso- + G. *odynē*, pain] A burning or painful tongue.

glossola'lia [glosso- + G. *lalia*, talk, chat] Unintelligible jargon.

glos'sopharyn'geal Relating to the tongue and the pharynx.

glos'soplasty [glosso- + G. *plassō*, to form] Reparative or plastic surgery of the tongue.

glos'sospasm Spasmodic contraction of the tongue.

glot'tic Relating to the tongue or to the glottis.

glot'tis, pl. **glot'tides** [G. *glōttis*, aperture of the larynx] [NA] The vocal apparatus of the larynx, consisting of the vocal folds of mucous membrane investing the vocal ligament and vocal muscle on each side, the free edges of which are the vocal cords, and of a median fissure, the rima glottidis.

glotti'tis Inflammation of the glottic portion of the larynx.

glu'cagon A polypeptide hormone secreted by pancreatic alpha cells. It activates hepatic phosphorylase, thereby increasing glycogenolysis; decreases gastric motility and gastric and pancreatic secretions; and increases urinary excretion of nitrogen and potassium.

glu'can A polyglucose.

gluco- Combining form denoting relationship to glucose. See also glyco-.

glu'cocor'ticoid **1.** Any steroid-like compound capable of significantly influencing intermediary metabolism and of exerting a clinically useful anti-inflammatory effect. **2.** Denoting an agent with this type of biological activity.

glucogen'esis [gluco- + G. *genesis*, production] Glycogenesis.

glu'coneogen'esis Glyconeogenesis.

glu'cose Dextrose; blood sugar; a dextrorotatory monosaccharide (hexose) found in the free state in fruits and other parts of plants, and combined in glucosides, disaccharides, oligosaccharides, and polysaccharides; the product of complete hydrolysis of cellulose, starch, and glycogen. Free g. occurs in the blood and in the urine in diabetes mellitus.

glu'coside A glycoside of glucose.

glucosu'ria The urinary excretion of glucose, usually in enhanced quantities.

glue-sniffing Inhalation of fumes from plastic cements, the solvents of which (toluene, xylene, and benzene) induce central nervous system stimulation followed by depression.

glu'tamate A salt or ester of glutamic acid.

glutam'ic acid (Glu) An amino acid occurring in proteins.

glu'tamine (Gln) The δ-amide of glutamic acid, derived by oxidation from proline in the liver or by the combination of glutamic acid with ammonia; present in proteins, in blood and other tissues, and an important source of urinary ammonia, being broken down in the kidney by the action of the enzyme glutaminase.

glutar'ic acid An intermediate in tryptophan catabolism.

glutathi'one A tripeptide of glycine, cystine, and glutamic acid. **Oxidized g. (GSSG)** acts in cells as a hydrogen acceptor and **reduced g. (GSH)** acts as a hydrogen donor; oxidized g. is reduced by **g. reductase,** which appears to be a ubiquitous reducing agent involved in many redox reactions.

glu'teal [G. *gloutos*, buttock] Relating to the buttocks.

glu'ten [L. *gluten*, glue] The insoluble protein constituent of wheat and other grains, a mixture of gliadin, glutenin, and other proteins.

glycae'mia [G. *glykys*, sweet, + *haima*, blood] Presence of glucose in the blood.

glyc'eride An ester of glycerol; usually used in combination with phospho-. Use of mono-, di-, and triglyceride is being replaced by the more precise mono-, di-, and triacylglycerol.

glyc'erol, glyc'erin A sweet, oily fluid, obtained by the saponification of fats and fixed oils. It is used as a solvent, as an emollient, by injection or in the form of suppository for constipation, orally to reduce ocular tension, and as a vehicle and sweetening agent.

gly'cine (Gly) Aminoacetic acid, used as a nutrient and dietary supplement, and in solution for irrigation.

glyco- [G. *glykys*, sweet] Combining form denoting relationship to sugars in general.

gly'cogen A glucosan of high molecular weight, resembling amylopectin in structure but more highly branched, found in most tissues of the body, especially those of the liver and muscular tissue; as the principal carbohydrate reserve, it is readily converted into glucose.

glycogen'esis [glyco- + G. *genesis*, production] Formation of glycogen from glucose by means of glycogen synthase and dextrin dextranase.

glycogenol'ysis The hydrolysis of glycogen to glucose.

glycogeno'sis Glycogen storage disease; any of the glycogen deposition diseases characterized by abnormal accumulation of glycogen in tissue. Six types (Cori classification) are recognized, depending on the enzyme deficiency involved, all of autosomal recessive inheritance, but with a different gene for each enzyme deficiency.

glycol'ysis [glyco- + G. *lysis*, a loosening] Energy-yielding anaerobic conversion of glucose to lactic acid in various tissues, notably muscle.

glycolyt'ic Relating to glycolysis.

glyconeogen'esis [glyco- + G. *neos*, new, + *genesis*, production] Formation of glycogen from noncarbohydrates, such as protein or fat, by conversion of the latter to glucose.

gly'copro'tein One of a group of protein-carbohydrate compounds (conjugated proteins), among which the most important are the mucins, mucoid and amyloid; sometimes restricted to proteins containing small amounts of carbohydrate, in contrast to mucoids or mucoproteins, usually measured as hexosamine.

gly'coside The condensation product of a sugar with any other radical involving the loss of the H of the hemiacetal OH of the sugar, leaving the O of this OH as the link.

glycosu'ria [glyco- + G. *ouron*, urine] **1.** Glucosuria. **2.** Urinary excretion of carbohydrates.

    alimentary g., g. developing after the ingestion of a moderate amount of sugar or starch, which normally is disposed of without appearing in the urine.

    renal g., recurring or persistent excretion of glucose in the urine, in association with blood levels that are in the normal range; results from the failure of renal tubules to reabsorb glucose at a normal rate from the glomerular filtrate.

gnath'ic [G. *gnathos*, jaw] Relating to the jaw or alveolar process.

gnatho-, gnath- [G. *gnathos*, jaw] Combining form relating to the jaw.

gnath'oplasty [gnatho- + G. *plassō*, to form] Reparative surgery of the jaw.

goi'tre [Fr. from L. *guttur*, throat] A chronic enlargement of the thyroid gland not due to a neoplasm.

    exophthalmic g., any of the various forms of hyperthyroidism in which the thyroid gland is enlarged and exophthalmos is present.

    lymphadenoid g., Hashimoto's disease.

    toxic g., g that forms an excessive secretion, causing signs and symptoms of hyperthyroidism.

goitrogen'ic Causing goitre.

goit'rous Denoting or characteristic of a goitre.

gold A yellow metallic element, symbol Au, atomic no. 79, atomic weight 196.97; compounds are used chiefly in treatment of arthritis.

gompho'sis [G. *gomphos*, bolt, nail, + *-osis*, condition] [NA] Peg-and-socket joint; a form of fibrous joint in which a peglike process fits into a hole, as the root of a tooth into the socket in the alveolus.

gon'ad [Mod. L. fr. G. *gonē*, seed] An organ that produces sex cells; the testis or ovary.

gon'adal Relating to a gonad.

gonadec'tomy [gonado- + G. *ektomē*, excision] Excision of an ovary or testis.

gonado-, gonad- [G. *gonē*, seed] Combining forms relating to the gonads.

gon'adop'athy [gonado- + G. *pathos*, suffering] Disease affecting the gonads.

gon'adotro'phic Gonadotropic.

gon'adotro'phin [gonado- + G. *trophē*, nourishment] Gonadotropin.

gon'adotro'pic [gonado- + G. *tropē*, a turning] **1.** Descriptive of or relating to the actions of a gonadotropin. **2.** Promoting the growth and/or function of the gonads.

gon'adotro'pin A hormone capable of promoting gonadal growth and function. Such effects, as exerted by a single hormone, are usually limited to discrete functions or histological components of a gonad; most g.'s exert their effects in both sexes, although the effect of a given g. will be very different in males and in females.

　anterior pituitary g., pituitary gonadotropic hormone; any g. of hypophyseal origin.

　chorionic g. (CG), human chorionic g. (HCG), chorionic gonadotropic hormone; a glycoprotein produced by the placental trophoblastic cells and excreted in the urine of pregnant women; its most important role appears to be stimulation, during the first trimester, of ovarian secretion of the oestrogen and progesterone required for the integrity of conceptus; used in the treatment of cryptorchidism and as an aid to conception in women by substituting for endogenous luteinizing hormone.

gon'aduct [gonado- + duct] **1.** Seminal *duct.* 2. Uterine *tube.*

gonio- [G. *gōnia*, angle] Combining form meaning angle.

goniom'eter [G. *gōnia*, angle, + *metron*, measure] **1.** An instrument for measuring angles, as of crystals. **2.** A calibrated device designed to measure the arc or range of motion of a joint.

go'niopunc'ture An operation for congenital glaucoma in which a puncture is made in the filtration angle of the anterior chamber.

go'nioscope [G. *gōnia*, angle + *skopeō*, to examine] A lens designed to study the angle of the anterior chamber of the eye or to view the retina using a biomicroscope.

goniot'omy [G. *gōnia*, angle, + *tomē*, incision] Surgical opening of Schlemm's canal by way of the angle of the anterior chamber in congenital glaucoma.

gonococ'cal Relating to gonococci.

gonococ'cus, pl. **gonococ'ci** [G. *gonē*, seed, + *kokkos*, berry] *Neisseria gonorrhoeae.*

gonococcae'mia [gonococcus + G. *haima*, blood]. Presence of gonococci in the circulating blood.

gonorrhoe'a [G. *gonorrhoia*, fr. *gonē*, seed, + *rhoia*, a flow] A contagious catarrhal inflammation of the genital mucous membrane transmitted chiefly by coitus and due to *Neisseria gonorrhoeae;* may involve the lower or upper genital tract, especially the uterine tubes, or spread to the peritoneum and other structures by the bloodstream.

Gonyau'lax catenel'la [G. *gony*, knee, + *aulakos*, a furrow] A marine dinoflagellate protozoan that produces a powerful toxin that accumulates in the tissues of mussels and other filter-feeding shellfish and may cause fatal mussel poisoning in man.

gon'ycamp'sis [G. *gony*, knee, + *kampsis*, a bending or curving] Ankylosis or any abnormal curvature of the knee.

gouge A strong curved chisel used in operation on bone.

goun'dou [native name] A disease, endemic in West Africa, characterized by exotoses from the nasal processes of the maxillary bones, producing a symmetrical swelling on each side of the nose; generally believed to be an osteitis connected with yaws.

gout [L. *gutta*, drop] An inherited metabolic disorder, occurring especially in men, characterized by raised but variable blood uric acid level, recurrent acute arthritis of sudden onset, deposition of crystalline sodium urate in connective tissues and articular cartilage, and progressive chronic arthritis.

graft [A.S. *graef*] **1.** Any free (unattached) tissue or organ for transplantation. **2.** To transplant such structures. See also flap; implant; transplant.

　autologous g., autoplastic g., autograft.

corneal g., keratoplasty.

free g., a g. transplanted without its normal attachments, or a pedicle, from one site to another.

full-thickness g., a g. of the full thickness mucosa and submucosa or of skin and subcutaneous tissue.

heterologous g., heteroplastic g., heterospecific g., heterograft.

homologous g., homoplastic g., homograft.

split-skin g., split-thickness g., partial-thickness g., a g. of portions of the skin or of part of the mucosa and submucosa, but not including the periosteum.

-gram [G. *gramma*, character, mark] Suffix denoting a recording, usually by an instrument.

gramici'din One of a group of polypeptides (two of which are known as q. D and q. S or g C) produced by *Bacillus brevis* and active against Gram-positive cocci and bacilli as a bacteriostatic.

Gram-neg'ative, Gram-pos'itive See Gram's *stain*.

grand mal Generalized *epilepsy*.

gran'ular **1.** Composed of or resembling granules or granulations. **2.** Denoting particles with strong affinity for nuclear stains, seen in many bacterial species.

granula'tion [L. *granulatio*] **1.** Formation into grains or granules; the state of being granular. **2.** A granular mass in or on the surface of any organ or membrane; or one of the individual granules forming the mass. **3.** Formation of minute, rounded, fleshy connective tissue projections on the surface of wound, ulcer, or inflamed tissue surface in the process of healing; one of the fleshy granules composing this surface.

gran'ule [L. *granulum*, dim of *granum*, grain] **1.** A grain; a granulation; minute discrete mass. **2.** A very small pill, usually gelatin coated or sugar coated.

granulo- [L. *granulum*, granule] Combining form meaning granular, or denoting relationship to granules.

gran'ulocyte [granulo- + G. *kytos*, cell] A mature granular leucocyte, including neutrophils, eosinophils, and basophils.

gran'ulocytope'nia [granulocyte + G. *penia*, poverty] Less than the normal number of granular leucocytes in the blood.

granulocyto'sis A condition characterized by more than the normal number of granulocytes in the circulating blood or in the tissues.

granulo'ma [granulo- + G. *-oma*, tumour] An indefinite term applied to nodular inflammatory lesions, usually small or granular, firm, persistent, and containing compactly grouped mononuclear phagocytes.

granulomato'sis Any condition characterized by multiple granulomas.

granulom'atous Having the characteristics of a granuloma.

-graph [G. *graphō*, to write] Suffix designating a recording instrument.

-graphy [G. *graphō*, to write] Suffix denoting a writing or description.

grattage' [Fr. scraping] Scraping or brushing to stimulate the healing process.

grav'el Small concretions, usually of uric acid, calcium oxalate, or phosphates, formed in the kidney and passed through the ureter, bladder, and urethra.

grav'id Pregnant.

grav'ida [L. *gravidus* (adj.), fem. *gravida*, fr. *gravis*, heavy] A pregnant woman, denoted by a Latin numerical prefix for each occurrence; *e.g.*, *pri'migrav'ida*, a woman in her first pregnancy; *secun'digrav'ida*, a woman in her second pregnancy, etc.

gravid'ity [L. *graviditas*, pregnancy] Number of pregnancies.

gravimet'ric Relating to or determined by weight.

grip **1.** Influenza. **2.** Grasp or clasp.

devil's g., epidemic *pleurodynia*.

grippe [Fr. *gripper*, to seize] Influenza.

groin Inguinal region; the topographical area of the abdomen related to the inguinal canal, lateral to the hypogastrium (pubic region).

group In chemistry, a radical.

prosthetic g., a non-amino acid compound attached to a protein, usually in a reversible fashion, that confers new properties upon the conjugated protein thus produced.

grypo'sis [G. *grypos*, hooked, + *-osis*, condition] An abnormal curvature, as of the nails.

guan'ine A major purine occurring in nucleic acids.

gubernac'ulum [L. a helm] A fibrous cord connecting two structures.

guide Any device or instrument by which another is led into its proper course, *e.g.*, a grooved director, a catheter g.

guil'lotine [Fr. instrument for decapitation] An instrument in the shape of a metal ring through which runs a sliding knifeblade, used in cutting off an enlarged tonsil.

gul'let [L. *gula*, throat] Throat (1).

gum 1. [A.S. *goma*, jaw] Gingiva. 2. [L. *gummi*] The dried exuded sap from a number of trees and shrubs, forming an amorphous brittle mass; usually forms a mucilaginous solution in water.

gum'boil A gingival abscess.

gum'ma, pl. **gum'mas** or **gum'mata** [L. *gummi*, gum, fr. G. *kommi*] An infectious granuloma characteristic of tertiary syphilis, but observed infrequently; may be solitary or multiple and diffusely scattered; characterized by an irregular central portion that is firm, sometimes partially hyalinized, and consisting of coagulative necrosis.

gum'matous Pertaining to or characterized by the features of a gumma.

gusta'tion [L. *gustatio*, fr. *gusto*, pp. -*atus*, to taste] 1. The act of tasting. 2. The sense of taste.

gus'tatory Relating to gustation, or taste.

gut [A.S.] 1. The intestine. 2. Embryonic digestive tube. 3. Catgut.

gut'ta-per'cha [Malay *gatah*, gum, + *percha*, tree] A temporary filing material in dentistry.

gut'tate Of the shape of, or resembling, a drop, characterizing certain cutaneous lesions.

gyn-, gynae-, gynaeco-, gyno- [G. *gyne*, woman] Combining forms denoting relationship to a woman.

gy'naecoid [gynaeco- + G. *eidos*, resemblance] Resembling a woman in form and structure.

gynaecolog'ic Relating to gynaecology.

gynaecol'ogist A specialist in gynaecology.

gynaecol'ogy [gynaeco- + G. *logos*, study] The medical specialty concerned with diseases of the female genital tract, as well as the endocrinology and reproductive physiology of the female.

gy'naecomas'tia [gynaeco- + G. *mastos*, breast] Excessive development of the male mammary glands, sometimes secreting milk.

gynand'rism [gyn- + G. *anēr* (*andr*-), man] A developmental abnormality characterized by hypertrophy of the clitoris and union of the labia majora, simulating in appearance the penis and scrotum.

gynan'dromor'phous Having both male and female characteristics.

gy'rate [L. *gyro*, pp. *gyratus*, to turn round in a circle, gyrus] 1. Of convoluted or ring shape. 2. To revolve.

gy'rospasm [G. *gyros*, circle, + *spasmos*, spasm] Spasmodic rotary movements of the head.

gy'rus, gen. and pl. **gy'ri** [L. fr. G. *gyros*, circle] [NA] Convolution; one of the prominent, rounded, folded elevations that form the cerebral hemispheres, each consisting of an exposed superficial portion and a portion hidden from view in the wall and floor of the sulcus separating it from the others.

H

habe'na, pl. **habe'nae** [L. strap] 1. A frenum or restricting fibrous band. 2. Habenula (2).

habe'nal, habe'nar Relating to a habena.

haben'ula, pl. **haben'ulae** [L. little strap] 1. A frenulum. 2. In neuroanatomy, originally the stalk of the pineal gland, but now the nucleus habenulae, a circumscript cell mass in the dorsomedial thalamus, embedded in the posterior end of the stria medullaris from which it received most of its afferent fibres.

haben'ular Relating to a habenula, especially the stalk of the pineal body.

hab'it [L. *habeo*, pp. *habitus*, to have] 1. An act, behavioural response, practice, or custom established by frequent repetition of the same act. See also addiction. 2. A basic variable in the study of conditioning and learning used to designate a new response learned either by association or by being followed by a reward or reinforced event.

habitua'tion 1. The process of forming a habit, referring generally to psychological dependence on the continued use of a substance to maintain a sense of well-being, which can result in addiction. 2. The method by which the nervous system reduces or inhibits responsiveness during repeated stimulation.

hab'itus [L. habit] Physical characteristics of a person.

haem Reduced haematin; the prosthetic, oxygen-carrying, colour-furnishing constituent of haemoglobin.

haem-, haema- [G. *haima*, blood] Combining forms meaning blood. See also haemat-, haemato-, haemo-.

haemadsorp'tion A phenomenon manifested by an agent or substance adhering to or being adsorbed on the surface of a red blood cell.

haem'agglutina'tion Agglutination of red blood cells which may be immune, as a result of specific antibody either for red blood cell antigens per se or other antigens which coat the red blood cells, or may be nonimmune, as in h. caused by viruses or other microbes.

haemagglu'tinin An antibody or other substance that causes haemagglutination.

haemago'gic Promoting a flow of blood.

haemangiec'tasis [G. *haima*, blood, + *angeion*, vessel, + *ektasis*, a stretching] Dilation of blood vessels.

haemangio- [G. *haima*, blood, + *angeion*, vessel] Combining form relating to the blood vessels.

haeman'gioblasto'ma A benign, slowly growing, cerebellar neoplasm composed of capillary vessel-forming endothelial cells.

haemangio'ma [haemangio- + G. *-oma*, tumour] A congenital anomaly in which a proliferation of vascular endothelium leads to a mass that resembles neoplastic tissue; most frequently seen in the skin and subcutaneous tissues.

haeman'giomato'sis Presence of numerous haemangiomas.

haemarthro'sis [G. *haima*, blood, + *arthron*, joint] Blood in a joint or its cavity.

haemat- [G. *haima* (*haimat-*), blood] Combining form meaning blood. See also haem-, haemato-, haemo-.

haematem'esis [haemat- + G. *emesis*, vomiting] Vomiting of blood.

haematidro'sis [hemat- + G. *hidrōs*, sweat] Excretion of blood or blood pigment in the sweat.

hae'matin An iron-protoporphyrin differing from haem in that the central iron atom is in the ferric (Fe^{3+}) rather than the ferrous (Fe^{2+}) state; the prosthetic group of methaemoglobin.

haemato- [G. *haima* (*haimat-*), blood] Combining form meaning blood. See also haem-, haemat-, haemo-.

haemat'ocele [haemato- + G. *kēlē*, tumour] 1. Haemorrhagic *cyst*. 2. An effusion of blood into a canal or a cavity of the body.

haematoche'zia [haemato- + G. *chezō*, to go to stool] Passage of bloody stools, in contradistinction to melaena, or tarry stools.

hae'matocolpome'tra [haemato- + G. *kolpos*, vagina, + *mētra*, womb] Accumulation of blood in the uterus and vagina.

hae'matocol'pos [haemato- + G. *kolpos*, vagina] Accumulation of menstrual blood in the vagina.

hae'matocrit [haemato- + G. *krinō*, to separate] 1. A centrifuge or device for separating cells and other particulate elements of the blood from the plasma. 2. (**Hct**) The percentage of the volume of a blood sample occupied by cells, as determined by a h.

hae'matocys'tis [haemato- + G. *kystis*, a bladder] An effusion of blood into the bladder.

haematol'ogist A physician specializing in haematology.

haematol'ogy [haemato- + G. *logos*, study] The medical specialty concerned with the anatomy, physiology, pathology, symptomatology, and therapeutics related to the blood and blood-forming tissues.

haemato'ma [haemato- + G. *-oma*, tumour] A localized mass of extravasated, usually clotted, blood confined within an organ, tissue, or space.

haematome'tra [haemato- + G. *mētra*, uterus] A collection or retention of blood in the uterine cavity.

hae'matomye'lia [haemato- + G. *myelos*, marrow] Haemorrhage into the substance of the spinal cord; usually a post-traumatic lesion but also encountered in instances of spinal cord capillary telangiectases.

hae'matopathol'ogy [haemato- + G. *pathos*, suffering, + *pathos*, suffering, + *logos*, study] The division of pathology concerned with diseases of the blood and of haemopoietic and lymphoid tissues.

haematop'sia [haemato- + G. *opsis*, vision] Haemorrhage into the eye.

hae'matosal'pinx [haemato- + G. *salpinx*, a trumpet] A collection of blood in a tube, often associated with a tubal pregnancy.

hae'matostat'ic 1. Haemostatic. **2.** Due to stagnation or arrest of blood in the vessels of the part.

haemature'sis Haematuria, especially with reference to unusually large amounts of blood in urine.

haematu'ria [haemato- + G. *ouron*, urine] Any condition in which the urine contains blood or red blood cells.

haemo- [G. *haima*, blood] Combining form signifying blood. See also haem-, haemat-, haemato-.

hae'mochromato'sis [haemo- + G. *chrōma*, colour, + *-osis*, condition] A disorder of iron metabolism characterized by increased absorption of ingested iron, saturation of iron-binding protein, and deposition of haemosiderin in tissue, particularly in the liver, pancreas, and skin.

haemoc'lasis [haemo- + G. *klasis*, a breaking] Rupture, dissolution (haemolysis), or other type of destruction of red blood cells.

hae'moclas'tic Pertaining to haemoclasis.

hae'moconcentra'tion Decrease in the volume of plasma in relation to the number of red blood cells; increase in the concentration of red blood cells in the circulating blood.

hae'mocyte [haemo- + G. *kytos*, a hollow (cell)] Any cell or formed element of the blood.

hae'mocytol'ysis [haemo- + G. *kytos*, cell, + *lysis*, dissolution] The dissolution of blood cells, including haemolysis.

hae'mocytom'eter [haemo- + G. *kytos*, cell, + *metron*, measure] An apparatus for estimating the number of blood cells in a quantitively measured volume of blood.

haemodi'alyser Artificial kidney; a machine for haemodialysis in acute or chronic renal failure; toxic substances in the blood are removed by exposure to dialysing fluid across a semipermeable membrane.

hae'modial'ysis Dialysis of soluble substances and water from the blood by diffusion through a semipermeable membrane; separation of cellular elements and colloids from soluble substances is achieved by pore size in the membrane and rates of diffusion.

hae'moglo'bin (Hb) The red respiratory protein of erythrocytes, consisting of approximately 6% haem and 94% globin, that transports oxygen (as oxyhaemoglobin, HbO_2) from the lungs to the tissues, where the oxygen is readily released and HbO_2 becomes Hb.

hae'moglobinae'mia Presence of free haemoglobin in the blood plasma.

hae'moglobinol'ysis [haemoglobin + G. *lysis*, dissolution] Destruction or chemical splitting of haemoglobin.

hae'moglobinop'athy [haemoglobin + G. *pathos*, disease] A disorder or disease caused by or associated with the presence of abnormal haemoglobins in the blood.

hae'moglobinu'ria [haemoglobin + G. *ouron*, urine] Presence of haemoglobin in the urine, including certain closely related pigments formed from slight alteration of the haemoglobin molecule; in sufficient quantities, they result in the urine being coloured from light red-yellow to fairly dark red.

hae'mogram [haemo- + G. *gramma*, a drawing] A record of the findings in an examination of the blood, especially with reference to the numbers, proportions, and morphologic features of the formed elements.

haemol'ysate The preparation resulting from the lysis of erythrocytes.

haemol'ysin 1. Any substance elaborated by a living agent and capable of causing lysis of red blood cells and liberation of their haemoglobin. **2.** A sensitizing (complement-fixing) antibody that combines with red blood cells of the antigenic type that stimulated formation of the h., affecting the cells in such a manner that complement fixes with the antibody-cell union and causes dissolution of the cells, with liberation of their haemoglobin.

haemol'ysis [haemo- + G. *lysis*, destruction] The alteration, dissolution, or destruction of red blood cells in such a manner that haemoglobin is liberated.

hae'molyt'ic Destructive to blood cells, resulting in liberation of haemoglobin.

haemop'athy [haemo- + G. *pathos*, suffering] Any abnormal condition or disease of the blood or haemopoietic tissues.

hae'mopericar'dium Blood in the pericardial sac.

haemophil'ia [haemo- + G. *philos*, fond] An inherited disorder of the blood marked by a permanent tendency to haemorrhages, spontaneous or traumatic, due to a defect in the coagulating power of the blood.

h. A., h. due to deficiency of factor VIII; an X-linked recessive condition occurring almost exclusively in males, characterized by prolonged clotting time, decreased formation of thromboplastin, and diminished conversion of prothrombin.

h. B., a clotting disorder resembling h. A, caused by the hereditary deficiency of factor IX.

vascular h., von Willebrand's *disease.*
haemophil'iac A person suffering from haemophilia.
Haemoph'ilus [G. *haima*, blood, + *philos*, fond] A genus of aerobic to facultatively anaerobic, parasitic bacteria (family Brucellaceae) containing minute, Gram-negative rod-shaped cells. The type species is *H. influenzae.*

H. ducrey'i, a species that causes soft chancre (chancroid)

H. influen'zae, Koch-Weeks bacillus; a species that causes acute respiratory infections, acute conjunctivitis, and purulent meningitis; originally considered to be the cause of influenza.
haemophthal'mia [haemo- + G. *ophthalmos*, eye] An effusion of blood into the eyeball.
hae'moplas'tic [haemo- + G. *plassō*, to form] Haemopoietic.
hae'mopneumotho'rax [haemo- + G. *pneuma*, air, + thorax] Accumulation of air and blood in the pleural cavity.
haemopole'sis [haemo- + G. *poiēsis*, a making] Formation and development of the various types of blood cells and other formed elements.
haemopoiet'ic Pertaining to or related to the formation of blood cells.
haemop'tysis [haemo- + G. *ptysis*, a spitting] The spitting of blood derived from the lungs or bronchial tubes.
haem'orrhage [G. *haima*, blood, + *rhēgnymi*, to burst forth] Bleeding; an escape of blood from the vessels.

cerebral h., h. into the substance of the cerebrum, usually in the region of the internal capsule by the rupture of the lenticulostriate artery.

postpartum h., h. from the birth canal in excess of 500 ml during the first 24 hours after birth.
haemorrhag'ic Relating to or marked by haemorrhage.
haem'orrhoid Denoting one of the tumours or varices constituting haemorrhoids.

haemorrhoi'dal 1. Relating to haemorrhoids. **2.** Denoting certain arteries and veins supplying the region of the rectum and anus.
haem'orrhoidec'tomy [haemorrhoids + G. *ektomē*, excision] Surgical removal of haemorrhoids, as by excision of haemorrhoidal tissues or by ligation to produce ischaemic necrosis and ultimate ablation of the h.
haem'orrhoids [G. *haimorrhois,* pl. *haimorrhoides,* veins likely to bleed] Piles; a varicose condition of the external haemorrhoidal veins causing painful swellings at the anus: **external h.,** when the dilated veins form tumours to the outer side of the external sphincter, or are covered by the skin of the anal canal; **internal h.,** when the swollen veins are beneath the mucous membrane within the sphincter.
haemosid'erin An insoluble protein produced by phagocytic digestion of haematin and found in most tissues, especially in the liver, in the form of granules much larger than ferritin molecules.
hae'mosidero'sis Abnormal accumulation of haemosiderin in tissue.
haemosper'mia [haemo- + G. *sperma*, seed] Presence of blood in the seminal fluid.
haemosta'sis [haemo- + G. *stasis*, a standing] **1.** The arrest of bleeding. **2.** The arrest of circulation in a part. **3.** Stagnation of blood.
hae'mostat 1. An antihaemorrhagic agent. **2.** An instrument for arresting haemorrhage by compression of the bleeding vessel.
hae'mostat'ic 1. Arresting the flow of blood within the vessels. **2.** Arresting haemorrhage.
haemother'apy Treatment of disease by the use of blood or blood derivatives, such as transfusion.
haemotho'rax Blood in the pleural cavity.
haemotox'ic 1. Causing blood poisoning. **2.** Haemolytic.
hae'motox'in Any substance that causes destruction of red blood cells; usually referring to substances of biologic origin in contrast to chemicals.
hair [A.S. *haer*] **1.** Pilus (1). **2.** One of the fine, hairlike processes of a sensory cell.
hair'ball Trichobezoar.
half-life The period during which the radioactivity of a radioactive substance, due to

disintegration, is reduced to half of its original value.

hal'ide A salt or compound of a halogen.

halito'sis [L. *halitus*, breath, + G. *-osis*, condition] Bad breath, especially a foul odour from the mouth.

hal'itus [L. fr. *halo*, to breathe] Any exhalation, as of a breath or vapour.

hal'lucal Relating to the hallux.

hallu'cina'tion [L. *alucinari*, to wander in mind] The apparent, often strong subjective sense perception of sight, sound, smell, taste, or touch without basis in external stimuli.

hallu'cinogen A substance whose most prominent pharmacologic action is on the central nervous system, eliciting hallucinations, depersonalization, perceptual disturbances, and disturbances of thought processes.

hal'lux, pl. **hal'luces** [a Mod. L. form for L. *hallex* (*hallic-*), great toe] [NA] The great toe, the first digit of the foot.

h. val'gus, deviation of the tip or main axis of the first toe, toward the outer side of the foot.

h. va'rus, deviation of the main axis of the great toe to the inner side of the foot.

ha'lo [G. *halōs*] **1.** A reddish yellow ring surrounding the optic disc, due to a widening out of the scleral ring permitting the deeper structures to show through. **2.** An annular flare of light surrounding a luminous body.

hal'ogen [G. *hals*, salt, + *-gen*, producing] One of the chlorine group (fluorine, chlorine, bromine, iodine, astatine) of elements which form monobasic acids with hydrogen.

hal'othane A widely used inhalation anaesthetic with rapid onset, rapid reversal, and benign odour.

hamar'toblasto'ma [hamartoma + blastoma] A malignant neoplasm of undifferentiated anaplastic cells thought to be derived from a hamartoma.

hamarto'ma [G. *hamartion*, a bodily defect, + *-oma*, tumour] A focal malformation that resembles a neoplasm but results from faulty development in an organ; composed of an abnormal mixture of tissue elements, or an abnormal proportion of a single element, normally present in that site which develop and grow at virtually the same rate as normal components, and are not likely to result in compression of adjacent tissue.

ham'mer Malleus.

ham'string One of the tendons bounding the popliteal space on either side: **medial h.,** comprises the tendons of the semimembranosus, semitendinosus, gracilis, and sartorius muscles; **lateral h.,** the tendon of the biceps femoris.

hand [A.S.] Manus.

accoucheur's h., obstetrical h., position of the h. in tetany or in muscular dystrophy; the fingers are flexed at the metacarpophalangeal joints and extended at the phalangeal joints, with the thumb flexed and adducted into the palm.

claw h., see clawhand.

cleft h., split h., a congenital deformity in which the division between the fingers, especially between the third and fourth, extends into the metacarpal region. See also lobster-claw *deformity*.

drop h., wrist-drop.

hand'edness Preference for the use of one hand, most commonly the right, associated with dominance of the opposite cerebral hemisphere; also the result of training or habit.

hand'icap A physical, mental, or emotional condition that interferes with one's functioning.

hang'nail A loose tag of epidermis attached at the proximal portion in the medial or lateral nail fold.

haplo- [G. *haplous*, simple, single] Combining form meaning simple or single.

hap'loid [haplo- + -ploid] Denoting the number of chromosomes in sperm or ova (23 in man); which is half the number in somatic (diploid) cells.

hare-lip Cleft *lip*.

hash'ish [Ar. hay] A form of cannabis that consists largely of resin from the flowering tops and sprouts of cultivated female plants; contains the highest concentration of cannabinols among the preparations derived from cannabis.

haustra'tion 1. Formation of a haustrum. **2.** An increase in prominence of the haustra.

haus'trum, pl. **haus'tra** [L. a machine for drawing water] One of a series of saccules or pouches (so-called because of a fancied resemblance to the buckets on a waterwheel), such as sacculations of the colon caused by longitudinal bands that are slightly shorter than the gut so that the latter is shaped into tucks or pouches.

head [A.S. *heāfod*] Caput.

head'ache Diffuse pain in various parts of the head, not confined to the area of distribution of any nerve.

cluster h., histaminic h., a migraine variant characterized by recurrent, severe, unilateral orbitotemporal h.'s associated with conjunctival injection.

migraine h., see migraine.

tension h., h. associated with nervous tension, anxiety, etc., often related to chronic contraction of the scalp muscles.

heal [A.S. *healan*] **1.** To restore to health, to cure; especially to cause an ulcer or wound to cicatrize or unite. **2.** To become well, to be cured; to cicatrize or close, said of an ulcer or wound.

heal'ing 1. Curing; restoring to health; promoting the closure of wounds and ulcers. **2.** The process of a return to health or closing of a wound.

h. by first intention, h. by fibrous adhesion, without suppuration or granulation tissue formation.

h. by second intention, union of two granulating surfaces accompanied by suppuration and delayed closure.

h. by third intention, the slow filling of a wound cavity or ulcer by granulations, with subsequent cicatrization.

health [A.S. haelth] The state of an organism when it functions optimally without evidence of disease or abnormality.

mental h., the absence of mental or behavioural disorder; a state of psychological well-being in which a person has achieved a satisfactory integration of his instinctual drives acceptable to both himself and his social milieu.

public h., the art and science of community health, concerned with statistics, epidemiology, hygiene, and the prevention and eradication of epidemic diseases.

hear'ing [A.S. *hēran*, hear] The ability to perceive sound; the sensation of sound as opposed to vibration.

hearing aid An electronic amplifying device designed to bring sound more effectively into the ear; consists of a microphone, amplifier, and receiver.

hearing impair'ment, hearing loss A reduction in the ability to perceive sound, ranging from partial to complete deafness.

heart [A.S. *heorte*] A hollow muscular organ that receives blood from the veins and propels it into the arteries; divided by a musculomembranous septum into two halves, venous and arterial, each of which consists of an atrium and a ventricle.

fatty h., (1) fatty degeneration of the myocardium; **(2)** accumulation of adipose tissue on the external surface of the h. with occasional infiltration of fat between the muscle bundles of the h. wall.

heart'burn Pyrosis.

heat [A.S. *haete*] A high temperature; the sensation produced by proximity to fire or an incandescent object, as opposed to cold.

prickly h., milaria rubra.

heat-la'bile Destroyed or altered by heat.

heat'stroke A condition produced by exposure to excessively high temperatures and characterized by headache, vertigo, confusion, and a slight rise in body temperature; collapse and coma, very high fever, tachycardia, and hot dry skin follow in severe cases.

hebephre'nia [G. *hēbē*, puberty, + *phrēn*, the mind] A syndrome characterized by shallow and inappropriate affect, giggling, and silly regressive behaviour and mannerisms.

hebet'ic [G. *hēbētikos*, youthful, fr. *hēbē*, youth] Pertaining to youth.

heb'etude [L. *hebetudo*, fr. *hebeo*, to be dull] Moria (1).

hed'rocele [G. hedra, a seat, the fundament, + *kēlē*, hernia] Prolapse of the intestine through the anus.

heel [A.S. *hēla*] Calx (2).

painful h., a condition in which bearing the weight on the h. causes pain of varying severity.

hel'ical [G. helix, a coil] **1.** Relating to a helix. **2.** Helicoid.

hel'icine [G. helix, a coil] **1.** Coiled. **2.** Helical (1).

hel'icoid [G. helix, a coil, + eidos, resemblance] Resembling a helix.

he'lium [G. *hēlios*, sun] A gaseous element, symbol He, atomic no. 2, atomic weight 4.0026; used as a diluent of medicinal gases.

he'lix, pl. **hel'ices** [L. fr. G. helix, a coil] **1.** [NA] The margin of the auricle; a folded rim of cartilage forming the upper part of the anterior, the superior, and the greater part of the posterior edges of the auricle. **2.** A line in the shape of a coil, (or a spring, or threads on a bolt (but mistakenly applied to a spiral), each point being equidistant from a straight line that is the axis of the cylinder in which each point of the h. lies.

Watson-Crick h., the helical structure assumed by two strands of deoxyribonucleic acid, held together throughout their length by hydrogen bonds between bases on opposite strands.

hel'minth [G. *helmins*, worm] An intestinal vermiform parasite.

helminthi'asis The condition of having intestinal vermiform parasites.

helmin'thic Anthelmintic (1).

helmintho'ma [G. *helmins*, worm, + *-oma*, tumour] A discrete nodule of granulomatous inflammation (including the healed stage) caused by a helminth or its products.

helo'ma [G. *hēlos*, nail, + *-oma*, tumour] Clavus (1).

helot'omy [heloma + G. *tomē*, cutting] The surgical treatment of corns.

hem'eralo'pia [G. *hēmera*, day, + *alaos*, obscure, + *ōps*, eye] Day blindness; night sight; inability to see as distinctly in a bright light as in a dim one.

hemi- [G.] Prefix signifying one-half. See also semi-.

hem'ianaesthe'sia Unilateral anaesthesia; loss of tactile sensibility on one side of the body.

alternate h., crossed h., h. affecting the head on one side and the body and extremities on the other side.

hemianop'sia, hemiano'pia [hemi- + G. *an-* priv. + *opsis*, vision] Loss of vision for one-half of the visual field of one or both eyes.

hemiat'rophy Atrophy of one lateral half of a part or of an organ.

hem'iballis'mus, hemibal'lism [hemi- + G. *ballismos*, jumping about] Violent writhing and choreic movements involving one side of the body, usually related to a lesion of the subthalamic nucleus of the opposite side of the brain.

hem'icephalal'gia [hemi- + G. *kephalē*, head, + *algos*, pain] The unilateral headache characteristic of typical migraine.

hemichore'a Chorea involving the muscles on one side of the body.

hem'icolec'tomy [hemi- + G. *kolon*, colon, + *ektomē*, excision] Removal of the right or left side of the colon.

hemicra'nia [hemi- + G. *kranion*, skull] **1.** Migraine. **2.** Hemicephalalgia.

hemiep'ilepsy Epilepsy in which the convulsive movements are confined to one side of the body.

hemifa'cial Pertaining to one side of the face.

hem'igastrec'tomy Excision of the distal half of the stomach.

hem'iglossec'tomy [hemi- + G. *glōssa*, tongue, + *ektomē*, excision] Surgical removal of one-half of the tongue.

hem'iglossi'tis [hemi- + G. *glōssa*, tongue, + *-itis*, inflammation] A vesicular eruption on one side of the tongue and the corresponding inner surface of the cheek.

hem'ilaminec'tomy [hemi- + L. *lamina*, layer, + G. *ektomē*, excision] Removal of a portion of a vertebral lamina; often used to denote unilateral laminectomy.

hem'ilaryngec'tomy [hemi- + G. *larynx* (*laryng-*), larynx, + *ektomē*, excision] Excision of a lateral half of the larynx.

hemilat'eral Relating to one lateral half.

hemipare'sis Slight paralysis affecting one side of the body.

hemiple'gia [hemi- + G. *plēgē*, a stroke] Paralysis of one side of the body.

alternating h., crossed h., h., as the result of a brainstem lesion, occurring on the contralateral side (with reference to the lesion) and a paralysis of a motor cranial nerve on the ipsilateral side.

hemiple'gic Relating to hemiplegia.

hem'ispasm A spasm affecting one or more muscles of one side of the face or body.

hem'isphere [hemi- + G. *sphaira*, ball, globe] Half of a spherical structure or organ.

cerebellar h., the large part of the cerebellum lateral to the vermis cerebelli.

cerebral h., the large mass of the telencephalon, on either side of the midline, consisting of the cerebral cortex and its associated fibre systems, together with the deeper-lying corpus striatum.

hemisys'tole Contraction of the left ventricle following every second atrial contraction only, so that there is but one pulse beat to every two heart beats.

hemizygos'ity The state of having unpaired genes in an otherwise diploid cell; males are normally hemizygous for genes on the X chromosome.

hemizy'gote [hemi- + G. *zytótos*, yoked (see zygote)] An individual hemizygous with respect to one or more specified genes.

he'par, gen. **he'patis** [L. borrowed fr. G. *hēpar*, gen. *hēpatos*, the liver] [NA] The liver.

hep'arin An anticoagulant principle that is a constituent of various tissues (especially liver and lung) and mast cells. In conjunction with a serum protein cofactor, h. is an antithrombin and an antiprothrombin by preventing platelet agglutination and thus prevents thrombus formation; also enhances activity of clearing factors.

hepat-, hepatico-, hepato- [G. *hēpar* (*hēpat-*), liver] Combining forms denoting the liver.

hepatec'tomy [hepat- + G. *ektomē*, excision] Excision of liver tissue.

hepat'ic [G. *hēpatikos*] Relating to the liver.

hepat'icoduodenos'tomy [hepatico- + duodenostomy] Establishment of a communication between the hepatic ducts and the duodenum.

hepat'icoenteros'tomy [hepatico- + enterostomy] Establishment of a communication between the hepatic ducts and the intestine.

hepa'ticogastros'tomy [hepatico- + gastrostomy] Establishment of a communication between the hepatic duct and the stomach.

hepat'icolith'otripsy [hepatico- + G. *lithos*, stone, + *tripsis*, a rubbing] Crushing a biliary calculus in the hepatic duct.

hepaticos'tomy [hepatico- + G. *stoma*, mouth] Establishment of an opening into the hepatic duct.

hepati'tis [hepat- + G. *-itis*, inflammation] Inflammation of the liver.

non-A, non-B h., h. caused by an infectious agents antigenically different from h viruses A and B; in the acute stage, it is generally milder than h. B, but a greater proportion of such infections become chronic.

viral h. type A, infectious h.; h. A; a virus disease with a short incubation period caused by h. virus A; occurs sporadically or in epidemics; transmission is by the faecal-oral route, with necrosis of liver cells characteristic and jaundice a common symptom.

viral h. type B, serum h.; h. B; a virus disease with a long incubation period caused by h. virus B, usually transmitted by injection of infected blood or blood derivatives or by contaminated instruments; clinically and pathologically, the disease is similar to viral h. type A; however, there is no cross-protective immunity and viral antigen (HBAg) is found in the serum.

hep'atiza'tion Conversion of a loose tissue into a firm mass like the substance of the liver macroscopically, denoting especially such a change in the lungs in the consolidation of pneumonia.

hepato- See hepat-.

hep'atoblasto'ma A malignant neoplasm, occurring in children, primarily in the liver, composed of tissue resembling fetal or mature liver cells or bile ducts.

hep'atocarcino'ma Malignant *hepatoma*.

hepat'ocele [hepato- + G. *kēlē*, hernia] Hernia of the liver; protrusion of part of the liver through the abdominal wall or the diaphragm.

hep'atocholangios'tomy Creation of an opening into the common bile duct to establish drainage.

hep'atocys'tic [hepato- + G. *kystis*, bladder] Relating to the gallbladder, or to both liver and gallbladder.

hep'atocyte A parenchymal liver cell.

hepatogen'ic, hepatog'enous Of hepatic origin; formed in the liver.

hepatog'raphy [hepato- + G. *graphē*, a writing] Radiography of the liver.

hep'atolith [hepato- + G. *lithos*, stone] A concretion in the liver.

hep'atolithec'tomy [hepato- + G. *lithos*, stone, + *oktomē*, excision] Removal of a calculus from the liver.

hep'atolithi'asis [hepato- + G. *lithiasis*, presence of a calculus] Presence of calculi in the liver.

hepatol'ogy [hepato- + G. *logos*, study] The branch of medical science concerned with the liver and its diseases.

hepato'ma [hepato- + G. *-oma*, tumour] See malignant h.

malignant h., a carcinoma derived from parenchymal cells of the liver.

hep'atomeg'aly [hepato- + G. *megas*, large] Enlargement of the liver.

hep'atopor'tal Relating to the portal system of the liver.

hep'atosplenog'raphy Use of contrast dyes to depict the liver and spleen radiographically.

hep′atosplenomeg′aly [hepato- + G. splēn, spleen, + megas, large] Enlargement of the liver and spleen.

hep′atotoxae′mia [hepato- + G. toxikon, poison, + haima, blood] Autointoxication originating in the liver.

hep′atotox′in A toxin that is destructive to parenchymal cells of the liver.

hepta- [G. hepta, seven] Prefix denoting seven.

herd An immunologic concept of an ecologic composite that includes susceptible animal species (including man), vectors, and environmental factors.

hered′itary Relating to heredity.

hered′ity [L. hereditas, inheritance, fr. heres (hered-), heir] 1. Genetic transmission of characters from parent to offspring. 2. One's genetic constitution.

heredo- [L. heres, an heir] Prefix denoting heredity.

her′edofamil′ial Denoting an inherited condition present in more than one member of a family.

heritabil′ity [See heredity] In genetics, the proportion of phenotypic variance due to variance in genotypes.

hermaph′rodite [G. Hermaphroditus, son of Hermēs + Aphroditē] An individual with hermaphroditism.

hermaph′roditism Presence in one individual of both ovarian and testicular tissue.

hermet′ic Denoting a container closed or sealed in such a way that it is airtight.

her′nia [L. rupture] Rupture; the protrusion of a part or structure through the tissues normally containing it.

  abdominal h., a h. protruding through or into any part of the abdominal wall.

  diaphragmatic h., protrusion of abdominal contents into the chest through a weakness in the respiratory diaphragm.

  inguinal h., a h. at the inguinal region: **direct i. h.** involves the abdominal wall between the deep epigastric artery and the edge of the rectus muscle; **indirect i. h.** involves the internal inguinal ring and passes into the inguinal canal.

  irreducible h., incarcerated h., a h. that cannot be reduced without an operation.

  reducible h., a h. in which the contents of the h. sac can be returned to their normal location by manipulation.

  strangulated h., an irreducible h. in which the circulation is arrested.

  umbilical h., a h. in which bowel or omentum protrudes through the abdominal wall under the skin at the umbilicus.

her′niated Denoting any structure protruded through a hernial opening.

hernia′tion Formation of a hernia.

hernio- [L. hernia, rupture] Combining form relating to hernia.

her′nioplasty hernio- + G. plassō, to form] Surgical correction of a hernia.

hernior′rhaphy [hernio- + G. rhaphē, a seam] Surgical correction of a hernia by suturing.

herniot′omy [hernio- + G. tomē, a cutting] Surgical correction of a hernia by cutting.

hero′ic [G. hērōikos, pertaining to a hero] Denoting an aggressive, daring procedure which in itself may endanger the patient but which also has a possibility of being successful, whereas lesser action would result in failure.

her′oin Diacetylmorphine; an addictive alkaloid, prepared from morphine by acetylation.

herpangi′na A disease caused by types of coxsackievirus and marked by a sudden onset of fever, loss of appetitie, dysphagia, pharyngitis, and sometimes abdominal pain, nausea, and vomiting; vesiculopapular lesions are present around the fauces and soon ulcerate.

her′pes [G. herpēs, a spreading skin eruption, shingles] An eruption of groups of deepseated vesicles on erythematous bases.

  genital h., h. genita′lis, herpetic lesions on the penis of the male or on the cervix, perineum, vagina, or vulva of the female, caused by herpesvirus (herpes simplex virus) type 2.

  h. sim′plex, fever blister; cold sore; a variety of infections caused by h. simplex virus (herpesvirus) types 1 and 2; type 1 infections are marked by the eruption of one or more groups of vesicles on the vermilion border of the lips or at the external nares, type 2 by such lesions on the genitalia; both types commonly are recrudescent and reappear during other febrile illnesses or certain physiologic states.

  h. zos′ter, shingles; an infection caused by a herpetovirus (varicella-zoster virus) and characterized by an eruption of groups of vesicles on one side of the body following the course of a nerve due to inflammation of ganglia and dorsal nerve roots resulting from activation of the virus which has been latent; the condition is self-limited but may be accompanied by or followed by severe pain.

her'pesvirus 1. Herpes simplex virus; a virus of the genus *Herpesvirus* (family Herpetoviridae), divided into two types: **h. type 1,** the pathogen of herpes simplex in humans, causing acute stomatitis, especially in children, and fever blisters, usually on the lips and external nares; also causes oozoma her peticum and herpetic gingivostomatitis, keratoconjunctivitis, and meningoencephalitis; **h. type 2,** the pathogen of genital herpes and neonatal herpes. 2. Formerly, any virus of the genus *Herpesvirus,* which then included those viruses now grouped in the family Herpetoviridae, now herpetovirus.

herpet'ic 1. Relating to or characterized by herpes. 2. Relating to a herpetovirus or herpesvirus.

herpet'iform Resembling herpes.

Her'petovi'ridae A family of morphologically similar viruses, all of which contain double-stranded DNA, whose infections produce type A inclusion bodies; only one genus, *Herpesvirus,* has been established. The family includes herpes simplex virus, varicella zoster virus, cytomegalovirus, and EB virus (which infect man), and many others.

hersage' [Fr. (from L. *hirpex,* a large rake), a harrowing] Surgical separation of the individual fibres of a nerve trunk.

hes'itancy An involuntary delay or inability in starting the urinary stream.

heterecious [heter- + G. *oikion,* home] Having more than one host, said of a parasite passing different states of its existence in different animals.

hetero-, heter- [G. *heteros,* other] Combining form meaning other, or different.

heteroan'tibody Antibody that is heterologous with respect to antigen.

het'erocel'lular Formed of cells of different kinds.

heterochro'mia [hetero- + G. *chrōma,* colour] A difference in coloration in two structures or two parts of the same structure which are normally alike in colour.

het'erogamet'ic [hetero- + G. *gametikos,* connubial] Relating to production of gametes of contrasting types with respect to sex chromosomes.

het'erogene'ic, het'erogen'ic Pertaining to different gene constitutions, especially with respect to different species.

het'erogene'ity The state of being heterogeneous.

heteroge'neous Composed of parts having various and dissimilar characteristics or properties.

het'erograft Heterologous graft; xenograft; a graft transferred from an animal of one species to one of another species.

heterol'ogous [hetero- + G. *logos,* ratio, relation] 1. Pertaining to cytologic or histologic elements occurring where they are not normally found. 2. Derived from a different species.

het'erometro'pia [hetero- + G. *metron,* measure, + *ōps,* eye] A condition in which the degree of refraction is unlike in the two eyes.

het'eromor'phous Differing from the normal type.

het'erophil, het'erophile [hetero- + G. *philos,* fond] 1. In man, the neutrophil leucocyte. 2. Pertaining to heterogenetic antigens and related antibody.

heteropho'ria [hetero- + G. *phora,* movement] A tendency for deviation of the eyes from parallelism, prevented by binocular vision.

het'eropla'sia [hetero- + G. *plasis,* a forming] 1. Development of cytologic and histologic elements that are not normal for the organ or part in question. 2. Malposition of tissue or a part that is otherwise normal.

het'eroplas'tic 1. Pertaining to or manifesting heteroplasia. 2. Relating to tissue transplantation from one species to another.

het'erosex'ual 1. Denoting or characteristic of heterosexuality. 2. One who practises heterosexuality.

het'erosexual'ity Erotic attraction, predisposition, or sexual behaviour between persons of the opposite sex.

het'erotax'ia [hetero- + G. *taxis,* arrangement] Abnormal arrangement of organs or parts of the body in relation to each other.

het'eroto'pia [hetero- + G. *topos,* place] 1. Ectopia. 2. In neuropathology, displacement of grey matter, typically into the deep cerebral white matter.

het'erotroph [hetero- + G. *trophē*, nourishment] A microorganism that obtains its carbon, as well as its energy, from organic compounds.

heterotro'pia [hetero- + G. *trope*, a turning] Strabismus.

het'erozygos'ity [hetero- + G. *zygon*, a yoke] The state of having different allelic genes at one or more paired loci in homologous chromosomes.

heterozy'gous Relating to heterozygosity.

hexa-, hex- [G. *hex*, six] Prefixes meaning six.

hexadac'tyly, hexadac'tylism [hexa- + G. *daktylos*, finger] Presence of six digits on one or both hands or feet.

hia'tus, pl. **hia'tus** [L. an aperture, fr. *hio*, pp. *hiatus*, to yawn] [NA] **1.** An aperture or fissure. **2.** A foramen.

hic'cup, hic'cough A diaphragmatic spasm causing sudden inhalation that is interrupted by a spasmodic closure of the glottis, producing the characteristic noise.

hidradeni'tis [G. *hidros*, sweat, + *aden*, gland, + *-itis*, inflammation] Inflammation of the sweat glands; more specifically, of the apocrine glands.

hidradeno'ma [G. *hidros*, sweat, + *aden*, gland, + *-oma*, tumour] A benign neoplasm derived from epithelial cells of sweat glands.

hidro-, hidr- [G. *hidros*, sweat] Combining forms relating to sweat or sweat glands.

hidro'sis [G. *hidros*, sweat, + *-osis*, condition] Production and excretion of sweat.

hidrot'ic Relating to or causing hidrosis.

hi'lar Pertaining to a hilus.

hil'lock In anatomy, any small elevation or prominence.

hi'lum, pl. **hi'la** [L. a small bit or trifle] [NA] Depression or slitlike opening in an organ where the nerves and vessels enter and leave.

hi'lus [an Eng. variant of L. *hilum*] Former incorrect NA designation for hilum.

hind'brain Rhombencephalon.

hind'gut 1. The large intestine, rectum, and anal canal. **2.** The caudal or terminal part of the embryonic gut.

hip [A.S. *hype*] Coxa; the lateral prominence of the pelvis from the waist to the thigh; more strictly the h. joint.

hippocam'pal Relating to the hippocampus.

hippocam'pus [G. *hippocampos*, seahorse] [NA] The complex, internally convoluted structure that forms the medial margin of the cortical mantle of the cerebral hemisphere, bordering the choroid fissure of the lateral ventricle, and composed of two gyri (Ammon's horn and the dentate gyrus), together with their white matter; it forms part of the limbic system and, by way of the fornix, projects to the septum, anterior nucleus of the thalamus, and mamillary body.

hippocrat'ic Relating to, described by, or attributed to Hippocrates.

hip'pus [G. *hippos*, horse, from a fancied suggestion of galloping movements] Spasmodic, rhythmical pupillary dilation and constriction, independent of illumination, convergence, or psychic stimuli.

hir'cus, gen. and pl. **hir'ci** [L. he-goat] **1.** The odour of the axillae. **2.** [NA] One of the hairs growing in the axillae. **3.** Tragus (1).

hir'sute [L. *hirsutus*, shaggy] Relating to or characterized by hirsutism.

hir'sutism [L. *hirsutus*, shaggy] Presence of excessive bodily and facial hair, especially in women.

hir'udin [L. *hirudo*, leech] An antithrombin substance extracted from the salivary glands of the leech that has the property of preventing coagulation of the blood.

Hiru'do [L. leech] A genus of leeches (class Hirudinea), including *H. medicinalis*, the species most commonly used in medicine.

his'taminae'mia Presence of histamine in the circulating blood.

his'tamine A depressor amine derived from histidine by decarboxylation; a powerful stimulant of gastric secretion, constrictor of bronchial smooth muscle, and vasodilator (capillaries and arterioles).

histamine-fast Indicating the absence of the normal response to histamine, especially in speaking of true gastric anacidity.

his'tidinae'mia Elevation of blood histidine level and excretion of histidine and related imidazole metabolites in urine due to deficiency of histidase activity; autosomal recessive inheritance.

his'tidine (His) A basic amino acid in proteins.

his'tidinu'ria Excretion of considerable amounts of histidine in the urine, as in histidinaemia.

histio- [G. *histion*, web (tissue)] Combining form relating to tissue.

his'tiocyte [histio- + G. *kytos*, cell] A macrophage present in connective tissue.

his'tiocyto'ma [histio- + G. *kytos*, cell, + -*ōma*, tumour] A tumour composed of histiocytes.

his'tiocyto'sis A generalized multiplication of histiocytes.

   kerasin h., Gaucher's *disease*.

   lipid h., h. with cytoplasmic accumulation of lipid, either cholesterol (Hand-Schüller-Christian disease), phospholipid (Niemann-Pick disease), or kerasin (Gaucher's disease).

   nonlipid h., Letterer-Siwe disease; an acute progressive generalized disease in young children, characterized by a purpuric rash, enlargement of lymph glands and spleen, and invasion of the spleen, liver, and bone marrow by histiocytes.

   h. X, histiocytic proliferation of undetermined type, possible Hand-Schüller-Christian d. or eosinophilic granuloma of bone.

histiogen'ic Histogenous.

histo- [G. *histos*, web (tissue)] Combining form relating to tissue.

his'tocompat'ibil'ity A state of immunologic similarity or identity of tissues sufficient to permit successful transplantation.

histocompatibility testing A testing system for HLA antigens, of major importance in transplantation.

his'tocyte Histiocyte.

his'toin'compatibil'ity State of immunologic dissimilarity of tissues sufficient to cause rejection of transplanted tissue.

histolog'ic, histolog'ical Pertaining to histology.

histol'ogy [histo- + G. *logos*, study] The science concerned with the minute structure of cells, tissues, and organs in relation to their function.

histol'ysis [histo- + G. *lysis*, dissolution] Disintegration of tissue.

his'tone One of a number of simple proteins that contains a high proportion of basic amino acids; *e.g.*, the proteins associated with nucleic acids in the nuclei of plant and animal tissues.

his'topathol'ogy The science concerned with the cytologic and histologic structure of abnormal or diseased tissue.

Histoplas'ma capsula'tum [histo- + G. *plasma*, something formed] A dimorphic fungus species that causes histoplasmosis in man and other mammals.

his'toplasmo'sis An infectious disease caused by *Histoplasma capsulatum* and manifested by a primary benign pneumonitis similar in clinical features to primary tuberculosis; occasionally, the primary disease progresses to produce localized lesions in lung, such as pulmonary cavitation, or the typical disseminated disease of the reticuloendothelial system manifested by fever, emaciation, splenomegaly, and leucopenia.

histotrop'ic [histo- + G. *tropikos*, turning] Attracted toward tissues; denoting certain parasites, stains, and chemical compounds.

HIV Human Immunodeficiency *virus*.

hives Urticaria.

hoarse [A.S. *hās*] Having a rough, harsh quality of voice.

ho'lism [G. *holos*, entire] In psychology, the approach to the study of a psychological phenomenon through the analysis of the phenomenon as a complete entity in itself.

holis'tic Pertaining to the characteristics of holism or h. psychologies.

holo- [G. *holos*, whole, entire, complete] Combining form denoting entirety or relationship to a whole.

homeo- [G. *homoios*, like] Combining form meaning the same, or alike. See also homo .

homeopath'ic Relating to homeopathy.

homeop'athist, ho'meopath A medical practitioner of the homeopathic school.

homeop'athy [homeo- + G. *pathos*, suffering] A system of therapy developed by Samuel Hahnemann on the theory that large doses of a certain drug given to a healthy person will produce certain conditions which, when occurring spontaneously as symptoms of a disease, are relieved by the same drug in small doses.

homeosta'sis [homeo- + G. *stasis*, a standing] **1.** The state of equilibrium in the body with respect to various functions and to the chemical compositions of the fluids and tissues. **2.** The processes through which such bodily equilibrium is maintained.

homo- [G. *homos*, the same] Combining form meaning the same or alike. See also homeo-.

ho'mogamet'ic [homo- + G. *gametikos*, connubial] Producing only one type of gamete with respect to sex chromosomes.

homoge'neous [homo- + G. *genos*, race] Of uniform structure or composition throughout.

homog'enous [homo- + G. *genos*, family, kind] Having a structural similarity because of descent from a common ancestor.

ho'mogentis'ic acid Alcapton; alkapton; an intermediate in tyrosine catabolism, accumulating in those persons suffering a congenital deficiency of the enzyme homogentisate 1,2-dioxygenase and occurring in the urine in alkaptonuria.

ho'mograft Homologous graft; a tissue or an organ transplanted from one individual to another of the same species, not identical twins; used generally or with respect to animal strains not isogeneic for histocompatibility genes.

  allogeneic h., allograft.

  isogeneic h., syngeneic h., isograft.

ho'molat'eral [homo- + L. *latus*, side] Ipsilateral.

homol'ogous [see homologue] Corresponding or alike in certain critical attributes; *e.g.*, of organs or parts corresponding in evolutionary origin and similar to some extent in structure, but not necessarily similar in function, of a single chemical series, differing by fixed increments, of chromosomes or chromosome parts identical with respect to their genetic loci, of serum or tissue derived from members of a single species, or of an antibody with respect to the antigen that produced it.

hom'ologue [homo- + G. *logos*, word, ratio, relation] A member of a homologous pair or series.

homomor'phic [homo- + G. *morphē*, shape, appearance] Denoting two or more structures of similar size and shape.

ho'moplasty Repair of a defect by a homograft.

homosex'ual 1. Denoting or characteristic of homosexuality. 2. One who practises homosexuality.

ho'mosexual'ity Erotic attraction, predisposition, or sexual behaviour between individuals of the same sex, especially past puberty.

homotyp'ic, homotyp'ical Of the same type or form; corresponding to the other one of two paired organs or parts.

homozygos'ity [homo- + G. *zygon*, yoke] The state of having identical genes at one or more paired loci in homologous chromosomes.

homozy'gous Relating to homozygosity.

hook'worm Common name for bloodsucking nematodes of the family Ancyclostomatidae, chiefly members of the genera *Ancylastoma*, *Necator*, and *Uncinaria*.

hordeo'lum [Mod. L. fr. L. *hordeolus*, a sty in the eye] Sty; suppurative infection of a marginal gland of the eyelid; may be external, inflammation of the sebaceous gland of an eyelash, or internal, acute purulent infection of a meibomian gland.

hormo'nal Pertaining to hormones.

hor'mone [G. *hormōn*, pres. part. of *hormaō*, to rouse or set in motion] A chemical substance, formed in one organ or part of the body and carried in the blood to another organ or part, with specific regulatory effect on functional activity, and sometimes the structure, of just one organ or of various numbers of them. For h.'s not listed below, see specific names.

  adrenocorticotropic h. (ACTH), corticotropin; adrenocorticotropin; the h. of the anterior lobe of the hypophysis that governs nutrition and growth of the adrenal cortex, stimulates it to functional activity, and also possesses extra-adrenal adipokinetic activity.

  androgenic h., any h. that produces a masculinizing effect.

  anterior pituitary-like h., chorionic *gonadotropin*.

  antidiuretic h. (ADH), vasopressin.

  follicle-stimulating h. (FSH), a glycoprotein h. of the anterior pituitary gland that stimulates the graafian follicles of the ovary and assists subsequently in follicular maturation and the secretion of oestradiol, and stimulates the epithelium of the seminiferous tubules and is partially responsible for inducing spermatogenesis.

  growth h. (GH), somatotropin.

  luteinizing h. (LH), a glycoprotein h. stimulating the final ripening of the follicles and the secretion of progesterone by them, their rupture to release the egg, and the conversion of the ruptured follicle into the corpus luteum.

horn [A.S.] Cornu.

Ammon's h. [G. *Ammon*, Egyptian deity] one of the two interlocking gyri composing the hippocampus, the other being the gyrus dentatus.

hos'pice [L. *hospes*, a host, a guest] An institution that provides a centralized program of palliative and supportive services to dying persons and their families, in the form of physical, psychological, social, and spiritual care.

hos'pital [L. *hospitalis*, for a guest, fr. *hospes*, a host, a guest] An institution for the treatment, care, and cure of the sick and wounded, for the study of disease, and for the training of health professionals.

hos'pitaliza'tion Confinement in a hospital as a patient for diagnostic study and treatment.

host [L. *hospes*, a host] The organism in or on which a parasite lives, deriving its body substance or nourishment from the h.

definitive h., final h., the h. in which a parasite reaches the adult or sexually mature stage.

intermediate h., intermediary h., the h. in which larval or developmental parasitic stages occur.

hot flash, hot flush A vasomotor symptom of the climacterium: sudden vasodilation with a sensation of heat, usually involving the face and neck, and upper part of the chest; sweats, often profuse, frequently follow.

hu'meral Relating to the humerus.

hu'merus, gen. and pl. **hu'meri** [L. shoulder] [NA] The bone of the arm, articulating with the scapula above and the radius and ulna below.

hu'mor, gen. **humo'ris** [L. correctly, *umor*, liquid] **1.** [NA] Any clear fluid or semifluid hyaline anatomical substance. **2.** One of the elemental body fluids that were the basis of the physiologic and pathologic teachings of the hippocratic school: blood, yellow bile, black bile, and phlegm.

h. aquo'sus, [NA], the watery fluid that fills the anterior and posterior chambers of the eye.

h. vit'reus [NA], the fluid component of the corpus vitreum.

hu'moral Relating to a humour.

hu'mour Humor.

aqueous h., humor aquosus.

vitreous h., humor vitreus.

hump'back, hunch'back Kyphosis.

hy'aline [G. *hyalos*, glass] Of a glassy, homogeneous, translucent appearance; a characteristic gross and microscopic appearance.

hyalino'sis Hyaline *degeneration*, especially that of relatively extensive degree.

hyali'tis Inflammation of the vitreous humour in which the inflammatory changes extend into the avascular vitreous from adjacent structures. See also hyalosis.

hyalo-, hyal- [G. *hyalos*, glass] Combining forms meaning glassy.

hyalo'sis [hyalo- + G. *-osis*, condition] Degenerative changes in the vitreous humour.

hybrido'ma [G. *hybris*, violation, wantonness, + *-oma*, tumour] A tumour of hybrid cells used in the *in vitro* production of specific monoclonal antibodies; produced by fusion of an established tissue culture line of lymphocyte tumour cells and specific antibody-producing cells.

hy'datid [G. *hydatis*, a drop of water, a hyatid] **1.** Hydatid *cyst*. **2.** A vesicular structure resembling an echinococcus cyst.

hydatid'iform Having the form or appearance of a hydatid.

hy'dragogue [hydr- + G. *agogos*, drawing forth] Producing a discharge of watery fluid; denoting a class of cathartics that retain fluids in the intestine and aid in the removal of oedematous fluids.

hydram'nion, hydram'nios [G. *hydor*, water, + amnion] Presence of an excessive amount of amniotic fluid.

hydrarthro'sis [hydr- + G. *arthron*, joint] Effusion of a serous fluid into a joint cavity.

hy'drate An aqueous solvate; a compound crystallizing with one or more molecules of water.

hydra'tion 1. Addition of water, differentiated from hydrolysis, where the union with water is accompanied by a splitting of the original molecule and the water molecule. **2.** Clinically, the taking in of water to correct a deficit, as in dehydration.

hydrae'mia [hydr- + G. *haima*, blood] An increase in blood volume as a result of an increase of plasma, with or without a reduction in the concentration of protein.

hydro-, hydr- [G. *hydōr*, water] Combining forms denoting water or association with water; hydrogen.

hydro'a [hydro + G. *ōon*, egg] Any bullous eruption.

hydrobleph'aron [hydro- + G. *blepharon*, eyelid] Oedematous swelling of the eyelid.

hydrocar'bon A compound containing only hydrogen and carbon.

hy'drocele [hydro- + G. *kēlē*, hernia] A collection of serous fluid in a sacculated cavity; specifically, such a collection in the tunica vaginalis testis.

hydroceph'alus [hydro- + G. *kephalē*, head] **1.** Excessive accumulation of fluid dilating the cerebral ventricles, thinning the brain, and causing a separation of cranial bones. **2.** In infants, an accumulation of fluid in the subarachnoid or subdural space.

hydrochlo'ric acid HCl; the acid of gastric juice.

hydrochlo'ride A compound formed by the addition of a hydrochloric acid molecule to an amine or related substance.

hydrocol'pocele, hydrocol'pos [hydro- + G. *kolpos*, vagina] Accumulation of mucus or other nonsanguineous fluid in the vagina.

hy'drocor'tisone Cortisol; a steroid hormone secreted by the adrenal cortex and the most potent of the naturally occurring glucocorticoids.

hy'drocyan'ic acid Prussic acid; hydrogen cyanide; HCN; a colourless liquid poison with the odour of bitter almonds.

hy'drocyst [hydro- + G. *kystis*, bladder] A cyst with clear, watery contents.

hy'drogen [hydro- + G. *-gen*, producing] A gaseous element, symbol H, atomic no. 1, atomic weight 1.0079.

hydro'gena'tion Addition of hydrogen to a compound, especially to an unsaturated fat or fatty acid; thus soft fats or oils are solidified or "hardened."

hydrol'ysis [hydro- + G. *lysis*, dissolution] A chemical process whereby a compound is cleaved into two or more simpler compounds with the uptake of the H and OH parts of a water molecule on either side of the chemical bond cleaved; effected by the action of acids, alkalies, or enzymes.

hydrom'eter [hydro- + G. *mēron*, measure] An instrument for determining the specific gravity of a liquid.

hydrome'tra [hydro- + G. *mētra*, uterus] Accumulation of thin mucus or other watery fluid in the cavity of the uterus.

hy'dromye'lia [hydro- + G. *myelos*, marrow] An increase of fluid in the dilated central canal of the spinal cord, or in congenital cavities elsewhere in the cord substance.

hy'dronephro'sis [hydro- + G. *nephros*, kidney, + *-osis*, condition] Dilation of the pelvis and calices of one or both kidneys resulting from obstruction to the flow of urine.

hy'dropericardi'tis Pericarditis with a large serous effusion.

hydropericar'dium Noninflammatory accumulation of fluid in the pericardial sac.

hy'droperitone'um [hydro- + peritoneum] Ascites.

hydrophil'ic Denoting the property of attracting or associating with water molecules, possessed by polar radicals or ions, as opposed to hydrophobic.

hydropho'bia [hydro- + G. *phobos*, fear] Rabies in man, so named from exaggerated folklore depictions.

hydropho'bic **1.** Relating to or suffering from hydrophobia. **2.** Repelling water, as opposed to hydrophilic.

hy'dropneu'moperitone'um [hydro- + G. *pneuma*, air, + peritoneum] Presence of gas and serous fluid in the peritoneal cavity.

hy'dropneumotho'rax [hydro- + G. *pneuma*, air, + thorax] Presence of both gas and fluids in the pleural cavity.

hy'drops [G. *hydrōps*] Excessive accumulation of clear, watery fluid in any of the tissues or cavities of the body as in ascites, anasarca, oedema, etc.

   endolymphatic h., Ménière's *disease*.

   fetal h., h. fetalis, abnormal accumulation of serous fluid in the fetal tissues, as in erythroblastosis fetalis.

hydrosal'pinx [hydro- + G. *salpinx*, trumpet] Accumulation of serous fluid in the fallopian tube.

hydrostat'ic Relating to the pressure of fluids or to their properties when in equilibrium.

hydrotax'is [hydro- + G. *taxis*, arrangement] Movement of cells or organisms in relation to water.

hydrotho'rax Presence of serous fluid in one or both pleural cavities, usually not associated with inflammatory reactions.

hy'drotuba'tion Injection of liquid medication or saline solution through the cervix into the uterine cavity and fallopian tubes for dilation and medication of the tubes.

hy'droure'ter Distension of the ureter with urine due to blockage.

hydrox'ide A compound containing a potentially ionizable hydroxyl group; particularly a compound that liberates OH- upon dissolving in water.

hydroxy- Prefix indicating addition or substitution of the —OH group to or in the compound whose name follows.

hydru'ria [hydro- + G. *ouron*, urine] Polyuria.

hy'giene [G. *hygieinos*, healthful, fr. *hygiēs*, healthy] The science of health.

   mental h., the science and practice of maintaining and restoring mental health; an interdisciplinary branch of psychiatry.

   oral h., cleaning of oral structures by means of brushing, flossing, irrigating, massaging, or the use of other devices.

hygien'ic Healthful; relating to hygiene, tending to preserve health.

hygro-, hygr- [G. *hygros*, moist] Combining forms meaning moist, relating to moisture or humidity.

hygro'ma [hygro- + G. *-oma*, tumour] A cystic swelling containing a serous fluid.

hy'men [G. *hymēn*, membrane] [NA] A thin crescentic or annular membranous fold partly occluding the vaginal external orifice of a virgin.

hymenec'tomy [G. *hymēn*, membrane, + *ektomē*, excision] Excision of the hymen.

hymenot'omy [G. *hymēn*, membrane, + *tomē*, incision] Surgical division of a hymen.

hyoglos'sal Relating to the hyoid bone and the tongue.

hy'oid [G. *hyoeidēs*, shaped like the letter upsilon, *υ*] U-shaped or V-shaped.

hy'oscine Scopolamine.

hyoscy'amine An alkaloid found in hyoscyamus, belladonna, duboisia (duboisine), and stramonium; the laevorotatory component of atropine; an antispasmodic, analgesic, and sedative.

hypacu'sis [hypo- + G. *akousis*, hearing] Hearing impairment attributable to deficiency in the peripheral organs of hearing; may be on a conductive or neurosensory basis.

hypaesthe'sia [G. *hypo*, under, + *aisthēsis*, feeling] Diminished sensitivity to stimulation.

hypalge'sia [G. *hypo*, under, + *algēsis*, sense of pain] Decreased sensibility to pain.

hyper- [G. *hyper*, above, over] Prefix denoting excessive or above the normal. See also super-.

hy'peracid'ity An abnormally high degree of acidity.

hy'peractiv'ity General restlessness or excessive movement such as that characterizing children with minimal brain dysfunction or hyperkinesis.

hy'peraou'sis [hyper- + G. *akousis*, a hearing] Abnormal acuteness of hearing due to increased irritability of the sensory neural mechanism.

hyperae'mia [hyper- + G. *haima*, blood] Presence of an increased amount of blood in a part or organ. See also congestion.

hy'peraesthe'sia [hyper- + G. *aisthēsis*, sensation] Abnormal acuteness of sensitivity to sensory stimuli.

hy'peralge'sia [hyper- + G. *algos*, pain] Extreme sensitiveness to painful stimuli.

hy'peralimenta'tion Administration or consumption of nutrients beyond normal requirements.

hyperbar'ic [hyper- + G. *baros*, weight] **1.** Pertaining to pressure of ambient gases greater than 1 atmosphere. **2.** With respect to solutions, more dense than the diluent or medium.

hyperbar'ism [hyper- + G. *baros*, weight, + *ismos*, condition] Disturbances in the body resulting from the pressure of ambient gases at greater than 1 atmosphere.

hy'perbetalip'oproteinae'mia Enhanced concentration of β-lipoproteins in the blood.

hy'perbilirubinae'mia An abnormally large amount of bilirubin in the circulating blood.

hy'percalcae'mia An abnormally high concentration of calcium compounds in the circulating blood; commonly used to indicate an elevated concentration of calcium ions in the blood.

hy′percalciu′ria Excretion of abnormally large amounts of calcium in the urine.

hypercap′nia [hyper- + G. *kapnos*, smoke, vapour] Presence of an abnormally large amount of carbon dioxide in the circulating blood.

hy′perchlorae′mia An abnormally large amount of chloride ions in the circulating blood.

hy′perchlorhy′dria [hyper- + chlorhydric (acid)] The presence of an abnormal amount of hydrochloric acid in the stomach.

hy′percholes′terolae′mia,
  hy′percholesterae′mia Presence of an abnormally large amount of cholesterol in the cells and plasma of the circulating blood.

hyperchy′lia [hyper- + G. *chylos*, juice] Excessive secretion of gastric juice.

hy′percryaesthe′sia [hyper- + G. *kryos*, cold, + *aisthēsis*, sensation] Extreme sensibility to cold.

hyperem′esis [hyper- + G. *emesis*, vomiting] Excessive vomiting.

hy′pererga′sia [hyper- + G. *ergasia*, work] Increased or excessive functional activity.

hy′perexten′sion Extension of a limb or part beyond the normal limit.

hy′perfibrinol′ysis Markedly increased fibrinolysis, as in subdural haematomas.

hy′perflex′ion Flexion of a limb or part beyond the normal limit.

hy′pergalacto′sis [hyper- + G. *gala*, milk, + -*osis*, condition] Excessive secretion of milk.

hy′pergammaglob′ulinae′mia An increased amount of the gamma globulins in the plasma, such as that frequently observed in chronic infectious diseases.

hypergen′esis [hyper- + G. *genesis*, production] Excessive development or redundant production of parts or organs of the body.

hypergen′italism Abnormally overdeveloped genitalia in adults or for the individual's age.

hypergeu′sia [hyper- + G. *geusis*, taste] Abnormal acuteness of the sense of taste.

hy′perglycae′mia [hyper- + G. *glykys*, sweet, + *haima*, blood] Abnormally high concentrations of glucose in the circulating blood, especially with reference to a fasting level.

hypergon′adism Enhanced secretion of gonadal hormones, with precocious sexual development.

hy′perhidro′sis [hyper- + hidrosis] Excessive or profuse sweating.

hyperin′sulinism Excessive secretion of insulin by the islets of Langerhans, resulting in hypoglycaemia; the symptoms are those of insulin shock, though more chronic in character.

hy′perinvolu′tion Superinvolution.

hy′perkalae′mia [hyper- + Mod. L. *kalium*, potash, + G. *haima*, blood] An abnormal concentration of potassium ions in the circulating blood.

hy′perkerato′sis, hyperker′atiniza′tion Hypertrophy of the horny layer of the epidermis.

hy′perkine′sis, hy′perkine′sia [hyper- + G. *kinēsis*, motion] Excessive motor function or activity.

hy′perkinet′ic Pertaining to or characterized by hyperkinesia.

hy′perlipae′mia,
  hy′perlipidae′mia [hyper- + G. *lipos*, fat, + *haima*, blood] Lipaemia.

hy′perlip′oproteinae′mia An increase in the lipoprotein concentration of the blood.

  acquired h., h. that develops as a consequence of some primary disease, such as thyroid deficiency.

  familial h., a group of diseases characterized by changes in concentration of β-lipoproteins and pre-β-lipoproteins and the lipids associated with them.

hy′perlipo′sis [hyper- + G. *lipos*, fat] **1.** Excessive adiposity. **2.** An extreme degree of fatty degeneration.

hy′perlysinae′mia Abnormal increase of lysine in the circulating blood; associated with mental retardation, convulsions, anaemia and asthenia; autosomal recessive inheritance.

hy′perlysinu′ria Abnormally high concentrations of lysine in the urine; a form of aminoaciduria.

hy′permas′tia [hyper- + G. *mastos*, breast] **1.** Polymastia. **2.** Excessively large mammary glands.

hy′permenorrhoe′a [hyper- + G. *mēn*, month, + *rhoia*, flow] Menorrhagia; excessively prolonged or profuse menses.

hy'permetro'pia [hyper- + G. *metron*, measure, + *ōps*, eye] Hyperopia.

hy'pernatrae'mia [hyper- + *natrium* (*q.v.*), + G. *haima*, blood] Abnormally high plasma concentration of sodium ions.

hy'peronyc'hia [hyper- + G. *onyx*, (*onych-*), nail] Hypertrophy of the nails.

hypero'pia (H) [hyper- + G. *ōps*, eye] Farsightedness; the refractive state of the eye in which parallel rays of light would come to focus behind the retina if not intercepted by it.

hypero'pic (H) Pertaining to hyperopia.

hyperos'mia [hypor- + G. *osmō*, sense of smell] An exaggerated or abnormally acute sense of smell.

hy'perosto'sis [hyper- + G. *osteon*, bone, + *-osis*, condition] **1.** Hypertrophy of bone. **2.** Exostosis.

hy'peroxalu'ria An unusually large amount of oxalic acid or oxalates in the urine

hy'perparathy'roidism An increase in the secretion of the parathyroids, causing generalized osteitis fibrosa cystica, elevated serum calcium, decreased serum phosphorus, and increased excretion of both calcium and phosphorus; due to neoplasms or idiopathic hyperplasia of the parathyroid glands (**primary h.**) or as a result of disordered metabolism (**secondary h.**)

hy'perperistal'sis Excessive rapidity of the passage of food through the stomach and intestine.

hy'perphenylal'aninae'mia Abnormally high blood levels of phenylalanine, which may or may not be associated with elevated tyrosine levels, in newborn infants, associated with the heterozygous state of phenylketonuria, maternal phenylketonuria, or transient deficiency of phenylalanine hydroxylase or p-hydroxyphenylpyruvic acid oxidase.

hy'perphosphatae'mia Abnormally high concentration of phosphates in the circulating blood.

hy'perphosphata'sia Elevated alkaline phosphatase, with dwarfism, macrocranium, blue sclerae, and expansion of the diaphyses of tubular bones with multiple fractures; autosomal recessive inheritance.

hy'perpigmenta'tion Excess pigment in a tissue or part.

hy'perpitu'itarism Excessive production of anterior pituitary hormones, especially somatotropin; may result in gigantism or acromegaly.

hyperpla'sia [hyper- + G. *plasis*, a moulding] An increase in number of cells in a tissue or organ, excluding tumour formation, whereby the bulk of the part or organ is increased.

hyperplas'tic Relating to hyperplasia.

hy'perploidy [hyper- + -ploid] The state of possessing one or more chromosomes in addition to the normal number.

hyperpnoe'a [hyper- + G. *pnoē*, breathing] Respiration that is deeper and more rapid than normal.

hyperprax'ia [hyper- + G. *praxis*, action] Excessive activity; restlessness.

hy'perprolac'tinae'mia An elevated level of prolactin in the blood, a normal physiological reaction during lactation, but pathological otherwise.

hy'perprolinae'mia A metabolic disorder characterized by enhanced plasma proline concentrations and urinary excretion of proline, hydroxyproline, and glycine; autosomal recessive inheritance.

hy'perpyrex'ia [hyper- + G. *pyrexis*, feverishness] Extremely high fever.

hy'perreflex'ia A condition in which the deep tendon reflexes are exaggerated.

hypersen'sitiveness,

hy'persensitiv'ity 1. Abnormal sensitiveness or sensitivity; a condition in which the response to a stimulus is excessive in degree. **2.** Allergy. "Hypersensitiveness" was introduced into immunologic terminology because of the original misconception that repeated inoculations of toxin-containing preparations produced an increase in the already existing sensitivity to the toxin.

hypersom'nia [hyper- + L. *somnus*, sleep] A condition in which one sleeps for an excessively long time, but is normal in the intervals; distinguished from somnolence, in which one is always inclined to sleep.

hypersple'nism A condition, or group of conditions, in which the haemolytic action of the spleen is greatly increased.

hypertel'orism [hyper- + G. *tele*, far off, + *horizō*, to separate] Abnormal distance between two paired organs.

ocular h., extreme width between the eyes due to an enlarged sphenoid bone; other congenital deformities and mental retardation may be associated.

hyperten'sive Characterized by or suffering from abnormally increased blood pressure.

hyperten'sion [hyper- + L. *tensio*, tension] Persistent high blood pressure.

essential h., h. without preexisting renal disease or known cause.

malignant h., severe h. that runs a rapid course, causing necrosis of arteriolar walls, haemorrhagic lesions, and a poor prognosis.

portal h., h. in the portal system as seen in cirrhosis of the liver and other conditions causing obstruction to the portal vein.

pulmonary h., h. in the pulmonary circulation; may be primary or secondary to pulmonary or cardiac disease.

hy'perther'mia [hyper- + G. *therme̅*, heat] Therapeutically induced hyperpyrexia.

malignant h., rapid onset of extremely high fever with muscle rigidity, precipitated in genetically susceptible persons, especially by halothane or succinylcholine.

hy'perthrombinae'mia An abnormal increase of thrombin in the blood, frequently resulting in a tendency to intravascular coagulation.

hyperthy'mism Excessive activity of the thymus gland, formerly postulated to be a causal factor in certain instances of unexpected and sudden death.

hyperthy'roidism An abnormality of the thyroid gland in which its secretion is usually increased and is no longer under regulatory control of hypothalamic-pituitary centres.

hyperto'nia [hyper- + G. *tonos*, tension] Extreme tension of the muscles or arteries.

hyperton'ic 1. Spastic; having a greater degree of tension. 2. Having a greater osmotic pressure than a reference solution.

hy'pertricho'sis [hyper- + G. *trichōsis*, a being hairy] Growth of hair in excess of the normal.

hy'pertriglyc'eridae'mia An elevated triglyceride concentration in blood.

hy'pertrophy [hyper- + G. *trophe̅*, nourishment] General increase in bulk of a part or organ, not due to tumour formation; may be restricted to denote greater bulk through increase in size, but not in number, of the individual tissue elements. See also hyperplasia.

hy'peruricae'mia Enhanced blood concentrations of uric acid.

hy'perventila'tion Increased alveolar ventilation relative to metabolic carbon dioxide production, so that alveolar carbon dioxide pressure tends to fall below normal.

hy'pervitamino'sis A condition resulting from the ingestion of an excessive amount of a vitamin preparation, the symptoms varying according to the particular vitamin implicated.

hy'pervolae'mia [hyper- + L. *volumen*, volume, + G. *haima*, blood] Abnormally increased volume of blood.

hy'pha, pl. **hy'phae** [G. *hyphe̅*, a web] A branching tubular cell characteristic of the growth of filamentous fungi; intercommunicating hyphae constitute a mycelium, the visible colony.

hyphae'ma Haemorrhage into the anterior chamber of the eye.

hypnago'gic [hypno- + G. *ago̅gos*, leading] Denoting a transitional state preceding the oncome of sleep; applied also to various hallucinations that may manifest themselves at that time.

hypno-, hypn- [G. *hypnos*, sleep] Combining forms relating to sleep or hypnosis.

hyp'nolepsy [hypno- + G. *le̅psis*, a seizing] Narcolepsy.

hypno'sis [G. *hypnos*, sleep, + *-osis*, condition] An artificially induced trancelike state resembling somnambulism in which the subject is highly susceptible to suggestion, oblivious to all else, and responds readily to the commands of the hypnotist.

hypnother'apy 1. Treatment of disease by inducing prolonged sleep. 2. Psychotherapeutic treatment by means of hypnotism.

hypnot'ic [G. *hypno̅tikos*, causing one to sleep] 1. Causing sleep. 2. Relating to hypnotism.

hyp'notism [G. *hypnos*, sleep] 1. The process or act of inducing hypnosis. 2. The practice or study of hypnosis.

hypo- [G. *hypo*, under] Prefix denoting a location beneath something else; a diminution or deficiency; the lowest, or least rich in oxygen, of a series of chemical compounds. See also sub-.

hy'poacid'ity A lower than normal degree of acidity.

hy'poaesthe'sia Hypaesthesia.

hy'poalge'sia Hypalgesia.

hypobar'ic [hypo- + G. *baros*, weight] 1. Pertaining to pressure of ambient gases below 1 atmosphere. **2.** With respect to solutions, less dense than the diluent or medium.

hy'pocalcae'mia Abnormally low levels of calcium in the circulating blood; commonly denotes subnormal concentrations of calcium ions.

hy'pocalcifica'tion Deficient calcification of bone or teeth.

hypocap'nia [hypo- + G. *kapnos*, smoke] Abnormally low tension of carbon dioxide in the circulating blood.

hy'pochlorae'mia An abnormally low level of chloride ions in the circulating blood.

hy'pochlorhy'dria An abnormally small amount of hydrochloric acid in the stomach.

hy'pocholes'terolae'mia Abnormally small amounts of cholesterol in the circulating blood.

hypochon'dria 1. Hypochondriasis. **2.** Plural of hypochondrium.

hypochon'driac 1. Hypochondriacal. **2.** A victim of hypochondriasis. **3.** Beneath the ribs; relating to the hypochondrium.

hypochondri'acal Relating to or suffering from hypochondriasis.

hypochondri'asis [hypochondrium, the site of hypochondria, + -*iasis*, condition] Morbid concern about one's own health and exaggerated attention to any unusual bodily or mental sensations; a false belief that one is suffering from some disease.

hypochon'drium, pl. **hypochon'dria** [L. fr. G. *hypochondrion*, abdomen, belly, from *hypo*, under, + *chondros*, cartilage (of ribs)] The area on each side of the abdomen covered by the costal cartilages, lateral to the epigastrium.

hypochro'mia [hypo- + G. *chrōma*, colour] An anaemic condition in which the percentage of haemoglobin in the red blood cells is less than the normal range.

hy'pocythae'mia [hypo- + G. *kytos*, cell, + *haima*, blood] Abnormally low numbers of red and white cells and other formed elements of the circulating blood, as in aplastic anaemia.

Hypoder'ma [hypo- + G. *derma*, skin] A genus of botflies whose larvae are the cause of cutaneous larva migrans of man.

hypoder'mic 1. Subcutaneous. **2.** Hypodermic *injection*. **3.** Hypodermic *syringe*.

hy'pofibrin'ogenae'mia Abnormally low concentration of fibrinogen in the circulating blood plasma.

hy'pogalac'tia [hypo- + G. *gala*, milk] Less than normal milk secretion.

hy'pogammaglob'ulinae'mia Decreased quantity of the gamma fraction of serum globulin; sometimes used loosely to denote a decreased quantity of immunoglobulins.

hypogas'tric Relating to the hypogastrium.

hypogas'trium [G. *hypogastrion*, lower belly, fr. *hypo*, under, + *gaster*, belly] [NA] Pubic region; the lower central area of the abdomen below the umbilicus.

hypogen'italism Partial or complete failure of maturation of the genitalia; commonly, a consequence of hypogonadism.

hypoglos'sal [L. *hypoglossus* fr. hypo- + *glossus*, tongue] Subglossal.

hypoglot'tis [G. *hypoglōsis*, or -*glōttis*, undersurface of tongue] The undersurface of the tongue.

hy'poglycae'mia An abnormally small concentration of glucose in the circulating blood, *i.e.*, less than the minimum of the normal range.

hypognath'ous [hypo- + G. *gnathos*, jaw] Having a congenitally defectively developed lower jaw

hypogo'nadism Inadequate gonadal function, as manifested by deficiencies in gametogenesis and/or the secretion of gonadal hormones.

hy'pohidro'sis Diminished perspiration.

hy'pokaiae'mia [hypo- + Mod. L. *kalium*, potassium, + G. *haima*, blood] An abnormally small concentration of potassium ions in the circulating blood.

hy'pokine'sis, hy'pokine'sia [hypo- + G. *kinēsis*, movement] Diminished or slow movement.

hy'pokinet'ic Relating to or characterized by hypokinesis.

hypomas'tia [hypo- + G. *mastos*, breast] Atrophy or congenital smallness of the breasts.

hy'pomenorrhoe'a [hypo- + G. *mēn*, month, + *rhoia*, flow] A diminution of the flow or a shortening of the duration of menstruation.

hy'pometab'olism Reduced metabolism; low metabolic rate.

hy'pome'tria [hypo- + G. *metron*, measure] A manifestation of ataxia characterized by underreaching an object or goal.

hy'ponatrae'mia [hypo- + L. *natrium*, sodium, + G. *haima*, blood] Abnormally low concentrations of sodium ions in the circulating blood.

hypopan'creatism A condition of diminished activity of the pancreas.

hy'poparathy'roidism A condition due to diminution or absence of the secretion of the parathyroid hormones.

hy'pophosphatae'mia Abnormally low concentrations of phosphates in the circulating blood.

hy'pophysec'tomy Excision or destruction of the pituitary gland.

hypophys'eal, hypophys'ial Relating to a hypophysis.

hypoph'ysis [G. an undergrowth] [NA] Pituitary gland; an unpaired compound gland suspended from the base of the hypothalamus by a short cordlike extension of the infundibulum; consists of two major subdivisions: 1) a posterior lobe that appears as the bulbous end of the stalk and stores and releases the hormone vasopressin and oxytocin, 2) the larger anterior lobe that, in response to releasing factors, releases into systemic circulation any one (or combination) of a variety of tropic hormones, each of which activates the corresponding endocrine gland and triggers the release of its hormone.

hy'popie'sis [hypo- + G. *piesis*, pressure] Hypotension (1).

hy'popitu'itarism A condition due to diminished activity of the anterior lobe of the hypophysis, with inadequate secretion of one or more anterior pituitary hormones.

hypopla'sia [hypo- + G. *plasis*, a moulding] **1.** Underdevelopment of tissue or an organ, usually due to a decrease in the number of cells. **2.** Atrophy due to destruction of some of the elements and not merely to their general reduction in size.

hypoplas'tic Pertaining to or characterized by hypoplasia.

hypopnoe'a [hypo- + G. *pnoē*, breathing] Respiration that is shallower, slower, or both, than normal.

hy'poprax'ia [hypo- + G. *praxis*, action, + -*ia*, condition] Deficient activity.

hy'poproteinae'mia Abnormally small amounts of total protein in the circulating blood plasma.

hy'poprothrom'binae'mia Abnormally small amounts of prothrombin in the circulating blood.

hypopty'alism [hypo- + G. *ptyalon*, saliva] Hyposalivation.

hy'poreflex'ia Diminished or weakened reflexes.

hy'posaliva'tion Reduced salivation.

hyposcle'ral Beneath the sclerotic coat of the eyeball.

hy'posecre'tion Diminished secretion, as by a gland.

hyposen'sitiveness, hy'posensitiv'ity Subnormal sensitiveness or sensitivity in which the response to a stimulus is unusually delayed or lessened in degree.

hypos'mia [hypo- + G. *osmē*, smell] Diminished sense of smell.

hypospa'dias [G. one having the orifice of the penis too low] A developmental anomaly characterized by a defect in the wall of the urethra so that a part of the canal is open on the undersurface of the penis; also a similar defect in the female in which the urethra opens into the vagina.

hypos'tasis [G. *hypo-stasis*, a standing under, sediment]. **1.** Formation of a sediment at the bottom of a liquid. **2.** Hypostatic *congestion*.

hypostat'ic **1.** Sedimentary; resulting from a dependent position. **2.** Relating to hypostasis.

hyposthe'nia [hypo- + G. *sthenos*, strength] Weakness.

hy'potel'orism [hypo- + G. *tēle*, far off, + *horizō*, to separate] Abnormal closeness of the eyes.

hypoten'sion [hypo- + L. *tensio*, a stretching] **1.** Subnormal arterial blood pressure. **2.** Reduced pressure or tension of any kind.

   orthostatic h., postural h., a form of low blood pressure that occurs when standing.

hypoten'sive Characterized by low blood pressure or causing a reduction in blood pressure.

hypothal'amus [hypo- + thalamus] [NA] The ventral and medial region of the diencephalon forming the walls of the ventral half of the third ventricle; its ventral surface is marked by, from before backward, the optic chiasma, the unpaired infundibulum, and the

paired mamillary bodies; prominently involved in the functions of the autonomic nervous system and, through its vascular link
with the anterior lobe of the hypophysis, in
endocrine mechanisms; also appears to play
a role in the nervous mechanisms underlying
moods and motivational states.

hypothe'nar [hypo- + G. *thenar*, the
palm] **1.** [NA] the fleshy mass at the medial
side of the palm. **2.** Denoting any structure in
relation with this part.

hypother'mia [hypo- + G. *therme*, heat]
A body temperature significantly below 98.6°F
(37°C).

  regional h., perfusion with cold blood or
local refrigeration to cool an organ being subjected to ischaemia in order to reduce its
metabolic requirements.

  total body h., deliberate reduction of
total body temperature to reduce the general
metabolism of the tissues.

hypoth'esis [L. fr. G. *hypotithenai*, to pro-
pose or suppose] A supposition or assumption advanced as a basis for reasoning or argument, or as a guide to experimental
investigation; a tentative theory unsupported
by the essential facts that would prove its
truth.

hy'pothrombinae'mia Abnormally
small amounts of thrombin in the circulating
blood, thereby resulting in bleeding tendency.

hypothy'mia [hypo- + G. *thymos*, mind,
soul] Depression of spirits; the "blues."

hypothy'roidism [hypo- + G. *thyreo-
eides*, thyroid] Diminished production of thyroid hormone, leading to thyroid insufficiency.

hypoto'nia [hypo- + G. *tonos*, tone] **1.**
Reduced tension in any part, as in the eyeball.
2. Relaxation of the arteries. **3.** A condition in
which there is diminution or loss of muscular
tonicity, in consequence of which the muscles
may be stretched beyond their normal limits.

hypoton'ic 1. Having a lesser degree of
tension. **2.** Having a lesser osmotic pressure
than a reference solution, ordinarily assumed
to be blood plasma or interstitial fluid.

hy'potricho'sis [hypo- + G. *trichosis*,
hairiness] A less than normal amount of hair
on the head and/or body.

hypotro'pia [hypo- + G. *trope*, turn]
Downward deviation of the visual axis of one
eye.

hy'poventila'tion Reduced alveolar
ventilation relative to metabolic carbon dioxide production, so that alveolar carbon dioxide pressure tends to rise above normal.

hy'povitamino'sis Insufficiency of one
or more essential vitamins.

hy'povolae'mia [hypo- + L. *volumen*,
volume, + G. *haima*, blood] Oligaemia.

hypoxae'mia [hypo- + oxygen, + G.
haima, blood] Subnormal oxygenation of arterial blood, short of anoxia.

hypox'ia Subnormal levels of oxygen in air,
blood, or tissue, short of anoxia.

hyster- See hystero-.

hysteral'gia [hystero- + G. *algos*, pain]
Pain in the uterus.

hys'teratre'sia Atresia of the uterine
cavity, usually resulting from inflammatory
endocervical adhesions.

hysterec'tomy [hystero- + G. *ektome*,
excision] Surgical removal of the uterus.

  abdominal h., removal of the uterus
through an incision in the abdominal wall.

  caesarean h., caesarean section followed by h.

  radical h., complete removal of the
uterus, upper vagina, and parametrium.

  supracervical h., subtotal h., removal of the fundus of the uterus, leaving the
cervix *in situ*.

  vaginal h., removal of the uterus
through the vagina without incising the wall of
the abdomen.

hystereu'rysis [hystero- + G. *eurynein*,
to dilate] Dilation of the lower segment and
cervical canal of the uterus.

hyste'ria [G *hystera*, womb, because formerly thought to be of uterine causation] A
diagnostic term, referable to a wide variety of
psychogenic symptoms involving disorder of
function which may be mental, sensory, motor, or visceral.

  conversion h., h. characterized by the
substitution through psychic transformation
of physical signs or symptoms for anxiety;
generally restricted to such major symptoms
as psychic blindness, deafness, or paralysis.

hyster'ical Relating to or suffering from
hysteria.

hystero-, hyster- 1. [G. *hystera*, womb
(uterus)] Combining forms denoting the
uterus (see also metra-, metro-, utero-) or
hysteria. **2.** [G. *hysteros*, later] Combining
forms meaning late or following.

hys'terocele [hystero- + G. *kēlē*, hernia]
1. An abdominal or perineal hernia containing part or all of the uterus. **2.** Protrusion of uterine contents into a weakened, bulging area of uterine wall.

hys'terodyn'ia [hystero- + G. *odynē*, pain] Hysteralgia.

hys'terogram **1.** A radiograph of the uterus, usually using contrast media. **2.** A record of the strength of uterine contractions.

hysterog'raphy [hystero- + G. *graphō*, to write] **1.** Radiography of a uterine cavity filled with contrast medium. **2.** The procedure of recording uterine contractions.

hy'stero-o'ophorec'tomy [hystero- + G. *ōon*, egg, + *phoros*, bearing, + *ektomē*, excision] Surgical removal of the uterus and ovaries.

hysterop'athy [hystero- + G. *pathos*, suffering] Any disease of the uterus.

hys'teropexy [hystero- + G. *pēxis*, fixation] Surgical fixation of a misplaced or abnormally movable uterus.

hys'teroplasty Uteroplasty.

hysteror'rhaphy [hystero- + G. *raphē*, suture] Sutural repair of a lacerated uterus.

hys'terorrhex'is [hystero- + G. *rhēxis*, rupture] Rupture of the uterus.

hys'terosal'pingec'tomy [hystero- + G. *salpinx*, a trumpet, + *ektomē*, excision] Surgical removal of the uterus and one or both uterine tubes.

hys'terosal'pingog'raphy [hystero- + G. *salpinx*, a trumpet, + *graphō*, to write] Radiography of the uterus and oviducts after the injection of radiopaque material.

hys'terosal'pingo-o'ophorec'tomy [hystero- + G. *salpinx*, trumpet, + *ōon*, egg, + *phoros*, bearing, + *ektomē*, excision] Excision of the uterus, oviducts, and ovaries.

hys'terosal'pingos'tomy [hystero- + G. *salpinx*, trumpet, + *stoma*, mouth] An operation to restore patency of a tube.

hys'terospasm Spasm of the uterus.

hysterot'omy [hystero- + G. *tomē*, incision] Incision of the uterus.

hys'terotrachelec'tomy [hystero- + G. *trachēlos*, neck, + *ektomē*, excision] Surgical removal of the cervix uteri.

hys'terotrachelor'rhaphy [hystero- + G. *trachēlos*, neck, + *rhaphē*, a seam] Sutural repair of a lacerated cervix uteri.

I

-ia [G. *-ia*, denoting action or an abstract] Suffix denoting a condition. *Cf.* -ism.

-iasis [G. verb-nominalizing suffix] Suffix denoting a condition or state, particularly morbid. See also -osis.

iatro- [G. *iatros*, physician] Combining form denoting relation to physicians, medicine, treatment.

iatrogen'ic [iatro- + G. *-gen*, producing] Denoting an unfavourable response to therapy, induced by the therapeutic effort itself; formerly used to imply autosuggestion resulting from the physician's discussion, examination, or suggestions.

ibupro'fen *dl-p*-Isobutylhydratropic acid; an anti-inflammatory agent.

ichthyo- [G. *ichthys*, fish] Combining form relating to fish.

ich'thyoid [ichthyo- + G. *eidos*, resemblance] Fish-shaped.

ichthyo'sis [ichthyo- + *-osis*, condition] A congenital disorder of keratinization characterized by dryness and fishskin-like scaling of the skin.

icter'ic [G. *ikterikos*, jaundiced] Relating to or marked by icterus (jaundice).

ictero- [G. *ikteros*, icterus, jaundice] Combining form relating to icterus.

ic'terogen'ic [ictero- + *-gen*, producing] Causing jaundice.

ic'terohepati'tis [ictero- + G. *hēpar*, liver, + *-itis*, inflammation] Inflammation of the liver with jaundice as a prominent symptom.

ic'teroid [ictero- + G. *eidos*, resemblance] Yellow-hued, or seemingly jaundiced.

ic'terus [G. *ikteros*] Jaundice.
  i. neonato'rum, jaundice of the newborn; either a mild temporary physiologic jaundice, or a severe and usually fatal form due to congenital occlusion of the common bile duct, erythroblastosis fetalis, congenital syphilitic cirrhosis of the liver, or septic pylephlebitis.

id [L. *id*, that] **1.** In psychoanalysis, a part of the "psychic or mental apparatus," that is completely in the unconscious realm, unorganized, the reservoir of psychic energy or libido, and under the influence of the primary processes. **2.** A single term for the total of all psychic energy available from the innate drives and impulses in a newborn infant. Through socialization this diffuse, undirected energy becomes channeled in less egocentric and more socially responsive directions (development of the ego from the id).

-id **1.** [G. -*eidēs*, resembling, through Fr. -*id*] Suffix indicating a state of sensitivity of the skin in which a part remote from the primary lesion reacts ("-id reaction") to substances of the pathogen, giving rise to a secondary inflammatory lesion; the lesion manifesting the reaction is designated by the use of -id as a suffix. **2.** [G. *idion*, a diminutive onding] Suffix indicating a small or young specimen.

-ide **1.** Suffix denoting a binary chemical compound; formerly denoted by the qualification, -ureted. **2.** Suffix to a sugar name indicating substitution for the H of the hemiacetal OH.

idea' [G. semblance] Any mental image or concept.

   autochthonous i.'s, thoughts that suddenly burst into awareness as if they are terribly important, often as if they have come from an outside source.

   compulsive i., a fixed and inappropriate i.

   dominant i., an i. that governs all the actions and thoughts of the individual.

   fixed i., an obsession; an exaggerated notion, belief, or delusion that persists, despite evidence to the contrary, and controls the mind.

   i. of reference, the misinterpretation that other people's statements or acts pertain to one's self when, in fact, they do not.

ideal'. A standard of perfection.

   ego i., the part of the personality that comprises the goals and aims of the self, usually refers to the emulation of significant persons with whom it has identified.

idea'tion The formation of ideas.

idea'tional Relating to ideation.

idée fixe [Fr. obsession] Fixed *idea.*

iden'tifica'tion [Mediev. L. *identicus*, fr. L. *idem*, the same, + *facio*, to make] **1.** In the behavioural sciences, an imitation, sense of oneness, or psychic continuity with another person or group. **2.** In psychoanalysis, an unconscious defence mechanism in which a person incorporates into himself the mental picture of another person and then patterns himself after this person, and thus sees himself as like that person.

ideo- [G. *idea*, form, notion] Combining form pertaining to ideas or ideation. *Cf.* idio-.

idio- [G. *idios*, one's own] Combining form meaning private, distinctive, peculiar to. *Cf.* ideo-.

id'iocy [G. *idiōteria*, awkwardness, uncouthness] Obsolete term for a subclass of mental *retardation.*

id'iopath'ic [idio- + G. *pathos*, suffering] **1.** Denoting a disease of unknown cause. **2.** Denoting a primary disease.

il'eac Relating to ileus or to the ileum.

il'eal Of or pertaining to the ileum.

ilei'tis Inflammation of the ileum.

   distal, regional, or **terminal i.,** regional *enteritis.*

ileo- [L. *ileum*] Combining form denoting relationship to the ileum.

ileocae'cal Relating to both ileum and caecum.

il'eocaecos'tomy Anastomosis of ileum to caecum.

il'eocoli'tis Inflammation of the mucous membrane of a greater or lesser extent of both ileum and colon.

il'eocolos'tomy [ileo- + colostomy] Surgical establishment of a new communication between the ileum and the colon.

ileocys'toplasty [ileo- + G. *kystis*, bladder, + *plastos*, moulded] Surgical reconstruction of the bladder involving the use of an isolated intestinal segment to augment bladder capacity.

il'eoileos'tomy [ileum + ileum + G. *stoma*, mouth] Surgical establishment of a communication between two segments of the ileum.

il'eopexy [ileo- + G. *pexis*, fixation] Surgical fixation of the ileum.

il'eoproctos'tomy [ileo- + G. *prōktos*, anus (rectum), + *stoma*, mouth] Surgical establishment of a communication between the ileum and the rectum.

il'eosigmoidos'tomy [ileo- + sigmoid, + G. *stoma*, mouth] Surgical establishment of a communication between the ileum and the sigmoid colon.

ileos'tomy [ileo- + G. *stoma*, mouth] Surgical establishment of a fistula through which the ileum discharges directly to the outside of the body.

ileot'omy [ileo- + G. *tomē*, incision] Incision into the ileum.

il'eum [L. fr. G. *eileō*, to roll up, twist] [NA] The third portion of the small intestine, extending from the junction with the jejunum to the ileocaecal opening.

il'eus [G. *eileos*, intestinal colic, from *eilō*, to roll up tight] Obstruction of the bowel attended with severe colicky pain, vomiting, and often fever and dehydration.

il'iac Relating to the ilium.

ilio- [L. *ilium*, *q.v.*] Combining form denoting relationship to the ilium.

il'iococcyg'eal Relating to the ilium and the coccyx.

ilioin'guinal Relating to the iliac region and the groin.

iliolum'bar Relating to the iliac and the lumbar regions.

il'ium, pl. **il'ia** [L. groin, flank] *Os* ilium.

ill'ness Disease (1).

   mental i., a broadly inclusive term, generally denoting one or all of the following: **1)** a disease of the brain, with predominant behavioural symptoms, as in paresis or acute alcoholism; **2)** a disease of the "mind" or personality, evidenced by abnormal behaviour; **3)** a disorder of conduct, evidenced by socially deviant behaviour.

illu'sion [L. *illusio*, to play at, mock] A false perception; the mistaking of something for what it is not.

illu'sional Relating to or of the nature of an illusion.

im'age [L. *imago*, likeness] The representation or picture of an object made by the rays of light emanating or reflected from it.

   body i., (1) the cerebral representation of all body sensation organized in the parietal cortex; **(2)** one's i. or concept of his own body, in contrast to his actual, anatomic body or to others' concept of it.

   mental i., a picture of an object not present, produced in the mind by memory or imagination.

immer'sion [L. *im-mergo*, pp. *-mersus*, to dip in] **1.** The placing of a body under water or other liquid. **2.** In microscopy, the use of a fluid medium (placed on the slide being examined) in order to exclude air from between the glass slide and the bottom lens of an immersion objective.

immis'cible [L. *im-misceo*, to mix in (*in* + *misceo*)] Incapable of mutual solution; *e.g.*, oil and water.

immo'bilize [L. *in-* neg. + *mobilis*, movable] To render fixed or incapable of moving.

immune' [L. *immunis*, free from service] **1.** Free from the possibility of acquiring a given infectious disease; resistant to an infectious disease. **2.** Pertaining to the mechanism of sensitization in which the reactivity is so altered by previous contact with an antigen that the responsive tissues respond quickly upon subsequent contact.

immu'nity [L. *immunitas* (see immune)] Insusceptibility; the status or quality of being immune (1).

   acquired i., resistance resulting from previous exposure of the individual in question to an infectious agent or antigen; it may be 1) *active* and *specific*, as a result of naturally acquired infection or intentional vaccination (*artificial active i.*) or 2) *passive*, being acquired from transfer of antibodies from another person or from an animal, either naturally, as from mother to fetus, or by intentional inoculation (*artificial passive i.*), and, with respect to the particular antibodies transferred, it is *specific*.

   cellular i., cell-mediated i. (CMI), i. associated with cellular elements (including T-lymphocytes).

   humoral i., i. associated with circulating antibodies.

   innate i., inherent i., natural i., resistance manifested by a species (or by races, families, and individuals in a species) that has not been immunized by previous infection or vaccination; nonspecific and is not stimulated by specific antigens.

im'muniza'tion The process or procedure by which an organism is rendered immune.

immuno- [L. *immunis*, immune] Combining form meaning immune, or relating to immunity.

im'munoas'say Detection and assay of hormones, or other substances, by serological (immunological) methods; in most applications the hormone (or other substance) in question serves as antigen, both in antibody production and in measurement of antibody by the test substance.

im'munocom'petence Normal capabilities of the immune system.

im'munocom'promised Denoting one whose immunologic mechanism is deficient either because of an immunodeficiency disorder or by immunosuppressive agents.

im'munodefic'iency Immune deficiency; a condition resulting from a defective immunological mechanism; may be *primary* (due to a defect in the immune mechanism *per se*) or *secondary* (dependent upon another disease process), *specific* (due to defect in either the B-lymphocyte or the T-lymphocyte system, or both) or *nonspecific* (due to defect in one or another component of the nonspecific immune mechanism).

im'munoglob'ulin (Ig) One of a class of structurally related proteins consisting of two pairs of polypeptide chains, one pair of light (L) [low molecular weight] chains (κ or λ) and one pair of heavy (H) chains (γ, α, or μ, and more recently, δ and ε), all four linked together by disulphide bonds. On the basis of the structural and antigenic properties of the H chains, Ig's are classified (in order of relative amounts present in normal human serum) as IgG (7S in size, 80%), IgA (10 to 15%), IgM (19S, a pentamer of the basic unit, 5 to 10%), IgD (less than 0.1%), and IgE (less than 0.01%). All of these classes are homogeneous and susceptible to amino acid sequence analysis. The large number of possible combinations of L and H chains make up the "libraries" of antibodies of each individual.

immunol'ogy [immuno- + G. *logos*, study] The science concerned with the various phenomena of immunity, induced sensitivity, and allergy.

im'munosuppres'sant Denoting an agent that effects immunosuppression.

im'munosuppres'sion Suppression of immunologic response, usually with reference to grafts or organ transplants, by use of chemical, pharmacologic, physical, or immunologic agents.

im'munotransfu'sion An indirect transfusion in which the donor is first immunized by means of injections of an antigen prepared from microorganisms isolated from the recipient; later, the donor's blood is administered to the patient who is then presumably passively immunized by means of antibody formed in the donor.

impac'ted [L. *impingo*, pp. -*pactus*, to strike at] Pressed closely together so as to be immovable; wedged and incapable of spontaneous advance or recession.

impair'ment Weakening, damage, or deterioration; *e.g.*, as a result of injury or disease.

impal'pable [L. *im*-; neg. + *palpabilis*, that can be felt] Not capable of being felt.

impa'tent Not patent; closed.

imper'forate Atretic.

imperfora'tion [L. *im*- neg. + *per-foro*, pp. -*auts*, to bore through] The condition of being atretic, occluded, or closed.

imper'meable [L. *im-permeabilis*, not to be passed through] Not permitting passage.

impeti'go [L. a scabby eruption, fr. *im-peto* (*inp*-), to rush upon, attack] A contagious superficial pyoderma, caused by staphylococci and streptococci, that begins with a superficial flaccid vesicle which ruptures and forms a thick yellowish crust.

implant [L. *im*-, in, + *planto*, pp. -*atus*, to plant, fr. *planta*, a sprout, shoot] **1.** (im-plant') To graft or insert. **2.** (im'plant) Material inserted or grafted into tissues.

implanta'tion 1. Attachment of the fertilized ovum (blastocyst) to the endometrium, and its subsequent embedding in the compact layer, occurring six or seven days after fertilization of the ovum. **2.** Grafting or inserting of material into tissues.

im'potence, im'potency [L. *impotentia*, inability] **1.** Weakness; lack of power. **2.** In the male, inability to achieve or maintain penile erection.

impreg'nate [L. *im*, in, + *praegnans*, with child] **1.** To fecundate; to cause to conceive. **2.** To diffuse or permeate with another substance.

impres'sion [L. *impressio*, to press upon] **1.** An indentation or depression made by the pressure of one organ on the surface of another. **2.** An effect produced upon the mind by some external object acting through the organs of sense. **3.** The negative form of the teeth and/or other tissues of the oral cavity made in a plastic material to reproduce a positive form or cast of the recorded tissues.

im'pulse [L. *im-pello*, pp. -*pulsus*, to push against, impel] **1.** A sudden pushing or driving force. **2.** A sudden, often unreasoning, determination to perform some act. **3.** The action potential of a nerve fibre.

impul'sive Relating to or actuated by an impulse, rather than controlled by reason.

in- [L.] **1.** Prefix conveying a sense of negation. **2.** Prefix denoting in, within, inside. **3.**

Prefix denoting an intensive action, appearing as im- before b, p, or m.

inac'tivate To destroy the activity or the effects of an agent or substance.

inani'tion [L. *inanis*, empty] Exhaustion from lack of food or defect in assimilation.

inap'petence [L. *in-* neg. + *ap-peto*, pp. *-petitus*, to strive after, long for] Lack of desire or of craving.

inassim'ilable Not assimilable; not capable of being appropriated for the nutrition of the body.

in'born Innate; inherited; implanted during development *in utero*.

incar'cerated [L. *in*, in, + *carcero*, pp. *-atus*, to imprison] Confined; imprisoned; trapped.

in'cest [L. *incestus*, unchaste, fr. *in-*, not, + *castus*, chaste] **1.** Sexual relations between persons so closely related by blood that such relations between them are prohibited by law or culture.

inces'tuous Pertaining to incest.

in'cidence [L. *incido*, to fall into or upon, to happen] The number of new cases of a disease in a population over a period of time.

inci'sal [L. *incido*, pp. *-cisus*, to cut into] Cutting; relating to the cutting edges of the incisor and cuspid teeth.

inci'sion [L. *incisio*] A cut; a surgical wound; a division of the soft parts made with a knife.

inci'sor [L. *incido*, to cut into] One of the cutting teeth, or i. teeth, four in number in each jaw at the apex of the dental arch.

inci'sure [L. *incisura*] Notch; an indentation at the edge of any structure.

inclina'tion [L. *inclinatio*, a leaning] **1.** A leaning or sloping, as of the pelvis, the angle which the plane of the pelvic inlet makes with the horizontal plane. **2.** In dentistry, the deviation of the long axis of a tooth from the perpendicular.

inclu'sion [L. *inclusio*, a shutting in] **1.** Any foreign or heterogenous substance contained in a cell or in any tissue or organ, not introduced as a result of trauma. **2.** The process by which a foreign or heterogenous structure is misplaced in another tissue.

incompa'tible [L. *in-* neg. + *con-*, with, + *patior*, pp. *passus*, to suffer] **1.** Not of suitable composition to be combined or mixed with another agent or substance, without resulting in an undesirable reaction (including

chemical alteration or destruction). **2.** Denoting persons who can not freely associate together without resulting anxiety and conflict.

incom'petence, incom'petency [L. *in-*, neg. + *com-peto*, strive after together] **1.** The quality of being incompetent or incapable of performing the allotted function. **2.** In psychiatry, the mental inability to distinguish right from wrong or to manage one's affairs.

incon'stant **1.** Variable; irregular. **2.** In anatomy, denoting a structure that normally may or may not be present.

incon'tinence [L. *in-continentia*, fr. *in-* neg. + *con-tineo*, to hold together] **1.** Inability to prevent the discharge of excretions, especially of urine or faeces. **2.** Lack of restraint; immoderation.

in'coordina'tion [L. *in-* neg. + coordination] Ataxia.

in'crusta'tion [L. *in-crusto*, pp. *-atus*, to incrust] **1.** Formation of a crust or a scab. **2.** A coating of some adventitious material or an exudate; a scab.

incuba'tion [L. *incubo*, to lie on] **1.** Maintenance of controlled environmental conditions for the purpose of favouring growth or development of microbial or tissue cultures or of an artificial environment for an infant, usually a premature or hypoxic one. **2.** Development, without sign or symptom, of an infection from the time it gains entry until the appearance of the first signs or symptoms.

in'cubator An apparatus in which controlled environmental conditions may be maintained, as for culturing microorganisms or for maintaining a premature infant.

in'cudal Relating to the incus.

in'curva'tion An inward curvature; a bending inward.

in'cus, gen. **incu'dis,** pl. **incu'des** [L. anvil] [NA] Anvil; the middle of the three ossicles in the middle ear; it has a body and two limbs or processes at the tip of the long limb is a small knob, processus lenticularis, which articulates with the head of the stapes.

in'dex, gen. **in'dicis,** pl. **in'dexes** or **in'dices** [L. one that points out, an informer] **1.** [NA] Forefinger; index finger; the second finger (the thumb as the first). **2.** A guide, standard, indicator, symbol, or number denoting the relation in respect to size, capacity, or function, of one part or thing to another.

in'dican A substance found (as its salts) in the sweat and in variable amount in the urine, indicative, when in quantity, of protein putrefaction in the intestine (indicanuria).

indicanu'ria An increased urinary excretion of indican.

indica'tion [L. fr. *in-dico*, to point out] A suggestion or pointer as to the proper treatment of a disease; it may be furnished by a knowledge of the cause (**causal i.**), by the symptoms present (**symptomatic i.**), or by nature of the disease (**specific i.**).

in'dicator [L. one that points out] In chemical analysis, a substance that changes colour within a certain definite range of pH or oxidation potential, or in any way renders visible the completion of a chemical reaction.

indiges'tion Failure of proper digestion and absorption of food in the alimentary tract, and the consequences thereof.

   acid i., thought to represent hyperchlorhydria; often used colloquially as a synonym for pyrosis.
   gastric i., dyspepsia.
   nervous i., i. caused by emotional factors.

in'dium [*indigo*, because it gives a blue line in the spectrum] A metallic element, symbol In, atomic no. 49, atomic weight 114.82. The radionuclide indium-111 (^{111}In) in chloride form is used as a bone marrow and tumour-localizing tracer; in chelate form, as a cerebrospinal fluid tracer.

in'dole 2,3-Benzopyrrole; basis of many biologically active substances.

in'dolent [L. *in-* neg. + *doleo*, pr. p. *dolens*, to feel pain] Inactive; sluggish; painless or nearly no

induc'tion [L. *inductio*, a leading in] **1.** Production or causation. **2.** The period from the start of anaesthesia to the establishment of a depth of anaesthesia adequate for operation.

in'durated [L. *in-duro*, pp. *-duratus*, to harden] Hardened, usually used with reference to soft tissues becoming extremely firm but not as hard as bone.

indura'tion [L. *induratio* (see indurated)] **1.** The process of becoming extremely firm or hard, or having such a quality. **2.** A focus or region of indurated tissue.

ine'bria'tion [L. *in-* intensive + *ebrietas*, drunkenness] Intoxication, as by alcohol.

inert' [L. *iners*, unskillful, sluggish] **1.** Slow in action; sluggish. **2.** Devoid of active chemical properties. **3.** Having no pharmacologic or therapeutic action.

iner'tia [L. want of skill, laziness] **1.** The state of a physical body in which it "resists" any force tending to move it from a position of rest or to change its uniform motion. **2.** Denoting inactivity or lack of force; lack of mental or physical vigour.

in extre'mis [L. *extremus*, last] At the point of death.

in'fant [L. *infans*, not speaking] A child under the age of 1 year; more specifically, a newborn baby.

   preterm i., an i. with gestational age of less than 37 completed weeks (259 completed days).
   stillborn i., an i. who shows no evidence of life after birth.

infan'ticide [infant + L. *caedo*, to kill] The killing of an infant.

in'fantile Relating to, or characteristic of, infants or infancy.

infan'tilism **1.** A state marked by extremely slow development of mind and body. **2.** Childishness as expressed by an adolescent or adult.

   sexual i., failure to develop secondary sexual characteristics after the normal time of puberty.

in'farct [L. *in-farcio*, pp. *-fartus*, to stuff into] An area of necrosis resulting from a sudden insufficiency of arterial or venous blood supply.

   anaemic i., an i. in which little or no bleeding into tissue occurs when the blood supply is obstructed.
   haemorrhagic i., red i., an i. red in colour from infiltration of blood from collateral vessels into the necrotic area.

infarc'tion **1.** Sudden insufficiency of arterial or venous blood supply due to emboli, thrombi, vascular torsion, or pressure that produces a macroscopic area of necrosis. **2.** Infarct.

   myocardial i., cardiac i., i. of an area of the heart muscle, usually as a result of occlusion of a coronary artery.

infect' [L. *in-ficio*, pp. *-fectus*, to corrupt, infect] **1.** To enter, invade, or inhabit another organism, causing infection or contamination. **2.** To dwell internally, endoparasitically, as opposed to infest.

infec'tion Multiplication of parasitic organisms within the body; multiplication of the "normal" flora of the intestinal tract is not considered an i.

infec'tious 1. Capable of being transmitted by infection, with or without actual contact. **2.** Infective. **3.** Denoting a disease due to the action of a microorganism.

infec'tive Producing or relating to an infection.

infe'rior [L. *lower*] **1.** Situated below or directed downward. **2.** [NA] In human anatomy, situated nearer the soles of the feet in relation to a specific reference point.

infe'rior'ity The condition or state of being or feeling inadequate or inferior, especially to others similarly situated.

in'fertil'ity [L. *in-* neg. + *fertilis*, fruitful] Relative sterility; diminished or absent fertility; does not imply (either in the male or the female) the existence of as positive or irreversible a condition as sterility. In the female, it indicates adequate anatomical structures and equivocal function, with the possibility of pregnancy that may or may not proceed to term.

infest' [L. *infesto*, pp. *-atus*, to attack] **1.** To infect, usually by macroscopic parasites; to invade parasitically. **2.** To dwell externally, ectoparasitically, as opposed to infect.

infesta'tion The act or process of infesting.

infiltra'tion 1. The act of passing into or interpenetrating a substance, cell, or tissue; said of gases, fluids, or matters held in solution. **2.** The gas, fluid, or dissolved matter that has entered any substance, cell, or tissue.

infirm' [L. *in-firmus*, fr. *in-* neg. + *firmus*, strong] Weak or feeble because of old age or disease.

infir'mary [L. *infirmarium;* see infirm] A small hospital, especially in a school or college.

infirm'ity A weakness; an abnormal, more or less disabling, condition of mind or body.

inflamma'tion [L. *inflammo*, pp. *-atus*, fr. *in*, in, + *flamma*, flame] A fundamental pathologic process consisting of a dynamic complex of cytologic and histologic reactions that occur in the affected blood vessels and adjacent tissues in response to an injury or abnormal stimulation caused by a physical, chemical, or biologic agent. The so-called cardinal signs of i. are: *rubor*, redness; *calor*, heat (or

warmth); *tumor*, swelling; and *dolor*, pain; a fifth sign, *functio laesa*, inhibited or lost function, is sometimes added. All may be observed in certain instances, but no one of them is necessarily always present.

acute i., any i. that has a fairly rapid onset and then relatively soon comes to a crisis, with clear and distinct termination.

catarrhal i., an inflammatory process that may occur in any mucous membrane and is characterized by hyperaemia of the mucosal vessels, oedema of the interstitial tissue, enlargement of the secretory epithelial cells, and an irregular layer of viscous, mucinous material on the surface.

chronic i., the antithesis of acute i. which may begin with a relatively rapid onset or in a slow, insidious, and even unnoticed manner, but tends to persist; termination of the pathologic process is indefinite and frequently not recognizable.

exudative i., i. in which the conspicuous or distinguishing feature is an exudate, which may be chiefly serous, serofibrinous, fibrinous, or mucous.

purulent i., suppurative i., an acute exudative i. in which the accumulation of polymorphonuclear leucocytes is sufficiently great that their enzymes cause liquefaction of the affected tissues; the purulent exudate is frequently termed pus.

inflam'matory Pertaining to, characterized by, resulting from, or becoming affected by inflammation.

influen'za [It. fr. L. *in-fluo*, pr. p. *influens*] The grippe (grip); the flu; an acute infectious respiratory disease, caused by orthomyxoviruses, in which the inhaled virus attacks the respiratory epithelial cells of susceptible persons and produces a catarrhal inflammation; commonly occurs in epidemics or pandemics which develop quickly, spread rapidly, and involve sizable proportions of the population; characterized by sudden onset, chills, fever of short duration, severe prostration, headache, muscle aches, and a dry cough.

Influen'zavirus The genus of Orthomyxoviridae that comprises the influenza viruses types A and B; each type has a stable nucleoprotein group antigen common to all strains of the type, but distinct from that of the other type.

infra- [L. below] Prefix denoting a position below the part denoted by the word to which it is joined. See also sub-.

infrac'tion [L. *infractio*, a breaking, fr. *in-fringere*, to break] A fracture, especially one without displacement.

inframax'illary Mandibular.

infrared' Beyond the red end of the spectrum; denoting that section of the electromagnetic spectrum, invisible to the eye, with wavelengths from 7700 nm upward to about 10,000,000 nm.

infrason'ic [infra- + L. *sonus*, sound] Pertaining to sounds with frequencies below the human range of hearing.

infundib'ular Relating to an infundibulum.

infundib'ulum, pl. **infundib'ula** [L. a funnel] **1.** [NA] A funnel or funnel-shaped structure or passage. **2.** I. tubae uterinae. **3.** The expanding portion of a calix as it opens into the pelvis of the kidney. **4.** [NA] Official alternative name for *conus* arteriosus. **5.** Termination of a bronchiole in the alveolus. **6.** Termination of the cochlear canal beneath the cupola. **7.** [NA] The funnel-shaped, unpaired prominence of the base of the hypothalamus behind the optic chiasm, enclosing the infundibular recess of the third ventricle and continuous below with the stalk of the hypophysis.

  i. tu'bae uteri'nae [NA], **i. of uterine tube,** the funnel-like expansion of the abdominal extremity of the uterine (fallopian) tube.

infu'sion [L. *infusio*, fr *in-fundo*, pp *-fusus*, to pour in] **1. The process of steeping a substance in water to extract its soluble principles. 2.** A medicinal preparation obtained by steeping the crude drug in water. **3.** The introduction of fluid other than blood into a vein.

Inges'ta [pl. of L. *ingestum*, ntr. pp. of *in gero, -gestus*, to carry in] Solid or liquid nutrients taken into the body.

inges'tion [L. *ingestio*, a pouring in] **1.** Introduction of food and drink into the stomach. **2.** The taking in of particles by a phagocytic cell.

in'guinal Relating to the groin.

in'guinocru'ral Relating to the groin and the thigh.

in'guinodyn'ia [L. *inguen* (inguin-), groin, + G. *odynē*, pain] Pain in the groin.

in'guinoper'itone'al Relating to the groin and the peritoneum.

in'guinoscro'tal Relating to the groin and the scrotum.

inha'lant [acc inhalation] **1.** That which is inhaled; a remedy given by inhalation. **2.** Finely powdered or liquid drugs that are carried to the respiratory passages by the use of special devices such as low pressure aerosol containers.

inhala'tion [L. *in-halo*, pp. *-halatus*, to breathe at or in] **1.** Inspiration; the act of drawing in the breath. **2.** Drawing a medicated vapour in with the breath. **3.** Denoting a solution of a drug or combination of drugs for administration as a nebulized mist intended to reach the repiratory tree.

inha'ler 1. Respirator (1). **2.** An apparatus for administering pharmacologically active agents by inhalation.

inher'itance [L. *heredito*, inherit, fr. *heres* (hered-), an heir] **1.** Characters or qualities that are transmitted from parent to offspring. **2.** That which is so transmitted.

inhibi'tion [L. *in-hibeo*, pp. *-hibitus*, to keep back] **1.** Depression or arrest of a function. **2.** In psychoanalysis, the restraining of instinctual or unconscious drives or tendencies, especially if they conflict with one's conscience or with the demands of society. **3.** In psychology, a generic term for a variety of processes associated with the gradual attenuation, masking, and extinction of a previously conditioned response.

inhib'itor 1. An agent that restrains or retards physiologic, chemical, or enzymic action. **2.** A nerve, stimulation of which represses activity.

  monoamine oxidase i. (MAOI), any of the hydrazine (-NHNH$_2$) and hydrazide (-CONHNH$_2$) derivatives that inhibit several enzymes and raise the brain noradrenaline and 5-hydroxytryptamine levels; used as antidepressant and hypotensive agents.

injec'tion [L. *injicio*, pp *-jactus*, to throw in] **1.** Introduction of a medicinal substance or nutrient material into the subcutaneous cellular tissue (*subcutaneous* or *hypodermic*), the muscular tissue (*intramuscular*), a vein (*intravenous*), the rectum (*rectal i.*, clyster, or enema), the vagina (*vaginal i.* or douche), the urethra, or other canals or cavities of the body. **2.** An injectable pharmaceutical preparation. **3.** Congestion or hyperaemia.

injury [L. *injuria*, fr. *in-* neg. + *jus* (jur), right] The damage or wound of trauma.

contrecoup i. of brain, an i. occurring beneath the skull opposite to the area of impact.

coup i. of brain, i. to the brain occurring directly beneath the area of impact.

hyperextension-hyperflexion i., violence to the body causing the unsupported head to hyperextend and hyperflex the neck rapidly.

open head i., a head i. in which there is a loss of continuity of scalp or mucous membranes; sometimes indicating a communication between the exterior and the intracranial cavity.

whiplash i., popular term for hyperextension-hyperflexion i.'s of the neck.

in'lay 1. In dentistry, a prefabricated restoration sealed in the cavity with cement. 2. A graft of bone, skin, or other tissue. 3. In orthopaedics, an orthomechanical device inserted into a shoe.

in'let A passage leading into a cavity.

innate' [L. *in-nascor,* pp. *-natus,* to be born in] Inborn.

innerva'tion [L. *in,* in, + *nervus,* nerve] The supply of nerve fibres functionally connected with a part.

innoc'uous [L. *innocuus*] Harmless.

innom'inate [L. *innominatus,* fr. *in-* neg. + *nomen* (*nomin-*), name] Nameless; applied to several anatomical structures.

inoc'ulable 1. Transmissible by inoculation. 2. Susceptible to a disease transmissible by inoculation.

inoc'ulate [L. *inoculo,* pp. *-atus,* to ingraft] 1. To introduce the agent of a disease or other antigenic material into the subcutaneous tissue or a blood vessel or through an abraded or absorbing surface for preventive, curative, or experimental purposes. 2. To implant microorganisms or infectious material into or upon culture media. 3. To communicate a disease by transferring its virus.

inop'erable Denoting that which cannot be operated upon, or cannot be corrected or removed by an operation.

in'organ'ic 1. Originally, not organic; not formed by living organisms; 2. In chemistry, refers to compounds not containing covalent bonds between atoms.

in'osine (Ino) A nucleoside formed by the deamination of adenosine.

inotrop'ic [ino- + G. *tropos,* a turning] Influencing the contractility of muscular tissue.

in'quest [L. *in,* in, + *quaero,* pp. *quaisitus,* to seek] A legal inquiry into the cause of sudden, violent, or mysterious death.

insan'ity [L. *in-* neg. + *sanus,* sound] 1. Now outmoded term, more or less synonymous with severe mental illness or psychosis. 2. In law, that degree of mental illness which negates the individual's legal responsibility or capacity.

inscrip'tion [L. *inscriptio*] 1. The main part of a prescription; that which indicates the drugs and the quantity of each to be used in the mixture. 2. A mark, band, or line.

insem'ina'tion [L. *in-semino,* pp. *-atus,* to sow or plant in] The deposit of seminal fluid within the vagina, as introduced during coitus.

artificial i., the introduction of semen of the husband (*homologous i.*) or of another (*heterologous i.*) into the vagina otherwise than through the act of coitus.

insen'sible [L. *in-sensibilis,* fr. *in,* neg. + *sentio,* pp. *sensus,* to feel] 1. Unconscious. 2. Not appreciable by the senses.

inser'tion [L. *insertio,* a planting in] 1. The attachment of a muscle to the more movable part of the skeleton, as distinguished from origin. 2. In dentistry, the intraoral placing of a dental prosthesis.

insid'ious [L. *insidiosus,* cunning, fr. *insidioe* (pl.), an ambush] Treacherous; stealthy; denoting a disease that progresses with few or no symptoms to indicate its gravity.

in si'tu [L. *in,* in, + *situs,* site] In position; confined to site or origin.

insol'uble Not soluble.

insom'nia [L. fr. *in-* priv. + *somnus,* sleep] Wakefulness, inability to sleep, in the absence of external impediments, during the period when sleep should normally occur.

insom'niac Exhibiting, suffering from, tending toward, or producing insomnia.

inspira'tion [L. *inspiratio,* fr. *in-spiro,* pp. *-atus,* to breathe in] Inhalation (1).

inspi'ratory Relating to or timed during inhalation.

inspis'sated [L. *in-* intensive + *spisso,* pp. *-atus,* to thicken] Thickened by evaporation or absorption of fluid.

in'step The arch, or highest part of the dorsum of the foot.

instilla'tion [L. *instillatio*, fr. *in-stillo*, pp. -*atus*, to pour in by drops] The dropping of a liquid on or into a part.

in'stinct [L. *instinctus*, impulse] 1. An enduring disposition or tendency of an organism to act in an organized and biologically adaptive manner characteristic of its species. 2. The unreasoning impulse to perform some purposive action without an immediate consciousness of the end to which that action will lead. 3. In psychoanalytic theory, the forces assumed to exist behind the tension caused by the needs of the id.

instinc'tive, instinc'tual Relating to instinct.

insuffi'ciency [L. *in-*, neg. + *sufficientia*, to suffice] 1. Lack of completeness of function or of power. 2. Incompetence (1).

   adrenocortical i., loss, to varying degrees, of adrenocortical function.

   cardiac i., heart *failure* (1).

   chronic adrenocortical i., Addison's disease; adrenocortical i. caused by idiopathic atrophy or destruction of both adrenal glands; characterized by fatigue, decreased blood pressure, weight loss, melanin pigmentation of the skin and mucous membranes, anorexia, and nausea or vomiting.

   coronary i., inadequate coronary circulation leading to anginal pain.

   myocardial i., heart *failure* (1).

   valvular i., failure of the cardiac valves to close perfectly, thus allowing regurgitation of blood past the closed valve; named, according to the valve involved: aortic, mitral, pulmonary, or tricuspid i.

insuf'flate [L. *in-sumo*, to blow on or into] To blow into; to fill the lungs of an asphyxiated person with air, or to blow a medicated vapour, powder, or anaesthetic into the lungs or into any cavity or orifice of the body.

insuffla'tion 1. The act or process of insufflating. 2. Inhalant (?)

in'sula, gen. and pl. **in'sulae** [L. island] 1. [NA] An oval region of the cerebral cortex overlying the capsula extrema, lateral to the lenticular nucleus, buried in the depth of the sylvian fissure. 2. Island. 3. Any circumscribed body or patch on the skin.

in'sulin A peptide hormone secreted by the pancreatic islets of Langerhans that promotes glucose utilization, protein synthesis, and the formation and storage of neutral lipids. Insulins, obtained from various animals

and available in a variety of preparation, are used parenterally in the treatment of diabetes mellitus.

in'sulinase An enzyme in liver, kidney, and muscle, capable of inactivating insulin

in'sulinae'mia [insulin + G. *haima*, blood] Abnormally large concentrations of insulin in the circulating blood.

in'sulino'ma An islet cell adenoma that secretes insulin.

insuli'tis [L. *insula*, island, + -*itis*, inflammation] A histologic change in which the islets of Langerhans are oedematous and contain small numbers of leucocytes.

in'sult [LL. *insultus*, fr. L. *insulto*, to spring upon] An injury, attack, or trauma.

integ'rity Soundness or completeness of structure; a sound or unimpaired condition.

integ'ument [L. *integumentum*, a covering] 1. Integumentum commune. 2. The rind, capsule, or covering of any body or part.

integumen'tum commu'ne [NA] The enveloping membrane of the body; includes, in addition to the epidermis and dermis, all of the derivatives of the epidermis, *i.e.*, hairs, nails, sudoriferous and sebaceous glands, and mammary glands.

intel'ligence [L. *intelligentia*] 1. An individual's aggregate capacity to act purposefully, think rationally, and deal effectively with his environment, especially in relation to the extent of his perceived effectiveness in meeting challenges. 2. An individual's relative standing on two quantitative indices, measured i. and effectiveness of adaptive behaviour.

inter- [L. *inter*, between] Prefix conveying the meaning of between, among.

in'terbod'y Between the bodies of two adjacent vertebrae

intercal'ary [L. *intercalarius*, concerning an insertion] Occurring between two others; as in a pulse tracing, an upstroke interposed between two normal pulse beats.

in'tercourse [L. *intercursus*, a running between] Communication or dealings between or among people; interchange of ideas.

   sexual i., coitus.

intercur'rent [inter- + L. *curro*, pr. p. *currens* (-*ent*-), to run] Intervening; said of a disease attacking a person already ill of another malady.

in'tercuspa'tion [L. *inter*, among, mutually, + *cusp*] 1. The cusp-to-fossa relation of the maxillary and mandibular posterior teeth to each other. **2.** The interlocking or fitting together of the cusps of opposing teeth.

interden'tal [inter- + L. *dens,* tooth] **1.** Between the teeth. **2.** Denoting the relationship between the proximal surfaces of the teeth of the same arch.

in'terdigita'tion [inter- + L. *digitus,* finger] **1.** The mutual interlocking of toothed or tonguelike processes. **2.** The processes thus interlocked. **3.** Infoldings or plicae of adjacent cell or plasma membranes. **4.** Intercuspation (2).

interfer'on (IFN) A glycoprotein induced in different cell types by appropriate stimuli. At least three types are recognized: **IFN-α** or **leucocyte i.,** elaborated by leucocytes in response to viral infection or stimulation with double-stranded RNA; **IFN-β** made by fibroblasts under the same conditions; **IFN-γ** or **immune i.,** produced by lymphocytes following mitogenic stimulation.

interic'tal [inter- + L. *ictus,* stroke] Denoting the interval between convulsions.

interleu'kin A class of lymphokine that acts as a T-lymphocyte growth factor.

interme'diate [L. *intermedius,* lying between] **1.** Between two extremes; interposed; intervening. **2.** A substance, formed in the course of chemical reactions, which then proceeds to participate rapidly in further reactions, so that at any given moment it is present in minute concentrations only.

intermit'tent Marked by intervals of complete quietude between two periods of activity.

inter'nal [L. *internus*] Interior; away from the surface; often incorrectly used to mean medial.

inter'naliza'tion Adopting as one's own the standards and values of another person or society.

International System of Units (SI) [Fr. *Système International d'Unités*] A system of weights and measures designed to cover both the coherent units (basic, supplementary, and derived units) and the decimal multiples and submultiples of these units formed by use of prefixes proposed for general international scientific and technological use. SI proposes seven basic units: metre (m), kilogram (kg), second (s), ampere (A), kelvin (K), candela (cd), and mole (mol) for the basic quantities, length, mass, time, electric current, temperature, luminous intensity, and amount of substance. Supplementary units proposed are radian (rad) for plane angle and steradian (sr) for solid angle. Derived units (*e.g.,* force, power, frequency) are stated in terms of the basic units. Multiples (prefixes) in descending order are: tera- (T, 10^{12}), giga- (G, 10^9), mega- (M, 10^6), kilo- (k, 10^3), hecto- (h, 10^2), deca- (da, 10^1), deci- (d, 10^{-1}), centi- (c, 10^{-2}), milli- (m, 10^{-3}), micro- (μ, 10^{-6}), nano- (n, 10^{-9}), pico- (p, 10^{-12}), femto- (f, 10^{-15}), atto- (a, 10^{-18}).

interneu'rones Combinations or groups of neurones between sensory and motor neurones which govern coordinated activity.

in'terocep'tive [inter- + L. *capio,* to take] Relating to the sensory nerve cells innervating the viscera (thoracic, abdominal and pelvic organs, and the cardiovascular system), their sensory end organs, or the information they convey to the spinal cord and the brain.

in'terocep'tor [inter- + L. *capio,* to take] One of the various forms of small sensory end organs (receptors) situated within the walls of the respiratory and gastrointestinal tracts or in other viscera.

in'terphase The stage between two successive divisions of a cell nucleus; the stage in which the biochemical and physiologic functions of the cell are performed.

interprox'imal Between adjoining surfaces.

intes'tinal Relating to the intestine.

intes'tine [L. *intestinus,* internal; as noun, the entrails] The digestive tract passing from the stomach to the anus.

   large i., the portion of the digestive tract extending from the ileocaecal valve to the anus; comprises the caecum, colon, rectum, and anal canal.

   small i., the portion of the digestive tract between the stomach and the caecum or beginning of the large intestine; consists of the duodenum, jejunum, and ileum.

in'tima [L. fem. of *intimus,* inmost] *Tunica intima.*

in'timal Relating to the intima or inner coat of a vessel.

intol'erance Abnormal metabolism, excretion, or other disposition of a given substance; term often used to indicate impaired disposal of dietary constituents.

intoxica'tion [L. *in*, in, + G. *toxicon*, poison] **1.** Poisoning. **2.** Acute *alcoholism*.

intra- [L. within] Prefix meaning within.

in'tracorpo'real [intra- + L. *corpus*, body] **1.** Within the body. **2.** Within any structure anatomically styled a corpus.

intrac'table [L. *in-tractabilis*, fr. *in-* neg. + *tracto*, to draw, haul] **1.** Refractory (1). **2.** Obstinate (1).

intrafi'lar [intra- + L. *filum*, thread] Lying within the meshes of a network.

in'tramedul'lary Within the bone marrow, the spinal cord, or the medulla ob longata.

intrapar'tum [intra- + L. *partus*, child birth] During labour and delivery or childbirth.

in'travasa'tion [intra- + L. *vas*, vessel] Entrance of foreign matter into a blood vessel.

intrin'sic [L. *intrinsecus*, on the inside] **1.** Inherent; belonging entirely to a part. **2.** In anatomy, denoting those muscles of the limbs whose origin and insertion are both in the same limb, distinguished from the extrinsic muscles which have their origin in some part of the trunk outside of the pelvic or shoulder girdle; applied also to the ciliary muscle as distinguished from the recti and other orbital muscles which are on the eyeball.

intro- [L. *intro*, into] Prefix meaning in or into.

introdu'cer [L. *intro-duco*, to lead into, introduce] An instrument or stylet for the introduction of a flexible instrument; *e.g.*, a catheter or an endotracheal tube.

intro'itus [L. entrance, fr. *intro-eo*, to go into] The entrance into a canal or hollow organ, as the vagina.

introjec'tion [intro- + L. *jacere*, to throw] A psychological defence mechanism involving appropriation of an external happening and its assimilation by the personality, making it a part of the self.

intromis'sion [intro- + L. *mitto*, to send] The insertion or introduction of one part into another.

introspec'tion [intro- + L. *spicere*, to look] Looking inward; self-scrutinizing; contemplating one's own mental processes.

introver'sion [intro- + L. *verto*, pp. *versus*, to turn] **1.** The turning of a structure into itself. **2.** A trait of preoccupation with oneself, in contrast to extraversion.

introvert **1.** (in'tro-vert) One who tends to be introspective and self-centred and who takes small interest in the affairs of others. **2.** (in-tro-vert') To turn a structure into itself.

intuba'tion The insertion of a tube into any canal or other part.

  endotracheal i. passage of a tube through the nose (**nasotracheal i.**) or mouth (**oratracheal i.**) into the trachea for maintenance of the airway during anaesthesia or in a patient with an imperilled airway.

intumesce' [L. *in-tumesco*, to swell up] To swell up; to enlarge.

intumes'cence **1.** An anatomical swelling, enlargement, or prominence. **2.** The process of enlarging or swelling.

in'tussuscep'tion [L. *intus*, within, + *sus-cipio*, to take up] The taking up or receiving of one part within another, especially the infolding of one segment of the intestine within another.

in'ulin A fructose polysaccharide from the rhizome of *Inula helenium* or *elecampane*, and other plants; a hygroscopic powder used by intravenous injection to determine the rate of glomerular filtration.

inunc'tion [L. *inunctio*, an anointing, fr. *inunguo*, pp. *-unctus*, to smear on] Anointing; the administration of a drug in ointment form applied with rubbing, with the purpose of causing absorption of the active ingredient.

in u'tero [L.] Within the womb; not yet born.

invag'inate [L. *in*, in, + *vagina*, a sheath] To ensheathe, infold, or insert a structure within itself or another.

invagina'tion **1.** The ensheathing, infolding, or insertion of a structure within itself or another. **2.** The state of being invaginated.

in'valid [L. *in-* neg. + *validus*, strong] **1.** Weak; sick. **2.** A sickly person suffering from a disabling but not necessarily completely incapacitating disease.

inva'sive **1.** Involving puncture, incision, or penetration of the body, as in a diagnostic technique. **2.** Denoting local spread of a malignant neoplasm by infiltration or destruction of adjacent tissue.

inver'sion [L. *inverto*, pp. *-versus*, to turn upside down, turn about] **1.** A turning inward, upside down, or in any direction contrary to the existing one. **2.** Conversion of a disaccharide or polysaccharide by hydrolysis into a monosaccharide. **3.** Alteration of a DNA molecule made by removing a fragment, reversing its orientation, and pulling it back into place.

i. of the uterus, a turning of the uterus inside out, usually following childbirth.

visceral i., situs inversus.

inver'tebrate **1.** Not possessed of a spinal, or vertebral, column. **2.** An invertebrate animal.

invert'or [see inversion] A muscle that inverts or causes inversion or turns a part, such as the foot, inward.

invet'erate [L. *in-vetero,* pp. *-atus,* to render old] Chronic; long seated; firmly established; said of a disease or of confirmed habits.

in vi'tro [L. in glass] In an artificial environment, referring to a process or reaction occurring therein, as in a test tube or culture media.

in vi'vo [L. in the living being] In the living body, referring to a process or reaction occurring therein.

involu'crum, pl. **involu'cra** [L. a wrapper, fr. *in-volvo,* to roll up] An enveloping membrane, *e.g.,* the sheath of new bone that forms around a sequestrum.

invol'untary [L. *in-* neg. + *voluntarius,* willing, fr. *volo,* to wish] **1.** Independent of the will; not volitional. **2.** Contrary to the will.

involu'tion [L. *in-volvo,* pp. *-volutus,* to roll up] **1.** The return of an enlarged organ, as the postpartum uterus, to normal size. **2.** The turning inward of the edges of a part. **3.** In psychiatry, the mental decline associated with later life.

i'odide The negative ion of iodine, I⁻.

io'dinate To treat or combine with iodine.

i'odine [G. *iōdēs,* violet-like] A nonmetallic chemical element, symbol I, atomic no. 53, atomic weight 126.91; used as a catalyst, a reagent and stain, a topical antiseptic, internally in thyroid disease, and as an antidote for alkaloidal poisons.

radioactive i., Usually refers to ¹³¹I, ¹²⁵I, or ¹²³I used as tracers in biology and medicine.

iodine-fast Denoting hyperthyroidism unresponsive to iodine therapy, which ultimately develops in most cases so treated.

i'odism Poisoning by iodine, a condition marked by severe coryza, an acneform eruption, weakness, salivation, and a foul breath.

i'odize To treat or impregnate with iodine.

io'dohip'purate **sodium** A radiopaque compound used intravenously, orally, or for retrograde urography; when tagged with iodine-131, used to measure renal function externally in radioisotopic renography.

iodop'sin A visual pigment found in the cones of the retina.

i'on [G. *iōn,* going] An atom or group of atoms carrying a charge of electricity by virtue of having gained or lost one or more valency electrons, usually constituting one of the parts of an electrolyte. Those charged with negative electricity, which travel toward a positive pole (anode) are *anions,* those charged with positive electricity, which travel toward a negative pole (cathode), are *cations.*

ion'ic Relating to an ion or ions.

i'oniza'tion **1.** Dissociation into ions, occurring when an electrolyte is dissolved in water. **2.** Iontophoresis.

ion'tophore'sis [ion + G. *phorēsis,* a being borne] Introduction into the tissues, by means of an electric current, of the ions of a chosen medicament.

ip'ecacuan'ha The dried root of *Uragoga* (*Cephaelis*) *ipecacuanha* (family Rubiaceae) which has expectorant, emetic, and antidysenteric properties.

ipsilat'eral [L. *ipse,* same, + *latus* (*later-*), side] With reference to a given point, on the same side.

irid- See irido-.

iridec'tomy [irido- + G. *ektomē,* excision] Excision of a portion of the iris.

ir'idenclei'sis [irido- + G. *enkleiō,* to shut in] Incarceration of a portion of the iris in a wound of the cornea as an operative measure in glaucoma to effect filtration; may also occur accidently.

ir'ides [G.] Plural of iris.

irido-, irid- [G. *iris* (*irid-*), rainbow] Combining forms relating to the iris.

irid'ocele [irido- + G. *kēlē,* hernia] Protrusion of a portion of the iris through a corneal defect.

ir'idoconstric'tor Causing contraction of the pupil; denoting especially the circular muscular fibres of the iris.

ir'idodial'ysis [irido- + G. *dialysis,* loosening] A colobomatous defect of the iris due to its separation from its ciliary attachment.

ir'idodila'tor Causing dilation of the pupil; applied to the radiating muscular fibres of the iris.

ir'idokine'sis, ir'idokine'sia [irido- + G. *kinēsis*, movement] The movement of the iris in contracting and dilating the pupil.

ir'idosclerot'omy [irido- + sclera + G. *tomē*, incision] An incision involving both sclera and iris.

iridot'omy [irido- + G. *tomē*, incision] Transverse division of some of the fibres of the iris, forming an artificial pupil.

i'ris, pl. **ir'ides** [G. rainbow] [NA] The anterior division of the vascular tunic of the eye, a disclike diaphragm, perforated in the centre (the pupil), attached marginally to the ciliary body; composed of stroma and a double layer of pigmented retinal epithelium from which are derived the sphincter and dilator muscles of the pupil.

iri'tis Inflammation of the iris.

iron (I) [A.S. *iren*] A metallic element, symbol Fe, atomic no. 26, atomic weight 55.85; occurs in the haem of haemoglobin, myoglobin, transferrin, ferritin, and iron-containing porphyrins, and is an essential component of enzymes such as catalase, peroxidase, and the various cytochromes; its ferric and ferrous salts are used medicinally.

irradia'tion [L. *ir-radio* (*in-r*), pp. *-radiatus*, to beam forth] **1.** Exposure or subjection to the action of radiant energy for diagnostic or therapeutic purposes. **2.** The spread of nervous effects (impulses) from one area in the brain or cord, or from a tract, to another tract.

irredu'cible **1.** Not reducible; incapable of being made smaller. **2.** In chemistry, incapable of being made simpler, or of being replaced or hydrogenated or reduced in positive charge.

ir'rigate [L. *ir-rigo*, pp. *-atus*, to irrigate] To wash out a cavity or wound with a fluid.

ir'ritabil'ity [L. *irritabilitas*, fr *irrito*, pp. *-atus*, to excite] The property inherent in protoplasm of reacting to a stimulus.

ir'ritable **1.** Capable of reacting to a stimulus. **2.** Tending to react immoderately to a stimulus.

ir'ritant Irritating; causing irritation.

irrita'tion [L. *irritatio*] **1.** Extreme incipient inflammatory reaction of the tissues to an injury. **2.** The normal response of nerve or muscle to a stimulus. **3.** Evocation of a normal or exaggerated reaction in the tissues by the application of a stimulus.

ischae'mia [G. *ischō*, to keep back, + *haima*, blood] Local anemia due to mechanical obstruction (mainly arterial narrowing) of the blood supply.

ischae'mic Relating to or affected by ischaemia.

ischial'gia [G. *ischion*, hip, + *algos*, pain] **1.** Pain in the hip; specifically, the ischium. **2.** Sciatica.

ischiat'ic Sciatic (1).

ischio- [G. *ischion*, hip-joint, haunch (ischium)] Combining form relating to the ischium.

is'chium, pl. **is'chia** [Mod. L. fr. G. *ischion*, hip] *Os* ischii.

is'land [A.S. *īgland*] In anatomy, any isolated part, separated from the surrounding tissues by a groove, or marked by difference in structure.
   i.'s of Langerhans, cellular masses varying from a few to hundreds of cells lying in the interstitial tissue of the pancreas; they are composed of different cell types which make up the endocrine portion of the pancreas, and are the source of insulin and glucagon.
   i. of Reil, insula (I).

is'let A small island.
   i.'s of Langerhans, islands of Langerhans.

-ism [G. *-isma, -ismos*, noun-forming suffix] Suffix denoting a condition or disease resulting from or involving, or a practice or doctrine. *Cf.* -ia.

-ismus [L. fr. G. *-ismos*, noun of action suffix] Suffix customarily used to imply spasm or contraction.

iso- [G. *isos*, equal] **1.** Prefix meaning equal, like. **2.** In chemistry, prefix indicating "isomer of." **3.** In immunology, prefix designating sameness with respect to species; recently, sameness with respect to genetic constitution of individuals.

i'soagglutina'tion [iso- + L. *ad*, to, + *gluten*, glue] Agglutination of red blood cells as a result of the reaction between an isoagglutinin and specific antigen in or on the cells.

i'soagglu'tinin An isoantibody that causes agglutination of cells.

isoan'tibody [G. *isos*, equal] **1.** An antibody that occurs only in some individuals of a species, and reacts specifically with the corresponding isoantigen; the latter does not occur naturally in the cells of the same individual who has the antibody.

isoan'tigen 1. An antigenic substance that occurs only in some individuals of a species, such as the blood group antigens of man. 2. Sometimes used as a synonym of alloantigen.

isobar'ic 1. Having equal weights or pressures. 2. With respect to solutions, having the same density as the diluent or medium.

i'sochromat'ic [iso- + G. *chrōma*, colour] 1. Of uniform colour. 2. Denoting two objects of the same colour.

isocor'tex See *cortex* cerebri.

isogen'ic Relating to a group of individuals or a strain of animals genetically alike with respect to specified gene pairs.

i'sograft [iso- + graft] Homograft; isologous graft; a tissue or organ transplanted between genetically identical individuals, or between syngeneic animals which are isogeneic with respect to histocompatibility genes.

i'soim'muniza'tion The development of a significant titre of specific antibody as a result of antigenic stimulation with material contained in or in the red blood cells of another individual of the same species.

i'solate [It. *isolare;* Mediev. L. *insulo,* pp. *-atus,* to insulate] 1. To separate; to set apart from others. 2. To free from chemical contaminants. 3. In psychoanalysis, to separate experiences or memories from the affects pertaining to them. 4. That which is isolated.

isol'ogous [iso- + G. *logos,* ratio] Relating to tissue transplant between identical twins or between syngeneic individuals, isogenic with respect to histocompatibility genes.

isom'erism The existence of a chemical compound in two or more forms that are identical with respect to percentage composition but differ as to the position of the atoms within the molecule, and also in physical and chemical properties.

isomet'ric [iso- + G. *metron,* measure] 1. Of equal dimensions. 2. In physiology, denoting the condition when the ends of a contracting muscle are held fixed so that contraction produces increased tension at constant overall length.

isomor'phic Isomorphous.

isomor'phism [iso- + G. *morphē,* shape] Similarity of form between two or more organisms or between parts of the body.

isomor'phous Having the same form or shape, or being morphologically equal.

isopro'pyl alcohol An isomer of propyl alcohol and a homologue of ethyl alcohol, similar in its properties, when used externally, to the latter, but more toxic when taken internally.

i'soproter'enol hydrochloride A sympathomimetic β-receptor stimulant possessing the inhibitory properties and the cardiac excitatory, but not the vasoconstrictor, actions of adrenaline.

Isos'pora [iso- + G. *sporos,* seed] A genus of coccidia (family Eimeriidae, class Sporozoa), with species parasitic chiefly in mammals. *I. hominis* is a rare species described only from man and capable of causing a mucous diarrhoea with anorexia, nausea, and abdominal pain; it is very similar to *I. bigemina* and may prove to be the same species.

isos'pori'asis Infection with coccidia of the genus *Isospora.*

isother'mal [iso- + G. *thermē,* heat] Having the same temperature.

isoto'nia [iso- + G. *tonos,* tension] A condition of tonic equality, in which tension or osmotic pressure in two substances or solutions is the same.

isoton'ic 1. Relating to isotonicity or isotonia. 2. Having equal tension; denoting solutions possessing the same osmotic pressure; more specifically, limited to solutions in which cells neither swell nor shrink. 3. In physiology, denoting the condition when a contracting muscle shortens against a constant load, as when lifting a weight.

i'sotonic'ity 1. The quality of possessing and maintaining a uniform tone or tension. 2. The property of a solution in being isotonic.

i'sotope [iso- + G. *topos,* part, place] Either of two or more nuclides that are chemically identical yet differ in mass number, since their nuclei contain different numbers of neutrons. Individual i.'s are named with the inclusion of their mass number; *e.g.,* carbon-12 (^{12}C).

    radioactive i., an i. with a nuclear composition that is unstable; nuclei of such an i. decompose spontaneously by emission of a nuclear electron (β-particle) or helium nucleus (α-ray) and radiation (γ-rays), thus achieving a stable nuclear composition; used as tracers.

stable i., a nonradioactive nuclide; an i. of an element that shows no tendency to undergo radioactive breakdown.

is'sue [Fr. a going out] **1.** A suppurating or discharging sore, acting as a counterirritant, sometimes maintained by the presence of a foreign body in the tissues. **2.** A discharge of pus, blood, or other matter.

isthmec'tomy [G. *isthmos*, isthmus, + *ektome*, excision] Excision of the midportion of the thyroid.

isth'mus, pl. **isth'muses, isth'mi** [G. *isthmos*] A constriction or narrow passage connecting two larger parts of an organ or other anatomical structure.

itch [A.S. *gikkan*] **1.** A peculiar irritating sensation in the skin that arouses the desire to scratch. **2.** Common name for scabies. **3.** Pruritus (2)

itch'ing An uncomfortable sensation of irritation of the skin or mucous membranes which causes scratching or rubbing of the affected parts.

-ite [G. *-ites*, fem. *itis*] **1.** Suffix denoting of the nature of, resembling. **2.** In chemistry, denoting a salt of an acid that has the termination -ous. **3.** In comparative anatomy, a suffix denoting an essential portion of the part to the name of which it is attached.

-ites [G. *itos*, m., or *-ites*, n.] An adjectival suffix to nouns, corresponding to the English -y, -like; the adjective so formed is used without the qualified noun. The feminine form, *-itis* (agreeing with *nosos*, disease), is so often associated with inflammatory disease that it has acquired in most cases the significance of inflammation.

-itis [G. fem of *-itus*] See Ites.

Ixo'des [G. *ixodes*, sticky, like bird-lime] A genus of hard ticks (family Ixodidae), many species of which are parasitic on man and animals; severe reactions frequently follow their bites.

ixodi'asis **1.** Skin lesions caused by the bites of certain ticks; the tick may burrow under the skin, causing some degree of irritation, but in most cases an urticarioid eruption is the only result. **2.** Any disease, such as Rocky Mountain fever, that is transmitted by ticks.

J

jack'et **1.** A fixed bandage applied around the body in order to immobilize the spine. **2.** In dentistry, a term commonly used in reference to an artificial crown composed of fired porcelain or acrylic resin.

jactita'tion [L. *jactatio*, a tossing] Extreme restlessness or tossing about from side to side.

jar'gon [Fr. gibberish] **1.** Language or terminology peculiar to a specific field, profession, or group. **2.** Paraphasia.

jaun'dice [Fr. *jaune*, yellow] Icterus; a yellowish staining of the integument, sclerae, and deeper tissues and the excretions with bile pigments, which are increased in the serum.

acholuric j., j. with excessive amounts of unconjugated bilirubin in the circulatory blood and without bile pigments in the blood.

haematogenous j., haemolytic j., j. resulting from excessive amounts of haemoglobin released by any process causing haemolysis of erythrocytes.

hepatocellular j., j. resulting from diffuse injury or inflammation or failure of function of the liver cells.

leptospiral j., j. associated with infection by various species of *Leptospira*.

obstructive j., mechanical j.; j. resulting from obstruction to the flow of bile into the duodenum.

jaw [A.S. *ceowan*, to chew] One of the two bony structures, maxillae or the mandible, in which the teeth are set, forming the framework of the mouth.

jejunec'tomy [jejunum + G. *ektome*, excision] Excision of all or a part of the jejunum.

jejuni'tis Inflammation of the jejunum.

jejuno-, jejun- [L. *jejunus*, empty] Combining forms relating to the jejunum.

jeju'nocolos'tomy [jejuno- + colon + G. *stoma*, mouth] Establishment of a communication between the jejunum and the colon.

jeju'noileos'tomy [jejuno- + G. *stoma*, mouth] Surgical establishment of a communication between the jejunum and the ileum.

jeju'nojejunos'tomy [jejuno- + jejuno- + G. *stoma*, mouth] An anastomosis between two portions of jejunum.

jeju'noplasty [jejuno- + G. *plastos*, moulded] A corrective surgical procedure on the jejunum.

jejunos'tomy [jejuno- + G. *stoma*, mouth] Surgical establishment of an opening from the abdominal wall into the jejunum, usually with creation of a stoma on the abdominal wall.

jejunot'omy [jejuno- + G. *tomē*, incision] Incision into the jejunum.

jeju'num [L. *jejunus*, empty] [NA] The portion of small intestine between the duodenum and the ileum.

jel'ly [L. *gelo*, to freeze] A semisolid resilient compound.

    Wharton's j., the mucous connective tissue of the umbilical cord.

jerk **1.** A sudden pull. **2.** Deep *reflex*.

jet lag A disturbance of normal circadian rhythm as a result of sub- or supersonic travel through a number of time zones, resulting in fatigue and varied constitutional symptoms.

jig'ger Common name for *Tunga penetrans*.

joint [L. *junctura*] Articulatio.

    ball-and-socket j., *articulatio* spheroidea.

    biaxial j., a j. in which there are two principal axes of movement situated at right angles to each other.

    hinge j., ginglymus.

    synovial j., *articulatio* synovialis.

    temporomandibular j., *articulatio* temporomandibularis.

ju'gal [L. *jugalis*, yoked together] **1.** Connecting; yoked. **2.** Relating to the zygomatic bone.

jug'ular [L. *jugulum*, throat] **1.** Relating to the throat or neck. **2.** Relating to the j. veins. **3.** A j. vein.

ju'gum, pl. **ju'ga** [L. a yoke] **1.** Yoke; a ridge or furrow connecting two points. **2.** A type of forceps.

juice [L. *jus*, broth] **1.** The tissue fluid of a plant or animal. **2.** A digestive secretion, such as that secreted by glands of the stomach and intestine.

junc'tion The point, line, or surface of union of two parts.

    dentinoenamel j., the surface at which the enamel and the dentine of the crown of a tooth are joined.

    gap j., a 20-Å gap between apposed cell membranes that contains subunits in the form of polygonal lattices; believed to mediate electrotonic coupling which allows ionic currents to pass from one cell to another.

    mucocutaneous j., the site of transition from epidermis to the epithelium of a mucous membrane.

    myoneural j., the synaptic connection of the axon of the motor neurone with a muscle fibre.

jux'taglomer'ular Close to or adjoining a renal glomerulus.

jux'tallocor'tex See *cortex* cerebri.

jux'taposi'tion [L. *juxta*, near to, + *positio*, a placing] A position side by side.

K

kal-, kali- [L. *kalium*, potassium] Combining forms relating to potassium; sometimes *kalio-*.

kal'a azar' [Hind. *kala*, black, + *azar*, poison] Visceral *leishmaniasis*.

ka'liope'nia [Mod. L. *kalium*, potassium, + G. *penia*, poverty] Insufficiency of potassium in the body.

kalure'sis [Mod. L. *kalium*, potassium, + G. *ouresis*, urination] The increased urinary excretion of potassium.

karyo- [G. *karyon*, nucleus] Combining form denoting nucleus.

kar'yocyte [karyo- + G. *kytos*, cell] A young, immature normoblast.

karyog'amy [karyo- + G. *gamos*, marriage] Fusion of the nuclei of two cells, as occurs in fertilization or true conjugation.

karyogen'esis [karyo- + G. *genesis*, production] Formation of the nucleus of a cell.

kar'yotype The chromosome characteristics of an individual or of a cell line, usually presented as a systemized array of metaphase chromosomes from a photomicrograph of a single cell nucleus arranged in pairs in descending order of size and according to the position of the centromere.

kata- [G. *kata*, down] Alternative spelling for *cata-*.

ke'loid [G. *kēlē*, a tumour (or *kēlis*, a spot), + *eidos*, appearance] A nodular linear mass of hyperplastic scar tissue, consisting of relatively wide and parallel bands of collagenous fibrous tissue; occurs in the dermis and adjacent subcutaneous tissue, usually after a traumatic injury, surgery, a burn, or severe cutaneous disease such as cystic acne.

ke'loido'sis Multiple keloids.

ke'loplasty [keloid + G. *plassō*, to fashion] Operative removal of a scar or keloid.

Kel'vin See K. *scale*.

ker'atecta'sia [kerato- + G. *ektasis*, extrusion] Herniation of the cornea.

keratec'tomy [kerato- + G. *ektomē*, excision] Excision of a portion of the cornea.

kerat'ic [G. *keras* (*kerat-*), horn] Horny.

ker'atin A scleroprotein or albuminoid that is present largely in cuticular structures and contains a relatively large amount of sulphur.

ker'atiniza'tion Keratin formation or development of a horny layer; may also apply to premature formation of keratin.

kerat'inous 1. Relating to keratin. 2. Horny.

kerati'tis [kerato- + -*itis*, inflammation] Inflammation of the cornea.

kerato-, kerat- [G *keras*, horn] Combining forms denoting the cornea or horny tissue or cells.

ker'atoacantho'ma A rapidly growing tumour usually occurring on exposed areas of the skin, with a central keratin mass that opens on the skin surface; it invades the dermis, but remains localized and usually resolves spontaneously.

ker'atocele [kerato- + G *kēlē*, hernia] Herniation of Descemet's membrane through a defect in the outer layer of the cornea.

ker'atoconjunctivi'tis Inflammation of the conjunctiva and of the cornea as a phlyctenular hypersensitivity reaction of corneal and conjunctival epithelium to endogenous toxin.

keratoco'nus [kerato- + G. *kōnos*, cone] A conical protrusion of the centre of the cornea due to noninflammatory thinning of the stroma; usually bilateral.

keratoder'ma [kerato- + G. *derma*, skin] 1. Any horny superficial growth. 2. A generalized thickening of the horny layer of the epidermis.

keratog'enous Causing a growth of cells that produce keratin and result in the formation of horny tissue.

ker'atoid [kerato- + G. *eidos*, resemblance] 1. Horny. 2. Resembling corneal tissue.

keratol'ysis [kerato- + G. *lysis*, loosening] 1. Separation or loosening of the horny layer of the epidermis. 2. A disease

characterized by a shedding of the epidermis recurring at more or less regular intervals.

kerato'ma [kerato- + G. -*oma*, tumour] 1. Callosity. 2. A horny tumour.

ker'atomala'cia [kerato- + G. *malakia*, softness] Dryness with ulceration and perforation of the cornea, with absence of inflammatory reactions, occurring in cachectic children.

ker'atome Keratotome.

keratom'eter [kerato- + G. *metron*, measure] An instrument for measuring the curvature of the anterior corneal surface.

ker'atopachyder'ma [kerato- + G. *pachys*, thick, + *derma*, skin] A syndrome of congenital deafness with development of hyperkeratosis of the skin of the palms, soles, elbows, and knees in childhood, and with bandlike constrictions of the fingers; autosomal dominant inheritance.

keratop'athy [kerato- + G. *pathos*, suffering, disease] A noninflammatory dystrophy of the cornea, as distinguished from keratitis.

ker'atoplasty [kerato- + G. *plassō*, to form] Corneal graft; the removal of a portion of the cornea containing an opacity and the insertion in its place of a piece of the same size and shape.

ker'atoscope [kerato- + G. *skopeō*, to examine] An instrument marked with lines or circles by means of which the corneal reflex can be observed.

keratos'copy [kerato- + G. *skopeō*, to examine] Examination of the reflections from the anterior surface of the cornea to determine the character and amount of corneal astigmatism.

kerato'sis [kerato- + G. -*osis*, condition] Any lesion on the epidermis marked by the presence of circumscribed overgrowths of the horny layer.

    k. follicula'ris, A familial eruption, beginning usually in childhood, in which keratotic papules originating from both follicles and intrafollicular epidermis of the trunk, face, scalp, and axillae become crusted and verrucous.

ker'atotome A knife used for incising the cornea.

keratot'omy [kerato- + G. *tomē*, incision] Incision through the cornea.

kernic'terus [Ger. *kern*, kernel (nucleus), + *ikteros*, jaundice] A grave form of icterus neonatorum in which a yellow pigment and degenerative lesions are found in the intracranial grey matter.

ket'amine hydrochloride A parenterally administered anaesthetic that produces catatonia, profound analgesia, increased sympathetic activity, and little relaxation of skeletal muscles.

ke'toacido'sis Acidosis, *e.g.*, diabetic acidosis, caused by the enhanced production of ketone bodies.

ketogen'ic Giving rise to ketones in metabolism.

ketonu'ria Enhanced urinary excretion of ketone bodies.

keto'sis [ketone + -*osis*, condition] A condition characterized by the enhanced production of ketone bodies, as in diabetes mellitus.

17-ketoste'roids (17-KS) Nominally, any steroid with a ketone group on C-17; commonly used to designate urinary C_{19} steroidal metabolites of androgenic and adrenocortical hormones that possess this structural feature.

kid'ney [A.S. *cwith*, womb, belly, + *neere*, kidney] One of the two organs in the lumbar region that filters blood and excretes urine.

  artificial k., haemodialyser.

  floating k., wandering k., the abnormally mobile k. in nephroptosia.

  horseshoe k., union of the lower or occasionally the upper extremities of the two k.'s by a band of tissue extending across the vertebral column.

  polycystic k., polycystic disease of the kidneys; a progressive disease characterized by formation of multiple cysts of varying size scattered diffusely throughout both k.'s resulting in compression and destruction of k. parenchyma, usually with hypertension, gross haematuria, and uraemia. There are two major types: one with onset in infancy or early childhood, usually with autosomal recessive inheritance; one with onset in adulthood, with autosomal dominant inheritance.

kin-, kine- [G. *kinēsis*, movement] Prefix denoting movement. See also cine-.

kinaesthe'sia [G. *kinēsis*, motion, + *aisthēsis*, sensation] **1.** The sense perception of movement; the muscular sense. **2.** An illusion of moving in space.

kin'anaesthe'sia [G. *kinēsis*, motion, + *an-* priv. + *aisthēsis*, sensation] A disturbance of deep sensibility in which there is

inability to perceive either direction or extent of movement, the result being ataxia.

ki'nase 1. An enzyme catalysing the conversion of a proenzyme to an active enzyme. **2.** An enzyme catalysing the transfer of phosphate groups to form triphosphates (ATP).

kinesal'gia [G. *kinēsis*, motion, + *algos*, pain] Pain caused by muscular movement.

kinesi-, kinesio-, kineso- [G. *kinēsis*, motion] Combining forms relating to motion.

kine'siol'ogy [G. *kinēsis*, movement, + *-logos*, study] The science or the study of movement, and the active and passive structures involved.

kine'sis [G.] Motion; as a suffix, used to denote movement or activation.

kinet'ic [G. *kinētikos*] Relating to motion or movement.

ki'nin One of a number of widely differing substances having pronounced and dramatic physiological effects. Some are plant growth regulators; others are polypeptides, formed in blood by proteolysis secondary to some pathological process, that stimulate visceral smooth muscle but relax vascular smooth muscle, thus producing vasodilation.

Klebsiel'la A genus of bacteria (family Enterobacteriaceae) containing Gram-negative, encapsulated rods which occur singly, in pairs, or in short chains. The type species, *K. pneumoniae*, occurs in the intestinal tract of man and other animals, and also in association with several pathologic conditions.

kleptoma'nia [G. *kleptō*, to steal, + *mania*, insanity] A morbid tendency to steal.

knee [A.S. *cneōw*] **1.** Genu. **2.** A geniculum.

  housemaid's k., inflammation and swelling of the bursa anterior to the patella, due to traumatism in those who are much on their k.'s.

  locked k., a condition in which the k. is prevented from full motion by an internal derangement of the joint.

knee'cap Patella.

knit'ting Nonmedical term denoting the process of union of the fragments of a broken bone or of the edges of a wound.

knock-knee Genu valgum.

koilonych'ia [G. *koilos*, hollow, + *onyx* (*onych-*), nail] A malformation of the nails in which the outer surface is concave.

krauro'sis vul'vae [G. *krauros*, dry, brittle] Atrophy and shrinkage of the skin of the vagina and vulva, often accompanied by a chronic inflammatory reaction in the deeper tissues.

ku'ru [to shiver from fear or cold] A progressive, fatal form of spongiform encephalopathy endemic to certain Melanesian tribes of New Guinea and probably due to a slow virus.

kwashior'kor [African, red boy or displaced child] A disease seen in African natives, particularly very young children, due to severe protein deficiency; characterized by anaemia, oedema, pot belly, depigmentation of the skin, loss or change in hair colour, marked hypoalbuminaemia, and bulky stools containing undigested food.

ky'mograph [G. *kyma*, wave, + *graphō*, to record] An instrument for recording wave-like motions or modulation, as of variations in blood pressure.

kymog'raphy Use of the kymograph.

ky'phoscolio'sis Kyphosis combined with scoliosis.

kypho'sis [G. *kyphōsis*, hump-back, fr. *kyphos*, bent, hump-backed] A deformity of the spine characterized by extensive flexion.

kyphot'ic Relating to kyphosis.

L

l- Prefix indicating a chemical compound to be laevorotatory.

L- Prefix indicating a chemical compound to be structurally (sterically) related to L-glyceraldehyde.

la belle indifférence [Fr.] A naive, inappropriate lack of emotion or concern for the implications of one's disability, typically seen in persons with conversion hysteria.

la'bial Relating to the lips or any labium.

la'bile [L. *labilis*, liable to slip] Unstable or unsteady; not fixed; characterized by adaptability to alteration or modification.

labio- [L. *labium*, lip] Combining form relating to the lips.

la'bioglos'solaryn'geal [labio- + G. *glōssa*, tongue, + larynx] Relating to the lips, tongue, and larynx.

la'bioglos'sopharyn'geal [labio- + G. *glōssa*, tongue, + pharynx] Relating to the lips, tongue, and pharynx.

la'bioplasty [labio- + G. *plassō*, to form] Plastic operation on a lip.

la'bium, gen. **la'bii,** pl. **la'bia** [L.] [NA] A lip or lip-shaped structure.

l. ma'jus puden'di, pl. **la'bia majo'ra** [NA], one of two rounded folds of integument forming the lateral boundaries of the rima pudendi.

l. mi'nus puden'di, pl **la'bia mino'ra** [NA], one of two narrow longitudinal folds of mucous membrane enclosed in the cleft within the labia majora.

la'bia o'ris [NA], the lips bounding the cavity of the mouth.

la'bour [L. toil, suffering] The process of expulsion of the fetus and the placenta from the uterus. The **stages of l.** are: **first,** the period of dilation of the os uteri; **second,** that stage of expulsive effort, beginning with the complete dilation of the cervix and ending with delivery of the infant; **third** (placental stage), the period beginning with the delivery of the baby and ending with more or less complete expulsion of the placenta; **fourth,** the period after the birth of the baby during which the membranes and placenta are extruded.

la'brum, pl. **la'bra** [L.] [NA] An edge, rim, or lip-shaped structure.

lab'yrinth [G. *labyrinthos*] **1.** The internal or inner ear, composed of the semicircular ducts, vestibule, and cochlea. **2.** Any group of communicating cavities, cells, or canals.

lab'yrinthec'tomy [labyrinth + G. *ektomē*, excision] Excision of the labyrinth of the ear.

lab'yrinthi'tis Otitis interna; inflammation of the labyrinth (the internal ear), sometimes accompanied by vertigo.

lab'yrinthot'omy [labyrinth + G. *tomē*, incision] Incision into the labyrinth of the ear.

lac, gen. **lac'tis** [L. milk] [NA] **1.** Milk. **2.** Any whitish, milky looking liquid.

lacera'tion [L. *lacero*, pp. -*atus*, to tear to pieces] **1.** A torn or jagged wound, or an accidental cut wound. **2.** The process or act of tearing the tissues.

lac'rimal [L. *lacrima*, a tear] Relating to tears, their secretion, and the organs concerned therewith.

lacrima'tion [L. *lacrimatio*] Secretion of tears, especially in excess.

lac'rimator [L. *lacrima*, tear] An agent (such as tear gas) that irritates the eyes and produces tears.

lacrimot'omy [L. *lacrima*, tear, + G. *tomē*, incision] Incision of the lacrimal duct or sac.

lact-, lacti-, lacto- [L. *lac, lactis,* milk] Combining forms denoting milk.

lactacido'sis Acidosis due to increased lactic acid.

lac'tase β-Galactosidase.

lacta'tion [L. *lactatio,* suckle] **1.** The production of milk. **2.** The period following childbirth during which milk is formed in the breasts.

lac'teal 1. Relating to or resembling milk; milky. **2.** Chyle or lacteal vessel; a lymphatic vessel that conveys chyle from the intestine.

lac'tic acid A liquid obtained by the action of the lactic acid bacillus on milk or milk sugar; a caustic in concentrated form, used internally to prevent gastrointestinal fermentation.

lactif'erous [lacti- + L. *fero,* to bear] Yielding milk.

lac'tifuge [lacti- + L. *fugo,* to drive away] Causing the arrest of the secretion of milk.

Lac'tobacil'lus A genus of bacteria (family Lactobacillaceae) containing Gram-positive rods which vary from long and slender cells to short coccobacilli. They ferment glucose, and at least half of the end product is lactic acid. Some organisms are parasitic in many warm-blooded animals, including man, but rarely are pathogenic. The type species is *L. delbrueckii.*

lac'togen [lacto- + -*gen,* producing] An agent that stimulates milk production or secretion.

lactogen'esis [lacto- + G. *genesis,* production] Milk production.

lac'tose A disaccharide present in mammalian milk and obtained from cow's milk; occurs naturally as α- and β-forms.

lactosu'ria [lacto- + G. *ouron,* urine] Excretion of lactose in the urine.

lacu'na, pl. **lacu'nae** [L. a pit] **1.** [NA] A small space, cavity, or depression. **2.** A gap or defect. **3.** An abnormal space between the strata or between the cellular elements of the epidermis.

lacu'nar 1. Relating to a lacuna. **2.** Denoting a hiatus or temporary lack of manifestation in a symptom.

la'cus, pl. **la'cus** [L. lake] A small collection of fluid.

laevo- [L. *laevus,* left]. Prefix denoting left, toward or on the left side.

laevodo'pa L-Dopa; the biologically active form of dopa; an antiparkinsonian agent.

laevocar'dia [levo- + G. *kardia,* heart]. Situs inversus of the viscera but with the heart normally situated on the left.

lae'vorota'tion [laevo- + L. *rotare,* to turn]. **1.** A turning or twisting to the left; in particular, the counterclockwise twist given the plane of plane-polarized light by solutions of certain optically active substances. **2.** Sinistrotorsion.

laevoro'tatory Denoting laevorotation, or certain crystals or solutions capable of doing so. As a chemical prefix, usually abbreviated *l-*.

lagophthal'mia, lagophthal'mos [G. *lagōs,* hare, + *ophthalmos,* eye] A condition in which complete closure of the eyelids over the eyeball is difficult or impossible.

lake [A.S. *lacu,* fr. L. *lacus,* lake] **1.** Lacus. **2.** To cause blood plasma to become red as a result of the release of haemoglobin from the erythrocytes, as when the latter are suspended in water.

lal'ling [G. *laleō,* to chatter] A form of stammering in which the speech is almost unintelligible.

lamb'doid [lambda + G. *eidos,* resemblance] Resembling the Greek letter lambda (Λ or λ).

Lam'blia intestina'lis Old term for *Giardia lamblia.*

lamblia'sis Giardiasis.

lamel'la, pl. **lamel'lae** [L. dim. of *lamina,* plate, leaf] **1.** A thin sheet or layer, as occurs in compact bone. **2.** A preparation in the form of a medicated gelatin disc, used as a means of making local applications to the conjunctiva in place of solutions.

lamel'lar 1. Scaly; arranged in thin plates or scales. **2.** Relating to lamellae.

lam'ina, pl. **lam'inae** [L.] [NA] A thin plate or flat layer.

   l. ar'cus ver'tebrae [NA], l. of the vertebral arch; neurapophysis; the flattened posterior portion of the vertebral arch from which the spinous process extends.

   l. lim'itans cor'neae [NA], **(1)** a basement membrane lying between the outer layer of stratified epithelium and the substantia propria of the cornea; **(2)** a basement membrane between the substantia propria and the endothelial layer of the cornea.

lam'inagraph A tomographic technique whereby tissues above and below the level of a suspected lesion are blurred out to emphasize a specific area.

lam'inar **1.** Laminated; arranged in plates or laminae. **2.** Relating to any lamina.

laminec'tomy [l. *lamina*, layer, + G *ektome*, excision] Excision of a vertebral lamina; commonly used to denote removal of the posterior arch.

laminot'omy [L. *lamina*, layer, + G. *tome*, incision] Division of one or more vertebral laminae.

lanat'osides A, B, and **C.** The cardioactive precursor glycosides obtained from *Digitalis lanata.*

lance [L. *lancea*, a slender spear] **1.** To incise a part, as an abscess or boil. **2.** A lancet.

lan'cet [Fr. *lancette*] A surgical knife with a small, sharp-pointed, two-edged blade.

lan'cinating [L. *lancino*, pp -*atus*, to tear] Denoting a sharp cutting or tearing pain.

lan'olin [L. *lana*, wool, + *oleum*, oil] A purified, fatlike substance from the wool of sheep, containing not less than 25% and not more than 30% of water, used as a water-adsorbable ointment base.

lanu'go [L. down, wooliness; fr. *lana*, wool] [NA] Fine, soft, unmedullated fetal or embryonic hair with minute shafts and large papillae.

laparo- [G. *lapara*, flank, loins] Combining form denoting the loins or, less properly, the abdomen in general.

lap'aroscope [laparo- + G. *skopeo*, to view] Peritoneoscope.

laparos'copy Peritoneoscopy.

laparot'omy [laparo- + G. *tome*, incision] **1.** Incision into the loin. **2.** Coeliotomy.

lar'va, pl **lar'vae** [L. a mask] **1.** The wormlike form of an insect or helminth upon issuing from the egg. **2.** The young of fishes or amphibians, often differing in appearance from the adult.

lar'val **1.** Relating to larvae. **2.** Larvate.

lar'va mi'grans [L. *larva*, mask, + *migrare*, to transfer, migrate] A larval worm, typically a nematode, that wanders in the host tissues but does not develop to the adult stage; usually occurs in abnormal hosts that inhibit normal development of the parasite.

lar'vate [L. *larva*, mask] Masked or concealed; applied to a disease with undeveloped, absent, or atypical symptoms.

laryn'geal Relating to the larynx.

laryngec'tomy [laryngo- + G. *ektome*, excision] Excision of the larynx.

lar'yngemphrax'is [G. *emphraxis*, a stoppage] Laryngeal obstruction or closure.

laryn'ges [L.] Plural of larynx.

laryngis'mus [L. fr. G. *larynx*, + -*ismos*, -ism] Spasmodic narrowing or closure of the rima glottidis.

    l. strid'ulus, a spasmodic closure of the glottis, lasting a few seconds, followed by noisy inspiration.

laryngi'tis [laryngo- + G. -*itis*, inflammation] Inflammation of the mucous membrane of the larynx.

laryngo-, laryng- Combining forms relating to the larynx.

laryn'gocele [laryngo- + G. *kele*, hernia] An air sac communicating with the larynx through the ventricle, often bulging outward into the tissue of the neck, especially during coughing.

laryngofis'sure Operative opening into the larynx, generally through the midline.

laryngol'ogy [laryngo- + G. *logos*, study] The branch of medical science concerned with the larynx; the specialty of diseases of the larynx.

laryn'goparal'ysis Paralysis of the laryngeal muscles.

laryn'gopharyn'geal Relating to both larynx and pharynx or to the laryngopharynx.

laryngophar'ynx The part of the pharynx lying below the aperture of the larynx and behind the larynx, extending from the vestibule of the larynx to the oesophagus at the level of the inferior border of the cricoid cartilage.

laryn'goplasty [laryngo- + G. *plasso*, to form] Reparative or plastic surgery of the larynx.

laryn'goscope [laryngo- + G. *skopeo*, to inspect] Any of several types of illuminated hollow tubes used in examining or operating upon the interior of the larynx through the mouth.

laryn'gospasm Spasmodic closure of the glottic aperture.

laryn'gosteno'sis [laryngo- + G. *stenosis*, a narrowing] Stricture or narrowing of the lumen of the larynx.

laryngos'tomy [laryngo- + G. *stoma*, mouth] Establishment of a permanent opening from the neck into the larynx.

laryngot'omy [laryngo- + G. *tomē*, incision] Laryngofissure.

laryngotra'cheal Relating to both larynx and trachea.

laryn'gotrachei'tis Inflammation of both larynx and trachea.

laryng'otra'cheobronchi'tis An acute respiratory infection involving the larynx, trachea, and bronchi. See croup.

laryn'gotracheot'omy laryngo- + trachea + G. *tomē*, incision] An incision through the cricoid cartilage and the upper tracheal rings.

lar'ynx, pl. **laryn'ges** [Mod. L. fr. G.] [NA] The organ of voice production; the part of the respiratory tract, between the pharynx and the trachea, consisting of a framework of cartilages and elastic membranes housing the vocal folds and the muscles which control the position and tension of these elements.

la'ser [*light a* mplification by *s*timulated *e*mission of *r*adiation] A device that concentrates high energies into a narrow beam of visible, coherent (nonspreading), monochromatic light; used in surgery to cut and dissolve tissue.

las'situde [L. *lassitudo*, fr. *lassus*; weary] A sense of weariness.

la'tah [Malay, ticklish] A nervous affection characterized by an exaggerated physical response to being startled or to unexpected suggestion.

la'tency 1. The state of being latent. **2.** In conditioning, the period of apparent inactivity between the time the stimulus is presented and the moment a response occurs.

la'tent [L. *lateo*, pres. p. *latens* (-*ent*-), to lie hidden] Not manifest, but potentially discernible.

lat'eral [L. *lateralis*, lateral, fr. *latus*, side] **1.** On the side. **2.** Farther from the median or midsagittal plane. **3.** In dentistry, a position either right or left of the midsagittal plane.

lateral'ity In voluntary motor acts, preferential use of members of one side of the body through right or left dominance of the cerebral cortex; **crossed l.** is right dominance of some members and left dominance of others.

latero- [L. *lateralis*, lateral, fr. *latus*, side] Combining form meaning lateral, to one side, or relating to a side.

lat'erodevia'tion [latero- + L. *devio*, to turn aside, fr. *via*, a way] A bending or a displacement to one side.

laterover'sion [latero- + L. *verto*, pp. *versus*, to turn] A turning to one side or the other, denoting especially a malposition of the uterus.

Latrodec'tus [L. *lactro*, servant, robber, + G. *dēktēs*, a biter] A genus of relatively small spiders, the "widow" spiders, capable of inflicting highly poisonous, neurotoxic, antagonizing bites; they are responsible, along with *Loxosceles* (the brown spider), for most of the severe reactions from spider envenomation.

la'tus, gen. **lat'eris**, pl. **lat'era** [L.] Flank; the side of the body between the pelvis and the ribs.

lau'danum [G. *lēdanon*, a resinous gum] A tincture containing opium.

lavage' [Fr. from L. *lavo*, to wash] The washing out of a hollow cavity or organ by copious injections and rejections of fluid.

law [A.S. *lagu*] A principle or rule; a formula expressing a fact or number of facts common to a group of processes or actions. See also theorem.

    Bowditch's l., all or none l.; any stimulus, however feeble, that will excite a cardiac contraction will produce as powerful a contraction as the strongest stimulus; "minimal stimuli cause maximal pulsations."

    Boyle's l., at constant temperature, the volume of a given quantity of gas varies inversely with its absolute pressure.

    l. of excitation, a motor nerve responds, not to the absolute value, but to the alteration of value from moment to moment, of the electric current.

    Hilton's l., the nerve supplying a joint supplies also the muscles which move the joint and the skin covering the articular insertion of those muscles.

    l. of independent assortment, Mendel's second l.; different hereditary factors are assorted independently when the gametes are formed (modified by the restriction that linked genes do not assort independently).

    l. of inverse square, intensity of radiation is inversely proportional to the square of the distance from the source.

    Pascal's l., fluids at rest transmit pressure equally in every direction.

    l. of segregation, Mendel's first l.; factors that affect development retain their individuality from generation to generation, do not become contaminated when mixed in a hybrid, and become sorted out from one another when the gametes are formed.

lax′ative [L. *laxo*, pp. *-atus*, to slacken, relax] **1.** Mildly cathartic; having the action of loosening the bowels. **2.** A mild cathartic; a remedy that moves the bowels slightly without pain or violent action.

lay′er A sheet of some substance lying upon another and distinguished from it.

    germ l., one of the three primordial cell l.'s (ectoderm, endoderm, mesoderm) established in an embryo during gastrulation and the immediately following stages.

    still l., the l. of the blood stream next to the wall in the capillary vessels that flows slowly and transports the white blood cells.

lead A metallic element, symbol Pb, atomic no. 82, atomic weight 207.21.

lead The electrical connection for taking records by means of the electrocardiograph.

    bipolar l., a record obtained with two electrodes placed on different regions of the body, each electrode contributing significantly to the record.

    unipolar l.'s, those in which the exploring electrode is on the chest in the vicinity of the heart or on one of the limbs, whereas the other or indifferent electrode is the central terminal.

lec′ithin [G. *lekithos*, egg yolk] Phospholipids that, on hydrolysis, yield two fatty acid molecules and a molecule each of glycerophosphoric acid and choline; under the microscope, they appear as irregular elongated particles known as myelin forms; found in nervous tissue, especially in myelin sheaths, in egg yolk and as essential constituents of animal and vegetable cells.

leech [A.S. *laece*, physician; a leech] **1.** A bloodsucking aquatic annelid worm (genus *Hirudo*, class Hirudinea formerly used in medicine for local abstraction of blood. **2.** To treat medically by applying leeches.

leg The segment of the inferior limb between the knee and the ankle; commonly used to mean the entire inferior limb.

    milk l., *phlegmasia* alba dolens.

    restless l.'s, restless legs *syndrome*.

-legia [L. *legere*, to read] Suffix that properly relates to reading, as distinguished from the -lexis and -lexy (G. *legein*, *lexai*, to speak).

Legionel′la A genus of Gram-negative bacilli that includes the species *L. pneumophila*, the aetiologic agent of Legionnaires' disease.

legionello′sis Legionnaires' *disease*.

leio- [G. *leios*, smooth] Combining form meaning smooth.

leiomyo′ma [leio- + G. *mys*, muscle, + *-oma*, tumour] A benign neoplasm derived from smooth muscle.

lei′omyosarco′ma [leio- + myosarcoma] A malignant neoplasm derived from smooth muscle.

Leishma′nia [W. B. *Leishman*] A genus of digenetic, asexual, protozoan flagellates (family Trypanosomatidae) whose species (*l braziliensis*, *L. donovani*, *L. tropica*) are indistinguishable morphologically, but may be separated serologically, on the basis of their sandfly host, by geographic occurrence, and by clinical manifestations of infection (leishmaniasis).

leishmani′asis Infection with a species of *Leishmania* resulting in a clinically ill-defined group of diseases traditionally divided into three major types: visceral l. (kala azar), cutaneous l. (Old World l.), and mucocutaneous l. (American or New World l.). Each is clinically and geographically quite distinct, aetiologic agents are morphologically identical, and transmission is by various species of sandfly of the genus *Phlebotomus* or *Lutzomyia*.

lemnis′cus, pl. **lemnis′ci** [L. from G. *lēmniskos*, ribbon or fillet] [NA] A bundle of nerve fibres ascending from sensory nuclei in the spinal cord and rhombencephalon to the thalamus.

lens [L. a lentil] **1.** A piece of glass or other transparent substance, with one or both surfaces curved, used for convergence or divergence of light. **2.** [NA] A transparent biconvex cellular body lying between the iris and the vitreous, one of the refracting media of the eye.

    bifocal l., a l. in which one portion is suited for distant vision, the other for reading and near work.

    contact l., a l. that fits over the cornea in direct contact with the sclera or cornea; used to correct refractive errors.

    photochromic l., a light-sensitive spectacle l. that automatically darkens in sunlight and clears in reduced light.

lensec′tomy [lens + G. *ektomē*, excision] Removal of the lens, usually done by puncture incision through the ciliary disc in the course of vitrectomy.

lentic'ular [L. *lenticula,* a lentil] **1.** Relating to or resembling a lens of any kind. **2.** Of the shape of a lentil.

len'tiform Lens-shaped.

lenti'go, pl. **lentig'ines** [L. fr. *lens (lent-),* a lentil] A brown macule resembling a freckle, except that the border is usually regular and microscopic proliferation of rete ridges is present.

   malignant l., l. malig'na, Hutchinson's or melanotic freckle; a brown or black mottled, slowly enlarging lesion usually occurring on the face of older persons; malignant change is frequent, but the resulting melanomas are not highly malignant.

   senile l., liver spot; a variably pigmented l. occurring on exposed skin of older Caucasians.

leonti'asis [G. *leōn (leont-),* lion] The ridges and furrows on the forehead and cheeks of patients with advanced lepromatous leprosy, giving a leonine appearance.

lep'er [G. *lepra*] One who has leprosy.

lepid'ic [G. *lepis (lepid-),* scale, rind] Relating to scales or a scaly covering layer.

lep'rechaunism [Irish *leprechaun,* elf] A congenital disorder characterized by extreme growth retardation and emaciation, with grotesque elfin facies and large, low-set ears; autosomal recessive inheritance.

lepro'ma [G. *lepros,* scaly, + *-oma,* tumour] A circumscribed discrete focus of granulomatous inflammation caused by *Mycobacterium leprae.*

lepro'matous Pertaining to, or characterized by, the features of a leproma.

lep'romin An extract of tissue infected with *Mycobacterium leprae* used in skin tests to classify the stage of leprosy.

lep'rostat'ic Inhibiting the growth of *Mycobacterium leprae.*

lep'rosy [G. *lepra,* from *lepros,* scaly] **1.** A name given in Biblical times to various cutaneous diseases, especially those of a chronic or contagious nature, that probably embraced psoriasis and leucoderma. **2.** Hansen's disease; chronic granulomatous infection caused by *Mycobacterium leprae* (Hansen's bacillus) which occurs in two principal types: lepromatous and tuberculoid.

   lepromatous l., l. in which nodular cutaneous lesions are infiltrated, have ill-defined borders, and are bacteriologically positive, but the lepromin test is negative.

   tuberculoid l., cutaneous l., nodular l., a benign, stable, and resistant form in which the lepromin reaction is strongly positive and in which the lesions are erythematous, insensitive, infiltrated plaques with clear-cut edges.

-lepsis, -lepsy [G. *lēpsis,* seizure] Combining forms denoting seizure.

lepto- [G. *leptos,* slender, delicate] A combining form meaning light, slender, thin, or frail.

lep'tomenin'ges [lepto- + G. *mēninges,* membranes] Collective term denoting the soft membranes enveloping brain and spinal cord, the pia mater and arachnoidea mater.

lep'tomeningi'tis Pia-arachnitis; inflammation of the leptomeninges.

Leptospi'ra [lepto- + G. *speira,* a coil] A genus of aerobic bacteria (order Spirochaetales) containing thin, tightly coiled organisms; type species is *L. interrogans,* with over 100 parasitic or saprophytic serovars.

leptospiro'sis Infection with species of *Leptospira.*

Leptotrich'ia [lepto- + G. *thrix,* hair] A genus of Gram-negative bacteria that occur in the oral cavity; type species is *L. buccalis.*

les'bianism [G. *lesbios,* relating to the island of Lesbos] Homosexual practices between women.

le'sion [L. *laedo,* pp. *laesus,* to injure] **1.** A wound or injury. **2.** A pathologic change in the tissues. **3.** One of the individual points or patches of a multifocal disease.

le'thal [L. *letalis,* death] Pertaining to or causing death; denoting especially the causal agent.

leth'argy [G. *lēthargis,* drowsiness] A state of deep and prolonged unconsciousness from which one can be aroused but into which one immediately relapses.

leuc-, leuco-, leuk- [G. *leukos,* white] Combining forms meaning white.

leu'cine An essential amino acid in protein.

leu'cocyte [leuco- + G. *kytos,* cell] White blood cell; a type of cell formed in the myelopoietic, lymphoid, and reticular portions of the reticuloendothelial system in various parts of the body, and normally present in those sites and in the circulating blood. L.'s represent three lines of development from primitive ele-

ments: myeloid, lymphoid, and monocytic series. On the basis of features observed with
various methods of staining, cells of the myeloid series are frequently termed granular
l.'s, or granulocytes and consist of three distinct types: neutrophils, eosinophils, and basophils, based on the staining reactions of the
cytoplasmic granules.

basophilic l., a polymorphonuclear l.
characterized by many large, coarse, metachromatic granules that usually fill the cytoplasm and may almost mask the nucleus;
unique in that they usually do not occur in
increased numbers as the result of acute infectious disease, and their phagocytic qualities are probably not significant.

eosinophilic l., eosinophil; a polymorphonuclear l. characterized by many large or
prominent, refractile, cytoplasmic granules
fairly uniform in size and with nuclei usually
larger than those of neutrophils.

neutrophilic l., a neutrophilic granulo-
cyte, the most frequent of the polymorphonuclear l.'s, and also the most active phagocyte
among the various types of white blood cells.

leu'cocytol'ysis [leucocyte + G. *lysis,*
dissolution] Dissolution or lysis of leucocytes.

leucocyto'ma [leucocyte + G. *-oma,* tu-
mour] A fairly well circumscribed, nodular,
dense accumulation of leucocytes.

leucocytope'nia Leucopenia.

leucocyto'sis [leucocyte + G. *-osis,* con-
dition] An abnormally large number of leucocytes, as observed in acute infections.

eosinophilic l., eosinophilia; a form of
relative l. in which the greatest proportionate
increase is in the eosinophils.

relative l., an increased proportion of
one or more types of leucocytes in the circulating blood, without an actual increase in the
total number of white blood cells.

leucoder'ma An absence of pigment, partial or total, in the skin.

leucodys'trophy [leuco- + G. *dys,* bad,
+ *trophē,* nourishment] Degeneration of the
white matter of the brain characterized by
demyelination and glial reaction, probably related to defects of lipid metabolism.

globoid cell l., Krabbe's disease; a
metabolic encephalopathy of infancy with
rapidly progressive cerebral degeneration,
massive loss of myelin, severe astrocytic gli-
osis, and infiltration of the white matter with
characteristic multinucleate globoid cells;

metabolically, there is gross deficiency of
cerebrosidase (galactosylceramide β-galactosidase); autosomal recessive inheritance.

leu'coencephali'tis Encephalitis restricted to the white matter.

acute epidemic l., a disease characterized by acute onset of fever, followed by
convulsions, delirium, and coma, and associated with perivascular demyelination and
haemorrhagic foci in the CNS.

leu'coencephalop'athy [leuco- + G.
enkephalos, brain, + *pathos,* suffering] Leu-
codystrophy.

leu'coerythroblasto'sis Any anaemic condition resulting from space-occupying
lesions in the bone marrow; the circulating
blood contains immature cells of the granulocytic series and nucleated red blood cells,
frequently in numbers disproportionately
large in relation to the degree of anaemia.

leuco'ma [G. whiteness] A dense, opaque,
white opacity of the cornea.

leuconyc'hia [leuco- + G. *onyx,* nail] Occurrence of white spots or patches under the
nails, due to the presence of air bubbles
between the nail and its bed.

leucope'nia [leucocyte + G. *penia,* pov-
erty] Any situation in which the total number of
leucocytes in the circulating blood is less than
normal.

leucopla'kia [leuco- + G. *plax,* plate] A
disturbance of keratinization of mucous membrane, variously present as small opalescent
patches or as extensive leathery plaques, occasionally ulcerated; may be precancerous.

leu'copoie'sis [leuco- + G. *poiēsis,* a
making] Formation and development of the
various types of white blood cells.

leucorrhoe'a [leuco- + G. *rhoia,* flow] A
discharge from the vagina of white or yellowish viscid fluid containing mucus and pus.

leu'cosarco'ma A variant of malignant
lymphoma in which abnormal immature
forms of the lymphocytic series are found in
large numbers in the circulating blood in lymphosarcoma.

leu'cosarcomato'sis A condition characterized by numerous widespread nodules
or masses of lymphosarcoma, and the presence of similar cells in the circulating blood.

leuco'sis Abnormal proliferation of one or
more of the leucopoietic tissues.

leucot'omy [leuco- + G. *tomē*, a cutting] Incision into the white matter of the frontal lobe of the brain.

leuk- See leuc-, leuco-.

leukae'mia [leuk- + G. *haima*, blood] Progressive proliferation of abnormal leucocytes found in haemopoietic tissues, other organs, and usually in the blood in increased numbers; classified by dominant cell type, and by duration from onset to death: duration of **acute l.** is a few months and is associated with symptoms that suggest acute infection, with severe anaemia, haemorrhages, and slight enlargement of lymph nodes or spleen; duration of **chronic l.** exceeds one year, with a gradual onset of symptoms of anaemia or marked enlargement of spleen, liver, or lymph nodes.

　granulocytic l., l. characterized by an uncontrolled proliferation of myelopoietic cells in the bone marrow and in extramedullary sites, and presence of large numbers of immature and mature granulocytic forms in various tissues (and organs) and in the circulating blood.

　lymphocytic l., lymphoid l., lymphatic l., l. characterized by an uncontrolled proliferation and conspicuous enlargement of lymphoid tissue in various sites and occurrence of increased numbers of cells of the lymphocytic series in the circulating blood and in various tissues and organs.

　myelocytic, myelogenic, myelogenous, or **myeloid l.,** granulocytic l.

leukae'mic Pertaining to, or having the characteristics of, leukaemia.

leva'tor [L. a lifter] **1.** A surgical instrument for prying up the depressed part in a fracture of the skull. **2.** One of several muscles whose action is to raise the part into which it is inserted.

-lexis, -lexy [G. *legein, lexai,* to speak] Suffix that properly relates to speech, although often confused with -legia (L. *legere,* to read).

libid'inous [L. *libidinosus,* pleasure, desire, fr. *libet,* it pleases] Lascivious; erotic; invested with or arousing sexual desire or energy.

libi'do [L. lust] Conscious or unconscious sexual desire.

lice Plural of louse.

li'chen [G. *leichēn*] A discrete flat papule or an aggregate of papules giving a patterned configuration resembling lichens growing on rocks.

　l. pla'nus, eruption of flat-topped, shiny, violaceous papules on flexor surfaces, male genitalia, and buccal mucosa; may form linear groups.

li'chenifica'tion [lichen + L. *facio,* to make] Leathery induration and thickening of the skin with hyperkeratosis, due to a chronic inflammation caused by scratching or long-continued irritation.

lie The relation which the long axis of the fetus bears to that of the mother.

lien-, lieno- [L. *lien,* spleen] Combining form relating to the spleen. See splen-; spleno-.

li'en [L.] [NA] Spleen.

　l. accesso'rius [NA], accessory spleen; one of the small globular masses of splenic tissue occasionally found in the area of the spleen, in one of the peritoneal folds, or elsewhere.

　l. mo'bilis, floating *spleen.*

li'entery [G. *leienteria,* fr. *leios,* smooth, + *enteron,* intestine] Passage of undigested food in the stools.

life [A.S. *lif*] **1.** Vitality, the essential condition of being alive; the state of existence characterized by active metabolism. **2.** The existence of organisms.

life'-span 1. The duration of existence of an individual. **2.** The normal or average duration of existence of a given species.

lig'ament [L. *ligamentum,* a band] Ligamentum.

ligamen'tous Relating to or of the form or structure of a ligament.

ligamen'tum, pl. **ligamen'ta** [L. a band, tie] [NA] Ligament. **1.** A band or sheet of fibrous tissue connecting two or more bones, cartilages, or other structures, or serving as support for fasciae or muscles. **2.** A fold of peritoneum supporting any of the abdominal viscera. **3.** The cordlike remains of a fetal vessel or other structure that has lost its original lumen.

li'gand [L. *ligo,* to bind] **1.** An organic molecule attached to a central metal ion by multiple coordination bonds. **2.** An organic molecule attached to a tracer element.

li'gase Generic term for enzymes catalysing the joining of two molecules coupled with the breakdown of a pyrophosphate bond in ATP or a similar compound.

liga'tion [L. *ligatio*, fr. *ligo*, to bind] Application of a ligature.

tubal l., interruption of the continuity of the oviducts, by cutting, cautery, or a device, to prevent future conception.

lig'ature [L. *ligatura*, a band or tie] **1.** A thread, wire, etc. tied tightly around a structure to constrict it. **2.** A wire or other material used to secure an orthodontic attachment or tooth to an archwire.

light [A.S. *leōht*] That portion of electromagnetic radiations to which the retina is sensitive.

polarized l., l. in which, as a result of reflection or transmission through certain media, the vibrations are all in one plane, transverse to the ray, instead of in all planes.

light'ening The feeling of decreased abdominal distension during the later weeks of pregnancy following the descent of the fetal head into the pelvic inlet.

lig'nocaine hydrochloride A local anaesthetic possessing pronounced antiarrhythmic and anticonvulsant properties.

limb [A.S. *lim*] **1.** An extremity; a member; an arm or leg. **2.** A segment of any jointed structure.

phantom l., the sensation that an amputated l. is still present, often associated with painful paraesthesia.

lim'bic Relating to a limbus or to the limbic system.

lim'bus, pl. **lim'bi** [L. a border] [NA] The edge, border, or fringe of a part.

l. cor'neae [NA], sclerocorneal junction; the margin of the cornea overlapped by the sclera.

lime 1. Fruit of the l. tree, *Citrus medica* (family Rutaceae). **2.** Calcium oxide; CaO; an alkaline earth which on exposure to the atmosphere it becomes converted into calcium hydrate and calcium carbonate.

li'men, pl. **lim'ina** [L.] [NA] Threshold; the external opening of a canal.

lim'inal [L. *limen* (*limin-*), a threshold] **1.** Pertaining to a threshold. **2.** Pertaining to a stimulus just strong enough to excite a tissue.

linc'ture, linc'tus [L. *lingo*, pp. *linctus*, to lick] An electuary or a confection; originally a medical preparation taken by licking.

line [L. *linea*, a linen thread, a string] A mark, strip, or streak. See also linea.

cell l., in tissue culture, the cells growing in the first or later subculture from a primary culture.

gum l., the position of the margin of the gingiva in relation to the teeth in the dental arch.

isoelectric l., the base line of the electrocardiogram.

white l., *linea alba.*

lin'ea, gen. and pl. **lin'eae** [L.] [NA] A line; a long narrow mark, strip, or streak distinguished from the adjacent tissues by colour, texture, or elevation.

l. al'ba [NA], white line; a fibrous band running vertically the entire length of the centre of the anterior abdominal wall, receiving the attachments of the oblique and transverse abdominal muscles.

lin'gua, gen. and pl. **lin'guae** [L. tongue] [NA] **1.** Glossa; tongue; a mobile mass of muscular tissue covered with mucous membrane, occupying the cavity of the mouth, forming part of its floor, bearing the organ of taste, and assisting in mastication, deglutition, and articulation. **2.** Any tongue-like anatomical structure.

lin'gual 1. Glossal; relating to the tongue or any tongue lilia part. **2.** Next to or toward the tongue.

lin'gula, pl. **lin'gulae** [L. dim. of *lingua*, tongue] [NA] Any of several tongue-shaped processes.

lin'iment [L. fr. *lino*, to smear] A liquid preparation for external application or application to the gums, frequently applied by friction to the skin; used as counterirritants, rubefacients, anodynes, or cleansing agents.

link'age 1. Chemical covalent bond. **2.** Association of genes in inheritance, due to the fact that they are in the same chromosome pair; may be between genes on the same chromosome (cis-l.) or on opposite chromosomes (trans-l.) of a homologous pair.

sex l., a form of inheritance related to sex as a result of the gene concerned being carried on the X chromosome.

linole'ic acid [L. *linum*, flax, + *oleum*, oil] An unsaturated fatty acid essential in nutrition.

lip- See lipo-.

lip [A.S. *lippa*] **1.** Labium oris; one of the two muscular folds with an outer mucosa having a stratified squamous epithelial surface layer which bound the mouth anteriorly. **2.** Any liplike structure bounding a cavity or groove. See also labium; labrum.

cleft l., harelip; a congenital facial deformity of the l. (usually the upper) due to a mesodermal deficiency or failure of merging in one or more of the embryologic processes that form the l.; frequently associated with cleft alveolus and cleft palate.

lipae'mia [lipid + G. haima, blood] Presence of an abnormally large amount of lipids in the circulating blood.

alimentary l., postprandial l., relatively transient l. occurring after the ingestion of foods with a large content of fat.

l. retina'lis, a creamy appearance of the retinal blood vessels when the lipoids of the blood are over 5%.

lip'ase Any fat-splitting or lipolytic enzyme that cleaves a fatty acid residue from the glycerol residue in a neutral fat or a phospholipid.

lipec'tomy [lipo- + G. ektomē, excision] Surgical removal of fatty tissue, as in cases of adiposity.

lip'id [G. lipos, fat] "Fat-soluble," denoting substances extracted from animal or vegetable cells by nonpolar or "fat" solvents; an operational term describing a solubility characteristic, not a chemical substance.

lipidae'mia Lipaemia.

lipido'sis, pl. **lipido'ses** [lipid + G. -osis, condition] Inborn or acquired disorder of lipid metabolism.

cerebral l., cerebral sphingolipidosis.
cerebroside l., Gaucher's disease.
sphingomyelin l., Niemann-Pick disease.

lipo-, lip- [G. lipos, fat] Combining forms relating to fat or lipid.

lip'oblast [lipo- + G. blastos, germ] An embryonic fat cell.

lip'ocele [lipo- + G. kēlē, tumour] Presence of fatty tissue, without intestine, in a hernia sac.

lip'ochon'drodys'trophy Hurler's syndrome.

lip'ochrome [lipo- + G. chroma, colour] 1. A pigmented lipid. 2. Yellow pigments that seem to be identical to carotene and xanthophyll, and frequently found in the serum, skin, adrenal cortex, corpus luteum, and arteriosclerotic plaques, as well as in the liver, spleen, and adipose tissue.

lipodys'trophy [lipo- + G. dys-, bad, difficult, + trophē, nourishment] Defective metabolism of fat.

lipogen'esis [lipo- + G. genesis, production] Production of fat, either fatty degeneration or fatty infiltration; also applied to the normal deposition of fat or to the conversion of carbohydrate or protein to fat.

lip'oid [lipo- + G. eidos, appearance] 1. Resembling fat. 2. Former term for lipid.

lipoido'sis Presence of anisotropic lipoids in the cells.

lipol'ysis [lipo- + G. lysis, dissolution] The splitting up (hydrolysis), or chemical decomposition, of fat.

lipo'ma [lipo- + G. -oma, tumour] A benign neoplasm of adipose tissue, composed of mature fat cells.

lipo'matoid Resembling a lipoma, said of accumulations of adipose tissue not thought to be neoplastic.

lipomato'sis Adiposis.

lipo'matous Pertaining to, manifesting the features of, or characterized by the presence of a lipoma.

lipopro'tein Complexes or compounds containing lipid and protein, the form of lipids in plasma. Plasma l.'s migrate electrophoretically with the α- and β-globulins, but are presently characterized by their flotation constants (densities) as follows: chylomicra (1.006), very low density (1.006–1.019), low density (1.019–1.063), high density (1.063–1.21), very high density (1.21); the last four are often abbreviated as VLD, LD, HD, VHD (followed by L for lipoprotein).

liposarco'ma [lipo- + G. sarx, flesh, + -oma, tumour] A malignant neoplasm consisting chiefly of immature, anaplastic lipoblasts of varying sizes (including giant forms), with bizarre nuclei and vacuoles of varying sizes in the cytoplasm, usually in association with a rich network of capillaries.

lipo'sis [lipo- + G. -osis, condition] 1. Adiposis. 2. Fatty infiltration, neutral fats being present in the cells.

lip'osuction Removal of subcutaneous fat by high-vacuum pressure; used in body contouring.

lip'otrop'ic 1. Pertaining to substances preventing or correcting the fatty liver of choline deficiency. 2. Relating to lipotropy.

lip'otropy [lipo- + G. tropē, turning] 1. Affinity of basic dyes for fatty tissue. 2. Prevention of accumulation of fat in the liver. **3.** Affinity of nonpolar substances for each other.

lip'ping Formation of a liplike structure, as at the articular end of a bone in osteoarthritis.

lipu'ria [lipo- + G. *ouron*. urine] Excretion of lipid in the urine.

liquefa'cient [L. *lique-facio*, pres. p. *-faciens*, to make fluid] Making liquid; causing a solid to become liquid.

liquefac'tion [see liquefacient] The act of becoming liquid; change from a solid to a liquid form.

liq'uid [L. *liquidus*] **1.** Flowing. **2.** An inelastic fluid, like water, that is neither solid nor gaseous.

liq'uor [L.] **1.** Any liquid or fluid. **2.** A term used for certain body fluids. **3.** Pharmacopoeial term for any aqueous solution (not a decoction or infusion) of a nonvolatile substance and for aqueous solutions of gases.

Liste'ria [Joseph *Lister*] A genus of parasitic bacteria (family Corynebacteriaceae) containing small, coccoid, Gram-positive rods; found in the faeces of man and other animals, on vegetation, and in silage. The type species is *L. monocytogenes*.

lith'agogue [litho- + G. *agōgos*, a drawing forth] Causing the dislodgment or expulsion of calculi, especially urinary calculi.

lithec'tomy [litho- + G. *ektomē*, excision] Lithotomy.

lithi'asis [litho- + G. *-iasis*, condition] Formation of calculi of any kind, especially of biliary or urinary calculi.

lith'ium [Mod. L. fr G. *lithos*, a stone] An element of the alkali metal group, symbol Li, atomic no. 3, atomic weight 6.940; some of its salts are used medicinally.

litho-, lith- [G. *lithos*, stone] Combining forms relating to a stone or calculus, or to calcification.

lith'oclast [litho- + G. *klastos*, broken] Lithotrite.

lithogen'esis [litho- + G. *genesis*, production] Formation of calculi.

litholapax'y [litho- + G. *lapaxis*, an emptying out] Crushing of a stone in the bladder and washing out the fragments through a catheter.

lithol'ysis [litho- + G. *lysis*, dissolution] Dissolution of urinary calculi.

lith'onephri'tis Interstitial nephritis associated with calculus formation.

lith'onephrot'omy [litho- + G. *nephros*, kidney, + *tomē*, incision] Incision of the kidney for the removal of a calculus.

lithopae'dion [litho- + G. *paidion*, small child] A retained fetus, usually extrauterine, that has become calcified.

lithot'omy [litho- + G. *tomē*, incision] Cutting for stone; surgical removal of a calculus, especially a vesical calculus.

lith'otripsy [litho- + G. *tripsis*, a rubbing] Crushing of a stone in the bladder or urethra.

lith'otrite [litho- + G. *tero*, pp. *tritus*, to rub] An instrument used to crush a stone in the bladder or urethra.

lithure'sis [litho- + G. *ourēsis*, urination] Passage of gravel in the urine.

lit'mus A blue colouring matter obtained from *Roccella tinctoria* and other species of lichens, the principal component of which is azolitmin; used as an indicator (reddened by acids and turned blue by alkalies).

live'do [L. lividness, fr. *liveo*, to be black and blue] A bluish discoloration of the skin, either in limited patches or general.

liv'er [A.S. *lifer*] Hepar; the largest gland of the body, lying beneath the diaphragm in the right hypochondrium and upper part of the epigastrium; it secretes the bile and is also of importance in both carbohydrate and protein metabolism.

liv'id [L. *lividus*, being black and blue] Having a black and blue or a leaden or ashy grey colour, as in discoloration from a contusion, congestion, or cyanosis.

load A departure from normal body content, as of water, salt, or heat; positive l.'s are quantities in excess of the normal, negative l.'s are deficits.

Loa loa The African eye worm, a species of the family Onchocercidae (superfamily Filarioidea) indigenous to the western part of equatorial Africa and the causal agent of loiasis; man is the only known definitive host, and parasites are transmitted by *Chrysops* or tabanid flies.

lo'bar Relating to any lobe.

lo'bate **1.** Divided into lobes. **2.** Lobe-shaped.

lobe [G. *lobos*, lobe] **1.** Lobus. **2.** A rounded projecting part, as the l. of the ear. See also lobule; lobulus. **3.** One of the larger divisions of the crown of a tooth, formed from a distinct point of calcification.

    frontal l., *lobus* frontalis cerebri.

occipital l., *lobus* occipitalis cerebri.

parietal l., *lobus* parietalis cerebri.

temporal l., *lobus* temporalis.

lobec'tomy [G. *lobos*, lobe, + *ektomē*, excision] Excision of a lobe of any organ or gland.

lobot'omy [G. *lobos*, lobe, + *tomē*, a cutting] **1.** Incision into a lobe. **2.** Division of one or more nerve tracts in a lobe of the cerebrum.

lob'ular Relating to a lobule.

lob'ule Lobulus.

lob'ulus, gen. and pl. **lob'uli** [Mod. L. dim. of *lobus*, lobe] [NA] A small lobe or subdivision of a lobe.

lo'bus, gen. and pl. **lo'bi** [LL. fr G. *lobos*] [NA] Lobe; one of the subdivisions of an organ or other part, bounded by fissures, connective tissue, septa, or other structural demarcations.

  l. fronta'lis cer'ebri [NA], frontal lobe; the portion of each cerebral hemisphere anterior to the central sulcus.

  l. occipita'lis cer'ebri [NA], occipital lobe; the posterior, somewhat pyramidal part of each cerebral hemisphere.

  l. parieta'lis cer'ebri [NA], parietal lobe; the middle portion of each cerebral hemisphere, separated from the fontal lobe by the central sulcus, from the temporal lobe by the lateral sulcus, and from the occipital lobe only partially by the parietooccipital sulcus on its medial aspect.

  l. poste'rior hypophys'eos [NA], neurohypophysis; the posterior lobe of the hypophysis. See hypophysis.

  l. tempora'lis [NA], temporal lobe; the lowest of the major subdivisions of the cortical mantle, forming the posterior two-thirds of the ventral surface of the cerebral hemisphere, separated from the frontal and parietal lobes above it by the fissure of Sylvius and arbitrarily delineated from the occipital lobe with which it is continuous posteriorly.

lo'cal [L. *localis*, fr. *locus*, place] Having reference or confined to a limited part; not general or systemic.

lo'caliza'tion **1.** Limitation to a definite area. **2.** The reference of a sensation to its point of origin. **3.** The determination of the location of a morbid process.

lo'cator An instrument or apparatus for finding the position of a foreign object in tissue.

lo'chia [G. neut. pl. of *lochios*, relating to childbirth, fr. *lochos*, childbirth] The discharge from the vagina of mucus, blood, and tissue debris, following childbirth.

lochiome'tra [G. *mētra*, womb] Distension of the uterus with retained lochia.

lock'jaw Trismus.

locomo'tor, locomo'tive [L. *locus*, place, + L. *moveo*, pp. *motus*, to move] Relating to locomotion, or movement from one place to another.

loc'ulate Containing numerous loculi.

locula'tion **1.** A loculate region in an organ or tissue, or a loculate structure formed between surfaces of organs, mucous or serous membranes, and so on. **2.** The process that results in the formation of a loculus or loculi.

loc'ulus, pl. **loc'uli** [L. dim. of *locus*, place] A small cavity or chamber.

lo'cus, pl. **lo'ci** [L.] A place; usually, a specific site.

-logia **1.** [G. *logos*, discourse, treatise] Suffix expressing in a general way the study of the subject noted in the body of the word, or a treatise on the same; also -logy, or, with the connecting vowel, -ology. **2.** [G. *legō*, to collect] A suffix signifying collecting or picking.

logo-, log- [G. *logos*, word, discourse] Combining forms relating to speech, or words.

logople'gia [logo- + G. *plēgē*, stroke] Paralysis of the organs of speech.

logorrhoe'a [logo- + G. *rhoia*, a flow] Garrulousness.

-logy See -logia.

loi'asis A chronic disease caused by infection with *Loa loa*, which provokes hyperaemia and exudation of fluid, and a "creeping" sensation in the tissues with intense itching.

loin [Fr. *longe*; E. *lumbus*] Lumbus.

loop [M.E. *loupe*] **1.** A curve or complete bend in a cord or other cylindrical body, forming an oval or circular ring. See also ansa.

  nephronic l., Henle'a l., the U-shaped part of the nephron extending from the proximal to the distal convoluted tubules and consisting of descending and ascending limbs.

lordo'sis [G. *lordōsis*, a bending backward] An abnormal extension deformity: anteroposterior curvature of the spine, generally lumbar with the convexity looking anteriorly.

lo'tion [L. *lotio*, a washing, fr. *lavo*, to wash] Wash; a class of pharmacopoeial preparations that are liquid suspensions or dispersions intended for external application.

loupe [Fr.] A magnifying lens.

louse pl. **lice** [A.S. *lūs*] Common name for members of the ectoparasitic insect orders Anoplura (sucking lice) and Mallophaga (biting lice).

loz'enge [Fr. *losange*, from *lozangé*, rhombic] Troche.

lucid'ity [L. *lucidus*, clear] Clarity, especially mental clarity.

lu'es [L. pestilence] A plague, or pestilence; specifically, syphilis.

luet'ic Syphilitic.

lumba'go [L. fr. *lumbus*, loin] Lumbar rheumatism; pain in mid and lower back; a descriptive term not specifying cause.

lum'bar [L. *lumbus*, a loin] Relating to the loins, or the part of the back and sides between the ribs and the pelvis.

lumbocos'tal [L. *lumbus*, loin, + *costa*, rib] Relating to the lumbar and the hypochondriac regions.

lumboin'guinal [L. *lumbus*, loin, + *inguen* (inguin-), groin] Relating to the lumbar and the inguinal regions.

lumbosa'cral Relating to the lumbar vertebrae and the sacrum.

lum'bricide [L. *lumbricus*, worm, + *caedo*, to kill] An agent that kills lumbricoid (intestinal) worms.

lum'bricus [L. earthworm] Common name for *Ascaris lumbricoides*.

lum'bus gen. and pl. **lum'bi** [L.] [NA] Loin; the part of the side and back between the ribs and the pelvis.

lu'men pl. **lu'mina** [L. light, window] The space in the interior of a tubular structure, such as an artery or the intestine.

lumpec'tomy Tylectomy.

lu'nar [L. *luna*, moon] **1.** Relating to the moon or to a month. **2.** Semilunar: resembling the moon in shape, especially a half moon.

lung [A.S. *lungen*] Either of the organs of respiration, occupying the cavity of the thorax, in which aeration of the blood takes place; the right l. is slightly larger than the left and is divided into three lobes (upper, middle, and lower or basal), whereas the left has but two lobes (upper and lower or basal).

black l., a form of pneumoconiosis common in coal miners; characterized by deposit of carbon particles in the lung.

farmer's l., an occupational disease characterized by fever and dyspnoea, caused by inhalation of organic dust from mouldy hay containing spores of actinomycetes and certain true fungi.

iron l., Drinker *respirator*.

miner's l., anthracosis.

lu'nula, pl. **lu'nulae** [L. dim. of *luna*, moon] **1.** [NA] The pale arched area at the proximal portion of the nail plate. **2.** A small semilunar structure.

lu'pus [L. wolf] A term originally used to depict erosion (as if gnawed) of the skin, now used with modifying terms designating various diseases.

systemic l. erythemato'sus (S.L.E.), an inflammatory connective tissue disease with variable features, frequently including fever, weakness and fatigability, joint pains or arthritis resembling rheumatoid arthritis, diffuse erythematous skin lesions on the face, neck, or upper extremities, with liquefaction degeneration of the basal layer and epidermal atrophy, lymphadenopathy, pleurisy or pericarditis, glomerular lesions, anaemia, hyperglobulinaemia, a positive L.E. cell test, and other evidence of an autoimmune phenomenon.

l. vulga'ris, cutaneous tuberculosis with characteristic nodular lesions on the face, particularly about the nose and ears.

lu'teal [L. *luteus*, saffron-yellow] Relating to the corpus luteum.

lu'teiniza'tion Transformation of the mature ovarian follicle and its theca interna into a corpus luteum after ovulation; the formation of luteal tissue.

lutro'pin Luteinizing *hormone*.

Lutzomy'ia A genus of New World sandflies or bloodsucking midges (family Psychodidae) that serve as vectors of leishmaniasis and Oroyo fever; formerly combined with the Old World sandfly genus *Phlebotomus*.

luxa'tion [L. *luxatio*] **1.** Dislocation. **2.** In dentistry, the dislocation or displacement of the condyle in the temporomandibular fossa, or of a tooth from the alveolus.

lying-in 1. Confinement. **2.** Relating to childbirth.

lymph- See lympho-.

lymph [L. *lympha*, clear spring water] A transparent, sometimes faintly yellow and slightly opalescent fluid that carries varying numbers of white blood cells (chiefly lymphocytes) and a few red blood cells, is collected from the tissues throughout the body, flows in the lymphatic vessels (through the lymph nodes), and is eventually added to the venous blood circulation.

lym'phadenec'tomy [lymphadeno- + G. *ektomē*, excision] Excision of lymph nodes.

lym'phadeni'tis [lymphadeno- + G. *-itis*, inflammation] Inflammation of one or more lymph nodes.

lymphadeno-, lymphaden- [L. *lympha*, spring water, + G. *adēn*, gland] Combining forms relating to the lymph nodes.

lym'phadenog'raphy [lymphadeno- + G. *graphō*, to write] Radiography after opaque (iodized) oil is injected into the centre of an enlarged lymph node.

lym'phadeno'ma [lymphadeno- + G. *-oma*, tumour] **1.** Obsolete term for an enlarged lymph node. **2.** Infrequently used term for Hodgkin's disease.

lym'phadenop'athy [lymphadeno- + G. *pathos*, suffering] Any disease process affecting lymph nodes.

lym'phangiec'tasis,
lym'phangiecta'sia [lymphangio- + G. *ektasis*, a stretching] Dilation of the lymphatic vessels.

lym'phangii'tis Lymphangitis.

lymphangio-, lymphangi- [L. *lympha*, spring water, + G. *angeion*, vessel] Combining forms relating to the lymphatic vessels.

lym'phangiog'raphy [lymphangio- + G. *graphō*, to write] Radiographic visualization of lymph vessels following injection of a contrast medium.

lym'phangio'ma [lymphangio- + G. *-oma*, tumour] A circumscribed nodule or mass of lymphatic vessels or channels that vary in size, are frequently greatly dilated, and are lined with normal endothelial cells; present at birth, or shortly thereafter, and probably represent anomalous development of lymphatic vessels rather than true neoplasms.

lym'phangiot'omy [lymphangio- + G. *tomē*, incision] Incision of lymphatic vessels.

lymphangi'tis [lymphangio- + G. *-itis*, inflammation] Inflammation of the lymphatic vessels.

lymphat'ic [L. *lymphaticus*, frenzied; Mod. L. use, of or for lymph] Pertaining to lymph, a vascular channel that transports lymph, or a lymph node.

lympho-, lymph- [L. *lympha*, spring water] Combining forms relating to lymph.

lym'phoblast [lympho- + G. *blastos*, germ] A young immature cell that matures into a lymphocyte.

lymphoblas'tic Pertaining to the production of lymphocytes.

lym'phoblasto'ma [lymphoblast + G. *-oma*, tumour] A form of malignant lymphoma in which the chief cells are lymphoblasts.

lym'phocyte [lympho- + G. *kytos*, cell] A white blood cell formed in lymphoid tissue; in normal adults, l.'s make up approximately 22 to 28% of the total number of leucocytes in the circulating blood.

  B l., B cell; an immunologically important l. that is not thymus-dependent, is of short life, and is responsible for the production of immunoglobulins.

  T l., T cell; an immunologically important l. that is thymocytic-derived, is of long life (months to years) and is responsible for delayed-type (cell-mediated) sensitivity.

lym'phocythae'mia Lymphocytosis.

lymphocyt'ic Pertaining to or characterized by lymphocytes.

lym'phocytope'nia Lymphopenia.

lym'phocyto'sis A form of actual or relative leucocytosis in which there is an increase in the number of lymphocytes.

lymphoede'ma [lymph + G. *oidēma*, a swelling] Swelling (especially in subcutaneous tissues) as a result of obstruction of lymphatic vessels or lymph nodes and the accumulation of large amounts of lymph in the affected region.

lym'phogranulo'ma 1. Old nonspecific term referring to a few basically dissimilar diseases in which the pathologic processes result in granulomas or granuloma-like lesions, especially in various groups of lymph nodes (which then become conspicuously enlarged). **2.** Old term for Hodgkin's disease.

  venereal l., l. vene'reum, a venereal infection usually caused by *Chlamydia*, and characterized by a transient genital ulcer and inguinal adenopathy in the male; in the female, perirectal nodes are involved and rectal stricture is a common occurrence.

lym'phoid [lympho- + G. *eidos*, appearance] **1.** Resembling lymph or lymphatic tissue, or pertaining to the lymphatic system. **2.** Adenoid (1).

lym'phokine'sis [lympho- + G. *kinēsis*, movement] **1.** Circulation of lymph in the lymphatic vessels and through the lymph nodes. **2.** Movement of lymph in the semicircular canals.

lympho'ma [lympho- + G. suffix *-oma*, tumour] General term for ordinarily malignant neoplasms of lymph and reticuloendothelial tissues which present as apparently circumscribed solid tumours composed of cells that appear primitive or resemble lymphocytes, plasma cells, or histiocytes; classified by cell type, degrees of differentiation, and nodular or diffuse pattern.

   Burkitt's l., a form of malignant l. frequently involving facial bones, ovaries, and abdominal lymph nodes, which are infiltrated by undifferentiated stem cells with scattered pale macrophages containing nuclear debris.

   nodular l., Brill-Symmers disease, malignant l. characterized by nodules resembling normal lymphoid follicles consisting of small lymphocytoid cells or with variable numbers of larger histiocyte-like cells.

lym'phomato'sis Any condition characterized by the occurrence of multiple, widely distributed sites of involvement with lymphoma.

lympho'matous Pertaining to or characterized by lymphoma.

lymphope'nia [lympho- + G. *penia*, poverty] A reduction, relative or absolute, in the number of lymphocytes in the circulating blood.

lym'phopoie'sis [lympho- + G. *poiesis*, a making] Formation of lymphocytes.

lym'phosarco'ma [lympho- + G. *sarkōma*, sarcoma] A diffuse lymphocytic lymphoma.

lymphosta'sis [lympho- + G. *stasis*, a standing still] Obstruction of the normal flow of lymph.

lyo- [G. *lyō*, to loosen, dissolve] Combining form relating to dissolution. See also lyso-.

lyoph'iliza'tion Freeze-drying; the process of isolating a solid substance from solution by freezing the solution and evaporating the ice under the vacuum.

ly'pressin Vasopressin containing lysine in position 8; an antidiuretic and vasopressor hormone.

lys- See lyso-.

ly'sate The material (cellular debris and fluid) produced by lysis.

lyser'gic acid diethylam'ide (LSD) A derivative of D-lysergic acid, a cleavage product of alkaline hydrolysis of ergot alkaloids; a hallucinogen and serotonin antagonist.

ly'sin **1.** A specific complement-fixing antibody that acts destructively on cells and tissues; various types are designated in accordance with the form of antigen that stimulates its production. **2.** Any substance that causes lysis.

lysinae'mia Increased concentration of lysine in the blood, associated with mental and physical retardation.

ly'sine (Lys) An α-amino acid found in many proteins; distinguished by an ε-amino group.

ly'sis [G. dissolution or loosening] **1.** Gradual subsidence of the symptoms of an acute disease, a form of curative process, distinguished from crisis. **2.** Destruction of red blood cells, bacteria, and other antigens, by a specific lysin.

lyso-, lys- [G. *lysis*, a loosening or dissolution] Combining forms relating to lysis, or dissolution. See also lyo-.

ly'sosome [lyso- + G. *soma*, body] A cytoplasmic, membrane-bound particle, 0.5 μm or less in diameter, containing hydrolysing enzymes.

ly'oozyme An enzyme destructive to cell walls of certain bacteria.

Lys'savirus A genus of viruses (family Rhabdoviridae) that includes the rabies virus group.

lyt'ic Pertaining to lysis.

M

macera'tion [L. *macero*, pp. *-atus*, to soften by soaking] **1.** Softening by the action of a liquid. **2.** Softening of tissues after death by nonputrefactive (sterile) autolysis.

macro-, macr- [G. *makros*, large] Combining form meaning large or long. See also mega-, megalo-.

macrocar'dia Cardiomegaly.

macrochei'lia, **macrochi'lia**
[macro- + G. *cheilos*, lip] **1.** Abnormally enlarged lips. **2.** Cavernous lymphangioma of the lip, a permanent swelling of the lip resulting from the presence of greatly distended lymphatic spaces.

macrochei'ria, **macrochi'ria**
[macro- + G. *cheir*, hand] Abnormally large hands.

macrocra'nium An enlarged skull, especially the bones containing the brain, as seen in hydrocephalus.

mac'rocyte [macro- + G. *kytos*, a hollow (cell)] A large erythrocyte, such as those observed in pernicious anaemia.

mac'rocythae'mia [macrocyte + G. *haima*, blood] Occurrence of unusually large numbers of macrocytes in the circulating blood.

macrocyto'sis [macrocyte + G. *-osis*, condition] Macrocythaemia.

macrodon'tia The state of having abnormally large teeth.

mac'roglos'sia [macro- + G. *glōssa*, tongue] Enlargement of the tongue.

macrognath'ia [macro- + G. *gnathos*, jaw, + *-ia*, condition] Enlargement or elongation of the jaw.

macromas'tia [macro- + G. *mastos*, breast] Abnormally large breasts.

macrome'lia [macro- + G. *melos*, limb] Abnormally large size of one or more of the extremities.

macromol'ecule A molecule of colloidal size, notably proteins, nucleic acids, and polysaccharides.

mac'rophage [macro- + G. *phagein*, to eat] Any large amoeboid mononuclear phagocytic cell, regardless of origin.

macrophthal'mia [macro- + G. *ophthalmos*, eye] Megalophthalmus.

macroscop'ic Visible to the naked eye.

macrosto'mia [macro- + G. *stoma*, mouth] Abnormally large size of the mouth.

macro'tia [macro- + G. *ous*, ear, + *-ia*, condition] Excessive enlargement of the auricle.

mac'ula, pl. **mac'ulae** [L. a spot]; macule. **1.** [NA] A small spot, perceptibly different in colour from the surrounding tissue. **2.** A small, discoloured patch or spot on the skin, neither elevated above nor depressed below the skin's surface.

m. lu'tea, m. ret'inae [NA], an oval area of the sensory retina, temporal to the optic disc, corresponding to the posterior pole of the eye; at its centre is the fovea centralis, which contains only retinal cones.

mac'ular, mac'ulate 1. Relating to or marked by macules. **2.** Denoting the retina, especially the macula retinae.

mac'ule [L. *macula*, spot] Macula.

mac'ulocer'ebral Denoting a type of nervous disease marked by degenerative lesions in both the retina and the brain.

mac'ulopap'ule A lesion with a sessile base, that slopes from a papule in the centre.

maculop'athy Any pathological condition of the macula lutea.

Madurel'la [*Madura*, India] A genus of the Fungi Imperfecti, including a number of species that cause maduromycosis, and two species, *M. grisea* and *M. mycetomi*, that cause mycetoma.

madur'omyco'sis A type of mycetoma caused by a varied group of filamentous or true fungi and characterized by the formation of tumefactions and sinuses, from which serosanguineous or "oily" exudate drains (containing characteristic granules of variable colours).

magne'sia [see magnesium] Magnesium oxide.

magne'sium [Mod. L. fr. G. *Magnēsia*, a region in Thessaly] A mineral element, symbol Mg, atomic no. 12, atomic weight 24.31, oxidizing to the alkaline earth magnesia; many of its salts are used medicinally.

m. sulphate, Epsom salts; the active ingredient of most of the natural laxative waters, and a promptly acting cathartic particularly useful in certain poisonings; when applied locally, it has anti-inflammatory action.

mal [Fr. fr. L. *malum*, an evil] A disease or disorder.

grand m., generalized *epilepsy*.

m. de mer, seasickness.

petit m., absence.

mal- [L. *malus*, bad] Combining form meaning ill or bad.

mal'absorp'tion Imperfect, inadequate or otherwise disordered gastrointestinal absorption.

mala'cia [G. *malakia*, a softness] A softening or loss of consistency and contiguity in any of the organs or tissues. Also used as combining form in suffix position.

mal'adjust'ment In the mental health professions, an inability to cope with the problems and challenges of everyday living.

mal'ady [Fr. maladie, illness] Disease; illness; especially a chronic, usually fatal, disease.

malaise' [Fr. discomfort] A feeling of general discomfort; an out-of-sorts feeling.

malalign'ment Displacement of a tooth or teeth from a normal position in the dental arch.

ma'lar Relating to the cheek or cheek bones.

malar'ia [It. malo (fem. mala), bad, + aria, air, referring to the old theory of the miasmatic origin of the disease] A disease caused by the presence of the sporozoan Plasmodium in human or other vertebrate red blood cells, and transmitted to humans by the bite of an infected female mosquito of the genus Anopheles, that previously sucked the blood from a person with m.

falciparum m., m. caused by Plasmodium falciparum; 48-hr malarial paroxysms of severe form occur with acute cerebral, renal, or gastrointestinal manifestations in severe cases, chiefly caused by the large number of red blood cells affected and the tendency for infected red cells to become sticky and clump, blocking capillaries.

malariae m., quartan m., m. with paroxysms that recur every 72 hours or every fourth day (reckoning the day of the paroxysm as the first); due to the schizogony and invasion of new red blood corpuscles by Plasmodium malariae.

vivax m., tertian m., m. with paroxysms that recur every 48 hours or every third day (reckoning the day of the paroxysm as the first); the fever is induced by release of merozoites and their invasion of new red blood corpuscles.

malar'ial Pertaining to or affected with malaria.

Malasse'zia [L. C. Malassez] A genus of fungi. M. furfur causes tinea versicolor (pityriasis versicolor).

male [L. masculus, fr. mas, male] **1.** In zoology, denoting the sex to which those belong that produce spermatozoa; an individual of the male sex. **2.** Masculine.

mal'erup'tion Faulty eruption of teeth.

mal'forma'tion Failure of proper or normal development; a primary structural defect

that results from a localized error of morphogenesis.

mal'function Disordered, inadequate or abnormal function.

malig'nant [L. maligno, pres. p. -ans (ant-), to do anything maliciously] **1.** Resistant to treatment; occurring in severe form, and frequently fatal; tending to become worse and lead to an ingravescent course. **2.** In reference to a neoplasm, having the property of locally invasive and destructive growth and metastasis.

malin'ger [Fr. malingre, poor, weakly] To sham; to feign an illness, usually in order to escape work, excite sympathy, or gain compensation.

mal'leoinc'udal Relating to the malleus and the incus in the tympanum.

malle'olus, pl. **malle'oli** [L. dim. of malleus, hammer] [NA] A rounded bony prominence such as those on either side of the ankle joint.

malleot'omy 1. [malleus + G. tomē, incision] Division of the malleus. **2.** [malleolus + G. tomē, incision] Division of the ligaments holding the mallooli in apposition, to permit their separation.

mal'leus, gen. and pl. **mal'lei** [L. a hammer] [NA] Hammer; the largest of the three auditory ossicles, resembling a club, which is attached to the tympanic membrane and articulates with the body of the incus.

malnutri'tion Faulty nutrition resulting from malassimilation, poor diet, or overeating.

malocclu'sion 1. Any deviation from a physiologically acceptable contact of opposing dentitions. **2.** Any deviation from a normal occlusion.

mal'prac'tice Mistreatment of a disease or injury through ignorance, carelessness, or criminal intent.

mal'presenta'tion Faulty presentation of the fetus; presentation of any part other than the occiput.

malrota'tion Failure during embryonic development of normal rotation of all or any portion of the intestinal tract.

mal'tose A disaccharide formed in the hydrolysis of starch and consisting of two glucose residues bound by a 1,4-α-glycoside link.

malu'nion Incomplete union, or union in a faulty position, after fracture or a wound of the soft parts.

mamil-, mamilli- [L. *mamilla*, nipple] Combining forms relating to the mamillae. See also mammil-. mammilli-.

mamil'la, pl. **mamil'lae** [L. nipple] **1.** A small rounded elevation resembling the female breast. **2.** *Papilla mammae.*

mam'illary Relating to or shaped like a nipple.

mam'ma, gen. and pl. **mam'mae** [L.] [NA] Breast; the organ of milk secretion; one of two hemispheric projections of variable size situated in the subcutaneous layer over the pectoralis major muscle on either side of the chest; rudimentary in the male. See *glandula* mammaria.

mam'maplasty [L. *mamma*, breast, + G. *plasso*, to form] Mammoplasty.

mam'mary Relating to the breasts.

mammil-, mammilli- [L. *mammilla (mamilla)*, nipple] Combining forms relating to the mamillae. See also mamil-, mamilli-.

mammo- [L. *mamma*, breast] Combining form relating to the breasts.

mam'mogram A radiograph of the breast.

mammog'raphy [mammo- + G. *grapho*, to write] Radiographic examination of the breast.

mam'moplasty [mammo- + G. *plasso*, to mould] Plastic surgery on the breast to alter its shape, size and/or position.

mandel'ic acid A urinary antibacterial agent (both bactericidal and bacteriostatic).

man'dible Mandibula.

mandib'ula, pl. **mandib'ulae** [L. a jaw, fr. *mando*, pp. *mansus*, to chew] [NA] Mandible; jaw bone; a U-shaped bone, forming the lower jaw, articulating by its upturned extremities with the temporal bone on either side.

mandib'ular Relating to the lower jaw.

mandib'ulofa'cial Relating to the mandible and the face.

mandib'ulo-oc'ulofa'cial Relating to the mandible and the orbital part of the face.

man'ganese [Mod. L. *manganesium, manganum*, an altered form of *magnesium*] A metallic element, symbol Mn, atomic no. 25, atomic weight 54.94.

ma'nia [G. frenzy] An emotional disorder characterized by great psychomotor activity, excitement, a rapid passing of ideas, exaltation, and unstable attention.

-mania [G. frenzy] Combining form used in the suffix position, usually referring to an abnormal love for, or morbid impulse toward, some specific object, place, or action.

man'ic-depres'sive Alternating between epidodes of mania and depression.

man'nitol The hexahydric alcohol, widespread in plants, derived by reduction of fructose; used in renal function testing to measure glomerular filtration, and intravenously as an osmotic diuretic.

manoeu'vre [Fr., from L. *manu operari*, to work by hand] A planned movement or procedure.

Heimlich m., expulsion of an obstructing bolus of food from the throat by suddenly thrusting the fist into the abdomen between the navel and the rib cage so as to force air up the trachea and dislodge the obstruction.

Sellick's m., pressure applied to the cricoid cartilage, to prevent regurgitation during endotracheal intubation in the anaesthetized patient.

Valsalva m., (1) forced expiratory effort with closed nose and mouth to inflate the eustachian tubes and middle ears, as used by persons descending from high altitudes; **(2)** any forced expiratory effort against a closed airway to increase intrathoracic pressure and thus impede venous return to the right atrium; used to study cardiovascular effects of raised peripheral venous pressure and decreased cardiac filling and cardiac output.

manom'eter [G. *manos*, thin, scanty, + *metron*, measure] An instrument for indicating the pressure of gases or vapour, or the tension of the blood.

Mansonel'la [P. *Manson*] Generic term for *M. ozzardi*, a filarial parasite occurring in areas of Central and South America, and causing mansonelliasis; the life cycle is similar to that of *Wuchereria bancrofti*, man is the only known definitive host, and the intermediate hosts are biting midges of the genus *Culicodes*.

man'sonelli'asis Infection with *Mansonella ozzardi*, transmitted to man by biting midges of the genus *Culicodes*, in the serous cavities, especially the peritoneal cavity, and in mesenteric and perivisceral adipose tissue.

manu'brium, pl. **manu'bria** [L. Handle] [NA] The portion of the sternum or of the malleus similar to a handle.

man'us, gen. and pl. **man'us** [L] [NA] Hand; the distal portion of the superior limb, comprising the carpus, metacarpus, and digits.

maran'tic, maras'mic Relating to or suffering from marasmus.

maras'mus [G. *marasmos*, withering] Cachexia, especially in young children, commonly due to prolonged dietary deficiency of protein and calories.

mar'ginoplasty Plastic or reparative surgery of the tarsal border of an eyelid.

mar'go, pl. **mar'gines** [L] [NA] Margin.

marihuan'a, marijuan'a [fr. Sp. *Maria-Juana*, Mary-Jane] Popular name for the dried flowering leaves of *Cannabis sativa*, which are smoked as cigarettes.

mar'row [A.S. *mearh*] **1.** The soft, fatty substance filling the medullary cavities and spongy extremities of the long bones. **2.** Any soft gelatinous or fatty material resembling the m. of bone. See also medulla.

marsu'pializa'tion [L. *marsupium*, pouch] Exteriorization of a cyst, or other such enclosed cavity, to create a pouch.

mask 1. Any of a variety of disease states producing alteration or discoloration of the skin of the face. **2.** The expressionless appearance seen in certain diseases. **3.** A covering for the mouth and nose to maintain antiseptic conditions. **4.** A device covering the mouth and nose for administration of inhalation anaesthetics or other gases. See also masking.

mask'ing 1. In hearing testing, the use of a noise applied to one ear while testing the hearing acuity of the other ear. **2.** In dentistry, an opaque covering used to camouflage the metal parts of a prosthesis.

mas'ochism [Leopold von Sacher-Masoch, Austrian novelist, 1836–1895] **1.** A form of perversion in which sexual pleasure is heightened in one who is beaten and maltreated. *Cf.* sadism. **2.** A general orientation in life that personal suffering relieves guilt and leads to a reward.

massage' [Fr. from G. *massō*, to knead] Manipulation of the body by rubbing, pinching, kneading, tapping, etc.

    closed chest m., external cardiac m., rhythmic compressiom of the heart between the sternum and spine.

    open chest m., rhythmic manual compression of the ventricles of the heart with the hand inside the thoracic cavity.

mast- See masto-.

Mastad'enovirus A genus of the family Adenoviridae, including adenoviruses, with at least 33 antigenic types (species) being infective for man; they can cause respiratory infections, acute follicular conjunctivitis, and epidemic keratoconjunctivitis, but many infections are inapparent.

mastal'gia [masto- + G. *algos*, pain] Mastodynia.

mastec'tomy [masto- + G. *ektomē*, excision] Excision of the breast.

    radical m., Halsted's operation; excision of the entire breast including the nipple, areola, and overlying skin, plus the pectoral muscles, lymphatic-bearing tissue in the axilla, and various other neighbouring tissue.

mastica'tion [L. *mastico*, pp. -*atus*, to chew] The process of chewing food in preparation for deglutition and digestion.

mas'ticatory Relating to mastication.

mas'tigote [G. *mastix*, a whip] An individual flagellate.

masti'tis [masto- + G. -*itis*, inflammation] Inflammation of the breast.

masto-, mast- [G. *mastos*, breast] Combining forms relating to the breast.

mastodyn'ia [masto- + G. *odynē*, pain] Pain in the breast.

mas'toid [masto- + G. *eidos*, resemblance] **1.** Resembling a mamma; breast shaped. **2.** Relating to the m. process, antrum, cells, etc.

mastoidec'tomy [mastoid (process) + G. *ektomē*, excision] Hollowing out of the mastoid process by curetting, gouging, drilling, or otherwise removing the bony partitions forming the mastoid cells.

mastoi'deocente'sis [mastoid + G. *kentēsis*, puncture] Drilling or chiseling into the mastoid cells and antrum.

mastoidi'tis Inflammation of any part of the mastoid process.

masturba'tion [L. *masturbatio*] Erotic stimulation of the genital organs usually resulting in orgasm, achieved by manual or other stimulation exclusive of sexual intercourse.

mate'ria [L. substance] Substance; matter.

m. al'ba [L. white matter], accumulation or aggregation of microorganisms, desquamated epithelial cells, blood cells and food debris loosely adherent to oral surfaces.

m. med'ica [L. medical matter], old term for: **(1)** that aspect of medical science concerned with the origin and preparation of drugs, their doses, and their mode of administration; **(2)** any agent used therapeutically.

mater'nal [L. *maternus*, fr. *mater*, mother] Relating to or derived from the mother.

matrilin'eal [L. *mater*, mother, + *linea*, line] Related to descent through the female line.

ma'trix, pl. **ma'trices** [L. womb; female breeding animal] **1.** The womb. **2.** [NA] The formative portion of a tissue. **3.** The intercellular substance of a tissue. **4.** A specially shaped device for holding and shaping the material used in filling a tooth cavity.

mat'ter [L. *materies*, substance] **1.** Substance. **2.** Pus.

  grey m., *substantia grisea*.

  white m., *substantia alba*.

matura'tion [L. *maturatio*, a ripening] **1.** A stage of cell division in the formation of sex cells during which the number of chromosomes in the germ cells is reduced to one-half the number characteristic of the species. **2.** Achievement of full development or growth. **3.** The developmental changes that lead to maturity.

matu'rity A state of full development or completed growth.

maxil'la, gen. and pl. **maxil'lae** [L. jawbone] [NA] Upper jaw bone; upppper jaw; an irregularly shaped bone supporting the superior teeth and taking part in the formation of the orbit, hard palate, and nasal cavity.

maxil'lary Relating to the maxilla.

maxil'loden'tal Relating to the upper jaw and its associated teeth.

maxil'lofa'cial Pertaining to the jaws and face, particularly with reference to specialized surgery of this region.

maxil'lomandib'ular Relating to the upper and lower jaws.

mea'sles [D. *maselen*] Rubeola; an acute exanthematous disease caused by measles virus and marked by fever and other constitutional disturbances, a catarrhal inflammation of the respiratory mucous membranes, and a generalized red maculopapular eruption followed by a branny desquamation.

  German m., three-day m., rubella.

mea'tal Relating to a meatus.

meato- Combining form relating to a meatus.

mea'toplasty Reparative or reconstructive surgery of a meatus or canal.

meatot'omy [meato- + G. *tomē*, incision] An incision made to enlarge a meatus, *e.g.*, of the urethra or ureter.

mea'tus, pl. **mea'tus** [L. a going, a passage] [NA] A passage or channel, especially the external opening of a canal.

  m. acus'ticus [NA], **acoustic m., (1)** external: auditory canal; the passage leading inward through the tympanic portion of the temporal bone, from the auricle to the membrana tympani; **(2)** internal: a canal running through the petrous portion of the temporal bone, giving passage to the facial and vestibulocochlear nerves and the labyrinthine artery and veins.

mech'anism [G. *mēchanē*, a contrivance] **1.** An arrangement or grouping of the parts of anything that has a definite action. **2.** The means by which an effect is obtained.

  defence m., (1) a psychological means of coping with conflict or anxiety, *e.g.*, conversion, denial, dissociation, rationalization, repression, and sublimation; **(2)** the psychic structure underlying a coping strategy; **(3)** immunological m.

  immunological m., the groups of cells (chiefly lymphocytes and cells of the reticuloendothelial system) that function in establishing active acquired immunity (induced sensitivity, allergy).

meco'nium [L. fr G. *mēkōnion*, dim. of *mēkōn*, poppy] **1.** The first intestinal discharges of the newborn infant, greenish in colour and consisting of epithelial cells, mucus, and bile. **2.** Opium.

me'dia [L. fem. of *medius*, middle] **1.** *Tunica media.* **2.** Plural of medium.

me'dian [L. *medianus*, middle] **1.** Central; middle; lying in the midline. **2.** The middle value in a set of measurements; like the mean, a measure of central tendency.

mediasti'nal Relating to the mediastinum.

mediasti'nopericardi'tis Inflammation of the pericardium and of the surrounding mediastinal cellular tissue.

mediasti'num [Mediev. L. *mediastinus*, medial] [NA] **1.** A septum between two parts of an organ or a cavity. **2.** Interpleural space; the median partition of the thoracic cavity, covered by the mediastinal pleura and containing all the thoracic viscera and structures except the lungs; divided arbitrarily into superior, middle, inferior, anterior, and posterior parts.

med'icable Treatable with hope of cure.

med'ical [L. *medicalis*, fr. *medicus*, physician] Relating to medicine or the practice of medicine.

medic'ament [L. *medicamentum*, medicine] A medicine; a medicinal application; a remedy.

med'icate [L. *medico*, pp. *-atus*, to heal] **1.** To treat disease by the giving of drugs. **2.** To imbue with a medical substance.

medic'inal Relating to medicine having curative properties.

med'icine [L. *medicina*, fr. *medicus*, physician] **1.** A drug or remedy. **2.** The art and science of preventing or curing disease. **3.** The study and treatment of general diseases or those affecting the internal parts of the body.

family m., the medical specialty concerned with providing continuous, comprehensive care to all age groups, from first patient contact to terminal care.

folk m., treatment of ailments in the home by remedies and simple measures based upon experience and knowledge passed from generation to generation.

forensic m., legal m., (1) the relation and application of medical facts to legal problems; **(2)** the law in its bearing on the practice of medicine.

internal m., the medical specialty concerned with nonsurgical diseases of a constitutional nature in adults.

nuclear m., the clinical discipline concerned with the diagnostic, therapeutic, and investigative uses of radionuclides, excluding the therapeutic use of sealed radiation sources.

physical m., the study and treatment of disease mainly by mechanical and other physical methods.

preventive m., the branch of medical science concerned with the prevention of disease and with promotion of physical and mental health, through study of the aetiology and epidemiology of disease processes.

veterinary m., the field concerned with the diseases and health of animal species other than man.

medico- [L. *medicus*, physician] Combining form meaning medical.

medicole'gal [medico- + L. *legalis*, legal] Relating to both medicine and the law.

medio-, medi- [L. *medius*, middle] Combining forms meaning middle, or median.

mediocar'pal 1. Relating to the central part of the carpus. **2.** Denoting the articulation between the two rows of carpal bones.

mediolat'eral Relating to the median plane and a side.

mediotar'sal Relating to the middle of the tarsus; denoting the articulations of the tarsal bones with each other.

me'dium, pl. **me'dia** [L. neuter of *medius*, middle] **1.** A means; anything through which an action is performed. **2.** A substance through which impulses or impressions are transmitted. **3.** Culture m. **4.** The liquid holding a substance in solution or suspension.

contrast m., any material relatively opaque to x-rays, such as barium, used in radiography to visualize the stomach, intestine, or other organ.

culture m., a substance used for the cultivation, isolation, identification, or storage of microorganisms.

me'dius [L.] [NA] Middle, denoting an anatomical structure that is between two other similar structures or that is midway in position.

modul'la, pl. **medul'lae** [L. marrow, fr. *medius*, middle] [NA] Any soft marrow-like structure, especially in the centre of a part.

m. oblonga'ta [NA], the lowest subdivision of the brainstem, immediately continuous with the spinal cord, extending from the lower border of the decussation of the pyramidal tracts up to the pons.

m. os'sium [NA], bone marrow; the tissue filling the cavities of bones, having a stroma of reticular fibres and cells.

m. spina'lis [NA], spinal cord; the elongated cylindrical portion of the central nervous system contained in the spinal or vertebral canal.

medul'lary Relating to the medulla or marrow.

med'ullated 1. Having a medulla or medullary substance. **2.** Myelinated.

medullo- [L. *medulla*] Combining form meaning medulla.

med'ulloblasto'ma A glioma consisting of neoplastic cells that resemble the undifferentiated cells of the primitive medullary tube.

mega- [G. *megas*, big] Combining form meaning large, oversize. See also macro-, megalo-.

megaceph'aly [mega- + G. *kephalē*, head] An abnormally large head.

megaco'lon Extreme dilation and hypertrophy of the colon.

congenital m., Hirschsprung's disease; congenital dilation and hypertrophy of the colon due to absence (aganglionosis) or marked reduction (hypoganglionosis) in the number of ganglion cells of the myenteric plexus of the rectum and a varying but continuous length of gut above the rectum.

megakar'yocyte [mega- + G. *karyon*, nut (nucleus), + *kytos*, hollow vessel (cell)] A large cell with a nucleus that is usually multilobed, normally present in bone marrow but not in the circulating blood; gives rise to blood platelets.

megalo-, megal-, -megaly [G. *megas* (*megal*-), large] Combining forms meaning large. See also macro-, mega-.

meg'aloblast [megalo- + G. *blastos*, germ, sprout] A large, nucleated, embryonic type of cell that is a precursor of erythrocytes in an abnormal erythropoietic process observed almost exclusively in pernicious anaemia.

meg'aloceph'aly Megacephaly.

megalocys'tis [megalo- + G. *kystis*, bladder] An enlarged or overdistended bladder.

megaloma'nia [megalo- + G. *mania*, frenzy] Morbid overevaluation of oneself or of some aspect of oneself.

meg'alophthal'mus [megalo- + G. *ophthalmos*, eye] Abnormally large eyes occurring as a developmental anomaly.

megalou'reter A congenitally enlarged ureter without evidence of obstruction or infection.

mega-oesoph'agus Enlargement of the lower portion of the oesophagus, as seen in patients with achalasia and Chagas disease.

meibomi'tis, meibo'miani'tis Inflammation of the meibomian glands.

meio'sis [G. *meiōsis*, a lessening] Meiotic division; the special process of cell division that results in the formation of gametes, consisting of two nuclear divisions in rapid succession that result in the formation of four gametocytes each containing half the number of chromosomes found in somatic cells.

mel-, melo- 1. [G. *melos*, limb] Combining form indicating limb. 2. [G. *mēlon*, cheek] Combining form indicating cheek. 3. [L. *mel*, *mellis*, honey; G. *meli*, *melitos*, honey] Combining form relating to honey or sugar. See also meli-.

melae'na [G. *melaina*, fem. of *melas*, black] Passage of dark coloured, tarry stools, due to the presence of blood altered by the intestinal juices.

melal'gia [G. *melos*, a limb, + *algos*, pain] Pain in a limb; specifically, burning pain in the feet extending up the leg and thickening of the walls of the blood vessels with obliteration of the vascular lumina.

melan-, melano- [G. *melas*, black] Combining forms meaning black or extreme darkness of hue.

melancho'lia [melan- + G. *cholē*, bile] Melancholy. 1. A mental disorder marked by apathy and indifference to one's surroundings, mental sluggishness, and depression, 2. A symptom occurring in other conditions, marked by depression of spirits and by a sluggish and painful process of thought.

mel'anin [G. *melas* (*melan*-), black] Any of the dark brown to black polymers of indole 5,6-quinone and/or 5,6-dihydroxyindole 2-carboxylic acid that normally occur in the skin, hair, pigmented coat of the retina, and inconstantly in the medulla and zona reticularis of the adrenal gland.

mel'anism Unusually marked, diffuse, melanin pigmentation of body hair.

mel'anocyte [melano- + G. *kytos*, cell] A cell located at the dermoepidermal junction having branching processes by means of which melanosomes are transferred to epidermal cells, resulting in pigmentation.

mel'anocyto'ma [melago + cyto- + G. *-oma*, tumour] 1. A pigmented tumour of the uveal stroma. 2. Usually benign melanoma of the optic disc, appearing in highly pigmented individuals as a small deeply pigmented tumour at the edge of the disc, sometimes extending into the retina and choroid.

mel'anoder'ma [melano- + G. *derma*, skin] An abnormal darkening of the skin by deposition of excess melanin or of metallic substances.

melano'ma [melano- + G. *ōma*, tumour] A malignant neoplasm derived from cells capable of forming melanin and which frequently metastasizes widely.

melano'sis [melano- + G. *-osis*, condition] **1.** Abnormal, dark brown or brown-black pigmentation of various tissues or organs, as the result of melanins or other substances that resemble melanin. **2.** Cachexia resulting from widespread metastases of melanoma.

mel'anosome [melano- + G. *sōma*, body] The generally oval pigment granule produced by melanocytes.

melanot'ic 1. Pertaining to the presence of melanin. **2.** Relating to or characterized by melanosis.

melanu'ria [melano- + G. *ouron*, urine] Excretion of urine of a dark colour, resulting from the presence of melanin or other pigments or from the action of coal tar derivatives.

melas'ma [G. a black colour, a black spot] A patchy or generalized pigmentation of the skin.

meli- [G. *meli*, honey] Combining form relating to honey or sugar. See also mel- (3).

mem'bra [L.] [NA] Plural of membrum.

membra'na, gen. and pl. **membra'nae** [L.] [NA] Membrane; a thin sheet or layer of pliable tissue, serving as a covering or envelope of a part, the lining of a cavity, as a partition or septum, or to connect two structures.

   m. decid'ua [NA], decidua; the mucous membrane of the pregnant uterus which has already undergone certain changes, under the influence of the ovulation cycle, to fit it for the implantation and nutrition of the ovum.

   m. synovia'lis [NA], synovial membrane; synovium; the connective tissue membrane that lines the cavity of a synovial joint and produces the synovial fluid.

   m. tym'pani [NA], tympanic membrane; eardrum; a thin tense membrane forming the greater part of the lateral wall of the tympanic cavity and separating it from the external acoustic meatus; constitutes the boundary between the external and middle ear.

mem'brane [L. *membrana*, skin or membrane that covers part of the body] Membrana.

   basement m., a thin layer that intervenes between epithelium and connective tissue.

   Descemet's m., *lamina limitans corneae* (2).

   fetal m., embryonic m., a structure or tissue developed from the fertilized ovum but which does not form part of the embryo proper.

   hyaline m., the thin, clear basement m. beneath certain epithelia.

   mucous m., see *tunica* mucosa.

   placental m., the semipermeable layer of tissue separating the maternal from the fetal blood.

   synovial m., *membrana* synovialis.

   tympanic m., drum m., *membrana* tympani.

mem'ory [L. *memoria*] **1.** General term for the recollection of that which was once experienced or learned. **2.** The mental information processing system that receives (registers), modifies, stores, and retrieves informational stimuli; composed of three stages: encoding, storage, and retrieval.

menar'che [G. *mēn*, month, + *archē*, beginning] The establishment of the menstrual function; the time of the first menstrual period or flow.

menin'geal Relating to the meninges.

menin'ges Plural of meninx.

meningio'ma [mening- + G. *-oma*, tumour] A benign encapsulated neoplasm of arachnoidal origin, occurring in adults; tends to occur along the superior sagittal sinus or the sphenoid ridge, or in the vicinity of the optic chiasm.

menin'gism A condition of irritation of the brain or spinal cord in which the symptoms simulate meningitis, but in which no actual inflammation is present.

meningi'tis pl. **meningit'ides** [mening- + G. *-itis*, inflammation] Inflammation of the membranes of the brain or spinal cord.

   meningococcal m., an acute infectious disease affecting children and young adults, caused by the meningococcus, *Neisseria meningitidis;* symptoms are headache, vomiting, convulsions, nuchal rigidity, photophobia, cutaneous hyperaesthesia, a purpuric or herpetic eruption, and the presence of Kernig's sign.

meningo-, mening- [G. *mēninx*, membrane] Combining forms relating to meninges.

menin'gocele [meningo- + G. *kēlē*, tumour] Protrusion of the membranes of the brain or spinal cord through a defect in the skull or spinal column.

meningococ'cus, pl. **meningococ'ci** [meningo- + G. *kokkos*, berry] *Neisseria meningitidis.*

menin'goencephali'tis [meningo- + G. *enkephalos*, brain, + *-itis*, inflammation] Inflammation of the brain and its membranes.

menin'goenceph'alomyeli'tis [meningo- + G. *enkephalos*, brain, + *myelos*, marrow, + *-itis*, inflammation] Inflammation of the brain and spinal cord together with their membranes.

menin'goencephalop'athy [meningo- + G. *enkephalos*, brain, + *pathos*, suffering] Any disorder affecting the meninges and the brain.

menin'gomyeli'tis [meningo- + G. *myelos*, marrow, + *-itis*, inflammation] Inflammation of the spinal cord and of its enveloping arachnoid and pia mater, less commonly also of the dura mater.

meningomy'elocele [meningo- + G. *myelos*, marrow, + *kēlē*, tumour] Protrusion of the spinal membranes and cord through a defect in the vertebral column.

men'inx, gen. **menin'gis,** pl. **menin'ges** [Mod. L. fr. G. *mēninx*, membrane] Any membrane; specifically, one of the membranous coverings of the brain and spinal cord: arachnoidea, dura mater, pia mater.

meniscec'tomy [G. *mēniskos*, crescent (meniscus) + *ektomē*, excision] Excision of a meniscus, usually from the knee joint.

menisci'tis [G. *mēniskos*, crescent (meniscus), + *-itis*, inflammation] Inflammation of a fibrocartilaginous meniscus.

menis'cus, pl. **menis'ci** [G. *mēniskos*, crescent] [NA] A crescent-shaped structure, as the fibrocartilage in certain joints.

meno- [G. *mēn*, month] Combining form denoting relationship to the menses.

men'opause [meno- + G. *pausis*, cessation] Permanent cessation of the menses.

menorrha'gia [meno- + G. *rhēgnymi*, to burst forth] Hypermenorrhoea.

men'ses [L. pl. of *mensis*, month] A periodic physiologic haemorrhage, occurring at approximately 4-week intervals, and having its source from the uterine mucous membrane; under normal circumstances, the bleeding is preceded by ovulation and predecidual changes in the endometrium. See also menstrual *cycle.*

men'strual [L. *menstrualis*] Relating to the menses.

menstrua'tion Cyclic endometrial shedding and discharge of a bloody fluid from the uterus during the catamenial period.

anovular m., menstrual bleeding without the discharge of an ovum.

retained m., haematocolpos.

vicarious m., bleeding from any surface other than the mucous membrane of the uterine cavity, occurring periodically at the time when the normal m. should take place.

men'tal 1. [L. *mens* (*ment-*), mind] Relating to the mind. **2.** [L. *mentum*, chin] Relating to the chin.

men'thol An alcohol obtained from peppermint oil or other mint oils, or prepared synthetically; used as an antipruritic and topical anaesthetic, and as a flavouring agent.

men'toplasty [L. *mentum*, chin + G. *plastos*, formed] Plastic surgery of the chin, whereby its shape or size is altered.

men'tum, gen. **men'ti** [L.] [NA] Chin.

mephit'ic [L. *mephitis*, a noxious exhalation] Foul; poisonous; noxious.

mepiv'acaine hydrochloride A local anaesthetic agent similar in action to lignocaine.

-mer 1. Suffix attached to a prefix such as mono-, di-, tri-, poly-, etc., to indicate the smallest unit of a repeating structure. See polymer. **2.** Suffix denoting a member of a particular group, as in isomer, enantiomer.

meral'gia [G. *mēros*, thigh, + *algos*, pain] Pain in the thigh.

m. paraesthet'ica, Paraesthesia in the outer side of the lower part of the thigh in the area of distribution of the external cutaneous branch of the femoral nerve.

mercu'rialism Mercury *poisoning.*

mer'cury [L. *Mercurius*, Mercury, Roman deity; Mediev. L. quicksilver, mercury] A liquid metallic element, symbol Hg, atomic no. 80, atomic weight 200.59; used in scientific instruments; some salts and organic mercurials are used medicinally.

mes- 219 mesovarium

mes- See meso-.

mesan'gium [mes- + G. *angeion*, vessel] A central part of the renal glomerulus between capillaries.

mesarteri'tis [mes- + arteritis] Inflammation of the middle (muscular) coat of an artery.

mes'caline The most active alkaloid present in the buttons of a small cactus, *Lophophora williamsii*, which produces psychotomimetic effects similar to those produced by LSD.

mes'encephal'ic Relating to the mesencephalon.

mesencephalon [mes- + G. *enkephalos*, brain] [NA] Midbrain; that part of the brainstem that develops from the middle of the three primary cerebral vesicles of the embryo; in the adult, characterized grossanatomically by the unique conformation of its roofplate, the lamina tecti mesencephali, and by the paired prominence of the crus cerebri at its ventral surface. Prominent cell groups of the m. include the motor nuclei of the trochlear and oculomotor nerves, the red nucleus, and the substantia nigra.

mes'enchyme [mes- + G. *enkyma*, infusion] 1. An aggregation of mesenchymal cells. 2. A primordial embryonic tissue consisting of mesenchymal cells, usually stellate in form, supported in a ground substance.

mesenter'ic Relating to the mesentery.

mesenteri'tis Inflammation of the mesentery.

mes'entery [Mod. L. *mesenterium*, fr. G. *mesenterion*, fr. G. *mesos*, middle + *enteron*, intestine] 1. A double layer of peritoneum attached to the abdominal wall and enclosing in its fold a portion or all of one of the abdominal viscera, conveying to it its vessels and nerves. 2. The fold of peritoneum encircling the greater part of the small intestines (jejunum and ileum) and attaching it to the posterior abdominal wall.

me'sial [G. *mesos*, middle] Proximal; toward the midline following the curvature of the dental arch.

mesio- [G. *mesos*, middle] Combining form meaning mesial.

mes'merism [F.A. *Mesmer*, Austrian physician, 1733–1815] A system of therapeutics from which were developed hypnotism and therapeutic suggestion.

meso-, mes- [G. *mesos*, middle] 1. Prefix meaning middle, or mean, or used to give an indication of intermediacy. 2. Prefix designating a mesentery or mesentery-like structure.

mes'oblast [meso- + G. *blastos*, germ] Mesoderm.

mesoblas'tic Relating to or derived from the mesoderm (mesoblast).

mes'oderm [meso- + G. *derma*, skin] The middle of the three primary germ layers of the embryo; gives origin to all connective tissues, all body musculature, blood, cardiovascular and lymphatic systems, most of the urogenital system, and the lining of the pericardial, pleural, and peritoneal cavities.

mesoil'eum The mesentery of the ileum.

mesojeju'num The mesentery of the jejunum.

mesome'trium [meso- + G. *metra*, uterus] [NA] The broad ligament of the uterus, below the mesosalpinx.

mes'omorph [meso- + G. *morphe*, form] A constitutional body type in which tissues that originate from the mesoderm prevail, with a proportional balance between trunk and limbs.

mes'oneph'ric Relating to the mesonephros.

mesoneph'ros, pl. **mesoneph'roi** [meso- + G. *nephros*, kidney] [NA] one of three excretory organs appearing in the evolution of vertebrates; it undergoes regression as an excretory organ but its duct system is retained in the male as the epididymis and ductus deferens.

mes'osal'pinx [meso- + G. *salpinx*, trumpet] [NA] The part of the broad ligament investing the fallopian tube.

mesothe'lial Relating to the mesothelium.

mes'othelio'ma [mesothelium + G. *-oma*, tumour] A rare neoplasm, derived from the lining cells of the pleura and peritoneum, which grows as a thick sheet covering the viscera and is composed of spindle cells or fibrous tissue.

mesothe'lium, pl. **mesothe'lia** [meso- + epithelium] A single layer of flattened cells forming an epithelium that lines serous cavities.

mesovar'ium, pl. **mesovar'ia** [meso- + L. *ovarium*, ovary] [NA] A short peritoneal fold connecting the anterior border of the ovary with the posterior layer of the broad ligament of the uterus.

meta- [G. after, between, over] **1.** Prefix denoting the concept of after, subsequent to, behind, or hindmost, corresponding to *post-*. **2.** Prefix denoting joint action or sharing. **3.** (**m-**) In chemistry, a prefix denoting that a compound is formed by two substitutions in the benzene ring separated by one carbon atom. For terms beginning with *meta-*, or *m-*, see the specific name.

metabol'ic Relating to metabolism.

metab'olism [G. *metabolē*, change] The sum of the chemical changes occurring in tissue, consisting of anabolism (those reactions that convert small molecules into large) and catabolism (those reactions that convert large molecules into small), including both endogenous large molecules as well as biodegradation of drugs and other xenobiotics.

    basal m., basal metabolic rate; heat production at the lowest level of cell chemistry in the waking state; the minimal amount of cell activity associated with the continuous organic functions of respiration, circulation, and secretion.

metab'olite Any product of metabolism, especially of catabolism.

metacar'pal Relating to the metacarpus.

metacar'pophalan'geal Relating to the metacarpus and the phalanges; denoting the articulations between them.

metacar'pus, pl. **metacar'pi** [meta- + G. *karpos*, wrist] [NA] The five bones of the hand between the carpus and the phalanges.

metal'lopro'tein A protein with a tightly bound metal ion or ions; *e.g.*, haemoglobin.

metal'lothione'in A small protein, rich in sulphur-containing amino acids, that is synthesized in the liver and kidney in response to the presence of divalent ions, and that binds these ions tightly; of importance in ion transport and detoxification.

met'amere [meta- + G. *meros*, part] One of a series of homologous body segments.

metam'erism A type of anatomic structure exhibiting serially homologous segments; are in vertebrates, evident in serially repeated vertebrae, ribs, intercostal muscles, and the spinal nerves.

metamor'phosis [G. transformation; *meta*, beyond, over, + *morphē*, form] A change in form, structure, or function.

met'aphase [meta- + G. *phasis*, an appearance] The stage of mitosis or meiosis in which the chromosomes become aligned on the equatorial plate of the cell with the centromeres mutually repelling each other.

metaphys'eal, metaphysi'al Relating to a metaphysis.

metaph'ysis, pl. **metaph'yses** [meta- + G. *physis*, growth] [NA] The growth zone between the epiphysis and diaphysis during development of a bone.

metaplas'tic Pertaining to metaplasia.

metapla'sia [G. *metaplasis*, transformation] Abnormal transformation of an adult, fully differentiated tissue of one kind into a differentiated tissue of another kind; an acquired condition.

    myeloid m., a syndrome characterized by anaemia, enlargement of the spleen, nucleated red blood cells and immature granulocytes in the circulating blood, and conspicuous foci of extramedullary haemopoiesis in the spleen and liver. It occurs in some persons who have another disease and is termed *secondary* or *symptomatic myeloid m.*; it also occurs as an apparently primary illness, and is then termed *primary* or *agnogenic myeloid m.,* or *myelofibrosis* or *myelosclerosis,* because of the presence of an associated fibrosis of the bone marrow of unknown cause.

metas'tasis, pl. **metas'tases** [G. a removing] **1.** The shifting of a disease, or its local manifestations, from one part of the body to another. **2.** In cancer, the appearance of neoplasms in parts of the body remote from the seat of the primary tumour. **3.** Transportation of bacteria from one part of the body to another, through the bloodstream or lymph channels.

metas'tasize To pass into or invade by metastasis.

met'astat'ic Relating to metastasis.

met'atar'sal Relating to the metatarsus or to one of the metatarsal bones.

metatarsal'gia [meta- + G. *algos*, pain] Pain in the forefoot in the region of the heads of the metatarsals.

metatar'sophalan'geal Relating to the metatarsal bones and the phalanges; denoting the articulations between them.

metatar'sus, pl. **metatar'si** [meta- + G. *tarsos*, tarsus] [NA] The distal portion of the foot between the instep and the toes, having as its skeleton the five metatarsal bones artic-

ulating posteriorly with the cuboid and cuneiform bones and distally with the phalanges.
Metazo'a [meta- + G. zōon, animal] A
subkingdom of the kingdom Animalia, including all multicellular animal organisms in
which the cells are differentiated and form
tissues.
met'encephal'ic Relating to the meten-
cephalon.
metenceph'alon [meta- + G. enkephalos, brain] [NA] The anterior of the two major
subdivisions of the rhombencephalon (the
posterior being the myelencephalon or medulla oblongata), composed of the pons and
the cerebellum.
meth-, metho- Chemical prefixes usually denoting a methyl or methoxy group.
meth'adone hydrochloride A synthetic narcotic analgesic similar in action to
morphine but with slightly greater potency
and longer duration; used orally as a replacement for morphine and heroin and during
withdrawal treatment in morphine and heroin
addiction.
met'haemalbu'min An abnormal compound formed in the blood as a result of haem
combining with plasma albumin.
met'haemoglo'bin (metHb) A
transformation product of oxyhaemoglobin
because of the oxidation of the normal FE^{2+} to
Fe^{3+}, thus converting ferroprotoporphrin to
ferriprotoporphyrin.
met'haemoglo'binae'mia
[methaemoglobin + G. haima, blood] Presence of methaemoglobin in the circulating
blood.
met'haemoglo'binu'ria
[methaemoglobin + G. ouron, urine] Presence of methaemoglobin in the urine.
**meth'amphet'amine hydrochlo-
ride** A sympathomimetic agent with
greater stimulating effects upon the CNS than
does amphetamine.
me'thane [meth(yl) + -ane] Marsh gas;
CH_4; an odourless combustible gas produced
by the decomposition of organic matter.
meth'anol Methyl alcohol.
methi'onine (Met) An essential amino
acid and an important natural source of "active methyl" groups in the body.
meth'od [G. methodos; fr. meta, after, +
hodos, way] The mode or manner or orderly
sequence of events of a process or procedure.

Lamaze m., a technique of psychopro-
phylactic preparation for childbirth, designed
to minimize the pain of labour.

rhythm m., a natural means of contra-
ception that spaces sexual intercourse to
avoid the fertile period of the menstrual cycle.
meth'yl (Me) [G. methy, wine, + hylē,
wood] The radical, $-CH_3$.
meth'ylate 1. To mix with methyl alcohol.
2. To introduce a methyl group. **3.** A compound of a metal ion with methyl alcohol.
meth'ylene The radical, $-CH_2-$.

m. blue, a basic dye used in histology
and microbiology, to track RNA and RNase in
electrophoresis, and as an antidote for met
haemoglobinaemia.

Loeffler's m. blue, a stain for diphtheria organisms.
meth'yltestos'terone A methyl derivative of testosterone, with the same actions
and uses.
metr-, metra- [G. mētra, uterus] Combining forms denoting the uterus. See also
hystero-, utero-.
me'tra [G. uterus] Uterus.
metrato'nia [metra- + G. a- priv. +
tonos, tension] Atony of the uterine walls after
childbirth.
me'tria [G. mētra, uterus] Pelvic cellulitis
or other inflammatory condition in the puerperal period.
metri'tis [G. mētra, uterus, + -itis, inflam-
mation] Inflammation of the uterus.
metro- [G. metra, uterus] Combining form
relating to the uterus. See also hystero-,
utero-.
me'trocysto'sis [metro- + G. kystis,
cyst, + -osis, condition] Formation of uterine
cysts.
metrodyn'ia [metro- + G. odynē, pain]
Hysteralgia.
metropath'ia [L.] Metropathy.

m. haemorrhag'ica, abnormal, excessive, often continuous uterine bleeding
due to persistence and exaggeration of the
follicular phase of the menstrual cycle.
metrop'athy [metro- + G. pathos, suffer-
ing] Any disease of the uterus.
me'troperitoni'tis [metro- + peritoni-
tis] Inflammation of the uterus involving the
peritoneal covering.
metrorrha'gia [metro- + G. rhēgnymi, to
burst forth] Any irregular, acyclic bleeding
from the uterus between periods.

me'trosalpingi'tis [metro- + G. *salpinx*, trumpet (oviduct), + *-itis*, inflammation] Inflammation of the uterus and of one or both fallopian tubes.

me'trosteno'sis [metro- + G. *stenosis*, a narrowing] A narrowing of the uterine cavity.

metyr'apone An inhibitor of adenocortical steroid administered to determine the ability of the pituitary gland to increase its secretion of corticotropin.

micrenceph'aly [micro- + G. *enkephalos*, brain] Abnormal smallness of the brain.

micro-, micr- [G. *mikros*, small] **1.** Prefix denoting smallness. **2.** Denoting that minimal quantities of the substance to be examined are used. **3.** Combining form meaning microscopic.

microab'scess A very small circumscribed collection of leucocytes in solid tissues.

microanat'omy Histology.

microan'eurysm Focal dilation of retinal capillaries occuring in diabetes mellitis, retinal vein obstruction, and absolute glaucoma, or of arteriolocapillary junctions in many organs in thrombotic thrombocytopenic purpura.

mi'crobe [Fr. fr. G. *mikros*, small, + *bios*, life] A microscopic or ultramicroscopic organism, including spirochaetes, bacteria, rickettsiae, and viruses; such organisms form a biologically distinctive group, in that the genetic material is not surrounded by a nuclear membrane, and mitosis does not occur during replication.

microbiol'ogy [Fr. *microbiologie*] The science concerned with microscopic and ultramicroscopic organisms.

microceph'aly [micro- + G. *kephalē*, head] Abnormal smallness of the head.

mi'crocir'cula'tion Circulation in the smallest vessels (arterioles, capillaries, and venules).

Micrococ'cus [micro- + G. *kokkos*, berry] A genus of bacteria (family Micrococcaceae) containing Gram-positive spherical cells that occur in irregular masses, and are saprophytic or parasitic but are not pathogenic. The type species is *M. luteus.*

microco'lon A small colon, often arising from a decreased functional state.

microcor'nea An abnormally thin and flat cornea.

mi'crocyte [micro- + G. *kytos*, cell] A small non-nucleated red blood cell.

microcythae'mia [microcyte + G. *haima*, blood] Presence of many microcytes in the circulating blood.

microcyto'sis [microcyte + G. *-osis*, condition] Microcythaemia.

mi'croenceph'aly Micrencephaly.

microdissec'tion Dissection of tissues under magnification, usually done by teasing the tissues apart with needles.

microfi'bril A very small fibril, which may be a bundle of still smaller elements, the microfilaments.

microfil'ament The finest of the fibrous elements of a cell or tissue.

mi'crofilar'ia, pl. **mi'crofilar'iae** Embryos of filarial nematodes in the family Onchocercidae.

microg'lia [micro- + G. *glia*, glue] Small neuroglial cells of mesodermal origin which may become phagocytic, hence are considered elements of the reticuloendothelial system.

microglos'sia [micro- + G. *glōssa*, tongue] Abnormal smallness of the tongue.

microgna'thia [micro- + G. *gnathos*, jaw] Abnormal smallness of the jaws, especially of the mandible.

mi'croinci'sion Destruction of cellular organelles by laser beam.

mi'cromanipula'tion Microdissection, microinjection, and other manoeuvres performed with the aid of a microscope.

micromas'tia [micro- + G. *mastos*, breast] A condition in which the breasts are rudimentary and functionless.

microme'lia [micro- + G. *melos*, limb] Disproportionately short or small limbs.

micronu'trients Essential food factors required in only small quantities by the body.

microor'ganism A microscopic organism.

mi'crophage [micro- + phag(ocyte)] A polymorphonuclear leukocyte that is phagocytic.

microphthal'mia, microphthal'mos [micro- + G. *ophthalmos*, eye] Abnormal smallness of one or both eyeballs.

microp'sia [micro- + G. *opsis*, sight] Subjective perception of objects as smaller than they actually are.

mi'cropuncture. Microincision.

mi′croscope [micro- + G. *skopeō*, to view] An instrument that gives an enlarged image of an object or substance that is minute or not visible with the naked eye.

   electron m., a visual and photographic m. in which electron beams with wavelengths thousands of times shorter than visible light are utilized in place of light, thereby allowing much greater magnification.

   scanning electron m., a m. in which the object is examined point by point directly by an electron beam, and an image is formed on a television screen

microscop′ic, microscop′ical 1. Of minute size; visible only with the aid of the microscope. **2.** Relating to a microscope.

micros′copy Investigation of minute objects by means of a microscope.

mioroso′mia [micro- + G. *sōma*, body] Abnormal smallness of body, as in dwarfism.

Microspo′rum [micro- + G. *sporos*, seed] A genus of pathogenic fungi causing dermatophytosis.

microsto′mia [micro- + G. *stoma*, mouth] Abnormal smallness of the oral aperature.

microsur′gery Surgical procedures performed under the magnification of a surgical microscope.

micro′tia [micro- + G. *ous*, ear, + *-ia*, condition] Abnormal smallness of the auricle or pinna of the ear.

mi′crotu′bule A cylindrical cytoplasmic element of variable length that increases in number during mitosis and meiosis, and occurs widely in plant and animal cells, where it may be related to movement of the chromosomes or chromatids on the nuclear spindle during nuclear division.

microvil′lus, pl. **microvil′li** One of the minute projections of cell membranes greatly increasing surface area.

mic′tion Urination.

micturi′tion [L. *micturio*, to desire to make water] **1.** Urination. **2.** The desire to urinate. **3.** Frequency of urination.

mid- [A.S. *mid, midd*] Combining form meaning middle.

mid′brain Mesencephalon.

mid′riff [A.S. *mid*, middle, + *hrif*, belly] Diaphragma (2).

mid′wife [A.S. *mid*, with, + *wif*, wife] A person qualified to practise midwifery, having specialized training in gynaecology and child care and the ability to carry out emergency measures in the absence of medical help.

midwif′ery Independent care of essentially normal, healthy women and infants by a midwife, antepartally, intrapartally, postpartally, and/or gynaecologically, including normal delivery of the infant, with medical consultation, collaborative management, and referral of cases in which abnormalities develop.

mi′graine [through O. Fr. fr. G. *hēmikrania*, pain on one side of the head] A symptom complex occurring periodically and characterized by pain in the head (usually unilateral), vertigo, nausea and vomiting, photophobia, and scintillating appearances of light. Classified as classic m., common m., cluster *headache*, hemiplegic m., ophthalmoplegic m., and ophthalmic m.

mi′grate [L. *migro*, pp. *-atus*, to move from place to place] To wander; to pass from one part to another, as in an organ or in the body.

migra′tion [L. *migratio* (see migrate)] **1.** Passing from place to place, said of certain morbid processes of symptoms. **2.** Diapedesis. **3.** Movement of a tooth or teeth out of normal position. **4.** Movement of molecules during electrophoresis.

miliar′ia [L. *miliarius*, relating to millet, fr. *milium*, millet] An eruption of minute vesicles and papules due to retention of fluid at the mouths of the sweat follicles.

   m. ru′bra, heat rash; prickly heat; an eruption of papules and vesicles at the mouths of the sweat follicles, accompanied by redness and inflammatory reaction of the skin.

mil′iary [see miliaria] **1.** Resembling a millet seed in size (about 2 mm). **2.** Marked by the presence of nodules of millet seed size on any surface.

mil′ium, pl. **mil′ia** [L. millet] Whitehead; a small subepidermal keratin cyst, usually multiple.

milk [A.S. *meolc*] **1.** A white liquid, containing proteins, sugar, lipids, secreted by the mammary glands and designed for nourishment of the young. **2.** Any whitish, milky fluid. **3.** A pharmacopoeial preparation that is a suspension of insoluble drugs in a water medium.

   m. of magnesia, an aqueous solution of magnesium hydroxide, used as an antacid and laxative.

mime'sis [G. *mimēsis*, imitation, fr. *mimeomai*, to mimic] **1.** Hysterical simulation of organic disease. **2.** Symptomatic imitation of one organic disease by another.

mimet'ic [G. *mimētikos*, imitative] Relating to mimesis.

min'eralocor'ticoid One of the steroid principles of the adrenal cortex that influences salt (sodium and potassium) metabolism.

min'eral oil A mixture of liquid hydrocarbons obtained from petroleum.

min'ilaparot'omy A technique for sterilization by surgical ligation of the fallopian tubes, performed through a small suprapubic incision.

mio- [G. *meiōn*, less] Combining form meaning less.

mio'sis [G. *meiosis*, a lessening] **1.** The period of decline of a disease in which the intensity of the symptoms begins to diminish. **2.** Contraction of the pupil.

miot'ic **1.** Relating to or characterized by miosis. **2.** An agent that causes the pupil to contract.

mis'carriage Spontaneous expulsion of the products of pregnancy before the middle of the second trimester.

mis'cible [L. *misceo*, to mix] Capable of being mixed and remaining so after the mixing process ceases.

mis'diagno'sis Wrong or mistaken diagnosis.

mite [A.S.] A minute arthropod of the order Acarina, a vast assemblage of parasitic and (primarily) free-living organisms of which only a small number are of importance as vectors or intermediate hosts of pathogenic agents by directly causing dermatitis or tissue damage, or by causing blood or tissue fluid loss.

mi'ticide [mite + L. *caedo*, to kill] An agent destructive to mites.

mit'igate [L. *mitigo*, pp. -*atus*, to make mild or gentle] Palliate.

mitochon'drial Relating to mitochondria.

mitochon'drion, pl. **mitochon'dria** [G. *mitos*, thread, + *chondros*, granule, grits] An organelle of the cell cytoplasm consisting of two sets of membranes, a smooth continuous outer coat and an inner membrane arranged in tubules or in folds that form platelike double membranes (cristae); the principal energy source of the cell, containing the cytochrome enzymes of terminal electron transport and the enzymes of the citric acid cycle, fatty acid oxidation, and oxidative phosphorylation.

mito'sis, pl. **mito'ses** [G. *mitos,* threat] The usual process of cell reproduction, consisting of a sequence of modifications of the nucleus (prophase, prometaphase, metaphase, anaphase, telophase) that result in the formation of two daughter cells with exactly the same chromosome and DNA content as that of the original cell.

mitot'ic Relating to or marked by mitosis.

mi'tral [L. *mitra*, a coif or turban] **1.** Relating to the mitral or bicuspid valve. **2.** Shaped like a bishop's mitre; denoting a structure resembling the shape of a headband or turban.

mit'telschmerz [Ger. middle pain] Abdominal pain occurring at the time of ovulation, resulting from irritation of the peritoneum by bleeding from the ovulation site.

mo'biliza'tion **1.** Making movable; restoring the power of motion in a joint. **2.** The act of mobilizing; exciting a hitherto quiescent process into physiologic activity.

modal'ity [Mediev. L. *modalitas*, fr. L. *modus*, a mode] **1.** Any form of therapeutic intervention. **2.** Various forms of sensation, *e.g.*, touch, vision.

mod'ifica'tion. A nonhereditary change in an organism; *e.g.*, one that is acquired from its own activity or environment.

    behaviour m., the systematic use of principles of conditioning and learning to teach simple skills or to alter undesirable behaviour.

modi'olus, pl. **modi'oli** [L., the nave of a wheel] [NA] The central cone-shaped core of spongy bone about which turns the spiral canal of the cochlea.

mo'lar **1.** [L. *molaris*, relating to a mill] Grinding. **2.** *Dens molaris*. **3.** [L. *moles*, mass] Massive; relating to a mass; not molecular. **4. (M,** *M*, **м).** Denoting a concentration of 1 gram-molecular weight (1 mole) of solute per litre of solution, the common unit of concentration in chemistry. **5.** Denoting specific quantity, *e.g.*, molar volume (volume of 1 mole). **6.** Relating to or associated with hydatidiform mole.

mole **1.** [A.S. *māēl* (L. *macula*), a spot] *Naevus pigmentosus.* **2.** [L. *moles*, mass] An intrauterine mass formed by the degeneration of the partly developed products of conception. **3. (mol).** The unit of "amount" of substance, one of the seven base SI units.

hydatidiform m., hydatid m., a vesicular or polycystic mass resulting from the proliferation of the trophoblast, with hydropic degeneration and avascularity of the chorionic villi.

molec'ular Relating to molecules.

mol'ecule [Mod. L. *molecula*, dim. of L. *moles*, mass] The smallest possible quantity of a di-, tri-, or polyatomic substance that retains the chemical properties of the substance.

mo'limen, pl. **molim'ina** [L. endeavor] An effort; the laborious performance of a normal function.

mollus'cous Relating to or resembling molluscum.

mollus'cum [L. *molluscus*, soft] A disease marked by the occurrence of soft rounded tumours of the skin.

m. contagio'sum, an infectious disease of the skin, caused by a virus of the family Poxviridae and characterized by the appearance of small, pearly, umbilicated, papular epithelial lesions which contain numerous inclusion bodies.

mon- See mono-.

mon'arthri'tis Arthritis of a single joint.

mon'artic'ular Relating to a single joint.

mon'golism [fancied facial appearance resembling that of a Mongol] Down's *syndrome*.

mon'goloid Relating to or characterized by mongolism.

Monil'ia [L. *monile*, necklace] Generic term for a large group of moulds or fungi commonly known as fruit moulds; a few closely related pathogenic organisms formerly classified in this genus are now properly termed *Candida*.

monill'asis Candidiasis.

monil'iform [L. *monile*, necklace, + *forma*, appearance] Shaped like a string of beads or beaded necklace.

mon'itor **1.** A device that records specified data for a given series of events, operations, or circumstances. **2.** To check constantly on a specific condition or situation.

mono-, mon- [G. *monos*, single] Prefix denoting the participation or involvement of a single element or part; equivalent of *uni-*.

monoba'sic Denoting an acid with only one replaceable hydrogen atom, or only one replaced hygrogen atom.

mon'ochorion'ic Relating to or having a single chorion; denoting monovular twins.

monochro'matism [mono- + G. *chrōma*, colour] **1.** The state of having or exhibiting only one colour. **2.** Achromatopsia.

monoclo'nal In immunochemistry, pertaining to a protein from a single clone of cells, all molecules of which are the same; *e.g.*, in the Bence-Jones protein, the chains are all κ or λ.

monoc'ular [mono- + L. *oculus*, eye] Relating to, affecting, or visible by, one eye only.

mon'ocyte [mono- + G. *kytos*, cell] A relatively large mononuclear leucocyte that normally constitutes 3 to 7% of the leucocytes of the circulating blood and is normally found in lymph nodes, spleen, bone marrow, and loose connective tissue.

mon'ocytope'nia [mono- + G. *kytos*, cell, + *penia*, poverty] Diminution in the number of monocytes in the circulating blood.

monoloc'ular [mono- + L. *loculus*, a small place] Having one cavity or chamber.

monoma'nia [mono- + G. *mania*, frenzy] An obsession or abnormally extreme enthusiasm for a single idea or subject, a psychosis marked by the limitation of symptoms to a certain group, as the delusion in paranoia.

mononu'clear Having only one nucleus.

mon'onucleo'sis Presence of abnormally large numbers of mononuclear leucocytes in the circulating blood, especially forms that are not normal.

infectious m., an acute febrile illness associated with the Epstein-Barr herpetovirus and characterized by fever, sore throat, enlargement of lymph nodes and spleen, and leucopenia that changes to lymphocytosis.

monopha'sic **1.** Characterized by only one phase **2.** Pertaining to a psychiatric disorder with one phase, as opposed to a diphasic disorder like manic-depressive psychosis.

mon'ophylet'ic [mono- + G. *phylē*, tribe] Having a single source of origin; derived from one line of descent.

monople'gia [mono- + G. *plēgē*, a stroke] Paralysis of one limb.

monosac'charide A carbohydrate that cannot form any simpler sugar by simple hydrolysis.

monoso'my State of an individual or cell that has lost one member of a pair of homologous chromosomes.

monozygot'ic [mono- + G. *zygōtos*, yoked] Denoting twins derived from a single fertilized ovum.

mons, pl. **mon'tes** [L. a mountain] [NA] An anatomical prominence or slight elevation above the general level of the surface.

m. pu'bis [NA], **m. ven'eris,** the prominence caused by a pad of fatty tisssue over the symphysis pubis in the female.

mood swing Oscillation of a person's emotional feeling tone between periods of euphoria and depression.

Moraxel'la [V. *Morax*] A genus of obligately aerobic, nonmotile bacteria, containing Gram-negative coccoids or short rods which usually occur in pairs, that are parasitic on the mucous membranes of man and other mammals. The type species, *M. lacunata*, causes conjunctivitis in man.

mor'bid [L. *morbidus*, ill, fr. *morbus*, disease] **1.** Diseased or pathologic. **2.** In psychology, abnormal or deviant.

morbid'ity 1. A diseased state. **2.** The ratio of sick to well in a community.

morbil'li [Mediev. L. *morbillus*, dim. of L. *morbus*, disease] Measles.

morbil'liform [see morbilli] Resembling measles.

mor'bus [L. disease] Disease (1).

morcella'tion [Fr. *morceler*, to subdivide] Division into and removal of small pieces, as of a tumour.

mo'ria [G. *mōria*, folly, fr. *mōros*, stupid, dull] **1.** Rarely used term denoting foolishness or dullness of comprehension. **2.** Rarely used term for a mental state marked by frivolity, joviality, and inveterate tendency to jest.

mo'ribund [L. *moribundus*, dying, fr. *morior*, to die] Dying; at the point of death.

mor'phine [L. *Morpheus*, god of dreams or sleep] The major phenanthrene alkaloid of opium; produces a combination of depression and excitation in the CNS and some peripheral tissues; repeated administration leads to the development of tolerance, physical dependence, and (if abused) psychic dependence; an analgesic that also produces sedation and allays anxiety.

morpho-, morph- [G. *morphē*, form, shape] Combining forms relating to form, shape, or structure.

morphoe'a [G. *morphē*, form, figure] Circumscribed or localized scleroderma; a cutaneous lesion characterized by indurated, slighty depressed plaques of thickened dermal fibrous tissue, of a whitish or yellowish white colour surrounded by a pinkish or purplish halo.

morphogen'esis [morpho- + G. *genesis*, production] Differentiation of cells and tissues in the early embryo which results in establishing the form and structure of the various organs and parts of the body.

mor'tal [L. *mortalis*, fr. *mors*, death] **1.** Pertaining to, or causing death. **2.** Destined to die.

mortal'ity [L. *mortalitus*, fr. *mors* (*mort*-), death] **1.** The state of being mortal. **2.** Mortality *rate*.

mor'tifica'tion [L. *mors* (*mort*-), death + *facio*, to make] Gangrene.

mor'ula [Mod. L. dim. of L. *morus*, mulberry] The mass of blastomeres resulting from the early cleavage divisions of the zygote.

mosa'ic [Mod. L. *mosaicus, musaicus*, pertaining to the Muses, artistic] Juxtaposition in an organism of genetically different tissues, resulting from somatic mutation (gene mosaicism), an anomaly of chromosome division resulting in two or more types of cells containing different numbers of chromosomes (chromosome mosaicism) or chimerism.

mosa'icism Condition of being mosaic.

mo'tile [L. *motio*, movement] **1.** Having the power of spontaneous movement. **2.** Denoting the type of mental imagery in which the person learns and recalls most readily that which he has felt.

motil'ity The power of spontaneous movement.

mo'tive [L. *moveo*, to move, to set in motion] **1.** Learned drive; a predisposition, need, or specific state of tension within an individual which arouses, maintains, and directs behaviour toward a goal. **2.** The reason attributed to or given by an individual for a behavioural act.

motoneu'rone Motor *neurone*.

mo'tor [L. a mover, fr. *movere*, to move] **1.** In anatomy and physiology, those neural structures which by the impulses generated and transmitted by them cause muscle fibres or pigment cells to contract, or glands to secrete. **2.** In psychology, the organism's overt reaction to a stimulus (motor response).

mot'tling [E. *motley*, variegated in colour] An area of skin comprised of macular lesions of varying shades or colours.

mould 1. A filamentous fungus, generally a circular colony with filaments not organized into large fruiting bodies, such as mushrooms. 2. A shaped receptacle into which material is pressed or poured in making a cast. 3. To shape a mass of plastic material according to a definite pattern. 4. To change in shape; denoting especially the adaptation of the fetal head to the pelvic canal. 5. In dentistry, the shape of an artificial tooth (or teeth).

mouth [A.S. *mūth*] 1. Oral cavity. 2. The opening, usually external, of a cavity or canal.

  tapir m., protrusion of the lips due to weakness of the oral muscle in certain forms of juvenile muscular dystrophy.

  trench m., necrotizing ulcerative *gingivitis*.

mouth'wash A medicated liquid used for cleaning the mouth and treating diseased states of its mucous membranes.

move'ment [L. *moveo*, pp. *motus*, to move] 1. The act of motion; said of the entire body or of one or more of its numbers or parts. 2. Stool. 3. Defaecation.

  passive m., m. of any joint effected by the hand of another person, or by mechanical means, without participation of the subject himself.

  rapid eye m.'s (REM), symmetrical quick m.'s occurring many times during a single night's sleep, in clusters far 5 ta 60 minutes, associated with dreaming.

  vermicular m., peristalsis.

muci- Combining form for mucus, mucous, or mucin. See also muco-, myxo-.

mu'cin A secretion containing mucopolysaccharides, such as that from mucous glandular cells; also present in the ground substance of connective tissue.

mu'cinase A term loosely applied to any enzyme that hydrolyses mucopolysaccharide substances (mucins).

mucin'ogen [mucin + G. -*gen*, producing] A glycoprotein that forms mucin through the imbibition of water.

mu'cinous Relating to or containing mucin.

muco- Combining form for mucus, mucous, or mucosa. See also muci-, myxo-.

mu'cocele [muco- + G. *kēlē*, tumor, hernia] 1. A mucous polypus. 2. A retention cyst of the lacrimal sac, paranasal sinuses, appendix, or gallbladder.

mu'cocuta'neous Relating to mucous membrane and skin; denoting the line of junction of the two at the nasal, oral, vaginal, and anal orifices.

mu'coid [mucus + G. *eidos*, appearance] 1. A mucin, mucoprotein, or mucopolysaccharide. 2. Mucinous.

mu'colipido'sis, pl. **mu'colipido'ses** Any of a group of metabolic storage diseases resembling Hurler's syndrome but with normal urinary mucopolysaccharides, in which symptoms of visceral and mesenchymal sphingolipid and/or glycolipid storage are present; autosomal recessive inheritance.

mucolyt'ic [muco- + G. *lysis*, dissolution] Capable of dissolving, digesting, or liquefying mucus.

mu'copolysac'charidase Mucinase.

mu'copolysac'charide A complex of protein and polysaccharide, usually implying that the polysaccharide component is a major part of the complex.

mu'copolysac'charido'sis Term embracing a group of diseases that have in common a disorder in metabolism of mucopolysaccharides, with various defects of bone, cartilage, and connective tissue.

mu'copu'rulent Pertaining to an exudate that is chiefly pus, but contains significant proportions of mucous material.

Mu'cor [L. mould] A genus of fungi (class Phycomycetes, family Mucoraceae), several species of which are pathogenic and may cause mucormycosis (phycomycosis) in man.

mu'cormyco'sis General term denoting conditions occasionally caused by, or associated with, various fungi species in the family Mucoraceae, *e.g.*, *Absidia*, *Mortierella*, *Mucor*, and *Rhizopus*.

muco'sa [L. fem. of *mucosus*, mucous] See *tunica* mucosa.

mu'cous [L. *mucosus*, mucous, fr. *mucus*] Relating to mucus or a m. membrane.

mu'coviscido'sis Cystic *fibrosis*.

mu'cus [L.] The clear viscid secretion of the mucous membranes, consisting of mucin, epithelial cells, leucocytes, and various inorganic salts suspended in water.

multi- [L. *multus*, much, many] Prefix denoting many, properly; equivalent of *poly-*. See also pluri.

mul'tiartic'ular [multi- + L. *articulus*, joint] Relating to or involving many joints.

multigrav'ida [multi- + L. *gravida*, pregnant] A pregnant woman who has been pregnant one or more times previously.

multilo'bar, multilo'bate, multilobed Having several lobes.

multilob'ular Having many lobules.

multiloc'ular Having many compartments or loculi.

multinu'clear, multinu'cleated Having two or more nuclei.

multip'ara [multi- + L. *pario*, to bring forth, to bear] A woman who has given birth at least two times to an infant, whether alive or dead.

multip'arous Relating to a multipara.

multipo'lar Having more than two poles; denoting a nerve cell in which the branches project from several points.

multiva'lent [multi- + L. *valentia*, power] **1.** In chemistry, having a combining power of more than one atom of hydrogen. **2.** Efficacious in more than one direction.

mumps [dialectic Eng. *mump*, a lump or bump] Epidemic *parotiditis*.

mu'ral [L. *muralis*; fr. *murus*, wall] Relating to the wall of any cavity.

mur'mur [L.] A soft sound heard on auscultation of the heart, lungs, or blood vessels. Also used for a variety of other-than-soft sounds, which may be loud, harsh, frictional, etc.

Mus'ca [L. fly] A genus of flies (family Muscidae, order Diptera) that includes the common housefly, *M. domestica*, a species involved in the mechanical transfer of numerous pathogens.

mus'cae volitan'tes [L. pl. of *musca*, fly; pres. p. pl. of *volito*, to fly to and fro] An appearance of moving spots before the eyes.

mus'carine A toxin with neurologic effects, isolated from *Amanita muscaria* (fly agaric mushroom) and also present in some other mushroom species; cholinergic substance whose pharmacologic effects resemble those of acetylcholine and postganglionic parasympathetic stimulation (cardiac inhibition, vasodilation, salivation, lacrimation, bronchoconstriction, gastrointestinal stimulation).

muscle [L. *musculus*] Tissue consisting predominantly of contractile cells and classified as skeletal, cardiac, or smooth, the latter lacking in transverse striations characteristic of the other varieties.

  antagonistic m.'s, m.'s having an opposite function, the contraction of one neutralizing that of the other.

  cardiac m., myocardium; m. of the heart, consisting of anastomosing transversely striated m. fibres formed of cells united at intercalated discs.

  involuntary m.'s, m.'s not under control of the will; except those of the heart, they are smooth m.'s.

  skeletal m., a m. connected at either or both extremities with a bone; consists of elongated, multinucleated, transversely striated skeletal muscle fibres, together with connective tissues, blood vessels, and nerves.

  smooth m., one of the m.'s of the internal organs, blood vessels, hair follicles, etc.; although transverse striations are lacking, fine myofibrils occur.

  sphincter m., see sphincter.

  striated m., skeletal or cardiac m. in which cross striations occur in the fibres.

  voluntary m., a m. whose action is under the control of the will; all the striated m.'s, except the heart, are voluntary m.'s.

mus'cular Relating to a muscle or the muscles.

mus'culature The arrangement of the muscles in a part or in the body as a whole.

mus'culocuta'neous Relating to or supplying both muscle and skin.

mus'culoskel'etal Relating to muscles and to the skeleton.

mus'culoten'dinous Relating to both muscular and tendinous tissues.

mus'culus, gen. and pl. **mus'culi** [L. a little mouse, a muscle] [NA] Muscle; one of the contractile organs of the body by which movements of the various organs and parts are effected; typically, a mass of muscle fibres attached at each extremity by means of a tendon to a bone or other structure. For histologic descriptions, see muscle.

  m. cilia'ris [NA], ciliary muscle; smooth muscle of the ciliary body, consisting of circular fibres and radiating fibres; *action*, changes shape of lens in process of accommodation.

m. deltoi'deus [NA], deltoid muscle; *origin*, lateral third of clavicle, lateral border of acromion process, lower border of spine of scapula; *insertion*, lateral side of shaft of humerus; *nerve supply*, axillary from fifth and sixth cervical through brachial plexus; *action*, abduction, flexion, extension, and rotation of arm.

m. gastrocne'mius [NA], *origin*, lateral and medial condyles of the femur; *insertion*, with soleus by tendo calcaneus (achillis) into lower half of posterior surface of calcaneus; *nerve supply*; tibial; *action*, plantar flexion of foot.

mu'tagen [L. *muto*, to change, + G. *-gen*, producing] Any agent that causes production of a mutation.

mutagen'ic Having the power to cause mutations.

mu'tant An organism possessing one or more genes that have undergone mutation.

muta'tion [L. *muto*, pp. -*atus*, to change] **1.** A change in the character of a gene that is perpetuated in subsequent divisions of the cell in which it occurs. **2.** Sudden production of a species, as distinguished from variation.

mute [L. *mutus*] **1.** Unable or unwilling to speak. **2.** One who does not have the faculty of speech.

mutila'tion [L. *mutilatio*, fr. *mutilo*, pp. -*atus*, to maim] Disfigurement or injury by removal or destruction of any conspicuous or essential part of the body.

mu'tism [L. *mutus*, mute] Organic or functional absence of the faculty of speech.

myal'gia [G. *mys*, muscle, + *algos*, pain] Pain in a muscle.

my'asthe'nia [G. *mys*, muscle, + *astheneia*, weakness] Muscular weakness.

m. gra'vis, a chronic progressive muscular weakness, beginning usually in the face and throat, unaccompanied by atrophy; due to a defect in myoneural conduction.

my'asthen'ic Relating to myasthenia.

myato'nia, myat'ony [G. *mys*, muscle, + *a*- priv. + *tonos*, tone] Abnormal extensibility of a muscle.

myce'lium, pl. **myce'lia** [G. *mykēs*, fungus, + *hēlos*, nail, wart] The mass of hyphae making up a colony of fungi.

my'cete [G. *mykēs*, fungus] A fungus.

mycet-, myceto-, myco- [G. *mykēs*, fungus] Combining forms relating to fungus.

myceto'ma 1. A chronic infection, usually involving the feet, characterized by the formation of localized lesions with tumefactions and multiple draining sinuses; the exudate contains granules that may be yellow, white, red, brown, or black, depending upon the causative agent. M. is caused by two principal groups of microorganisms: actinomycetes and true fungi. **2.** Any tumour produced by filamentous fungi.

my'cobacte'ria Organisms belonging to the genus *Mycobacterium*.

My'cobacte'rium [myco- + bacterium] A genus of aerobic, nonmotile bacteria (family Mycobacteriaceae) containing Gram-positive rods; parasitic and saprophytic species occur. The type species is *M. tuberculosis*.

M. bal'nei, *M. marinum*.

M. kansas'ii, a species causing a tuberculosis-like pulmonary disease, and various infections.

M. lep'rae, Hansen's bacillus; an obligately parasitic species of man which causes leprous lesions.

M. mari'num, a species causing swimming pool granuloma.

M. scrofula'ceum, a species frequently associated with cervical adenitis in children.

M. tuberculo'sis, Koch's bacillus; tubercle bacillus (human); a species that causes tuberculosis in man.

mycol'ogy [myco- + G. *logos*, study] The science and study of fungi.

Mycoplas'ma [myco- + G. *plasma*, something formed (plasm)] A genus of aerobic to facultatively anaerobic bacteria (family Mycoplasmataceae) containing Gram-negative cells that do not possess a true cell wall, but are bounded by a three-layered membrane; they are parasitic to pathogenic. The type species is *M. mycoides*.

M. hom'inis, a species found in the genital tract and anal canal of man.

M. mycoi'des, a species containing two subspecies, *M. mycoides* subsp. *mycoides*, the type subspecies, and *M. mycoides* subsp. *capri*, which cause pleuropneumonia in cattle and goats; the type species of the genus *M.*

M. pharyn'gis, a species occurring as a commensal in human oropharynx.

M. pneumo'niae, a species causing primary atypical pneumonia in man.

mycoplas'ma, pl. **mycoplas'mata** Any member of the genus *Mycoplasma*.

myco'sis [myco- + G. -*osis*, condition] Any disease caused by fungi.

m. fungoi'des, a chronic progressive lymphoma arising in the skin (so-called because tumours in the late stage resemble mushrooms); initially, the disease simulates eczema or other inflammatory dermatoses.

mycot'ic Relating to a mycosis or to a fungus.

mydri'asis [G.] Dilation of the pupil.

mydriat'ic Causing mydriasis or dilation of the pupil.

myec'tomy [G. *mys*, muscle, + *ektome*, excision] Exsection of a portion of muscle.

myel-, myelo- [G. *myelos*, medulla, marrow] Combining form denoting relationship to the bone marrow, the spinal cord and medulla oblongata, or the myelin sheath of nerve fibres.

my'elenceph'alon [myel- + G. *enkephalos*, brain] [NA] *Medulla* oblongata.

my'elin 1. The lipoproteinaceous material enveloping the axon of myelinated nerve fibres, composed of regularly alternating layers of lipids and protein. **2.** Droplets of lipid formed during autolysis and postmortem decomposition.

my'elinated Having a myelin sheath.

myeli'tis [myel- + G. -*itis*, inflammation] Inflammation of the spinal cord, or of the bone marrow.

my'eloblast [myelo- + G. *blastos*, germ] An immature cell in the granulocytic series, occurring normally in bone marrow but not in the circulating blood, which matures into a promyelocyte and then a myelocyte.

my'elocele [myelo- + G. *kele*, hernia] Protrusion of the spinal cord in spina bifida.

my'elocyte [myelo- + G. *kytos*, cell] **1.** A young cell of the granulocytic series, occurring normally in bone marrow but not in circulating blood, which matures into a metamyelocyte. **2.** A nerve cell of the grey matter of the brain or spinal cord.

myelocyt'ic Pertaining to or characterized by myelocytes.

my'elodyspla'sia [myelo- + G. *dys-*, difficult, + *plasis*, a moulding] An abnormality in development of the spinal cord.

myelogen'esis Development of bone marrow.

myelog'raphy [myelo- + G. *graphe*, a drawing] Radiography of the spinal cord after injection of a radiopaque substance into the spinal arachnoid space.

my'eloid 1. Pertaining to, derived from, or manifesting certain features of the bone marrow. **2.** Sometimes used with reference to the spinal cord. **3.** Pertaining to certain characteristics of myelocytic forms, not necessarily implying origin, in the bone marrow.

myelo'ma [myelo- + G. -*oma*, tumour] A tumour composed of cells derived from haemopoietic tissues of the bone marrow.

endothelial m., Ewing's *tumour*.

multiple m., a clinically characteristic monoclonal gammopathy that occurs more frequently in men than in women and is associated with anaemia, haemorrhages, recurrent infections, and weakness; ordinarily regarded as a malignant neoplasm that originates in bone marrow and involves chiefly the skeleton; clinical features are attributable to the sites of involvement and to abnormalities in formation of plasma protein, the most frequent being: occurrence of Bence Jones proteinuria, great increase in γ-globulin in the plasma, occasional formation of cryoglobulin, and a form of primary amyloidosis.

plasma cell m., (1) multiple m.; **(2)** plasmacytoma of bone, usually a solitary lesion and not associated with the occurrence of Bence Jones protein or other disturbances in the metabolism of protein.

my'elomato'sis The occurrence of myelomas in various sites.

myelon'ic [G. *myelon*, fr. *myelos*, marrow] Relating to the spinal cord.

myelop'athy [myelo- + G. *pathos*, suffering] **1.** Disturbance or disease of the spinal cord. **2.** A disease of the myelopoietic tissues.

myeloph'thisis [myelo- + G. *phthisis*, a wasting away] **1.** Wasting or atrophy of the spinal cord. **2.** Replacement of haemopoietic tissue in the bone marrow by abnormal tissue, usually fibrous tissue or malignant tumours that are most commonly metastatic carcinomas.

my'elopoie'sis [myelo- + G. *poiesis*, a making] Formation of the tissue elements of bone marrow, any of the types of blood cells derived from bone marrow, or both processes.

my'elopoiet'ic Relating to myelopoiesis.

my'eloprolif'erative Pertaining to or characterized by unusual proliferation of myelopoietic tissue.

myelo'sis 1. Abnormal proliferation of tissue or cellular elements of bone marrow. 2. Abnormal proliferation of medullary tissue in the spinal cord.

erythremic m., a neoplastic process involving the erythropoietic tissue, characterized by anaemia, irregular fever, splenomegaly, hepatomegaly, haemorrhagic disorders, and numerous erythroblasts in all stages of maturation in the circulating blood. Acute and chronic forms are recognized, the former is also called Di Guglielmo's disease and acute erythraemia.

myi'asis [G. *myia*, fly] Any infection due to invasion of tissues or cavities of the body by larvae of dipterous insects by larva migrans.

myo- [G. *mys*, muscle] Combining form relating to muscle.

myocar'dial Relating to the myocardium.

myocardi'tis Inflammation of the muscular walls of the heart.

myocar'dium, pl. **myocar'dia** [myo- + G. *kardia*, heart] [NA] The middle layer of the heart, consisting of cardiac muscle.

my'ocele [myo- + G. *kēlē*, hernia] Protrusion of muscle substance through a rent in its sheath.

myoclon'ic Showing myoclonus.

myoclo'nus [myo- + G. *klonus*, tumult] Clonic spasm or twitching of a muscle or group of muscles.

m. mul'tiplex, Friedreich's disease; a disorder marked by rapid contractions occurring simultaneously or consecutively in various unrelated muscles.

nocturnal m., frequently repeated muscular jerks occurring at the moment of dropping off to sleep.

my'ocuta'neous 1. Musculocutaneous. 2. Denoting a parcel comprising a muscle and its investments and vascular supply, the overlying skin, and the intervening tissues.

myodys'trophy [myo- + G. *dys-*, difficult, poor, + *trophē*, nourishment] Muscular dystrophy.

myofi'bril [myo- + Mod. L. *fibrilla*, fibril] One of the fine longitudinal fibrils occurring in a skeletal or cardiac muscle fibre; in striated muscle, the fibril is made up of ultramicroscopic thick and thin myofilaments.

myofibro'sis Chronic myositis with diffuse hyperplasia of the interstitial connective tissue pressing upon and causing atrophy of the muscular tissue.

myofil'aments Ultramicroscopic threads making up myofibrils in striated muscle.

myogenet'ic, myogen'ic,

myog'enous 1. Originating in or starting from muscle. 2. Relating to the origin of muscle cells or fibres.

myoglo'bin (Mb) The oxygen-transporting protein of muscle, resembling blood haemoglobin in function, but containing only one haem as part of the molecule and with one-fourth of the molecular weight.

my'oglobinu'ria Excretion of myoglobin in the urine.

my'ograph [myo- + G. *graphō*, to write] A recording instrument by which tracings are made of muscular contractions.

myog'raphy The recording of muscular movements by the myograph.

myoky'mia [myo- + G. *kyma*, wave] A benign condition, often familial, characterized by an irregular twitching of most of the muscles.

myo'ma [myo- + G. *-oma*, tumour] A benign neoplasm of muscular tissue.

myomec'tomy [myoma + G. *ektomē*, excision] Operative removal of a myoma, specifically of a uterine myoma.

myome'trium [myo- + G. *mētra*, uterus] [NA] The muscular wall of the uterus

myoneu'ral [myo- + G. *neuron*, nerve] Denoting the synapse of the motor neurone with striated muscle fibres; myoneural junction or motor endplate

myoneural'gia [myo- + G. *neuron*, nerve, + *algos*, pain] Neuralgic pain in a muscle.

myo-oede'ma [myo- + G. *oidēma*, swelling] Localized contraction of a degenerating muscle, occurring at the point of a sharp blow; the response is independent of the nerve supply.

myopal'mus [myo- + G. *palmos*, a quivering] Muscle twitching.

myop'athy [myo- + G. *pathos*, suffering] Any abnormal conditions or disease of the muscular tissues, especially involving skeletal muscle.

my'opericardi'tis [myo- + pericarditis] Inflammation of the muscular wall of the heart and of the enveloping pericardium.

myo'pia (M, my.) [G. fr. *myo*, to shut, + *ōps*, eye] Shortsightedness; nearsightedness; an error in refraction or of elongation of the globe of the eye, causing parallel rays to be focused in front of the retina.

myop'ic Relating to myopia.

my'oplasm [myo- + G. *plasma*, a thing formed] The contractile portion of the muscle cell.

myoplas'tic Relating to the plastic surgery of the muscles, or to the use of muscular tissue in correcting defects.

myorrhex'is [myo- + G. *rhēxis*, a rupture] Tearing of a muscle.

my'osarco'ma A malignant neoplasm derived from muscular tissue.

my'osin A globulin in muscle that in combination with actin forms actomyosin, the fundamental contractile unit of muscle.

myosi'tis [myo- + G. *-itis*, inflammation] Inflammation of a muscle.

   m. ossif'icans, ossification or deposit of bone in muscle with fibrosis, causing pain and swelling muscles.

my'ospasm Spasmodic muscular contraction.

my'otome [myo- + G. *tomos*, a cut] **1.** A knife for dividing muscle. **2.** In embryos, that part of the somite that gives rise to skeletal muscle. **3.** All muscles derived from one somite and innervated by one segmental spinal nerve.

myot'omy [myo- + G. *tomē*, excision] **1.** Anatomy or dissection of the muscles. **2.** Surgical division of a muscle.

myoto'nia [myo- + G. *tonos*, tension, stretching] Delayed relaxation of a muscle after an initial contraction.

   m. congen'ita, An hereditary disease marked by momentary tonic spasms occurring when a voluntary movement is attempted.

myoton'ic Pertaining to or exhibiting myotonia.

myot'onus [myo- + G. *tonos*, tension, stretching] A tonic spasm or temporary rigidity of a muscle or group of muscles.

myot'ony [myo- + G. *tonos*, tension] Muscular tonus or tension.

myringec'tomy [myring- + G. *ektomē*, excision] Excision of the tympanic membrane.

myringi'tis [myring- + G. *-itis*, inflammation] Tympanitis; inflammation of the tympanic membrane.

myringo-, myring- [Mod. L. *myringa*] Combining forms denoting the membrana tympani.

myrin'goplasty [myringo- + G. *plassō*, to form] Surgical repair of a damaged tympanic membrane.

myringot'omy [myringo- + G. *tomē*, excision] Paracentesis of the tympanic membrane.

myr'inx [Mod. L. *myringa*, drum membrane] *Membrana* tympani.

myxadeno'ma An adenoma, in which the loose connective tissue of the stroma has a resemblance to relatively primitive mesenchymal tissue.

myxo-, myx- [G. *myxa*, mucus] Combining forms relating to mucus. See also muci-, muco-.

myxoede'ma [myx- + G. *oidema*, swelling] Hypothyroidism characterized by a relatively hard oedema of subcutaneous tissue; caused by removal or loss of functioning thyroid tissue.

   congenital m., cretinism.

myxofibro'ma [myxo- + L. *fibra*, fibre, + G. *-ōma*, tumour] A benign neoplasm of fibrous connective tissue in which focal or diffuse degenerative changes result in portions that resemble primitive mesenchymal tissue.

myx'oid [myxo- + G. *eidos*, resemblance] Resembling mucus.

myxo'ma [myxo- + G. *-ōma*, tumour] A neoplasm derived from connective tissue, consisting chiefly of polyhedral and stellate cells that are loosely embedded in a soft, mucoid matrix, thereby resembling primitive mesenchymal tissue.

myxo'matous 1. Pertaining to or characterized by the features of a myxoma. **2.** Said of tissue that resembles primitive mesenchymal tissue.

myxosarco'ma [myxo- + G. *sarx*, flesh, + *-ōma*, tumour] A sarcoma characterized by immature, relatively undifferentiated, and primitive gross cells that grow rapidly and invade extensively, resulting in tissue that resembles primitive mesenchyme in its gross features.

myx'ovirus Term formerly used for viruses with an affinity for mucins, now included in the families Orthomyxoviridae and Paramyxoviridae, which include influenza virus, parainfluenza virus, respiratory syncytial virus, and measles virus.

N

nae'vus, pl. **nae'vi** [L. *naevus*, mole, birthmark] **1.** Birthmark, a circumscribed malformation of the skin, especially if coloured by hyperpigmentation or increased vascularity. **2.** A benign localized overgrowth of melanin-forming cells arising in the skin early in life.

  n. pigmento'sus, mole; a congenital pigmented lesion of varying size, raised or level with the skin.

  n. pilo'sus, hairy mole; a mole covered with an abundant growth of hair.

  spider n., arterial spider.

  strawberry n., a small n. vascularis resembling a strawberry in size, shape, and colour.

  n. vascula'ris, n. vasculo'sus, a congenital irregular red discoloration of the skin caused by an overgrowth of the cutaneous capillaries.

nail [A.S. *naegel*] **1.** Unguis. **2.** A slender rod used in operations to fasten together the divided extremities of a broken bone.

  ingrown n., ingrown toenail; a toenail, one edge of which is overgrown by the nailfold, producing a pyogenic granuloma.

  spoon n., koilonychia.

nal'orphine An antagonist of most of the depressant and stimulatory effects of morphine and related narcotic analgesics.

nalox'one hydrochloride A potent antagonist of all narcotics, unique because of the absence of pharmacologic action when administered without narcotics.

nano- [G. *nānos*, dwarf] Combining form relating to dwarfism (nanism).

nan'ism [G. *nanos*; L. *nanus*, dwarf] Dwarfism.

nape Nucha.

nar'cissism [*Narkissos*, G. myth. char.] **1.** Self-love; sexual attraction toward one's own person. **2.** A state in which the individual regards everything in relation to himself and not to other persons or things.

narco- [G. *narkoun*, to benumb, deaden] Combining form relating to stupor or narcosis.

narcoanal'ysis Psychotherapeutic treatment under light anaesthesia.

narcohypno'sis [narco- + G. *hypnos*, sleep] Stupor or deep sleep induced by hypnosis.

nar'colepsy [narco- + G. *lēpsis*, seizure] A sudden uncontrollable disposition to sleep occurring at irregular intervals, with or without obvious predisposing or exciting cause, usually involving an abnormality in sleep-stage sequencing.

narco'sis [G. a benumbing] An obsolete synonym for anaesthesia; now used to denote general and nonspecific reversible depression of neuronal excitability, produced by a number of physical and chemical agents, usually resulting in stupor rather than in anaesthesia.

narcother'apy Psychotherapy conducted with the patient under the influence of a sedative or narcotic drug.

narcot'ic [G. *narkōtikos*, benumbing] **1.** Any substance producing stupor associated with analgesia; specifically, a drug derived from opium or opium-like compounds, with potent analgesic effects associated with significant alteration of mood and behaviour, and with the potential for dependence and tolerance following repeated administration. **2.** Capable of inducing a state of stuporous analgesia.

na'ris, pl. **na'res** [L.] [NA] Nostril; the anterior opening on either side of the nasal cavity.

na'sal [L. *nasus*, nose] Rhinal; relating to the nose.

nas'cent [L. *nascor*, pres. p. *nascens*, to be born] **1.** Beginning; being born or produced. **2.** Denoting the state of a chemical element at the moment it is set free from one of its compounds.

naso- [L. *nasus*, nose] Combining form relating to the nose.

nasofron'tal Relating to the nose and the forehead, or to the nasal cavity and the frontal sinuses.

nasolac'rimal Relating to the nasal and the lacrimal bones, or to the nasal cavity and the lacrimal ducts.

nasopal'atine Relating to the nose and palate.

nasopharyn'geal   Relating to the nose or the nasal cavity and the pharynx, or to the rhinopharynx or nasopharynx.

na'sopharyngi'tis   [naso- + pharynx, + G. *-itis*, inflammation] Inflammation of the mucous membrane of the posterior nares and upper part of the pharynx.

nasophar'ynx   The part of the pharynx that lies above the soft palate, anteriorly opening into the nasal cavity.

na'sosinusi'tis   Inflammation of the nasal cavities and of the accessory sinuses.

na'sus   [L.] [NA] Nose; the external portion of the respiratory pathway which forms a prominent feature of the face and contains the nasal cavity perforated inferiorly by two nostrils separated by a septum.

na'tal   **1.** [L. *natalis*, fr. *nascor*, pp. *natus*, to be born] Relating to birth. **2.** [L. *nates*, buttocks] Relating to the buttocks or nates.

natal'ity   [see natal (1)] The birth rate; the ratio of births to the general population.

na'tes   [L. pl. of *natis*] [NA] The buttocks; breech; the prominence formed by the gluteal muscles on either side.

natrae'mia   [natrium (sodium) + G. *haima*, blood] Presence of sodium in the circulating blood.

na'trium   [Ar. *natrūm*, fr. G. *nitron*, carbonate of soda] Sodium.

naturop'athy   A system of therapeutics in which neither surgical nor medicinal agents are used, dependence being placed only on natural (nonmedicinal) forces.

nau'sea   [L. fr. G. *nausia*, seasickness, fr. *naus*, ship] Sickness at the stomach; an inclination to vomit.

   n. gravida'rum, morning *sickness*.

na'vel   [A.S. *nafela*] Umbilicus.

navic'ular   [L. *navicularis*, relating to shipping] Scaphoid.

near'sight'edness   Myopia.

neb'ula, pl. **neb'ulae** [L. fog, cloud, mist] **1.** A faint, foglike opacity of the cornea. **2.** A class of oily preparations, intended for application by atomization.

neb'ulizer   [L. *nebula*, mist] A device used to reduce liquid medication to an extremely fine cloud; useful in delivering medication to the deep part of the respiratory tract.

Neca'tor   [L. a murderer] A genus of nematode hookworms (family Ancylostomatidae, subfamily Necatorine) distinguished by two chitinous cutting plates in the buccal cavity and fused male copulatory spicules. Species include *N. americanus* (New World hookworm), the adults of which attach to villi in the small intestine and suck blood, causing abdominal discomfort, diarrhoea (usually with melaena) and cramps, anorexia, loss of weight, and anaemia. See also *Ancylostoma*.

necatori'asis   Hookworm disease caused by *Necator*, the resulting anaemia being usually less severe than that from ancylostomiasis.

neck   [A.S. *hnecca*] **1.** Collum. **2.** Any constricted part of a structure having a fancied resemblance to the n. of an animal.

   stiff n., wry n., torticollis.

necro-, necr-   [G. *nekros*, corpse] Combining forms relating to death or to necrosis.

nec'robio'sis   [necro- + G. *biōs*, life] **1.** Physiologic or normal death of cells or tissues as a result of changes associated with development, aging, or use. **2.** Necrosis of a small area of tissue.

necrogen'ic, necrog'enous   [necro- + G. *genesis*, origin] Relating to, living in, or having origin in dead matter.

nec'ropsy   [necro- + G. *opsis*, view] Autopsy.

necro'sis   [G. *nekrōsis*, death] Pathologic death of one or more cells, or of a portion of tissue or organ, resulting from irreversible damage.

necrot'ic   Pertaining to or affected by necrosis.

necrot'omy   [necro- + G. *tomē*, cutting] **1.** Dissection. **2.** Surgical removal of a sequestrum or necrosed portion of bone.

nee'dle   **1.** A slender, usually sharp-pointed, instrument used for puncturing tissues, suturing, or passing a ligature around an artery, or for injection or aspiration. **2.** To separate tissues by means of one or two n.'s in the dissection of small parts. **3.** To perform discission of a cataract by means of a knife n.

needle-holder, -carrier, -driver   An instrument for grasping a needle in suturing.

need'ling   Discission of a soft or of a secondary cataract.

nega'tion   Denial.

neg'ative (-)   [L. *negativus*, fr. *nego*, to deny] **1.** Not affirmative; refutative; not positive. **2.** Denoting failure of response, absence of a reaction, or absence of an entity or condition in question.

neg'ativism A tendency to do the opposite of what one is requested to do, or to stubbornly resist for no apparent reason.

Neisse'ria [A. *Neisser*] A genus of aerobic to facultatively anaerobic bacteria (family Neisseriaceae) containing Gram-negative cocci which occur in pairs with the adjacent sides flattened. The type species is *N. gonorrhoeae*.

   N. gonorrhoe'ae, gonococcus; a species that causes gonorrhoea and other infections in man.

   N. meningiti'dis, meningococcus; a species that is the causative agent of meningococcal meningitis; groups are characterized by serologically specific capsular polysaccharides (A, B, C, and D).

nema-, nemat-, nemato- [G. *nēma*, thread] Combining forms meaning thread, threadlike.

Nemato'da [nemat- + G *eidos*, form] A class in the phylum Aschelminthes, including species parasitic in man and plant-parasitic and free-living soil or aquatic nonparasitic species; may be classified in two groups, based on their habitat in the human body; **1)** intestinal roundworms (*Ascaris, Trichuris, Ancylostoma, Necator, Strongyloides, Enterobius,* and *Trichinella*); **2)** filarial roundworms of the blood, lymphatic tissues, and viscera (*Wuchereria, Mansonella, Dipetalonema, Loa, Onchocerca,* and *Dracunculus*).

nem'atode Any parasitic worm of the class Nematoda.

neo- [G. *neos*, new] Prefix meaning new or recent.

neoblas'tic [neo- + G *blastos*, germ, offspring] Developing in or characteristic of new tissue.

ne'ocerebel'lum [NA] The large lateral portion of the cerebellar hemisphere receiving its dominant input from the pontine nuclei which, in turn, are dominated by afferent nerves originating from all parts of the cerebral cortex.

neocor'tex See *cortex* cerebri.

neol'ogism [neo- + G. *logos*, word] A new word or phrase, or an old word used in a new sense.

neomy'cin sulphate The sulphate of an antibacterial substance produced by the growth of *Streptomyces fradiae*, active against a variety of Gram-positive and Gram-negative bacteria.

neona'tal [neo- + L. *natalis*, relating to birth] Newborn; relating to the period immediately succeeding birth and continuing through the first 28 days of life.

ne'onate [L. *neonatus*, newborn] A neonatal infant.

ne'onatol'ogy [neo- + L. *natus*, pp. born, + G. *logos*, theory] The specialty concerned with disorders of the neonate.

neopal'lium See *cortex* cerebri.

neopla'sia [neo- + G. *plasis*, a moulding] The pathologic process that results in the formation and growth of a neoplasm.

ne'oplasm [neo- + G. *plasma*, thing formed] Tumour; an abnormal tissue that grows by cellular proliferation more rapidly than normal, continues to grow after the stimuli that initiated the new growth cease, shows partial or complete lack of structural organization and functional coordination with the normal tissue, and usually forms a distinct mass of tissue which may be either benign or malignant.

neoplas'tic Pertaining to or characterized by neoplasia, or containing a neoplasm.

nephr- See nephro-.

nephral'gia [nephr- + G. *algos*, pain] Pain in the kidney.

nephrec'tasis [nephr- + G. *ektasis*, a stretching] Dilation or distention of the pelvis of the kidney.

nephrec'tomy [nephr- + G. *ektomē*, excision] Surgical removal of a kidney.

neph'ric Renal; relating to the kidney.

nephrit'ic Relating to nephritis.

nephri'tis, pl. **nephrit'ides** [nephr- + G. *itis*, inflammation] Inflammation of the kidneys.

   glomerular n., glomerulonephritis.

   suppurative n., focal glomerulonephritis with abscess formation in the kidney.

nephro-, nephr- [G. *nephros*, kidney] Combining forms denoting the kidney. See also reno-.

neph'roblasto'ma Wilms *tumour*.

neph'rocalcino'sis [nephro- + calcinosis] Renal lithiasis characterized by diffusely scattered foci of calcification in the kidneys.

neph'rocapsec'tomy [nephro- + L. *capsula*, a small box, + G. *ektomē*, excision] Decortication, or decapsulation, of the kidney.

neph'rocele [nephro- + G. *kēlē*, hernia] Hernial displacement of a kidney.

neph'rocystanastomo'sis [nephro- + G. *kystis*, bladder, + *anastomo̅sis*, an outlet] Establishment of a connection between the kidney and the bladder, for correction of a permanent obstruction of the ureter.

nephrocysto'sis [nephro- + G. *kystis*, cyst, + *-osis*, condition] Formation of renal cysts.

neph'rogenet'ic, neph'rogen'ic [nephro- + G. *gene̅sis*, origin] Giving rise to kidney tissue.

nephrog'enous Arising from kidney tissue.

neph'rogram Radiograph of the kidney after the intravenous injection of a radiopaque substance.

neph'rolith [nephro- + G. *lithos*, stone] A renal calculus; a calculus occurring within the kidney.

neph'rolithi'asis The presence of renal calculi.

neph'rolithot'omy [nephro- + G. *lithos*, stone, + *tome̅*, incision] Incision into the kidney for the removal of a renal calculus.

nephrol'ogy [nephro- + G. *logos*, study] The branch of medical science concerned with the kidneys.

nephrol'ysis [nephro- + G. *lysis*, dissolution] **1.** Freeing of the kidney from inflammatory adhesions, with preservation of the capsule. **2.** Destruction of renal cells.

nephrolyt'ic Pertaining to, characterized by, or causing nephrolysis.

nephro'ma [nephro- + G. *-oma*, tumour] A tumour arising from renal tissue.

neph'ron [G. *nephros*, kidney] The functional unit of the kidney, consisting of the renal corpuscle, the proximal convoluted tubule, the nephronic loop, and the distal convoluted tubule.

nephrop'athy [nephro- + G. *pathos*, suffering] Any disease of the kidney.

neph'ropexy [nephro- + G. *pe̅xis*, fixation] Surgical fixation of a floating or mobile kidney.

nephropto'sis [nephro- + G. *pto̅sis*, a falling] Prolapse of the kidney.

nephropy'eloplasty [nephro- + G. *pyelos*, trough (pelvis), + *plasso̅*, to form] A plastic procedure on the kidney and renal pelvis.

nephropyo'sis [nephro- + G. *pyo̅sis*, suppuration] Suppuration of the kidney.

neph'rosclero'sis [nephro- + G. *skle̅rosis*, hardening] Induration of the kidney from overgrowth and contraction of the interstitial connective tissue.

arterial n., patchy atrophic scarring of the kidney due to arteriosclerotic narrowing of the lumens of large branches of the renal artery, occurring in old or hypertensive persons and occasionally causing hypertension.

arteriolar n., renal scarring due to arteriolar sclerosis resulting from longstanding hypertension.

neph'rosclerot'ic Pertaining to or causing nephrosclerosis.

nephro'sis [nephro- + G. *-osis*, condition] **1.** Nephropathy. **2.** Degeneration of renal tubular epithelium. **3.** Nephrotic *syndrome*.

nephros'tomy [nephro- + G. *stoma*, mouth] Establishment of an opening between the pelvis of the kidney through its cortex to the exterior of the body.

nephrot'ic Relating to, caused by, or similar to nephrosis.

nephroto'mogram A sectional radiograph of the kidneys following intravenous administration of contrast material to improve visualization of the renal parenchyma.

nephrot'omy [nephro- + G. *tome̅*, incision] Incision into the kidney.

nephrotox'ic **1.** Pertaining to nephrotoxin. **2.** Nephrolytic.

nephrotox'in A cytotoxin specific for cells of the kidney.

neph'roureterec'tomy [nephro- + ureter + G. *ektome̅*, excision] Surgical removal of a kidney and its ureter.

neph'roure'terocystec'tomy [nephro- + ureter + G. *kystis*, bladder, + *ektome̅*, excision] Surgical removal of kidney, ureter, and part or all of the bladder.

nerve [L. *nervus*] Microscopically, a bundle composed of one or more fascicles of myelinated or unmyelinated n. fibres, or both, together with accompanying connective tissue and blood vessels.

afferent n., a n. conveying impulses from the periphery to the CNS.

efferent n., a n. conveying impulses from the central nervous system to the periphery.

mixed n., a n. containing both afferent and efferent fibres.

motor n., an efferent n. conveying an impulse that excites muscular contraction.

parasympathetic n., one of the n.'s of the parasympathetic nervous system.

pressor n., an afferent n., stimulation of which excites a reflex vasocontriction, thereby raising the blood pressure.

sensory n., an afferent n. conveying impulses that are processed by the CNS so as to become part of the organism's perception of self and its environment.

somatic n., one of the n.'s of sensation or motion.

sympathetic n., one of the n.'s of the sympathetic nervous system.

trigeminal n., *nervus* trigeminus.

vagus n., *norvus* vagus.

vasomotor n., a motor n. effecting dilation (**vasodilator n.**) or contraction (**vasoconstrictor n.**) of the blood vessels.

ner'vous [L. *nervosus*] **1.** Relating to a nerve or the nerves **2.** Easily excited or agitated; suffering from instability.

ner'vus, pl. **ner'vi** [L.] [NA] Nerve; a whitish cord, made up of nerve fibres arranged in fascicles held together by a connective tissue sheath, through which stimuli are transmitted from the CNS to the periphery or the reverse.

ner'vi crania'les [NA], cranial nerves; twelve paired nerves that emerge from, or enter, the brain: olfaotory (I), optic (II), oculomotor (III), trochlear (IV), trigeminal (V), abducent (VI), facial (VII), vestibulocochlear (VII), glossopharyngeal (IX), vagus (X), accessory (XI), and hypoglossal (XII).

n. op'ticus [NA], optic nerve, second cranial nerve; originating from retina, it passes out of orbit through optic canal to chiasm, where part of its fibres cross to opposite side and pass through optic tract to geniculate bodies and superior colliculus.

ner'vi spina'les [NA], spinal nerves; 31 pairs of nerves emerging from the spinal cord, each attached to the cord by two roots, anterior and posterior (ventral and dorsal), the latter provided with a spinal ganglion.

n. trigem'inus [NA], trigeminal nerve; fifth cranial nerve; chief sensory nerve of face and motor nerve of muscles of mastication.

n. va'gus [NA], vagus or pneumogastric nerve; tenth cranial nerve; a mixed nerve that arises by numerous small roots from side of medulla oblongata; supplies pharynx; larynx, lungs, heart, oesophagus, stomach, and most of abdominal viscera.

neur-, neuri-, neuro- [G. *neuron*, nerve] Combining form denoting a nerve or relating to the nervous system.

neu'ral [G. *neuron*, nerve] **1.** Relating to any structure composed of nerve cells or their processes, or that on further development will give rise to nerve cells. **2.** Referring to the dorsal side of the vertebral bodies or their precursors, where the spinal cord is located.

neural'gia [neur- + G. *algos*, pain] Pain of a severe throbbing, or stabbing character in the course or distribution of a nerve.

trigeminal n., severe paroxysmal bursts of pain in one or more branches of the trigeminal nerve, often induced by touching trigger areas in or about the mouth.

neuraprax'ia [neur- + apraxia] Injury to a nerve resulting in paralysis without degeneration and followed by rapid and complete recovery of function.

neurasthe'nia [neur- + G. *asthenela*, weakness] An ill-defined condition, commonly accompanying or following depression, characterized by vague functional fatigue.

neurasthen'ic Relating to neurasthenia.

neurax'is The axial unpaired part of the CNS: spinal cord, rhombencephalon, mesencephalon, and diencephalon.

neurec'tomy [neur- + G. *ektomē*, excision] Excision of a segment of a nerve.

neurilem'ma Neurolemma.

neu'rilemo'ma [neurilemma + G. *-oma*, tumour] A benign encapsulated neoplasm in which the fundamental component is structurally identical to Schwann cells; neoplastic cells proliferate within the endoneurium, and the perineurium forms the capsule; may originate from a peripheral or sympathetic nerve, or from various cranial nerves, particularly the eighth nerve.

neuri'tis, pl. **neurit'ides** [neuri- + G. *-itis*, inflammation] Inflammation of a nerve, marked by neuralgia, hyperaesthesia, anaesthesia or parasthesia, paralysis, muscular atrophy in the region supplied by the affected nerve, and by abolition of the reflexes.

neu'roanat'omy The anatomy of the nervous system.

neu'roblast [neuro- + G. *blastos*, germ] An embryonic nerve cell.

neu'roblasto'ma A malignant neoplasm characterized by immature, only slightly differentiated nerve cells of embryonic type arranged in sheets, irregular clumps, cordlike groups, individually, and in pseudorosettes; occurs frequently in infants and children in the mediastinal and retroperitoneal regions, and widespread metastases are common.

neurocra'nium [neuro- + G. *kranion*, skull] The part of the skull enclosing the brain, as distinguished from the bones of the face.

neu'rodermati'tis [neuro- + G. *derma*, skin, + *-itis*, inflammation] A chronic lichenified skin lesion, localized or disseminated.

neu'roepithe'lium [NA] Epithelial cells specialized for the reception of external stimuli.

neurofi'bril A filamentous aggregation microfilaments and microtubules in the nerve cell's body, dendrites, axon, and sometimes synaptic endings.

neu'rofibro'ma A moderately firm, benign, nonencapsulated tumour resulting from proliferation of Schwann cells in a disorderly pattern that includes portions of nerve fibres.

neu'rofibromato'sis (von) Recklinghausen's disease; small, discrete, pigmented skin lesions (café-au-lait spots, pigmented naevi) that develop into multiple slow-growing neurofibromas, usually subcutaneous, along the course of a peripheral nerve; sometimes associated with acoustic neurinomas or other intracranial neoplasms; autosomal dominant inheritance with marked clinical variability.

neurogen'ic, neurogenet'ic Originating in, or caused by, the nervous system or nerve impulses.

neurog'lia [neuro- + G. *glia*, glue] Glia; non-neuronal cellular elements of the central and peripheral nervous system.

neurohor'mone A hormone liberated by nerve impulses formed by neurosecretory cells.

neu'rohypoph'ysis [neuro- + hypophysis] [NA] *Lobus posterior hypophyseos.* See also hypophysis.

neurolem'ma [neuro- + G. *lemma*, husk] A cell that enfolds one or more axons of the peripheral nervous system.

neurolep'tic [neuro- + G. *lēpsis*, taking hold] Denoting an agent producing analgesia, sedation, and tranquilization or a condition similar to that produced by such an agent.

neurol'ogy [neuro- + G. *logos*, study] The branch of medical science concerned with the nervous system and its disorders.

neuroly'sin An antibody causing destruction of ganglion and cortical cells.

neuro'ma [neuro- + G. *-oma*, tumour] Old general term for any neoplasm derived from cells of the nervous system; such neoplasms are now classified in more specific categories, . *e.g.*, ganglioneuroma, neurilemoma, pseudoneuroma.

neuromus'cular Referring to the relationship between nerve and muscle.

neu'romyeli'tis [neuro- + G. *myelos*, marrow, + *-itis*, inflammation] Neuritis combined with spinal cord inflammation.

   n. op'tica, a demyelinating disorder associated with transverse myelopathy and optic neuritis.

neu'romyop'athy [neuro- + G. *mys*, muscle, + *pathos*, disease] A disorder of muscle that directly reflects a disease or disorder of nerve supplying the muscle.

neu'romyosi'tis [neuro- + G. *mys*, muscle, + *-itis*, inflammation] Neuritis with inflammation of the muscles with which the affected nerve or nerves are in relation.

neu'rone, neu'ron [G. *neuron*, a nerve] Nerve cell; the morphologic and functional unit of the nervous system, consisting of the nerve cell body, the dendrites, and the axon.

   motor n., motoneurone; a nerve cell in the spinal cord, rhombencephalon, or mesencephalon characterized by having an axon that leaves the CNS to establish a functional connection with an effector tissue; **somatic motor n.'s** directly synapse with striated muscle fibres by motor endplates; **visceral** or **autonomic motor n.'s (preganglionic motor n.'s)** innervate smooth muscle fibres or glands only by the intermediary of a second, peripheral, n. (**postganglionic** or **ganglionic motor n.**) located in an autonomic ganglion.

neu'ronal Pertaining to a neurone.

neu'roparal'ysis Paralysis resulting from disease of the nerve supplying the affected part.

neuropath'ic Relating in any way to neuropathy.

neu'ropathol'ogy Pathology of the nervous system.

neurop'athy [neuro- + G. *pathos*, suffering] Any disorder affecting any segment of the nervous system; specifically, a disease involving the cranial or spinal nerves.

diabetic n., a combined sensory and motor n., typically symmetric and segmental, and involving autonomic fibres, seen frequently in older diabetic persons.

entrapment n., a region of traumatic neuritis in which the nerve is maintained in an irritated state by external pressure created by encroachment or impingement from a nearby structure.

segmental n., demyelination of scattered segments of peripheral nerves, with relating sparing of axons; noted in diabetes, arsenic poisoning, lead poisoning, diphtheria, and leprosy.

neu'rophysiol'ogy Physiology of the nervous system.

neu'ropil, neu'ropile [neuro- + G. pilos, felt] The complex net of axonal, dendritic, and glial arborizations that forms the bulk of the CNS grey matter, and in which the nerve cell bodies lie embedded.

neu'roplasty [neuro- + G. plassō, to form] Plastic surgery of the nerves.

neu'ropsychi'atry The specialty concerned with organic and functional diseases of the nervous system.

neuror'rhaphy [neuro- + G. rhaphē, suture] Joining together, usually by suture, of a divided nerve.

neuro'sis, pl. **neuro'ses** [neuro- + G. -osis, condition] **1.** A psychological or behavioural disorder in which anxiety is the primary characteristic; in contrast to the psychoses, persons with a n. do not exhibit gross distortion of reality or disorganization of personality. **2.** A functional nervous disease, or one which is dependent upon no evident lesion. **3.** A peculiar state of tension or irritability of the nervous system; any form of nervousness.

anxiety n., chronic abnormal distress and worry to the point of panic.

obsessive-compulsive n., disorder characterized by the persistent and repetitive intrusion of unwanted thoughts, urges, or actions that the individual is unable to prevent; anxiety or distress is the underlying emotion or drive state, and ritualistic behaviour is a learned method of reducing the anxiety.

occupation or **professional n.,** a functional disorder of a group of muscles used chiefly in one's occupation, marked by the occurrence of spasm, paresis, or incoordina-

tion on attempt to repeat the habitual movements.

neurosur'geon A surgeon specializing in neurosurgery.

neurosur'gery Surgery of the nervous system.

neurosu'ture Neurorrhaphy.

neurosyph'ilis Nervous system manifestations of syphilis, including tabes dorsalis, general paresis, and meningovascular syphilis.

neurot'ic Relating to a neurosis.

neurotme'sis [neuro- + G. tmēsis, a cutting] The condition in which there is complete division of a nerve.

neurot'omy [neuro- + G. tomē, a cutting] Surgical division of a nerve.

neurotox'ic Poisonous to nervous substance.

neurotox'in Neurolysin.

neurotrans'mitter [neuro- + L. transmitto, to send across] Any specific chemical agent released by a presynaptic cell, upon excitation, which crosses the synapse to stimulate or inhibit the postsynaptic cell.

neurotrip'sy [neuro- + G. tripsis, a rubbing] Surgical crushing of a nerve.

neurotro'pic Having an affinity for the nervous system.

neurovas'cular Relating to both nervous and vascular systems; relating to the nerves supplying the walls of the blood vessels.

neutro-, neutr- [L. neutralis, fr. neuter, neither] Combining forms meaning neutral.

neutrope'nia [neutrophil + G. penia, poverty] Presence of abnormally small numbers of neutrophils in the circulating blood

neu'trophil, neu'trophile [neutro- + G. philos, fond] **1.** A mature white blood cell in the granulocytic series, formed by myelopoietic tissue of the bone marrow and released into the circulating blood; characterized by a lobated nucleus with a coarse network of fairly dense chromatin and a cytoplasm that contains numerous fine granules. **2.** Any cell or tissue that manifests no special affinity for acid or basic dyes.

neutrophil'ic 1. Pertaining to or characterized by presence of neutrophils. **2.** Characterized by a lack of affinity for acid or basic dyes.

ni'acin Nicotinic acid.

nicotin'amide Biologically active amide of nicotinic acid.

nic'otine A poisonous volatile alkaloid, derived from tobacco and responsible for many of its effects; it first stimulates (small doses) then depresses (large doses) at autonomic ganglia and myoneural junctions.

nicotin'ic acid Niacin; a part of the vitamin B complex; is used in the prevention and treatment of pellagra, as a vasodilator, and as a cholesterol-lowering agent.

nictita'tion [L. *nicto*, pp. *-atus*, to wink, fr. *nico*, to beckon] Winking.

nida'tion [L. *nidus*, nest] Embedding of the early embryo in the uterine mucosa.

ni'dus, pl. **ni'di** [L. nest] **1.** The nucleus or central point of origin of a nerve. **2.** A focus or point of lodgment and development of a pathogenic organism. **3.** The coalescence of molecules or small particles that is the beginning of a crystal or similar solid deposit.

night'-terrors A disorder allied to nightmare in which a child awakes screaming with fright, the alarm persisting for a time during a state of semiconsciousness.

ni'hilism [L. *nihil*, nothing] **1.** In psychiatry, the delusion of the nonexistence of everything especially of the self or part of the self. **2.** Engagement in acts which are totally destructive to one's own purposes and those of one's group.

nip'ple [dim. of A.S. *neb*, beak, nose] *Papilla mammae.*

nit [A.S. *knitu*] The ovum of a body, head, or crab louse attached to human hair or clothing by a layer of chitin.

ni'trate A salt of nitric acid.

ni'tric acid HNO_3; a strong acid oxidant.

ni'trite A salt of nitrous acid.

ni'trofuranto'in An antimicrobial effective against Gram-positive and Gram-negative organisms.

ni'trogen [L. *nitrum*, nitre, + *-gen*, to produce] **1.** A gaseous element, symbol N, atomic no. 7, atomic weight 14.007, forming about 77 parts by weight of the atmosphere. **2.** Pharmaceutical grade N_2; contains not less than 99.0% by volume of N_2; used as a diluent for medicinal gases, and for air replacement in pharmaceutical preparations.

nitrogen lag The length of time after the ingestion of a given protein before the amount of nitrogen equal to that in the protein has been excreted in the urine.

nitrogen mustards Compounds of the general formula $R-N(CH_2CH_2Cl)$, the proto-

type of which is HN2 nitrogen mustard (mechlorethamine) in which R is CH_3; some have been used as antineoplastics.

nitroglyc'erin An explosive yellowish oily fluid formed by the action of sulphuric and nitric acids on glycerin; used as a vasodilator, especially in angina pectoris.

nitros'amines Compounds that can be formed by direct combination of an amine and nitrous acid (which can be formed from nitrites in the acidic gastric juice); some are mutagenic and/or carcinogenic.

ni'trous acid HNO_2; a standard biologic and clinical laboratory reagent.

ni'trous oxide Laughing gas; N_2O; a rapidly acting and reversible, nondepressant, and nontoxic inhalation analgesic to supplement other anaesthetics and analgesics.

noci- [L. *noceo*, to injure, hurt] Combining form relating to hurt, pain, or injury.

nocicep'tor [noci- + L. *capio*, to take] A peripheral nerve organ or mechanism for the appreciation and transmission of painful or injurious stimuli.

noct- [L. *nox*, night] Combining form meaning night, nocturnal. See also nycto-.

noctu'ria [noct- + G. *ouron*, urine] Urinating at night, often because of increased nocturnal secretion of urine.

noctur'nal [L. *nocturnus*, of the night] Pertaining to the hours of darkness; the opposite of diurnal.

no'dal Relating to any node.

node [L. *nodus*, a knot] **1.** A knob; nodosity; a circumscribed swelling. **2.** A circumscribed mass of differentiated tissue. See nodus. **3.** A knuckle, or finger joint.

    atrioventricular n., *nodus* atrioventricularis.

    Heberden's n.'s, small exostoses found on the terminal phalanges of the fingers in osteoarthritis, which are enlargements of the tubercles at the articular extremities of the distal phalanges.

    lymph n., lymph gland; one of numerous round, oval, or bean-shaped bodies located along the course of lymphatic vessels, usually presenting a depressed area, the hilum, on one side through which blood vessels enter and efferent lymphatic vessels emerge; afferent vessels enter at many points of its periphery.

    Ranvier's n., a short interval in the myelin sheath of a nerve fibre, occurring between each two successive segments of the myelin sheath; at the n., the axon is invested only by short, finger-like cytoplasmic processes of the two neighbouring Schwann cells or, in the CNS, oligodendroglia cells.

sinoatrial n., sinus n., *nodus* sinuatrialis.

nod'ule [L. *nodulus,* dim. of *nodus,* knot] A small node.

no'dus, pl. **no'di** [L. a knot] [NA] Node; in anatomy, a circumscribed mass of tissue.

n. atrioventricula'ris [NA], a small node of specialized cardiac muscle fibres, located near the ostium of the coronary sinus, that gives rise to the atrioventricular bundle of the conduction system of the heart.

n. lymphat'icus, lymph *node.*

n. sinuatria'lis [NA], the mass of specialized cardiac muscle fibres that normally acts as the "pacemaker" of the cardiac conduction system; it lies under the epicardium at the upper end of the sulcus terminalis.

no'ma [G. *nomē,* a spreading (sore)] A gangrenous stomatitis, usually beginning in the mucous membrane of the corner of the mouth or cheek, and then progressing fairly rapidly to involve the entire thickness of the lips, cheek, or both, with conspicuous necrosis and complete sloughing of tissue. A similar process (**n. pudendi, n. vulvae**) may also involve the labia majora.

nom'ogram [G. *nomos,* law, + *gramma,* something written] A series of scales arranged so that calculations can be performed graphically.

non com'pos men'tis [L. *non,* not + *compos,* participating, competent, + *mēns,* gen. *mentis,* mind] Not of sound mind; mentally incapable of managing one's affairs.

noninva'sive Denoting diagnostic procedures that do not involve penetration of the skin.

non'union Failure of normal healing of a fractured bone.

noradren'aline A catecholamine hormone of which the natural form is D, although the L form has some activity. The base is considered to be the postganglionic adrenergic mediator present in the adrenal medulla which possesses the excitatory actions of adrenaline but has minimal inhibitory effects.

nor'epineph'rine Term preferred in the U.S. for noradrenaline.

nor'mal [L. *normalis,* according to pattern] **1.** Typical; usual; healthy; according to the rule or standard. **2.** In bacteriology, nonimmune; untreated; denoting an animal, or the serum or substance contained therein, that has not been experimentally immunized against any microorganism or its products. **3.** In psychiatry and psychology, denoting a state of effective function satisfactory to both the individual and his social milieu.

normo- [L. *normalis,* normal, according to pattern] Combining form meaning normal, usual.

nor'moblast [normo- + G. *blastos,* sprout, germ] A nucleated red blood cell, the immediate precursor of a normal erythrocyte in man.

normocap'nia [normo- + G. *kapnos,* vapour] A state in which the arterial carbon dioxide pressure is normal, about 40 mm Hg.

normochro'mia [normo- + G. *chrōma,* colour] Normal colour; referring to blood in which the amount of haemoglobin in the red blood cells is normal.

nor'moglycae'mia Euglycaemia.

normoten'sive Indicating a normal arterial blood pressure.

normoton'ic 1. Relating to or characterized by normal muscular tone. **2.** Normotensive.

nos'capine An isoquinoline alkaloid, occurring in opium, with papaverine-like action on smooth muscle.

nose [A.S. *nosu*] Nasus.

saddle n., a n. with markedly depressed bridge.

noso- [G. *nosos,* disease] Combining form relating to disease.

nosoco'mial [G. *nosokomeian,* hospital] **1.** Relating to a hospital. **2.** Denoting a new disorder (unrelated to the patient's primary condition) associated with being treated in a hospital.

nosol'ogy [noso- + G. *logos,* study] The science of classification of diseases.

nostal'gia [G. *nostos,* a return (home), + *algos,* pain] Homesickness; the longing to return home or to familiar surroundings.

nos'tril Naris.

nox'ious [L. *noxius,* injurious, fr. *noceo,* to injure] Injurious.

nu'cha [Fr. *nuque*] [NA] Nape; the back of the neck.

nu'clear Relating to a nucleus.

nu'clease General term for enzymes that catalyse the hydrolysis of nucleic acid.

nu'cleated Provided with a nucleus, a characteristic of all true cells.

nu'clei Plural of nucleus.

nu'cleic acid A family of substances of large molecular weight, found in chromosomes, nucleoli, mitochondria, and cytoplasm of all cells, and in viruses; in combination with proteins they are called nucleoproteins. On hydrolysis they yield purines, pyrimidines, phosphoric acid, and a pentose, either D-ribose or D-deoxyribose; from the last, the n.a.'s derive their more specific names, ribonucleic acid and deoxyribonucleic acid.

nucleo-, nucl- Combining forms for nucleus or nuclear.

nucleo'lus, pl. **nucleo'li** [L. dim of *nucleus*, a nut, kernel] A small, usually single, rounded mass within the cell nucleus where ribonucleoprotein is produced.

nu'cleopro'tein A complex of protein and nucleic acid, the form in which essentially all nucleic acids exist in nature.

nu'cleotide Originally a combination of a (nucleic acid) purine or pyrimidine, one sugar (usually ribose or deoxyribose), and a phosphate group.

nu'cleotox'in A toxin acting upon the cell nuclei.

nu'cleus, pl. **nu'clei** [L. a little nut, a kernel] **1.** In cytology, a rounded or oval mass of protoplasm within the cytoplasm of a cell, which undergoes mitosis during cell division. **2.** [NA] In neuroanatomy, a group of nerve cells in the brain or spinal cord that can be demarcated from neighbouring groups on the basis of either differences in cell type or the presence of a surrounding zone of nerve fibres or cell-poor neuropil. **3.** Any substance around which a urinary or other calculus is formed. **4.** The central portion of an atom (composed of protons and neutrons) where most of the mass and all of the positive charge are concentrated.

amygdaloid n., *corpus* amygdaloideum.

n. cauda'tus [NA], **caudate n.,** an elongated curved mass of grey matter, consisting of an anterior thick portion that projects into the anterior horn of the lateral ventricle, a portion extending along the floor of the body of the lateral ventricle, and an elongated curved thin portion that curves downward and backward in the temporal lobes to the wall of the descending horn.

n. lentifor'mis [NA], **lentiform n., lenticular n.,** the large cone-shaped mass of grey matter forming the central core of the cerebral hemisphere; its convex base is formed by the putamen which together with the caudate n. composes the corpus striatum, the apical part consists of the large-celled globus pallidus.

n. pulpo'sus [NA], the soft fibrocartilage central portion of the intervertebral disc.

n. ru'ber [NA], **red n.,** a large, well defined, somewhat elongated cell mass of reddish-grey hue, located in the rostral part of the mesencephalic tegmentum.

nullip'ara [L. *nullus*, none, + *pario*, to bear] A woman who has never borne any children.

nullip'arous Never having borne children.

num'mular [L. *nummus*, coin] **1.** Discoid or coin-shaped; denoting the thick mucous or mucopurulent sputum in certain respiratory diseases, so called because of the disc shape assumed when it is flattened on the bottom of a sputum mug containing water or transparent disinfectant. **2.** Arranged like stacks of coins, denoting the association of the red blood corpuscles with flat surfaces apposed, forming rouleaux.

nurse [O. Fr. *nource*, fr. L. *nutrix*, wet-nurse, fr. *nutrio*, to suckle, to tend] **1.** To suckle; to give suck to an infant. **2.** To perform all the necessary offices in the care of the sick. **3.** A woman who has the care of an infant or young child. **4.** One who is professionally trained in the care of a sick person.

n. anaesthetist, a person who, after completing basic educational requirements as a nurse, is additionally trained in the administration of anaesthetics, in order to function thereafter as an anaesthetist under the direction of a physician.

registered n. (R.N.), a n. who has been graduated from an accredited school of nursing, and has been registered and licensed to practise by a government authority.

wet n., a woman who suckles a child not her own.

nurse-mid'wife A person formally educated and certified to practise in the two disciplines of nursing and midwifery.

nurse practi'tioner A registered n. with special skills in assessing the physical and psychosocial status of patients, often as a colleague of a physician.

nurs'ing 1. Feeding an infant at the breast; tending and taking care of a child. **2.** Caring for the ill or infirm; performing the duties of a nurse. **3.** The scientific care of the sick by a professional nurse.

nuta'tion [L. *annuere*, to nod] The act of nodding, especially involuntary nodding.

nu'trient [L. *nutriens*, fr. *nutrio*, to nourish] An item of food; may be essential or nonessential.

nutri'tion [L. *nutritio*, fr. *nutrio*, to nourish] **1.** A function of living organisms, consisting in the taking in and assimilation through chemical changes (metabolism) of material whereby tissue is built up and energy liberated; its successive stages are: digestion, absorption, assimilation, and excretion. **2.** The study of the food and drink requirements of human beings or animals for maintenance, growth, activity, reproduction, and lactation.

nyctal'gia [nyct- + G *algos*, pain] Night pain, denoting especially the osteoscopic pains of syphilis occurring at night.

nyctalo'pia [nyct- + G. *alaos*, obscure, + *ōps, eye*] Night blindness, decreased ability to see in reduced illumination.

nycto-, nyct- [G. *nyx*, night] Combining forms denoting night, nocturnal. See also noct-.

nym'pha, pl. **nym'phae** [Mod. L. fr. G. *nymphē*, a bride] One of the labia minora.

nymphi'tis [nymph- + G. -*itis*, inflammation] Inflammation of the labia minora.

nympho-, nymph- Combining forms denoting the nymphae (labia minora).

nym'phoma'nia [nympho- + G. *mania*, frenzy] Extreme eroticism or sexual desire in women.

nystag'mograph An apparatus for measuring the amplitude and velocity of ocular movements in nystagmus, by measuring the change in the resting potential of the eye as the eye moves.

nystagmog'raphy The technique of recording nystagmus.

nystag'mus [G. *nystagmos*, a nodding, fr. *nystazō*, to be sleepy, nod] Rhythmical oscillation of the eyeballs, either pendular or jerky.

O

o- ortho- (2).

obese' [L. *obesus*, fat] Extremely fat or corpulent.

obe'sity [see obese] Fatness; corpulence; an abnormal increase of fat in the subcutaneous connective tissues.

  morbid o., the condition of weighing at least twice the ideal weight.

objec'tive [L. *ob-jicio*, pp. -*jectus*, to throw before] **1.** The lens or lenses in the lower end of a microscope, by means of which the image of the object examined is brought to a focus. **2.** Viewing events or phenomena as they exist in the external world, impersonally or in an unprejudiced way.

ob'ligate [L. *ob-ligo*, pp. -*atus*, to bind to] Without an alternative pathway.

oblique' [L. *obliquus*] Slanting; deviating from the perpendicular or the horizontal.

oblit'era'tion [L. *oblittero*, to blot out] Blotting out, especially by filling of a natural space or lumen by fibrosis or inflammation.

oblonga'ta [L. fem. of *oblongatus*, from *oblongus*, rather long] Medulla oblongata.

obses'sion [L. *obsideo*, pp. -*sessus*, to besiege] A condition, usually associated with anxiety and dread, in which one idea constantly fills the mind despite one's efforts to ignore or dislodge it.

obses'sive-compul'sive Having a tendency to perform certain repetitive acts or ritualistic behaviour to relieve anxiety.

obstet'ric, obstet'rical Relating to obstetrics.

ob'stetri'cian A specialist in obstetrics.

obstet'rics [L. *obstetrix*, a midwife] The medical specialty concerned with the care of the pregnant woman during pregnancy, parturition, and the puerperium.

ob'stinate [L. *obstinātus*, determined]. **1.** Firmly adhering to one's own purpose, opinion, etc., not yielding to argument, persuasion, or entreaty. **2.** Refractory (1).

obstipa'tion [L. *ob*, against, + *stipo*, pp. -*atus*, to crowd] Intestinal obstruction; severe constipation.

obstruc'tion [L. *obstructio*] Blockage or clogging as by occlusion or stenosis.

obtund' [L. *ob-tundo*, to beat against, blunt] To dull or blunt, especially sensation or pain.

ob'turator [L. *obturo*, pp. *-atus*, to occlude or stop up] **1.** Any structure that occludes an opening. **2.** A prosthesis used to close an opening of the hard palate, usually a cleft palate. **3.** The stylus or removable plug used during the insertion of many tubular instruments.

obtu'sion Dulling or deadening of sensibility.

occip'ital Relating to the occiput.

occipito- Combining form for occiput, occipital.

occip'itofron'tal **1.** Relating to the occiput and the forehead. **2.** Relating to the occipital and frontal lobe of the cerebral cortex.

oc'ciput, gen. **occip'itis** [L.] [NA] The back of the head.

occlude' [see occlusion] **1.** To close or bring together. **2.** To inclose, as in an occluded virus.

occlu'sal **1.** Pertaining to occlusion or closure. **2.** In dentistry, pertaining to the contacting surfaces of opposing occlusal units (teeth or occlusion rims), or the masticating surfaces of the posterior teeth.

occlu'sion [L. *oc-cludo*, pp. *-clusus*, to shut up] **1.** The act of closing or the state of being closed. **2.** In chemistry, the absorption of a gas by a metal or the inclusion of one substance within another. **3.** Any contact between the incising or masticating surfaces of the upper and lower teeth. **4.** The relationship between the occlusal surfaces of the maxillary and mandibular teeth when they are in contact.

  balanced o., the simultaneous contacting of the upper and lower teeth on the right and left and in the anterior and posterior occlusal areas in centric and eccentric positions within the functional range.

  coronary o., blockage of a coronary vessel, usually by thrombosis or atheroma, and often leading to infarction of the myocardium.

occlu'sive Serving to close; denoting a bandage or dressing that closes a wound and excludes it from the air.

oc'cult [L. *oc-culo*, pp. *-cultus*, to cover, hide] **1.** Hidden; concealed. **2.** Denoting a concealed haemorrhage, the blood being so changed as not to be readily recognized. **3.** In oncology, a clinically unidentified primary tumour with recognized metastases.

oct-, octa-, octi-, octo- [G. *oktō*, L. *octo*, eight] Combining forms meaning eight.

oc'tan [L. *octo*, eight] Applied to fever, the paroxysms of which recur every eighth day, the day of each paroxysm being included in the count.

oc'ular [L. *oculus*, eye] **1.** Ophthalmic. **2.** The eyepiece of a microscope, the lens or lenses at the upper end of a microscope by means of which the image focused by the objective is viewed.

oc'ulist [L. *oculus*, eye] Ophthalmologist.

oculo- [L. *oculus*, eye] Combining form denoting eye, ocular. See also ophthalmo-.

oc'ulocuta'neous Relating to the eyes and the skin.

oculofa'cial Relating to the eyes and the face.

oculogy'ric Referring to rotation of the eyeballs.

oculomo'tor [oculo- + L. *motorius*, moving] Relating to or causing movements of the eyeball.

oc'ulus, gen. and pl. **oc'uli (O)** [L.] [NA] Eye; the organ of vision, consisting of the eyeball and the optic nerve.

-odes [G. *eidos*, form, resemblance] Suffix denoting having the form of, like, resembling.

odont-, odonto- [G. *odous* (*odont-*), tooth] Combining forms denoting a tooth or teeth.

odontal'gia [odont- + G. *algos*, pain] Toothache.

odontogen'esis [odonto- + G. *genesis*, production] The process of development of the teeth.

odon'toid [odont- + G. *eidos*, resemblance] Shaped like a tooth.

odontol'ogy [odonto- + G. *logos*, study] Dentistry.

odonto'ma [odonto- + G. *-oma*, tumour] **1.** A tumour of odontogenic origin. **2.** A developmental anomaly of odontogenic origin composed of enamel, dentine, cementum, and pulp tissue.

o'dour [L.] Scent; smell; emanation from any substance that stimulates the olfactory cells in the organ of smell.

odyn-, odyno- [G. *odyne*, pain] Combining forms meaning pain.

oede'ma [G. *oidēma*, a swelling] An accumulation of an excessive amount of watery fluid in cells, tissues, or serous cavities.

angioneurotic o., periodically recurring episodes of noninflammatory swelling of skin, mucous membranes, viscera, and brain, of sudden onset and occasionally with arthralgia, purpura, or fever.

cardiac o., o. resulting from congestive heart failure.

cerebral o., brain swelling due to increased volume of the extravascular compartment from the uptake of water in the neuropile and white matter.

o. neonato′rum, a diffuse, firm o. occuring in the newborn, beginning usually in the legs and spreading upward.

pulmonary o., o of lungs usually resulting from mitral stenosis or left ventricular failure.

oedem′atous Marked by oedema.

oesophagal′gia [oesophagus + G. algos, pain] Pain the the oesophagus.

oesophage′al Relating to the oesophagus.

opesophagec′tasis

oesoph′agecta′sia [oesophagus + G. ektasis, a stretching] Dilation of the oesophagus.

oesophagec′tomy [oesophagus + G. ektomē, excision] Excision of any part of the oesophagus.

oesoph′agism Oesophageal spasm causing dysphagia.

oesophagi′tis Inflammation of the oesophagus.

peptic o., inflammation of the lower oesophagus from regurgitation of acid gastric contents, producing substernal pain.

oesoph′agocar′dioplasty A reconstructive operation on the oesophagus and cardiac end of the stomach.

oesoph′agocele [oesophagus + G. kēlē, hernia] Protrusion of the mucous membrane of the oesophagus through a rent in the muscular coat.

oesophagodyn′ia [oesophagus + G. odynē, pain] Oesophagalgia.

oesoph′agoenteros′tomy [oesophagus + G. enteron, intestine, + stoma, mouth] Operative formation of a direct communication between the oesophagus and intestine.

oesoph′agogas′troplasty Surgical repair of the cardiac sphincter of the stomach.

oesoph′agoplasty [oesophagus + G. plassō, to form] Surgical repair of a defect in the wall of the oesophagus.

oesoph′agoscope [oesophagus + G. skopeō, to examine] An endoscope for inspecting the interior of the oesophagus.

oesophagos′copy [oesophagus + g. skopeō, to examine] Inspection of the interior of the oesophagus by means of an endoscope.

oesoph′agospasm Spasm of the walls of the oesophagus.

oesoph′agosteno′sis [oesophagus + G. stenōsis, a narrowing] Stricture or a general narrowing of the oesophagus.

oesophagos′tomy [oesophagus + G. stoma, mouth] The operative formation of an opening directly into the oesophagus from without.

oesophagot′omy [oesophagus + G. tomō, an incision] An incision through the wall of the oesophagus.

oesoph′agus, pl. **oesoph′agi** [G. oisophagos, gullet] [NA] The portion of the digestive canal between the pharynx and stomach. It is about 25 cm long and consists of three parts: cervical, from the cricoid cartilage to the thoracic inlet; thoracic from thoracic inlet to the diaphragm; and abdominal, below the diaphragm to the cardiac opening of the stomach.

oestradi′ol The most potent naturally occurring oestrogen in mammals, formed by the ovary, the placenta, the testis, and possibly the adrenal cortex; therapeutic indications for o. are those typical of an oestrogen.

oes′trogen Generic term for any substance, natural or synthetic, that exerts biological effects characteristic of oestrogenic hormones, such as oestradiol; formed by the ovary, placenta, testes, possibly the adrenal cortex, and certain plants. Besides stimulation of secondary sexual characteristics, they also exert systemic effects, such as growth and maturation of long bones, and are used therapeutically in any disorder attributable to o. deficiency, to prevent or stop lactation, to suppress ovulation, and to ameliorate carcinoma of the breast and of the prostate.

-oid [G. eidos, form, resemblance] Suffix denoting resemblance to; equivalent to -form.

oint′ment [O. Fr. oignement; L. unguo, pp. unctus, to smear] Salve; unguent; a semisolid preparation usually containing medicinal substances and intended for external application.

olec'ranon [G. the head or point of the elbow] [NA] Tip or point of the elbow; the prominent curved proximal extremity of the ulna.

olfac'tion [L. ol-facio, pp. -factus, to smell] **1.** The sense of smell. **2.** The act of smelling.

olfac'tory [see olfaction] Relating to the sense of smell.

oligae'mia [oligo- + G. haima, blood] A deficiency in the amount of blood in the body.

oligo-, olig- [G. oligos, few] **1.** Combining form denoting a few or a little. **2.** In chemistry, used in contrast to "poly-" in describing polymers.

oligoam'nios [oligo- + amnion] Deficiency in the amount of the amniotic fluid.

ol'igocar'dia [oligo- + G. kardia, heart] Bradycardia.

ol'igohydram'nios [oligo- + G. hydōr, water, + amnion] Oligoamnios.

ol'igomenorrhoe'a [oligo- + menorrhoea] Scanty menstruation.

ol'igopty'alism [oligo- + G. ptyalon, saliva] Scanty secretion of saliva.

ol'igosac'charide A compound made up of the condensation of a small number of monosaccharide units.

ol'igosper'mia [oligo- + G. sperma, seed] A subnormal concentration of spermatozoa in the penile ejaculate.

oligu'ria [oligo- + G. ouron, urine] Scanty urination.

oli'va, pl. **oli'vae** [L.] [NA] A smooth oval prominence of the ventrolateral surface of the medulla oblongata lateral to the pyramidal tract, corresponding to the nucleus olivaris.

ol'ivary **1.** Relating to the oliva. **2.** Relating to or shaped like an olive.

ol'ive [L. oliva] Oliva.

-ology See -logia.

-oma [G. -ōma] Suffix denoting a tumour or neoplasm.

omen'tal Relating to the omentum.

omentec'tomy [oment- + G. ektomē, excision] Resection or excision of the omentum.

omento-, oment- Combining forms relating to the omentum. See also epiplo-.

omen'topexy [omento- + G. pēxis, fixation] **1.** Suture of the great omentum to the abdominal wall to induce collateral portal circulation. **2.** Suture of the omentum to another organ to increase arterial circulation.

omen'toplasty [omento- + G. plassō, to form, manipulate] Use of the great omentum to cover or fill a defect, augment arterial or portal venous circulation, absorb effusions, or increase lymphatic drainage.

omen'tum, pl. **omen'ta** [L. the membrane that encloses the bowels] [NA] A fold of peritoneum passing from the stomach to another abdominal organ.

  o. ma'jus [NA], **greater o.,** a peritoneal fold passing from the greater curvature of the stomach to the transverse colon, hanging like an apron in front of the intestines.

  o. mi'nus [NA], **lesser o.,** a peritoneal fold passing from the margins of the porta hepatis and the bottom of the fossa ductus venosi to the lesser curvature of the stomach and to the upper border of the duodenum.

omniv'orous [L. omnis, all, + voro, to eat] Living on food of all kinds, upon both animal and vegetable food.

omphal-, omphalo- [G. omphalos, navel (umbilicus)] Combining form denoting relationship to the umbilicus.

omphal'ic [G. omphalos, umbilicus] Umbilical.

omphali'tis Inflammation of the umbilicus and surrounding parts.

om'phalocele [omphalo- + G. kēlē, hernia] Congenital herniation of viscera into the base of the umbilical cord, with a covering membranous sac of peritoneum-amnion.

om'phalophlebi'tis [omphalo- + G. phleps, vein, + -itis, inflammation] Inflammation of the umbilical veins.

o'nanism [Onan, son of Judah, who practised it. Genesis 38:9] **1.** Coitus interruptus; withdrawal of the penis before ejaculation, in order to prevent insemination and fecundation of the ovum. **2.** Incorrectly used when synonymous with masturbation.

oncho- For words beginning thus, and not found here, see onco-.

Onchocer'ca [G. onkos, a barb, + kerkos, tail] A genus of elongated filariform nematodes (family Onchocercidae) that inhabit the connective tissue of their hosts, usually within firm nodules in which these parasites are coiled and entangled. O. volvulus is a species that causes onchocerciasis in man.

on'chocerci'asis,
on'chocerco'sis Infection with Oncho-

cerca (especially *O. volvulus*), marked by nodular swellings forming a fibrous cyst enveloping the coiled parasites. Ocular complications may develop, with blindness in advanced cases, as a result of the sensitization of the cornea to the microfilariae.

onco- [G. *onkos*, bulk, mass] Combining form denoting a tumour, some relation to a tumour, bulk, or volume.

on'cocyte [onco- + G. *kytos*, cell]. A large, granular, acidophilic tumour cell containing numerous mitochondria; a neoplastic oxyphil cell.

on'cogene A viral gene, found in certain retroviruses, that may transform the host cell to a neoplastic phenotype but is not required for viral replication.

oncogen'esis [onco- + G. *genesis*, production] Origin and growth of a neoplasm.

oncogen'ic, oncog'enous Causing, inducing, or being suitable for the formation and development of a neoplasm.

oncol'ogist A specialist in oncology.

oncol'ogy [onco- + G. *logos*, study] The science dealing with the physical, chemical, and biologic properties and features of neoplasms, including causation, pathogenesis, and treatment.

oncot'ic Relating to or caused by oedema or any swelling.

on'covi'rus Any virus of the subfamily Oncovirinae; *i.e.*, an RNA tumour virus.

Oncovir'inae A subfamily of viruses (family Retroviridae) composed of the RNA tumour viruses which contain RNA-dependent DNA polymerases (reverse transcriptases) that can be integrated into the DNA of the host cell where it serves as a cellular gene.

ontogen'esis Ontogony.

on'togenet'ic Relating to ontogeny

ontog'eny [G. *ōn*, being, + *genesis*, origin] Development of the individual, as distinguished from phylogenesis, evolutionary development of the species.

onych'ia [onycho- + G. *-ia*, condition] Inflammation of the nail matrix.

onycho-, onych- [G. *onyx*, nail] Combining forms denoting a fingernail or toenail.

on'ychodys'trophy [onycho- + G. *dys-*, bad, + *trophē*, nourishment] Dystrophic changes in nails occuring as a congenital defect or due to any illness or injury that may cause a malformed nail.

on'ychogrypo'sis, on'ychogrypho'sis [onycho- + G. *grypōsis*, a curvature] Enlargement with increased thickening and curvature of the fingernails or toenails.

onychol'ysis [onycho- + G. *lysis*, loosening] Loosening of the nails, beginning at the free border, and usually incomplete.

on'ychomala'cia [onycho- + G. *malakia*, softness] Abnormal softness of the nails.

on'ychomyco'sis [onycho- + G. *mykes*, fungus, + *-ōsis*, condition] Ringworm of the nails: a fungus infection of the nails, causing thickening, roughness, and splitting, usually caused by *Trichophyton rubrum* or *T. mentagrophytes*.

onychop'athy [onycho- + G. *pathos*, suffering] Any disease of the nails.

onychoph'agy, on'ychopha'gia [onycho- + G. *phagein*, to eat] Nailbiting.

onycho'sis Onychopathy.

oo- [G. *ōon*, egg] Combining form denoting egg, ovary. See also oophor-, ovario-, ovi-, ovo-.

o'ocyte [G. *ōon*, egg, + *kytos*, a hollow (cell)] The immature ovum.

oogen'esis [G. *ōon*, egg, + *genesis*, origin] Formation and development of the ovum.

oophor-, oophoro- [Mod. L. *oophoron*, ovary, fr. G. *ōophoros*, egg-bearing] Combining forms denoting the ovary. See also oo-, ovario-.

o'ophorec'tomy [G. *ōon*, egg, + *phoros*, bearing, + *ectomē*, excision] Ovariectomy.

o'ophori'tis [G. *ōon*, egg, + *phoros*, a bearing, + *-itis*, inflammation] Inflammation of an ovary.

oophoro- See oophor-.

ooph'orocystec'tomy Excision of an ovarian cyst.

ooph'orohysterec'tomy Ovariohysterectomy.

ooph'oron [Mod. L. ovary, fr. G. *ōon*, egg, + *phoros*, bearing] Ovary.

ooph'oropexy [oophoro- + G. *pēxis*, fixation] Surgical fixation or suspension of an ovary.

oophoros'tomy [oophoro- + G. *stoma*, mouth] Ovariostomy.

opac'ifica'tion [L. *opacus*, shady] **1.** The process of making opaque. **2.** The formation of opacities.

opac'ity [L. *opacitas*, shadiness] A lack of transparency; an opaque or nontransparent area.

opaque' [Fr. fr. L. *opacus*, shady] Impervious to light; not translucent.

op'erable Denoting a patient or condition on which a surgical procedure can be performed with a reasonable expectation of cure or relief.

op'erant In conditioning, any behaviour or specific response chosen by the experimenter.

op'erate [L. *operor*, pp. *-atus*, to work] To work upon the body by the hands or by means of cutting or other instruments to correct a surgical problem.

opera'tion 1. Any surgical procedure. 2. The act, manner, or process of functioning.

oper'culum, pl. **oper'cula** [L. cover or lid] 1. Anything resembling a lid or cover. 2. [NA] In anatomy, the portions of the frontal, parietal, and temporal lobes bordering the lateral sulcus and covering the insula. 3. A bit of mucus sealing the endocervical canal of the uterus after conception has taken place. 4. The attached flap in tear of retinal detachment. 5. The mucosal flap partially or completely covering an unerupted tooth.

ophthal'mia [G.] 1. Severe, often purulent, conjunctivitis. 2. Inflammation of the deeper structures of the eye.

    gonorrhoeal o., acute purulent conjunctivitis due to gonococcal infection.

    o. neonato'rum, a conjunctival inflammation occurring within the first 10 days of life; causes include *Neisseria gonorrhoeae*, *Staphylococcus*, *Streptococcus pneumoniae*, and *Chlamydia oculogenitalis*.

    sympathetic o., a serous or plastic uveitis caused by a perforating wound of the uvea followed by a similar severe reaction in the other eye that may eventuate to bilateral blindness.

ophthal'mic [G. *ophthalmikos*] Relating to the eye.

ophthalmo-, ophthalm- [G. *ophthalmos*, eye] Combining forms denoting relationship to the eye. See also oculo-.

ophthalmol'ogist Oculist; a specialist in ophthalmology.

ophthalmol'ogy [ophthalmo- + G. *logos*, study] The medical specialty concerned with the eye, its diseases, and refractive errors.

ophthal'mople'gia [ophthalmo- + G. *plēgē*, stroke] Paralysis of one or more of the motor nerves of the eye.

ophthal'moscope [ophthalmo- + G. *skopeō*, to examine] A device for studying the interior of the eyeball through the pupil.

-opia [G. *ōps*, eye] Suffix meaning vision.

o'piate Any preparation or derivative of opium.

o'pioid Any synthetic narcotic that resembles opiates in action but is not derived from opium.

opis'thenar [G. back of the hand] Dorsum of the hand.

opistho- [G. *opisthen*, at the rear, behind] Combining form denoting backward, behind, dorsal.

o'pisthorchi'asis Infection with the Asiatic liver fluke, *Opisthorchis viverrini*, or other opisthorchids.

Opisthor'chis [opistho- + G. *orchis*, testis] A genus of digenetic trematodes (family Opisthorchiidae) found in the bile ducts or gallbladder of fish-eating mammals, birds, and fish.

    O. felin'eus, the cat liver fluke, a parasitic species whose ingested eggs hatch in *Bithynia* snails and cercariae encyst on various species of fish; man acquires the infection by ingesting raw or inadequately cooked fish.

    O. viverri'ni, a species closely related to O. *felineus* which also causes opisthorchiasis.

opisthot'onos [opistho- + G. *tonos*, tension, stretching] A tetanic spasm in which the spine and extremities are bent with convexity forward, the body resting on the head and the heels.

o'pium [L. fr. G. *opion*, poppy-juice] The air-dried milky exudation obtained by incising the unripe capsules of *Papaver somniferum* or its variety *P. album* (family Papaveraceae); contains some 20 alkaloids, including morphine, 9 to 16%; noscapine, 4 to 8%; codeine, 0.8 to 2.5%; papaverine, 0.5 to 2.5%; and thebaine, 0.5 to 2%.

op'portunis'tic 1. Denoting an organism capable of causing disease only in a host whose resistance is lowered. 2. Denoting a disease caused by an o. organism.

op'sonin [G. *opsonein*, to cater, prepare food] A substance that enhances phagocytosis.

normal o., o. normally present in the blood, without stimulation by a known specific antigen, that reacts with various organisms

specific o., o. formed in response to stimulation by a specific antigen, either as a result of a disease or of injections with a suitably prepared suspension of the specific microorganism; it reacts only with microorganisms that contain the specific antigens that stimulated formation of the antibody.

opsoniza'tion The process by which bacteria are altered in such a manner that they are more readily and more efficiently engulfed by phagocytes.

op'tic, op'tical [G. *optikos*] Relating to the eye, vision, or optics.

opti'cian One who practises opticianry.

opti'cianry The professional practice of filling prescriptions for ophthalmic lenses, dispensing spectacles, and making and fitting contact lenses.

op'tics [G. *optikos*, fr. *ops*, eye] The science concerned with the properties of light, its refraction and absorption, and the refracting media of the eye in that relation.

opto-, optico- [G. *optikos*, optical, from *ops*, eye] Combining forms relating to the eye.

optom'eter [opto- + G. *metron*, measure] An instrument for determining the refraction of the eye.

optom'etry 1. The profession concerned with the examination of the eyes and related structures to determine the presence of vision problems and eye disorders, and with the prescription and adaptation of lenses and other optical aids. **2.** Use of an optometer.

u'ra [ ] Plural of t *os*, the mouth

o'ra, pl. **o'rae** [L.] [NA] An edge or a margin.

o'ral [L. *os* (*or-*), mouth] Relating to the mouth.

oral'ity A term used to denote the psychic organization derived from, and characteristic of, the oral period of psychosexual development.

orbic'ular [L. *orbiculus*, a small disc, dim. of *orbis*, circle] Circular.

or'bit Orbita.

or'bita, pl. **or'bitae** [L. a wheel-track, fr. *orbis*, circle] [NA] Orbital cavity; eye socket; the bony cavity containing the eyeball and its adnexa, formed of parts of seven bones: frontal, maxillary, sphenoid, lacrimal, zygomatic, ethmoid, and palatine.

Orbivi'rus [L. *orbis*, ring, + virus] A genus of viruses of vertebrates (family Reoviridae) that multiply in insects, including the Colorado tick fever virus of man and certain viruses formerly included with the arboviruses. They are antigenically distinct from other groups of viruses and are characterized by an indistinct but rather large outer layer of capsomeres which give the appearance of rings.

orchi-, orchido-, orchio- [G. *orchis*, testis] Combining forms denoting relationship to the testes.

orchial'gia [orchi- + G. *algos*, pain] Pain in the testis.

orchidec'tomy Orchiectomy.

orchid'ic Relating to the testis.

orchiec'tomy [orchi- + G. *ektome*, excision] Removal of one or both testes.

or'chiepididymi'tis [orchi- + epididymis, + G. -*itis*, inflammation] Inflammation of the testis and epididymis

or'chiocele [orchio- + G. *kele*, hernia tumour] **1.** A tumour of the testis. **2.** A testis retained in the inguinal canal. ·

orchiop'athy [orchio- + G. *pathos*, suffering] Any disease of a testis.

or'chiopexy [orchio- + G. *pexis*, fixation] Surgical treatment of an undescended testicle by freeing it and implanting it into the scrotum.

or'chioplasty [orchio- + G. *plasso*, to form] Plastic surgery of the testis.

orchiot'omy [orchio- + G. *tome*, incision] Incision into a testis.

orchi'tis [orchi- + G. -*itis*, inflammation] Inflammation of the testis.

or'der [L. *ordo*, regular arrangement] In biological classification, the division just below the class (or subclass) and above the family.

or'gan [G. *organon*, a tool, organ] Any part of the body exercising a specific function.

Corti's o., spiral o., a prominent ridge of highly specialized epithelium in the floor of the cochlear duct overlying the basilar membrane; containing one inner row and three or four outer rows of hair cells supported by various columnar cells.

target o., a tissue or o. upon which a hormone exerts its action; may be an endocrine gland, a nonendocrine gland; or a type of tissue.

vestigial o., a rudimentary structure in man corresponding to a functional structure or o. in the lower animals.

or'gana Plural or organum.

organelle' [Mod. L. dim. of G. *organon*, organ] One of the specialized parts of a cell, including mitochondria, the Golgi apparatus, cell centre and centrioles, granular and agranular endoplasmic reticulum, vacuoles, microsomes, lysosomes, plasma membrane, and certain fibrils, as well as plastids of plant cells.

organ'ic [G. *organikos*] **1.** Relating to an organ. **2.** Relating to an animal or vegetable organism. **3.** Organized; structural. **4.** In chemistry, relating to those compounds in which the atoms are linked by covalent bonds, chiefly the compounds of carbon; originally, relating to compounds of natural origin.

or'ganism Any living individual, whether plant or animal, considered as a whole.

or'gasm [G. *orgaō*, to swell, be excited] The acme or climax of the sexual act.

or'ifice [L. *orificium*] Any aperture or opening. See also ostium, foramen, meatus.

or'igin [L. *origo*, source, beginning] **1.** The less movable of the two points of attachment of a muscle, that which is attached to the more fixed part of the skeleton. **2.** The starting point of a cranial or spinal nerve.

ornitho'sis [G. *ornis* (ornith-), bird, + *-osis*, condition] A disease of birds and fowl caused by *Chlamydia psittaci* and contracted by man by contact with these birds; generally milder than psittacosis.

oro- [L. *os, oris*, mouth] Combining form relating to the mouth.

o'rodigitofa'cial Relating to the mouth, fingers, and face.

orona'sal Relating to the mouth and the nose.

oropharynx [L. *os* (or-), mouth] The portion of the pharynx that lies posterior to the mouth and is continuous above with the nasopharynx and below with the laryngopharynx.

orthe'sis An orthopaedic brace or appliance.

ortho- [Gr. *orthos*, correct, straight] **1.** Prefix denoting straight, normal, or in proper order. **2. (o-)** In chemistry, denoting that a compound has two substitutions on adjacent carbon atoms in a benzene ring.

orthodon'tics, orthodon'tia [ortho- + G. *odous*, tooth] That branch of dentistry concerned with the correction and prevention of irregularities and malocclusion of the teeth.

Or'thomyxovi'ridae The family of viruses that comprises the three groups of influenza viruses (types A, B, and C). The only recognized genus is *Influenzavirus*, which comprises the strains of virus types A and B. Influenza virus type C differs somewhat from types A and B and probably belongs to a separate genus.

orthopae'dic Relating to orthopaedics.

orthopae'dics [ortho- + G. *pais* (paid-), child] The medical specialty concerned with the preservation, restoration, and development of form and function of the extremities, spine, and associated structures by medical, surgical, and physical methods.

orthopnoe'a [ortho- + G. *pnoē*, a breathing] Discomfort on breathing which is partly or wholly relieved by the erect sitting or standing position.

orthopnoe'ic Relating to or suffering from orthopnoea.

Orthopox'virus The genus of the family Poxviridae which comprises the viruses of alastrim, vaccinia, variola, cowpox, ectromelia, monkeypox, and rabbitpox.

or'thopsychi'atry The science relating to the study and treatment of disorders of behaviour, especially in children.

orthop'tics [ortho- + G. *optikos*, relating to sight] The study and treatment of defective binocular vision, of defects in the action of the ocular muscles, or of faulty visual habits.

ortho'sis, pl. **ortho'ses** [G. *orthōsis*, a making straight] The straightening of a deformity, often by use of orthopaedic appliances.

orthostat'ic Relating to an erect posture or position.

orthot'ics The science concerned with the making and fitting of orthopaedic appliances.

orthot'onos, orthot'onus [ortho- + G. *tonos*, tension] A form of tetanic spasm in which the neck, limbs, and body are held fixed in a straight line.

os, pl. **o'ra** [L. mouth] **1.** [NA] The mouth. **2.** An opening into a hollow organ or canal, especially one with thick or fleshy edges.

os, gen. **os'sis,** pl. **os'sa** [L. bone] [NA] Bone; a portion of osseous tissue of definite shape and size, forming a part of the animal skeleton and consisting of a dense outer layer of compact or cortical substance covered by the periosteum, and an inner, loose, spongy substance; the central portion of a long bone is filled with marrow. See also bone.

o. coc'cygis [NA], coccyx; the small bone at the end of the vertebral column, formed by the fusion of four rudimentary vertebrae, that articulates above with the sacrum.

o. cox'ae [NA], hip or innominate bone; a large flat bone formed by the fusion of ilium, ischium, and pubis (in the adult), constituting the lateral half of the pelvis; articulates with its fellow anteriorly, with the sacrum posteriorly, and with the femur laterally.

o. ethmoida'le [NA], ethmoid bone; an irregularly shaped bone lying between the orbital plates of the frontal bone and anterior to the sphenoid bone.

o. fem'oris [NA], thigh bone; femur; the long bone of the thigh, articulating with the hip bone proximally and the tibia and patella distally.

o. fronta'le [NA], frontal bone; the large single bone forming the forehead and the upper margin and roof of the orbit on either side.

o. il'ium [NA], ilium; iliac bone; the broad flaring portion of the hip bone, distinct at birth but later becoming fused with the ischium and pubis; its body joins the pubis and ischium to form the acetabulum and the ala or wing.

o. is'chii [NA], ischium; ischial bone; the lower and posterior part of the hip bone.

o. occipita'le [NA], occipital bone; a bone at the lower and posterior part of the skull, consisting of three parts (basilar, condylar, and squamous) enclosing the foramen magnum; articulates with the parietal and temporal bones on either side, the sphenoid bone anteriorly, and the atlas below.

o. parieta'le [NA], parietal bone; a flat curved bone of irregular quadrangular shape at either side of the vault of the cranium; articulates with its fellow medially, with the frontal bone anteriorly, the occipital bone posteriorly, and the temporal and sphenoid bones inferiorly.

o. pu'bis [NA], pubis; anteroinferior portion of the hip bone, distinct at birth but later becoming fused with the ilium and ischium.

o. sa'crum [NA], sacrum; the segment of the vertebral column forming part of the pelvis and closing in the pelvic girdle posteriorly; formed by the fusion of five originally separate sacral vertebrae; articulates with the last lumbar vertebra, the coccyx, and the hip bone on either side.

o. sphenoida'le [NA], sphenoid bone; a bone of irregular shape occupying the base of the skull.

o. tempora'le [NA], temporal bone; a large irregular bone situated in the base and side of the skull, articulating with the sphenoid, parietal, occipital, and zygomatic bones, and by a synovial joint with the mandible.

o. zygomat'icum [NA], zygomatic bone; a quadrilateral bone that forms the prominence of the cheek.

oscilla'tion [L. *oscillatio*, fr. *oscillo*, to swing] **1.** A to and fro movement. **2.** A stage in the vascular changes in inflammation in which the accumulation of leucocytes in the small vessels arrests the passage of blood and there is simply a to-and-fro movement at each cardiac contraction.

os'culum, pl. **os'cula** [L. dim.of *os*, mouth] A pore or minute opening.

-ose 1. In chemistry, a termination usually indicating a carbohydrate. **2.** [L. *-osus*, full of, abounding] Suffix with significance of the commoner -ous (2).

-osis [G.] Suffix meaning a process, condition, or state, usually abnormal or diseased; denotes primarily any production or increase, physiologic or pathologic, and secondarily an invasion, and increase within the organism of parasites (in the latter sense, similar to and often interchangeable with -iasis).

osmo- 1. [G. *osmos*, impulsion] Combining form denoting osmosis. **2.** [G. *osme*, smell] Combining form denoting smell or odour.

os'morecep'tor 1. [G. *osmos*, impulsion] A receptor in the CNS that responds to changes in the osmotic pressure of the blood. **2.** [G. *osmē*, smell] A receptor that receives olfactory stimuli.

os'moreg'ulatory Influencing the degree and the rapidity of osmosis.

osmo'sis [G. *ōsmos*, a thrusting, an impulsion] The phenomenon of the passage of certain fluids and solutions through a membrane or other porous substance; the net passage of fluid from the less concentrated to the more concentrated side of the membrane.

osmot'ic Relating to osmosis.

os'sa [L.] Plural of os (bone).

osseo- [L. *osseus*, bony] Combining form denoting bony. See also ossi-, osteo-.

os'seous [L. *osseus*] Osteal; bony.

ossi- [G. *os*, bone] Combining form denoting bone. See also osseo-, osteo-.

os'sicle [L. *ossiculum*, dim of *os*, bone] Ossiculum.

ossic'ular Pertaining to an ossicle.

ossiculec'tomy [L. *ossiculum*, ossicle, + G. *ektomē*, excision] Removal of the ossicles of the middle ear.

ossiculot'omy [L. *ossiculum*, ossicle, + G. *tomē*, incision] Division of one of the processes of the ossicles of the middle ear, or of a fibrous band causing ankylosis between any two ossicles.

ossic'ulum, pl. **ossic'ula** [L. dim. of *os*, bone] [NA] Ossicle; a small bone; specifically, one of the bones of the middle ear: the malleus, incus, and stapes which are articulated to form a chain for the transmission of sound from the tympanic membrane to the oval window (fenestra vestibuli).

ossifica'tion [L. *ossificatio*, fr. *os*, bone, + *facio*, to make] **1.** Formation of bone. **2.** A change into bone.

os'sify [ossi- + L. *facio*, to make] To form bone or change into bone.

os'teal [G. *osteon*, bone] Osseous.

osteal'gia [osteo- + G. *algos*, pain] Pain in a bone.

ostei'tis [osteo- + G. *-itis*, inflammation] Inflammation of bone.

   central o., **(1)** osteomyelitis; **(2)** endosteitis.

   o. defor'mans, Paget's disease (1).

   o. fibro'sa cys'tica or **generalisa'ta,** increased osteoclastic resorption of calcified bone with replacement by fibrous tissue, due to primary hyperparathyroidism or other causes of the rapid mobilization of mineral salts.

osteo-, ost-, oste- [G. *osteon*, bone] Combining forms denoting bone. See also osseo-, ossi-.

os'teoarthri'tis Degenerative joint disease; degeneration of articular cartilage, either primary or secondary to trauma or other conditions, especially affecting weight-bearing joints.

os'teoarthrop'athy [osteo- + G. *arthron*, joint, + *pathos*, suffering] Any disorder affecting bones and joints.

os'teoblast [osteo- + G. *blastos*, germ] A bone-forming cell derived from mesenchyme to form the osseous matrix in which it becomes enclosed as an osteocyte.

osteoblas'tic Relating to osteoblasts.

os'teochondri'tis [osteo- + G. *chondros*, cartilage, + *-itis*, inflammation] Inflammation of a bone with its cartilage.

   o. defor'mans juveni'lis, Legg-Calvé-Perthes *disease*.

   o. defor'mans juveni'lis dor'si, Scheuermann's *disease*.

os'teochondro'ma [osteo- + G. *chondros*, cartilage, + *-oma*, tumour] A benign cartilaginous neoplasm that consists of a pedicle of normal bone (protruding from the cortex) covered with a rim of proliferating cartilage cells; multiple o.'s are inherited and referred to as hereditary multiple exostoses.

os'teochondro'sis [osteo- + G. *chondros*, cartilage, + *-osis*, condition] Any of a group of disorders of one or more ossification centres in children, characterized by degeneration or aseptic necrosis followed by reossification.

osteoc'lasis, osteocla'sia [osteo- + G. *klasis*, fracture] Intentional fracture of a bone to correct deformity.

os'teoclast [osteo- + G. *klastos*, broken] **1.** A large multinucleated cell with abundant acidophilic cytoplasm, functioning in the absorption and removal of osseous tissue. **2.** An instrument used to break a misshapen bone to correct the deformity.

os'teocyte [osteo- + G. *kytos*, cell] A cell of osseous tissue which occupies a lacuna and has processes which extend into canaliculi and make contact by means of gap junctions with other processes.

os'teodyn'ia [osteo- + G. *odynē*, pain] Ostealgia.

os'teodys'trophy [osteo- + G. *dys*, difficult, imperfect, + *trophē*, nourishment] Defective formation of bone.

   Albright's hereditary o., pseudohypoparathyroidism or pseudo-pseudohypoparathyroidism with diabetes, hypertension, arteritis, and polyarthrosis.

   renal o., generalized bone changes resembling osteomalacia and rickets or osteitis fibrosa, occurring in children or adults with chronic renal failure.

os'teofibro'ma A benign lesion of bone, consisting chiefly of fairly dense, moderately cellular, fibrous connective tissue in which there are small foci of osteogenesis.

os'teofibro'sis Fibrosis of bone, mainly involving red bone marrow.

osteogen'esis [osteo- + G. *genesis*, production] The formation of bone.

   o. imperfec'ta, brittle bones; a condition of abnormal fragility and plasticity of bone, with recurring fractures on minimal trauma, deformity of long bones, usually bluish colour of sclerae, and, in many cases, the development of otosclerosis; inheritance is autosomal dominant in most families, but a rare autosomal recessive type also exists. In **o. i. congenita,** a more severe form, the fractures occur before or at birth; in **o.i. tarda,** a less severe form, the fractures occur later in childhood.

os'teogen'ic, os'teogenet'ic Relating to osteogenesis.

osteo'ma [osteo- + G. *-oma*, tumour] A benign slow-growing mass of mature, predominantly lamellar bone, usually arising from the skull or mandible.

os'teomala'cia [osteo- + G. *malakia*, softness] A disease characterized by a gradual and painful softening and bending of the bones; due to the bones containing osteoid tissue which has failed to calcify because of a lack of vitamin D or renal tubular dysfunction.

   infantile o., juvenile o., rickets.

os'teomyeli'tis [osteo- + G. *myelos*, marrow, + *-itis*, inflammation] Inflammation of the marrow and adjacent bone.

os'teopath A practitioner of osteopathy.

osteop'athy [osteo- + G. *pathos*, suffering] 1. Any disease of bone. 2. A school of medicine based upon the idea that the normal body when in "correct adjustment" is a vital machine capable of making its own remedies against infections and other toxic conditions; employs the diagnostic and therapeutic measures of ordinary medicine in addition to manipulative measures.

osteope'nia [osteo- + G. *penia*, poverty] 1. Decreased calcification or density of bone. 2. Reduced bone mass due to inadequate osteoid synthesis.

os'teoperiosti'tis Inflammation of the periosteum and of the underlying bone.

osteopetro'sis [osteo- + G. *petra*, stone, + *-osis*, condition] Albers-Schönberg disease; excessive formation of dense trabecular bone and calcified cartilage, especially in long bones, leading to obliteration of marrow spaces and to anaemia, with myeloid metaplasia and hepatosplenomegaly, beginning in infancy and with progressive deafness

and blindness; autosomal recessive inheritance.

os'teophlebi'tis [osteo- + G. *phleps*, vein, + *-itis*, inflammation] Inflammation of the veins of a bone.

os'teophyte [osteo- + G. *phyton*, plant] A bony outgrowth.

os'teoplasty [osteo- + G. *plassō*, to form] 1. Bone grafting; reparative or plastic surgery of the bones. 2. In dentistry, resection of osseous structure to achieve acceptable gingival contour.

os'teoporo'sis [osteo- + G. *poros*, pore, + *-osis*, condition] Reduction in the quantity of bone or atrophy of skeletal tissue; occurs in postmenopausal women and elderly men, resulting in bone trabeculae that are scanty, thin, and without osteoelastic resorption.

os'teoporot'ic Pertaining to, characterized by, or causing a porous condition of the bones.

osteor'rhaphy [osteo- + G. *rhaphē*, suture] Wiring together of the fragments of a broken bone.

os'teosarco'ma Osteogenic *sarcoma*.

os'teosclero'sis [osteo- + G. *sklērōsis*, hardness] Abnormal hardening or eburnation of bone.

   o. congen'ita, achondroplasia.

osteo'sis [osteo- + G. *-osis*, condition] 1. A morbid process in bone. 2. Osteogenesis.

os'teotome [osteo- + G. *tomē*, incision] A chisel-like instrument for use in cutting bone.

osteot'omy [osteo- + G. *tomē*, incision] Cutting a bone, usually by means of a saw or chisel, for any purpose.

os'tia [L.] Plural of ostium.

os'tial Relating to any orifice, or ostium.

osti'tis Osteitis.

os'tium, pl. **os'tia** [L. door, entrance, mouth] [NA] A small opening, especially as an entrance into a hollow organ or canal.

os'tomy [L. *ostium*, mouth] 1. An artificial stoma or opening into the urinary or gastrointestinal canal, or the trachea. 2. Any operation by which an opening is created between two hollow organs or between a hollow viscus and the abdominal wall.

ot-, oto- [G. *ous*, ear] Combining form denoting the ear. See also auri-.

otal'gia [ot- + G. *algos*, pain] Earache.

o'tic [G. *otikos*, fr. *ous*, ear] Relating to the ear.

oti'tis [ot- + G. *-itis*, inflammation] Inflammation of the ear.

   o. exter'na, inflammation of the external auditory canal.

   o. inter'na, labyrinthitis.

   o. me'dia, inflammation of the middle ear.

   serous o., inflammation of middle ear mucosa, often accompanied by accumulation of fluid, secondary to eustachian tube obstruction.

o'toantri'tis Inflammation of the mastoid antrum.

otodyn'ia [oto- + G. *odynē*, pain] Earache.

otogen'ic, otog'enous [oto- + G. *-gen*, producing] Originating within the ear, especially from inflammation of the ear.

o'tolaryngol'ogist A specialist in otolaryngology.

o'tolaryngol'ogy [oto- + G. *larynx*, *logos*, study] The medical specialty concerned with diseases of the ear and larynx, often including the upper respiratory tract and many diseases of the head and neck, tracheobronchial tree, and oesophagus.

o'tolith [oto- + G. *lithos*, stone] Statoconium. See statoconia.

otol'ogy [oto- + G. *logos*, study] The branch of medical science that embraces the study, diagnoses, and treatment of diseases of the ear and related structures.

-otomy See -tomy.

otomyco'sis [oto- + G. *mykēs*, fungus] An infection due to a fungus in the external auditory canal.

otop'athy [oto- + G. *pathos*, suffering] Any disease of the ear.

o'toplasty [oto- + G. *plassō*, to form] Reparative or plastic surgery of the auricle of the ear.

otorhi'nolaryngol'ogy [oto- + G. *rhis*, nose, + *larynx*, larynx, + *logos*, study] The medical specialty concerned with diseases of the ear, nose, and larynx.

otorhinol'ogy [oto- + G. *rhis*, nose, + *logos*, study] The branch of medicine concerned with disease of the ear and nose.

otorrhoe'a [oto- + G. *rhoia*, flow] A discharge from the ear.

otosclero'sis [oto- + G. *sklērosis*, hardening] A new formation of spongy bone about the stapes and fenestra vestibuli, resulting in progressively increasing deafness, without signs of disease in the auditory tube or tympanic membrane.

o'toscope [oto- + G. *skopeō*, to view] An instrument for examining the drum membrane or auscultating the ear.

otos'copy [oto- + G. *skopeō*, to view] Inspection of the ear, especially of the drum membrane.

otos'teal [oto- + G. *osteon*, bone] Relating to the ossicles of the ear.

otot'omy [oto- + G. *tomē*, incision] Dissection of the ear.

oua'bain A glycoside from ouabaio, obtained from the wood of *Acocanthera ouabaio* or from the seeds of *Strophanthus gratus;* its action is qualitatively identical to that of the digitalis glycosides; used for rapid digitalization.

-ous 1. A chemical suffix denoting that the element to the name of which it is attached is in one of its lower valencies. **2.** [L. *-osus*, full of, abounding] Suffix for forming an adjective from a noun.

out'patient A patient treated in a hospital, dispensary, or clinic and released in the same day.

o'va [L.] Plural of ovum.

ovar'ian Relating to the ovary.

o'variec'tomy [ovario- + G. *ektomē*, excision] Excision of one or both ovaries.

ovario-, ovari- [L. *ovarium*, ovary] Combining forms denoting ovary. See also oo-, oophor-, oophoro-.

ovar'iohysterec'tomy [ovario- + G. *hystera*, uterus, + *ektomē*, excision] Removal of ovaries and uterus.

ovar'iosalpingi'tis [ovario- + salpingitis] Inflammation of ovary and oviduct.

ovarios'tomy [ovario- + G. *stoma*, mouth] Establishment of a temporary fistula for drainage of a cyst of the ovary.

ovariot'omy [ovario- + G. *tomē*, incision] Incision into an ovary.

ovari'tis Oophoritis.

o'vary [Mod. L. *ovarium*, fr. *ovum*, egg] One of the paired female reproductive glands whose stroma is a vascular connective tissue containing numbers of ovarian follicles enclosing the ova; surrounding this is a more condensed layer of stroma called the tunica albuginea.

   polycystic o., enlarged cystic o.'s, pearl white in colour, thickened tunica albuginea, characteristic of the Stein-Leventhal syndrome; clinical features are abnormal menses, obesity, and evidence of masculinization, such as hirsutism and clitoromegaly.

o'verbite Extension of the upper teeth over the lower teeth in a vertical direction when the opposing posterior teeth are in contact.

o'vercompensa'tion 1. An exaggeration of personal capacity to overcome a real or imagined inferiority. 2. The process in which a psychologic deficiency inspires exaggerated correction.

o'verdose 1. An excessive dose. 2. To administer an excessive dose.

ovi-, ovo-, [L. ovum, egg] Combining forms denoting egg. See also oo-.

o'viduct [ovi | L. ductus, a leading] Uterine tube.

ovigen'esis Oogenesis.

ovula'tion Release of an ovum from the ovarian follicle.

o'vum, pl. o'va [L. ogg] The female sex cell that, when fertilized by a spermatozoon, is capable of developing into a new individual of the same species.

oxalae'mia [oxalate + G. haima, blood] The presence of an abnormally large amount of oxalates in the blood.

ox'alate A salt of oxalic acid.

oxal'ic acid An acid found in many plants and vegetables which is toxic when ingested by man; used as a general reducing agent.

oxalo'sis Widespread deposition of calcium oxalate crystals in the kidneys, bones, arterial media, and myocardium, with increased urinary excretion of oxalate.

oxalu'ria [oxalate | G. ouron, urine] Excretion of an abnormally large amount of oxalates, especially calcium oxalate, in the urine.

oxida'tion 1. Combination with oxygen or increasing the valency of an atom or ion by the loss from it of hydrogen or of one or more electrons, thus rendering it more electropositive. 2. In bacteriology, the aerobic dissimilation of substrates with the production of energy and water; in contrast to fermentation, the transfer of electrons is accomplished via the respiratory chain, which utilizes oxygen as the final electron acceptor.

oxida'tion-reduc'tion Any chemical oxidation or reduction reaction, which must, in toto, comprise both oxidation and reduction; often shortened to "redox."

ox'ide A compound of oxygen with another element or a radical.

oxy- [G. oxys, keen] Combining form denoting: sharp, pointed; acid; acute; shrill; in chemistry, the presence of oxygen, either added or substituted, in a substance.

oxyceph'aly [G. oxys, pointed. + kephalē, head] Craniosynostosis in which there is premature closure of the lambdoid and coronal sutures, resulting in an abnormally high, peaked, or conically shaped skull.

ox'ygen 1. A gaseous element, symbol O, atomic no. 8, atomic weight 16.000; combines with most of the other elements to form oxides. 2. A medicinal gas that contains not less than 99.0%, by volume, of O_2.

oxygena'tion Addition of oxygen to any chemical or physical system.

ox'yhaemoglo'bin (HbO₂) Haemoglobin in combination with oxygen, the form of haemoglobin present in arterial blood.

oxyphil'ic Having an affinity for acid dyes.

ox'ytetracy'cline An antibiotic produced by Streptomyces rimosus, with actions and uses similar to those of tetracycline.

oxyto'cic Hastening childbirth.

oxyto'cin [G. okytokos, first birth, prompt delivery] A nonapeptide hormone of the neurohypophysis that causes myometrial contractions at term and promotes milk release during lactation; used for the induction or stimulation of labour, in the management of postpartum haemorrhage and atony, and to relieve painful breast engorgement.

oxyuri'asis Disease manifestations from infection with seatworms or pinworms (oxyurids).

oxyu'rid [see Oxyuris] Common name for members of the family Oxyuridae

Oxyu'ridae A family of parasitic nematodes (superfamily Oxyuroidea), found in the large intestine or caecum of vertebrates and the intestine of invertebrates, including the genera Aspiculuris, Enterobius, Oxyuris, Passalurus, Syphacia, and Thelandros.

Oxyu'ris [G. oxys, sharp, + oura, tail] A genus of nematodes commonly called seatworms or pinworms; the pinworm of man is the closely related form, Enterobius vermicularis.

ozae'na [G. ozaina, a fetid polypus, fr. ozō, to smell] A disease characterized by intranasal crusting, atrophy, and fetid odour.

o'zone [G. ozō, to smell] O_3; air containing a perceptible amount of O_3 formed by an electric discharge or by the slow combustion of phosphorus, with an odour suggestive of Cl or SO_2; a powerful oxidizing agent.

P

p- para- (3).

pace'maker Biologically, any rhythmic centre that establishes a pace of activity; also used to mean an artificial p.

    artificial p., any device that substitutes for an anatomic p. to control the rhythm of the organ; especially a cardiac p.

    demand p., a form of artificial p. usually implanted into cardiac tissue because its output of electrical stimuli can be inhibited by endogenous cardiac electrical activity.

    fixed-rate p., an artificial p. that emits electrical stimuli at a constant frequency.

pachy- [G. *pachys*, thick] Prefix denoting thick.

pachydac'tyly [pachy- + G. *daktylos*, finger or toe] Enlargement of the fingers or toes, especially extremities.

pachyder'ma [pachy- + G. *derma*, skin] Abnormally thick skin. See also elephantiasis.

pachyder'moperiosto'sis [pachy- + G. *derma*, skin, + periostosis]. A syndrome characterized by clubbing of the digits, periosteal new bone formation especially over the distal ends of the long bones, and coarsening of the facial features with thickening, furrowing, and oiliness of the skin of the face and forehead; probably of autosomal dominant inheritance, usually more severe in males.

pach'ymeningi'tis [pachy- + G. *mēninx*, membrane, + -*itis*, inflammation] Inflammation of the dura mater.

pach'ymeningop'athy [pachy- + G. *mēninx* (*mēning-*), membrane, + *pathos*, disease] Any disease of the dura mater.

pachymen'inx [pachy- + G. *mēninx*, membrane] The dura mater.

pachyonych'ia [pachy- + G. *onyx*, nail] Abnormal thickness of the fingernails or toenails.

pack'ing 1. Filling a natural cavity or a wound with some material. 2. The material so used.

pad 1. Soft material forming a cushion, to apply or relieve pressure on a part, or fill a depression. 2. A body of fat or some other tissue serving to fill a space or act as a cushion in the body.

    laparotomy p., a p. made from several layers of gauze folded into a rectangular shape; used as a sponge, for packing off the viscera in abdominal operations, etc.

paed-, paedi-, paedo- [G. *pais*, child] Combining forms denoting child.

pae'derasty [G. *paiderastia;* fr. *pais* (*paid-*), boy, + *eraō*, to long for] Anal intercourse, especially when practised on boys.

paediat'ric [paed- + G. *iatrikos*, relating to medicine] Relating to paediatrics.

pae'diatri'cian A specialist in paediatrics.

paediat'rics [paed- + G. *iatreia*, medical treatment] The medical specialty concerned with the development and care of children and the diagnosis and treatment of their diseases.

paedodon'tics, paedodon'tia [ped- + G. *odous*, tooth] The branch of dentistry concerned with dental care and treatment of children.

paedophil'ia [G. *pais*, child, + *philos*, fond] Fondness of children by an adult for sexual purposes.

-pagus [G. *pagos*, something fixed] A termination denoting conjoined twins, the first element of the word denoting the parts fused. See also -didymus, -dymus.

pain [L. *poena*, a fine, a penalty] 1. An unpleasant sensory and emotional experience associated with, or described in terms of, actual or potential tissue damage. 2. One of the uterine contractions occurring in childbirth.

    after-p.'s, see afterpains.

    bearing-down p., a uterine contraction accompanied with straining and tenesmus; usually appearing in the second stage of labour.

    expulsive p.'s, p.'s associated with contraction of the uterine muscle.

    false p.'s, ineffective uterine contractions, preceding and sometimes resembling true labour, but distinguishable from it by the lack of progressive effacement and dilation of the cervix.

    growing p.'s, p.'s, frequently felt at night, in the limbs of growing children.

    hunger p., cramp in the epigastrium associated with hunger.

    intermenstrual p., (1) pelvic discomfort occurring at midpoint of the menstrual cycle; **(2)** mittelschmerz.

labour p.'s, rhythmical uterine contractions that under normal conditions increase in quality, frequency, and duration, culminating in vaginal delivery of the infant.

phantom limb p., see phantom *limb*.

referred p., p. perceived as coming from an area or situation remote from its actual origin.

pal'atal Relating to the palate or the palate bone.

pal'ate [L. *palatum*, palate] The roof of the mouth; the bony and muscular partition between the oral and nasal cavities.

bony p., a concave elliptical bony plate, constituting the roof of the oral cavity, formed by the palatine process of the maxilla and the horizontal plate of the palatine bone on either side.

cleft p., a congenital fissure in the median line of the p., often associated with cleft lip.

hard p., the anterior part of the palate, consisting of the bony palate covered above by the mucous membrane of the floor of the nose and below by the mucoperiosteum of the roof of the mouth which contains the palatine vessels, nerves, and mucous glands.

soft p., the posterior muscular portion of the palate, forming an incomplete septum between the mouth and the oropharynx, and between the oropharynx and the nasopharynx.

pal'atine Palatal.

palato- [L. *palatum*, palate] Combining form meaning palate.

pal'atopharyn'geal Relating to palate and pharynx.

pal'atoplasty [palato- + G. *plasso*, to form] Surgery of the palate to restore form and function.

palatople'gia [palato- + G. *plege*, stroke] Paralysis of the muscle of the soft palate.

palator'rhaphy [palato- + G. *rhaphe*, suture] Suture of a cleft palate.

paleo-, pale- [G. *palaios*, old, ancient] Combining forms denoting old, primitive, primary, early.

pal'eocor'tex The phylogenetically oldest part of the cortical mantle of the cerebral hemisphere, represented by the olfactory cortex.

palindrom'ic Relapsing; recurring.

pallaesthe'sia [G. *pallo*, to quiver, + *aisthesis*, sensation] The appreciation of vi-

bration, a form of pressure sense most acute when a vibrating tuning fork is applied over a bony prominence.

pal'liate [L. *palliatus*, cloaked] Mitigate; to reduce the severity of; to relieve somewhat.

pal'liative Reducing the severity of; denoting the alleviation of symptoms without curing the underlying disease.

pallidec'tomy [pallidum + G. *ektome*, excision] Excision or destruction of the globus pallidus.

pallidot'omy [pallidum + G. *tome*, incision] A lesion-producing operation on the globus pallidus to relieve involuntary movements or muscular rigidity.

pal'lidum [L. *pallidus*, pale] *Globus pallidus.*

pal'lium [L. cloak] [NA] Brain mantle, the cerebral cortex with the subjacent white substance.

pal'lor [L.] Paleness, as of the skin.

pal'ma, pl. **pal'mae** [L.] [NA] Palm.

pal'mar [L. *palmaris*, fr. *palma*] Referring to the palm of the hand.

pal'mus, pl. **pal'mi** [G. *palmos*, pulsation, quivering] 1. Facial *tic.* 2. Rhythmical fibrillary contractions in a muscle.

pal'pable [see palpation] 1. Perceptible to touch; capable of being palpated. 2. Evident; plain.

pal'pate To examine by feeling and pressing with the palms of the hands and the fingers.

palpa'tion [L. *palpatio*, fr. *palpo*, pp. -*atus*, to touch, stroke] 1. Examination by means of the hands, to outline the organs or tumours of the abdomen, to determine the degree of resistance of various parts, to feel the heart beat, the vibrations in the chest, etc. 2. Touching, feeling or perceiving by the sense of touch.

palpe'bra, pl. **palpe'brae** [L.] [NA] Eyelid; one of the two movable folds of skin, lined with conjunctiva, in front of the eyeball.

pal'pebral Relating to an eyelid or the eyelids.

palpita'tion [L. *palpitatio*, to throb] Perceptible forcible pulsation of the heart, usually with an increase in frequency or force, with or without irregularity in rhythm.

pal'sy [a corruption thru O. Fr. fr. L. and G. *paralysis*] Paralysis; often used to connote paresis.

birth p., paralysis due to cerebral haemorrhage occurring at birth or to anoxic injury of the fetal brain *in utero.*

cerebral p., defect of motor power and coordination related to damage of the brain.

Erb's p., birth p. in which there is paralysis of the muscles of the upper arm due to a lesion of the brachial plexus or of the roots of the fifth and sixth cervical nerves.

facial p., Bell's p., unilateral paralysis of the facial muscles supplied by the seventh cranial nerve.

pan- [G. *pas,* all] Prefix denoting all, entire. See also pant-.

panace'a [G. *panakeia,* universal remedy (fr. *Panacea,* G. myth. char.] A cure-all; a remedy claimed to be curative of all problems or disorders.

panarthri'tis 1. Inflammation involving all the tissues of a joint. **2.** Inflammation of all the joints of the body.

pancardi'tis Diffuse inflammation of the heart.

pan'creas, pl. **pancrea'ta** [G. *pankreas,* the sweetbread] [NA] A lobulated gland, devoid of capsule, extending from the concavity of the duodenum to the spleen and consists of a flattened head within the duodenal concavity, an elongated three-sided body extending transversely across the abdomen, and a tail in contact with the spleen; it secretes pancreatic juice, discharged into the intestine, and the internal secretions, insulin and glucagon.

pancreat-, pancreatico-, pancreato-, pancreo- [G. *pankreas,* pancreas] Combining forms denoting the pancreas.

pancreatec'tomy [pancreat- + G. *ektome,* excision] Excision of the pancreas.

pancreat'ic Relating to the pancreas.

pancreati'tis Inflammation of the pancreas.

acute haemorrhagic p., acute inflammation of the pancreas accompanied by the formation of necrotic areas on the surface of the pancreas and in the omentum due to the action of the escaped pancreatic enzymes, and, frequently, haemorrhages into the substance of the gland.

pancreatog'enous Of pancreatic origin; formed in the pancreas.

pancreatog'raphy [pancreato- + G. *grapho,* to write] Radiographic visualization

of the pancreatic ducts after injection of radiopaque material into the collecting system.

pancreat'olith [pancreato- + G. *lithos,* stone] A pancreatic calculus; a concretion, usually multiple, in the pancreatic duct, associated with chronic pancreatitis.

pancreatot'omy [pancreato- + G. *tome,* incision] Incision of the pancreas.

pancytope'nia [pan- + G. *kytos,* cell, + *penia,* poverty] Pronounced reduction in the number of erythrocytes, all types of white blood cells, and the blood platelets in the circulating blood.

congenital p., Fanconi's p., Fanconi's *anaemia.*

pandem'ic [pan- + G. *demos,* the people] A widespread epidemic.

pan'encephali'tis A diffuse inflammation of the brain.

panhy'popitu'itarism A state in which the secretion of all anterior pituitary hormones is inadequate or absent, as a result of destruction of substantially all of the anterior pituitary gland.

pan'ic [fr. G. god *Pan,* presumed to inspire terror] A violent and unreasoning anxiety and fear.

pannic'uli'tis [panniculus + G. *-itis,* inflammation] Inflammation of the panniculus adiposus of the abdominal wall.

pannic'ulus, pl. **pannic'uli** [L. dim. of *pannus,* cloth] [NA] A sheet or layer of tissue.

p. adipo'sus [NA], the superficial fascia which contains a fatty deposit in its areolar substance.

pan'nus, pl. **pan'ni** [L. cloth] A membrane of granulation tissue covering a normal surface, particularly the articular cartilages in rheumatoid arthritis and the cornea in trachoma, where it occurs in three forms: **p. crassus,** thick, with many blood vessels and very dense opacity; **p. siccus,** dry, with a dry glossy surface; **p. tenuis,** thin, with few blood vessels and slight opacity.

panophthal'mia,
pan'ophthalmi'tis [pan- + G. *ophthalmos,* eye] Purulent inflammation of all parts of the eye.

panoti'tis [pan- + G. *ous,* ear, + *-itis,* inflammation] General inflammation of the entire ear.

pan'sinusi'tis Inflammation of all paranasal sinuses on one or both sides.

pant-, panto- [G. *pas*, all] Prefix denoting all, entire. See also pan-.

pantal'gia [pant- + G. *algos*, pain] Pain involving the entire body.

pan'tomograph A panoramic radiographic instrument that permits visualization of the entire dentition, alveolar bone, and contiguous structures on a single extraoral film.

pantothen'ic acid A growth substance widely distributed in plant and animal tissues, and in part of the vitamin B_2 complex part of coenzyme A.

papav'erine A benzylisoquinoline alkaloid of opium; not narcotic but has mild analgesic action, and is a powerful spasmolytic.

papil'la, pl. **papil'lae** [L. a nipple, dim. of *papula*, a pimple] [NA] Any small nipple-like process.

   papillae fungifor'mes [NA], **fungiform papillae,** numerous minute elevations on the dorsum of the tongue, of a fancied mushroom shape; the epithelium of many of these papillae have taste buds.

   p. inci'siva [NA], **incisive p.,** a slight elevation of the mucosa at the anterior extremity of the raphe of the palate.

   interdental p., the gingiva that fills the interproximal space between two adjacent tooth.

   p. mam'mae [NA], nipple; teat; the projection at the apex of the mamma, on the surface of which the lactiferous ducts open, surrounded by a circular pigmented area, the areola.

   optic p., discus nervi optici

   tactile n., one of the papillae of the skin containing a tactile cell or corpuscle.

pap'illary Relating to, resembling, or provided with papillae.

papilli'tis [papilla + G. -*itis*, inflammation] Inflammation of the optic disc or renal papilla.

papillo- [L. *papilla*] Combining form denoting papilla, papillary.

papilloede'ma [papilla + oedema] Oedema of the optic disc.

papillo'ma [papilla + G. -*oma*, tumour] A benign epithelial neoplasm consisting of villous or arborescent outgrowths of fibrovascular stroma covered by neoplastic cells.

pap'illomato'sis 1. The development of numerous papillomas. 2. Papillary projections of the epidermis forming a microscopically undulating surface.

Papillo'mavirus A genus of viruses (family Papovaviridae) containing DNA, including the papilloma and warts viruses of man and other animals.

Papo'vavi'ridae [pa(pilloma) + po(lyoma) + va(cuolating)] A family of small antigenically distinct viruses, comprising the genera *Papillomavirus* and *Polyomavirus*, that replicate in nuclei of infected cells; most have oncogenic properties.

papo'vavirus Any virus of the family Papoviridae.

pap'ular Relating to papules.

pap'ule [L. *papula*, pimple] A small, circumscribed, solid elevation on the skin.

papulo- [L. *papula*, papule] Combining form denoting papule.

pap'ulopus'tular Denoting an eruption composed of papules and pustules.

papulo'sis The occurrence of numerous widespread papules.

pap'ulovesic'ular Denoting an eruption composed of papules and vesicles.

para- [G. alongside of, near] 1. Prefix denoting departure from the normal. 2. Prefix denoting involvement of two like parts or a pair. 3. (*p-*) In chemistry, a prefix designating two substitutions in the benzene ring arranged symmetrically. For words so beginning, see the specific name.

par'a [L. *pario*, to bring forth] A woman who has given birth to an infant or infants, denoted either by a Latin numerical prefix or by a Roman numeral for each occurrence; *e.g.*, **primipara** or **para I,** first infant(s); **secundipara** or **para II,** second infant(s).

par'acente'sis [G *parakentēsis*, a tapping for dropsy] The passage into a cavity of a trocar and cannula, needle, or other hollow instrument to remove fluid; variously designated according to the cavity punctured.

Par'acoccidioi'des brasilie'nsis A dimorphic fungus that causes paracoccidioidomycosis; grows as large spherical or oval cells which bear single or several buds, occasionally covering the entire surface.

par'acoccidioi'domyco'sis A chronic mycosis caused by *Paracoccidioides brasiliensis* and characterized by primary pulmonary lesions with dissemination to many visceral organs, conspicuous ulcerative granulomas of the buccal and nasal mucosa with extensions to the skin, and generalized lymphangitis.

paracu'sis, paracu'sia [para- + G. akousis, hearing] **1.** Impaired hearing. **2.** Auditory illusion or hallucination.

paracysti'tis [para- + G. kystis, bladder, + -itis, inflammation] Inflammation of the connective tissue and other structures about the urinary bladder.

paradip'sia [para- + G. dipsa, thirst] Perverted appetite for fluids ingested without relation to bodily need.

paraesthe'sia [para- + G. aisthēsis, sensation] An abnormal sensation, such as of burning, pricking, tickling, or tingling.

paraesthet'ic Relating to or marked by paraesthesia; denoting numbness and tingling in an extremity which usually occurs on the resumption of the blood flow to a nerve following temporary pressure or mild injury.

paraffino'ma A tumefaction, usually a granuloma, caused by the prosthetic or therapeutic injection of paraffin; sometimes referring to similar lesions resulting from the injection of any oil, wax, etc.

paragang'lion, pl. **paragan'glia** A small, roundish body containing chromaffin cells; a number of such bodies may be found retroperitoneally near the aorta and in organs such as the kidney, liver, heart, and gonads.

parageu'sia [para- + G. geusis, taste] Disordered or perverted sense of taste.

paragonimi'asis Infection with a worm of the genus Paragonimus, especially P. westermani.

Paragon'imus [para- + G. gonimos, with generative power] A genus of lung flukes, parasitic in man and a wide variety of mammals, that feed upon crustaceans carrying the metacercariae.

　　P. westerman'i, a species that causes paragonimiasis, found chiefly in Asia in man, excysted worms invade the wall of the gut and migrate through the diaphragm into the lungs, causing an intense inflammatory reaction and eventually forming fibrous-walled nodules that usually contain a pair of adult worms, exudate, eggs, and remains of red blood cells; the fibroparasitic nodules may become contiguous and form multiloculated cystlike structures.

paragraph'ia [para- + G. graphō, to write] **1.** Loss of the power of writing from dictation, although the words are understood. **2.** Writing one word when another is intended.

parala'lia [para- + G. lalia, talking] Any speech defect; especially one in which one letter is habitually substituted for another.

paral'ysis, pl. **paral'yses** [G. fr. para- + lysis, a loosening] **1.** Palsy; loss of power of voluntary movement in a muscle through injury or disease of its nerve supply. **2.** Loss of any function.

　　acute ascending p., Landry's p., a p. of rapid course beginning in the legs and involving progressively the trunk, arms, and neck.

　　bulbar p., progressive bulbar p.

　　compression p., p. due to compression of a nerve, as by prolonged pressure.

　　Duchenne-Erb p., Erb's p., Erb's palsy.

　　Klumpke's p., atrophic p. of the forearm and small muscles of the hand together with paralysis of the eighth cervical and first dorsal nerves.

　　periodic p., term for a group of diseases characterized by recurring episodes of muscular weakness or flaccid p. without loss of consciousness, speech, or sensation; attacks begin when the patient is at rest, and there is apparent good health between attacks.

　　progressive bulbar p., progressive atrophy and p. of the muscles of the tongue, lips, palate, pharynx, and larynx, occurring in later life and due to atrophic degeneration of the neurones innervating these muscles.

　　sleep p., a condition in which upon waking in the morning the person is aware of his surroundings but is unable to move.

paralyt'ic Relating to paralysis.

Parame'cium [G. paramēkēs, rather long, fr. mēkos, length] A genus of freshwater holotrichous ciliates, characteristically slipper-shaped, commonly used for genetic and other studies.

paramed'ical Relating to the medical profession in an adjunctive capacity, e.g., denoting allied fields such as physical therapy.

parametri'tis [parametrium + G. -itis, inflammation] Inflammation of the cellular tissue adjacent to the uterus.

parame'trium, pl. **parame'tria** [para- + G. mētra, uterus] [NA] The connective tissue of the pelvic floor extending from the fibrous subserous coat of the supracervical portion of the uterus laterally between the layers of the broad ligament.

paramne'sia [para- + G. *amnēsia*, forgetfulness] False recollection, events being recalled which have never occurred.

paramu'cin A glycoprotein found in ovarian and certain other cysts, insoluble in water like mucin, but unlike mucin precipitated by tannin.

paramyoto'nia An atypical form of myotonia.

 congenital p., p. congen'ita, a nonprogressive disease characterized by myotonia induced by exposure to cold, with episodes of intermittent flaccid paralysis, but no atrophy or hypertrophy of muscles; autosomal dominant inheritance.

Paramyx'ovirus A genus of viruses (family Paramyxoviridae) that includes Newcastle disease, mumps, and parainfluenza viruses (types 1 to 5); all have haemagglutinating and haemadsorbing activities.

paranol'a [G. derangement, madness, fr. para- + *noeō*, to think] A mental disorder characterized by the presence of systematized delusions, often of a persecutory character, in an otherwise intact personality; when symptoms are relatively mild and mental illness is not present, the condition is called paranoid *personality*.

par'anoid Relating to, or characterized by, paranoia.

parapare'sis [para- + paresis] A slight degree of paralysis, affecting the lower extremities.

parapha'sia [para- + G. *phasis*, speech] Aphasia in which the patient has lost the power of speaking correctly, substituting one word for another, and jumbling words and sentences in such a way as to make speech unintelligible.

paraphil'ia [para- + G. *philos*, fond] Sexual practices that are socially prohibited.

paraphimo'sis [para- + G. phimosis] **1.** Painful constriction of the glans penis by a phimotic foreskin, which has been retracted behind the corona. **2.** A retraction of the lid behind a protruding eyeball.

paraple'gia [G. a stroke on one side, fr. para, beside, + *plēgē*, a stroke] Paralysis of both lower extremities and, generally, the lower trunk.

paraple'gic Relating to or suffering from paraplegia.

par'apsychol'ogy The study of extrasensory perception, such as thought transference (telepathy) and clairvoyance.

par'areflex'ia A condition characterized by abnormal reflexes.

par'asite [G. *parasitos*, a guest, fr. para, beside, + *sitos*, food] **1.** An organism that lives on or in another and draws its nourishment therefrom. **2.** In the case of a fetal inclusion or conjoined twins, the more or less incomplete twin that derives its support from the more nearly normal autosite.

parasit'ic 1. Relating to or of the nature of a parasite. **2.** Denoting organisms that normally grow only in or on the living body of a host.

parasit'icide [parasite + L. *caedo*, to kill] An agent that destroys parasites.

par'asitism A symbiotic relationship in which one species (the parasite) benefits at the expense of the other (the host).

parasitol'ogy [parasite + G. *logos*, study] The branch of biology and of medicine concerned with parasitism.

par'asympathet'ic Pertaining to a division of the autonomic nervous system.

parasym'patholyt'ic Relating to an agent that annuls or antagonizes the effects of the parasympathetic nervous system.

parasym'pathomimet'ic [para- + G. *sympatheia*, sympathy, + *mimētikos*, imitative] Relating to an agent having an action resembling that caused by stimulation of the parasympathetic nervous system.

parathi'on A highly poisonous organic phosphate insecticide; an irreversible inhibitor of cholinesterases.

parathy'roid *Glandula* parathyroidea.

par'athyroidec'tomy [parathyroid + G. *ektomē*, excision] Excision of the parathyroid glands.

paraty'phoid Resembling in some respects, yet not the same as, typhoid.

parax'ial By the side of the axis of any body or part.

paregor'ic [G. *parēgorkos*, soothing] An antiperistaltic containing powdered opium, anise oil, benzoic acid, camphor, glycerin, and diluted alcohol.

paren'chyma [G. anything poured in beside] [NA] The distinguishing or specific cells of a gland or organ, contained in and supported by the connective tissue framework, or stroma, as of the testis, consisting of the seminiferous tubules located within the lobules.

paren'teral [para- + G. *enteron*, intestine] By some other means than through the gastrointestinal tract or lungs; referring particularly to the introduction of substances into an organism; *i.e.*, by intravenous, subcutaneous, intramuscular, or intramedullary injection.

pare'sis [G. a letting go, slackening] **1.** Partial or incomplete paralysis. **2.** A disease of the brain, syphilitic in origin, marked by progressive dementia, tremor, speech disturbances, and increasing muscular weakness.

par'ies, pl. **pari'etes** [L. wall] [NA] A wall, as of the chest, abdomen, or any hollow organ.

pari'etal Relating to the wall of any cavity.

parieto- [L. *paries*, wall] Combining form denoting relationship to a wall (paries) or to the parietal bone.

par'ity [L. *pario*, to bear] The state of having given birth to an infant or infants, alive or dead; multiple birth is considered as a single parous experience.

parkinso'nian Relating to parkinsonism.

park'insonism **1.** Parkinson's disease; a neurological syndrome usually resulting from arteriosclerotic changes in the basal ganglia and characterized by rhythmical muscular tremors, rigidity of movement, festination, droopy posture, and masklike facies. **2.** A syndrome similar to p. appearing as a side effect of certain antipsychotic drugs.

paronych'ia [para- + G. *onyx*, nail] Inflammation of the nail fold with separation of the skin from the proximal portion of the nail.

paros'mia [para- + G. *osmē*, the sense of smell] Any disorder of the sense of smell, especially the subjective perception of odours that do not exist.

parot'id [G. *parōtis* (*parōtid-*), the gland beside the ear, fr. *para*, beside, + *ous* (*ōt-*), ear] Situated near the ear; usually refers to the p. salivary gland.

parotidi'tis, paroti'tis Inflammation of the parotid gland.

   epidemic p., mumps; an acute infectious and contagious disease caused by Paramyxovirus and characterized by inflammation and swelling of the parotid gland, sometimes of other salivary glands, and occasionally by inflammation of the testis, ovary, pancreas, or meninges.

par'ous [L. *pario*, to bear] Pertaining to parity.

par'oxysm [G. *paroxysmos*, fr. *paroxynō*, to sharpen, irritate] **1.** A sharp spasm or convulsion. **2.** A sudden onset of a symptom or disease, especially one with recurrent manifestations such as the chills and rigor of malaria.

paroxys'mal Relating to or occurring in paroxysms.

pars, pl. **par'tes** [L. *pars* (*part-*) a part] [NA] A part or portion of a structure.

par'thenogen'esis [G. *parthenos*, virgin, + *genesis*, product] A form of asexual reproduction in which the female reproduces its kind without fecundation by the male.

partic'ulate Relating to or occurring in the form of fine particles.

partu'rient [L. *parturio*, to be in labour] Relating to or being in the process of parturition or childbirth.

parturifa'cient]L. *parturio*, to be in labour, + *facio*, to make] Inducing or accelerating labour.

parturi'tion [L. *parturitio*, fr. *parturio*, to be in labour] Childbirth.

Par'vovirus A genus of viruses (family Parvoviridae), of which the Kilham rat virus is the type species, whose members replicate autonomously in suitable cells.

pas'sive [L. *passivus*, fr. *patior*, to endure] Not active; submissive.

pas'sivism [see passive] **1.** An attitude of submission. **2.** A form of sexual perversion in which the subject, usually male, is submissive to the will of his partner in sexual practices.

Pasteurel'la [L. *Pasteur*] A genus of aerobic to facultatively anaerobic, nonmotile bacteria (family Brucellaceae) containing small Gram-negative, rods; parasites of man and other animals. The type species is *P. multocida*.

   P. multoci'da, a species that causes fowl cholera and haemorrhagic septicaemia in warm-blooded animals; it is the type species of the genus *P.*

   P. pes'tis, *Yersinia pestis.*

   P. pseudotuberculo'sis, *Yersinia pseudotuberculosis.*

   P. tularen'sis, *Francisella tularensis.*

pasteuriza'tion [L. *Pasteur*] The heating of milk or other liquids for about 30 minutes at 68°C. (154.4°F.) whereby the living bacteria are destroyed, but the flavour or bouquet is preserved; the spores are unaffected, but are kept from developing by immediately cooling the liquid to 10°C (50°F) or lower.

patel'la, pl. **patel'lae** [L. a small plate, the kneecap, dim. of *patina*, a shallow disc, fr. *pateo*, to lie open] [NA] Kneecap; the large sesamoid bone, in the combined tendon of the extensors of the leg, covering the anterior surface of the knee

patel'lar Relating to the patella.

patellec'tomy [patella + G. *ektomē*, excision] Excision of the patella.

pa'tent [L. *patens*, pres. p. of *pateo*, to lie open] Open; exposed.

path-, patho-, -pathy [G. *pathos*, suffering, disease] Combining forms meaning disease.

path'ogen [patho- + G. *-gen*, to produce] Any virus, microorganism, or other substance causing disease.

pathogenesis [patho- + G. *genesis*, production] The mode of origin or development of any disease or morbid process.

pathogen'ic   **pathogenet'ic**
Causing disease.

pathogenic'ity The condition of being pathogenic or of causing disease.

path'ognomon'ic [patho- + G. *gnōmē*, a mark, a sign] Characteristic or indicative of a disease; denoting especially one or more typical symptoms.

patholog'ic, patholog'ical Pertaining to pathology; morbid; diseased; resulting from disease

pathol'ogy [patho- + G. *logos*, study, treatise] The medical science and specialty practice concerned with all aspects of disease, but with special reference to the essential nature, cause, and development of abnormal conditions, as well as the structural and functional changes that result from the disease processes.

  clinical p., (1) in a strict sense, any part of the medical practice of p. as it pertains to the care of patients; **(2)** the subspecialty in p. concerned with the theoretical and technical aspects of laboratory technology as pertains to the diagnosis and prevention of disease.

  speech p., the science concerned with functional and organic speech defects and disorders.

path'ophysiol'ogy Derangement or alteration of function seen in disease.

path'way 1. A collection of axons establishing a conduction route for nerve impulses from one group of nerve cells to another group or to an effector organ composed of muscle or gland cells. **2.** Any sequence of chemical reactions leading from one compound to another; if taking place in living tissue, usually referred to as a **biochemical p.**

-pathy See path-.

pa'tient [L. *patiens*, pres. p. of *patior*, to suffer] One who is suffering from a disease or disorder and is under treatment for it; not to be confused with "case."

patrilin'eal L. *pater*, father, + *linea*, line] Related to descent through the male line.

pec'cant [L. *peccans* (*-ant-*), pres. p. of *pecco*, to sin] Morbid; unhealthy; producing disease.

pec'ten [L. comb] [NA] A structure with comblike processes or projections.

  p. ana'lis [NA], **anal p.,** the middle third of the anal canal.

  p. os'sis pu'bis [NA], pectineal line of the pubis, the continuation on the superior pubic ramus of the terminal line, forming a sharp ridge.

pectin'eal Ridged; relating to the os pubis or to any comblike structure.

pec'toral [L. *pectoralis*; fr. *pectus*, breast bone] Relating to the chest.

pec'tus, pl. **pec'tora** [L.] [NA] The thorax; the chest; especially the anterior wall, the breast

  p. carina'tum, a flattening of the chest on either side with forward projection of the sternum resembling the keel of a boat.

  p. excava'tum, p. recurva'tum, a hollow at the lower part of the chest caused by a backward displacement of the xiphoid cartilage.

ped-, pedi-, pedo- [L. *pes*, foot] Combining forms denoting feet.

ped'al [L. *pedalis*, fr. *pes* (*ped-*), a foot] Relating to the feet, or to any structure called pes.

ped'icle [L. *pediculus*, dim. of *pes*, foot] **1.** Pediculus. **2.** A stalk by which a nonsessile tumour is attached to normal tissue. **3.** A stalk through which a skin flap receives nourishment until its transfer to another site results in the nourishment coming from that site.

pedic'ulate [L. *pedicutatus*] Not sessile, having a pedicle or peduncle.

pedicula'tion [L. *pediculus*, louse] Infestation with lice.

pedic'uli [L.] Plural of pediculus.

pedic'ulicide [L. *pediculus*, louse, + *caedo*. to kill] An agent used to destroy lice.

pediculo'sis [L. *pediculus*, louse, + G. *-osis*, condition] The state of being infested with lice.

Pedic'ulus [L.] A genus of parasitic lice (family Pediculidae) that live in the hair and feed periodically on blood, including *P. humanus*, the species infecting man; *P. humanus* var. *capitis*, the head louse of man; *P. humanus* var. *corporis* (also called *P. vestimenti* or *P. corporis*), the body louse or clothes louse, which lives and lays eggs (nits) in clothing and feeds on the human body; and *P. pubis* (see *Pthirus pubis*).

pedic'ulus, pl. **pedic'uli** [L. pedicle] [NA] A constricted portion or stalk.

pedun'cle [Mod. L. *pedunculus*, dim. of *pes*, foot] **1.** Pedunculus. **2.** Pedicle (2).

pedun'cular Relating to a pedicle or peduncle.

pedun'culus, pl. **pedun'culi** [Mod. L. dim. of *pes*, foot] [NA] A stalk or stem; in neuroanatomy, a variety of stalklike connecting structures in the brain, composed either exclusively of white matter or of white and grey matter.

pellag'ra [It. *pelle*, skin, + *agro*, rough] An affection characterized by gastrointestinal disturbances, erythema followed by desquamation, and nervous and mental disorders; may occur because of a poor diet, alcoholism, or some other disease upsetting nutrition; main cause is a deficiency of niacin.

pel'let [Fr. *pelote*; L. *pila*, a ball] **1.** A pilule, or minute pill. **2.** A small rod-shaped or ovoid dosage form that is sterile and is composed essentially of pure steroid hormones in compressed form, intended for subcutaneous implantation in body tissues as a depot providing slow release of the hormone over an extended period of time.

pelvi-, pelvio-, pelvo- Combining forms relating to the pelvis.

pel'vic Relating to a pelvis.

pel'vicephalom'etry [pelvi- + G. *kephalē*, head, + *metron*, measure] Measurement of the pelvic diameters in relation to those of the fetal head.

pel'vifixa'tion Surgical attachment of a floating pelvic organ to the wall of the cavity.

pel'vilithot'omy [pelvi- + G. *lithos*, stone, + *tomē*, incision] Operative removal of a calculus from the kidney through an incision in the renal pelvis.

pelvim'eter An instrument shaped like calipers for measuring the diameters of the pelvis.

pelvim'etry [pelvi- + G. metron, measure] Measurement of the diameters of the pelvis.

pel'vis, pl. **pel'ves** [L. basin] **1.** [NA] The cup-shaped ring of bone, with its ligaments, at the lower end of the trunk, formed of the os coxae (the pubic bone, ilium, and ischium) on either side and in front, and the sacrum, and coccyx posteriorly. **2.** Any basin-like or cup-shaped cavity, as the p. of the kidney.

p. rena'lis [NA], **renal p.,** a flattened funnel-shaped expansion of the upper end of the ureter receiving the calices of the kidney, the apex being continuous with the ureter.

pel'vospondyli'tis ossif'icans [L. *pelvis*, basin, + G. *spondylos*, vertebra, + *-itis*; L. *os*, bone, + *facere*, to make] Deposit of bony substance between the vertebrae of the sacrum.

pem'phigoid [G. *pemphix*, blister, + *eidos*, resemblance] **1.** Resembling pemphigus. **2.** A disease resembling pemphigus but significantly distinguishable histologically and clinically (generally benign course).

pem'phigus [G. *pemphix*, a blister] General term used to designate the chronic bullous diseases: p. foliaceus, p. erythematosus, or p. vegetans; also used with a modifying adjective to designate a variety of blistering skin diseases.

p. erythemato'sus, an eruption involving the scalp, face, and trunk; the lesions are scaling erythematous macules and blebs, combining the clinical features of both lupus erythematosus and p. vulgaris.

p. folia'ceus, a generally chronic form of p. in which extensive exfoliative dermatitis, with no perceptible blistering, may be present in addition to the bullae.

p. veg'etans, (1) a form of p. vulgaris in which vegetations develop on the eroded surfaces left by ruptured bullae; new bullae continue to form; **(2)** a chronic benign vegetating form of p., with lesions commonly in the axillae and perineum.

p. vulga'ris, p. in which cutaneous flaccid bullae and oral mucosal erosions may be localized before becoming generalized; the blisters break easily, leaving new non-breaking areas; results from the action of autoimmune antibodies that localize to intercellular sites of stratified squamous epithelium.

-penia [G. *penia*, poverty] Suffix denoting deficiency.

penicil'lamine A degradation product of penicillin; a chelating agent used in the treatment of lead poisoning, hepatolenticular degeneration, and cystinuria, and in the removal of excess copper in Wilson's disease.

penicil'lin [L. *penicillus*, paint brush] **1.** Originally, an antibiotic substance obtained from cultures of the moulds *Penicillium notatum* or *P. chrysogenum*. **2.** One of a family of natural or synthetic variants, mainly bacteriostatic in action, but also slightly bactericidal, especially active against Gram-positive organisms, and with a particularly low toxic action on animal tissue.

penicil'linase **1.** An enzyme that brings about the hydrolysis of penicillin to penicilloic acid; found in most staphylococcus strains that are naturally resistant to penicillin. **2.** A purified enzyme preparation obtained from cultures of a strain of *Bacillus cereus;* formerly used in the treatment of slowly developing or delayed penicillin reactions.

Penicil'lium [see penicillin] A genus of fungi (class Ascomycetes, order Aspergillales), species of which yield several antibiotic substances and biologicals.

pe'nile Relating to the penis.

pe'nis [L. tail] [NA] Phallus; the male organ of copulation, formed by three columns of erectile tissue, two arranged laterally on the dorsum (corpora cavernosa) and one median below (corpus spongiosum); the extremity (glans p.) is formed by an expansion of the corpus spongiosum, covered by a free fold of skin (preputium).

penta- [G. *pente*, five] Combining form denoting five.

pen'tose A monosaccharide containing five carbon atoms in the molecule.

pentosu'ria The excretion of one or more pentoses in the urine.

pep'sin [G. *pepsis*, digestion] Former term for **pepsin A,** the principal digestive enzyme (protease) of the gastric juice, formed from pepsinogen.

pepsin'ogen [pepsin + G. *-gen*, producing] A proenzyme formed and secreted by the chief cells of the gastric mucosa; acidity of gastric juice and pepsin itself remove 42 amino acid residues from p. to form active pepsin.

pep'tic [G. *peptikos*, fr. *peptō*, to digest] Relating to the stomach, to gastric digestion, or to pepsin A.

pep'tidase An enzyme capable of hydrolysing one of the peptide links of a peptide.

pep'tide A compound of two or more amino acids in which the α-carboxyl group of one is united with the α-amino group of the other, with the elimination of a molecule of water, thus forming a p. bond, $-CO-NH-$.

pep'tone Descriptive term applied to intermediate polypeptide products formed in partial hydrolysis of proteins; generally soluble in water, diffusible, and not coagulable by heat.

per- [L. through, throughout, extremely] **1.** Prefix denoting through, conveying intensity. **2.** In chemistry, a prefix denoting: 1) more or most, with respect to the amount of a given element or radical contained in a compound; 2) the degree of substitution for hydrogen.

per a'num [L.] By or through the anus.

per'cept [L. *perceptum*, a thing perceived] **1.** That which is perceived; the complete mental image, formed by the process of perception, of an object present in space. **2.** In clinical psychology, a single unit of perceptual report, such as one of the responses to an inkblot in the Rorschach test.

percep'tion The mental process of becoming aware of or recognizing an object; primarily cognitive rather than affective or conative, although all three aspects are manifested.

percus'sion [L. *percussio*, fr. *per-cutio*, pp. *-cussus*, to beat, fr. *quatio*, to shake, beat] A diagnostic procedure designed to determine the density of a part by means of tapping the surface with the finger or a plessor.

percuta'neous Denoting the passage of substances through unbroken skin, as in absorption by inunction.

per'forated [L. *perforatus,* fr. *per-foro,* pp. *-atus,* to bore through] Pierced with one or more holes.

perfora'tion [see perforated] An abnormal opening in a hollow organ or viscus.

perfu'sion [L. *perfusio*, fr. per- + *fusio*, a pouring] Passage of blood or other fluid through a vascular bed.

peri- [G. around] Prefix denoting around, about.

periadeni'tis [peri- + G. *adēn*, gland, + *itis*, inflammation] Inflammation of the tissues surrounding a gland.

   p. muco'sa necrot'ica recur'rens, a severe form of recurrent aphthous stomatitis, marked by recurrent attacks of aphtha-like lesions that begin as small, firm nodules which then enlarge, ulcerate, and heal by scar formation, leaving numerous atrophied scars on the oral mucosa.

periangi'tis [peri- + G. *angeion*, a vessel, + -*itis*, inflammation] Inflammation of the adventitia of a blood vessel or of the tissues surrounding it or a lymphatic vessel.

peria'pical 1. At or around the apex of a root of a tooth. 2. Denoting the periodontal membrane and adjacent bone.

periarteri'tis Inflammation of the outer coat, or adventitia, of an artery.

periarthri'tis Inflammation of the parts surrounding a joint.

periartic'ular Surrounding a joint.

pericar'diac, pericar'dial 1. Surrounding the heart. 2. Relating to the pericardium.

per'icardiec'tomy [pericardium + G. *ektomē*, excision] Excision of a portion of the pericardium.

pericar'diocente'sis [peri- + G. *kardia*, heart, + *kentēsis*, puncture] Paracentesis of the pericardium.

per'icardi'tis Inflammation of the pericardium.

   adhesive p., p. with adhesions between the two pericardial layers, between the pericardium and heart, or between the pericardium and neighbouring structures.

   constrictive p., tuberculous or other infection of the pericardium, with thickening of the membrane and constriction of the cardiac chambers.

   fibrinous p., acute p. with fibrinous exudate.

   internal adhesive p., concretio cordis.

   p. oblit'erans, inflammation of the pericardium leading to adhesion of the two layers, obliterating the sac.

pericar'dium, pl. **pericar'dia** [L. fr. G. *pericardion*, the membrane around the heart] [NA] The fibroserous membrane covering the heart and beginning of the great vessels; consists of two layers: visceral (epicardium), immediately surrounding the heart, and the outer parietal layer, forming the sac, composed of strong fibrous tissue (**p. fibrosum**) lined with serous membrane (**p. serosum**).

perichon'drium [peri- + G. *chondros*, cartilage] [NA] The dense, irregular connective tissue membrane around cartilage.

pericoli'tis, pericoloni'tis Inflammation of the connective tissue or peritoneum surrounding the colon.

pericra'nium [peri- + G. *kranion*, skull] [NA] The periosteum of the skull.

perienteri'tis Inflammation of the peritoneal coat of the intestine.

per'ifolliculi'tis The presence of an inflammatory infiltrate surrounding hair follicles, frequently in conjunction with folliculitis.

per'ilymph Perilympha.

perilym'pha [peri- + L. *lympha*, a clear fluid (lymph)] [NA] The fluid contained within the osseus labyrinth, surrounding and protecting the membranous labyrinth.

perilymphat'ic 1. Surrounding a lymphatic structure (node or vessel). 2. The spaces and tissues surrounding the membranous labyrinth of the inner ear.

perim'eter [G. *perimetros*, circumference, fr. *peri*, around, + *metron*, measure] 1. A circumference, edge, or border. 2. An instrument used to measure field of vision.

perime'trium, pl. **perime'tria** [peri- + G. *mētra*, uterus] [NA] The serous (peritoneal) coat of the uterus.

perim'etry [G. *perimetros*, circumference] The determination of the limits of the visual field.

perina'tal [peri- + L. *natus*, pp. of *nascor*, to be born] Occurring during, or pertaining to, the periods before, during, or after the time of birth; *i.e.*, before delivery from the 28th week of gestation through the first 7 days after delivery.

per'inatol'ogy Subspecialty of obstetrics concerned with care of the mother and fetus during pregnancy, labour, and delivery, especially when the mother and/or fetus are ill or at risk of becoming ill.

perine'al Relating to the perineum.

perineo- [L. fr. G. *perineon, perinaion*] Combining form denoting the perineum.

perineot'omy Incision into the perineum as in external urethrotomy, lithotomy, etc., or to facilitate childbirth.

perineph'rium, pl. **perineph'ria** [peri- + G. *nephros,* kidney] The connective tissue and fat surrounding the kidney.

perine'um, pl. **perine'a** [L. fr. G. *perineon, perinaion*] 1. [NA] The area between the thighs extending from the coccyx to the pubis and lying below the pelvic diaphragm. 2. The external surface of the central tendon of the perineum, lying between the vulva and the anus in the female and the scrotum and the anus in the male.

period'ic Recurring at regular intervals, denoting a disease with regularly recurring exacerbations or paroxysms.

periodic'ity The tendency to recurrence at regular intervals.

periodon'tal [peri- + G. *odous,* tooth] Around a tooth; relating to the periodontium.

periodon'tics [peri- + G. *odous,* tooth] The branch of dentistry concerned with the study of the normal tissues and the treatment of abnormal conditions of the tissues immediately about the teeth.

per'iodonti'tis [periodontium + G. *-itis,* inflammation] A disease of the periodontium characterized by inflammation of the gingivae, resorption of the alveolar bone, degeneration of the periodontal membrane (ligament), migration of the epithelial attachment apically, and formation of periodontal pockets.

periodon'tium, pl. **periodon'tia** [L. fr. peri + G. *odous,* tooth] [NA] Alveolodental or peridental membrane; the tissues that surround and support the teeth; includes the gingivae, cementum, periodontal ligament, and alveolar and supporting bone.

periop'erative Denoting an event that occurs during the period of an operation.

perios'teal Relating to the periosteum.

perios'teum, pl. **perios'tea** [Mod. L. fr. G. *periosteon,* fr. *peri,* around, + *osteon,* bone] [NA] The thick fibrous membrane covering the entire surface of a bone except its articular cartilage. In young bones it consists of two layers: an inner which is osteogenic, forming new bone tissue, and an outer connective tissue layer conveying the blood vessels and nerves supplying the bone; in older bones the osteogenic layer is reduced.

periosti'tis Inflammation of the periosteum.

periph'eral 1. Relating to or situated at the periphery. 2. Situated nearer the periphery of an organ or part of the body in relation to a specific reference point.

periph'ery [G. *periphereia,* fr. *peri,* around, + *phero,* to carry] The part of a body away from the centre; the outer part or surface.

peristal'sis [peri- + G. *stalsis,* constriction] The movement of the intestine or other tubular structure; the waves of alternate circular contraction and relaxation of the tube by which the contents are propelled onward.

   reversed p., a wave of intestinal contraction in a direction the reverse of normal, by which the contents of the tube are forced backward.

peristal'tic Relating to peristalsis.

peritec'tomy [peri- + G. *ektome,* excision] The removal of a paracorneal strip of the conjunctiva to correct pannus.

perit'omy [G. *peritome,* fr. *peri,* around, + *tome,* incision] 1. Peritectomy. 2. Circumcision (1).

peritone'al Relating to the peritoneum.

peritoneo- Combining form denoting the peritoneum.

peritone'oscope [peritoneum + G. *skopeo,* to view] An endoscope for examining the peritoneal cavity.

per'itoneos'copy Examination of the contents of the peritoneum with a peritoneoscope passed through the abdominal wall.

peritone'um, pl. **peritone'a** [Mod. L. fr. G. *peritonaion,* fr. *periteino,* to stretch over] [NA] The serous sac, consisting of mesothelium and a thin layer of irregular connective tissue, that lines the abdominal cavity (**parietal p.**) and covers most of the viscera contained therein (**visceral p.**); forms two sacs, the peritoneal (or greater) sac and the omental bursa (lesser sac) connected by the foramen epiploicum (of Winslow).

peritoni'tis Inflammation of the peritoneum.

peritrich'ous [peri- + G. *thrix,* hair] 1. Relating to cilia or other appendicular organs projecting from the periphery of a cell. 2. Having flagella uniformly distributed over a cell; especially referring to bacteria.

permeabil'ity The property of being permeable.

per'meable [L. *permeabilis* (see permeation)] Permitting the passage of substances through a membrane or other structure.

permea'tion [L. *per-meo*, pp. *-meatus*, to pass through] The extension of a malignant neoplasm by proliferation of the cells continuously along the blood vessels or lymphatics.

perni'cious [L. *perniciosus*, destructive] Destructive; harmful; denoting a disease of severe character and usually fatal without specific treatment.

pero- [G. *pēros*, maimed] Combining form meaning maimed or malformed.

perome'lia [pero- + G. *melos*, limb] Severe congenital malformations of extremities, including absence of hand or foot.

per os [L.] By mouth.

perox'ide That oxide of any series that contains the greatest number of oxygen atoms; applied to compounds containing an —O—O— link.

per rec'tum [L.] By rectum.

persevera'tion [L. *persevero*, to persist] **1.** Constant repetition of a meaningless word or phrase. **2.** In clinical psychology, the repetition of a previously appropriate or correct response, even though the repeated response has since become inappropriate or incorrect.

persis'tence [L. *persisto*, to abide, stand firm] Obstinate continuation of characteristic behaviour, or of existence in spite of opposition or adverse environmental conditions.

per'sonal'ity **1.** The unique self; the organized system of attitudes and behavioural predispositions by which one impresses and establishes relationships with others. **2.** An individual with a particular p. pattern.

perspira'tion [L. *per-spiro*, pp. *-atus*, to breathe everywhere] **1.** Sweating; excretion of fluid by the sweat glands of the skin. **2.** All fluid loss through normal skin, whether by sweat gland secretion or by diffusion through other skin structures. **3.** The fluid excreted by the sweat glands; it consists of water containing sodium chloride and phosphate, urea, ammonia, ethereal sulphates, creatinine, fats, and other waste products.

per tu'bam [L.] Through a tube.

pertus'sis [L. *per*, very (intensive), + *tussis*, cough] Whooping cough; an acute infectious disease caused by *Bordetella pertussis*, and characterized by an inflammation of the larynx, trachea, and bronchi producing recurrent bouts of spasmodic coughing that continue until the breath is exhausted, then ending in a noisy inspiratory stridor ("whoop") caused by laryngeal spasm.

perver'sion [L. *perversio*, fr. *per-verto*, pp. *-versus*, to turn about] A deviation from a societal norm, especially concerning sexual interest or behaviour considered medically abnormal, morally wrong, or legally prohibited.

per vi'as natura'les [L.] Through the natural passages; *e.g.*, denoting a normal delivery, as opposed to caesarean section, or the passage in stool of a foreign body instead of its surgical removal.

pes, pl. **pe'des** [L.] **1.** [NA] The foot. **2.** Any footlike or basal structure or part. **3.** Talipes. In this sense, p. is qualified by a modifier expressing the specific type.

pes'sary [L. *pessarium*, fr. G. *pessos*, an oval stone used in certain games] **1.** An appliance of varied form, introduced into the vagina to support the uterus or to correct any displacement. **2.** A medicated vaginal suppository.

pes'ticide An agent that destroys fungi, insects, rodents, or any other pest.

pes'tilence [L. *pestilentia*] An epidemic of any infectious disease.

pete'chiae, sing. **pete'chia** [Mod. L. form of It. *petecchie*] Minute haemorrhagic spots in the skin.

petit mal Absence.

pétrissage' [Fr. kneading] A manipulation in massage, consisting in a kneading of the muscles.

petro- [L. *petra*, rock; G. *petros*, stone] Combining form denoting stone, stone-like hardness.

petrola'tum Petroleum jelly; a mixture of the softer members of the paraffin or methane series of hydrocarbons, obtained from petroleum as an intermediate product in its distillation; used as a soothing application to burns and abrasions of the skin, and as a base for ointments.

petro'leum benzine Benzin; benzine; naphtha; purified low boiling fractions distilled from petroleum consisting of hydrocarbons, chiefly of the methane series; highly flammable, and its vapours, when mixed with air and ignited, may explode; used as a solvent.

petro'sa, pl. **petro'sae** [L. fr. *petra,* rock] The petrous portion of the temporal bone.

petro'sal Relating to the petrosa.

petrosi'tis Inflammation involving the petrous portion of the temporal bone and its air cells.

pet'rous [L. *petrosus,* fr. *petra,* a rock] **1.** Of stony hardness. **2.** Petrosal.

-pexy [G. *pēxis,* fixation] Suffix meaning fixation, usually surgical.

phaco- [G. *phakos,* lentil (lens), anything shaped like a lentil] Combining form usually meaning lens-shaped, or relating to a lens.

phac'oanaphylax'is Hypersensitiveness to protein of the lens.

phac'oemulsifica'tion A method of emulsifying and aspirating a cataract with the use of a low-frequency ultrasonic needle.

phaoo'ma [phaco- + G. *-oma,* tumour] A hamartoma found in phacomatosis.

phacomato'sis [Van der Hoeve's coinage fr. G. *phakos,* mother-spot] A group of hereditary diseases characterized by hamartomas involving multiple tissues: Lindau's disease, neurofibromatosis, Sturge-Weber syndrome, tuberous sclerosis.

phaeo- [G. *phaios,* dusky] Combining form meaning dusky, grey, or dun.

phae'ochromocyto'ma A functional chromaffinoma, usually benign, derived from cells in the adrenal medullary tissue and characterized by the secretion of catecholamines, resulting in hypertension which may be paroxysmal.

phage Bacteriophage.

-phage, -phagia, -phagy [G. *phagein,* to eat] Suffixes meaning eating or devouring.

phagedae'na [G *phagedaina,* a canker] An ulcer that rapidly spreads peripherally, destroying the tissues as it increases in size.

phago- [G. *phagein,* to eat] Prefix denoting eating, devouring.

phag'ocyte [phago- + G. *kytos,* cell] A cell possessing the property of ingesting bacteria, foreign particles, and other cells; divided into two general classes: microphages and macrophages.

phagocyt'ic Relating to phagocytes or phagocytosis.

phagocyto'sis [phagocyte + G. *-osis,* condition] The process of ingestion and di-

gestion by phagocytes of solid substances, such as other cells, bacteria, bits of necrosed tissue, foreign particles.

phako- See phaco-.

phako'ma Phacoma.

phalan'geal Relating to a phalanx.

phal'anx, pl. **phalan'ges** [L. fr. G. *phalanx* (*-ang-*), line of soldiers] [NA] One of the long bones of the fingers or toes, 14 in number for each hand or foot, two for the thumb or great toe, and three each for the other four digits; designated as proximal, middle, and distal, beginning from the metacarpus.

phall-, phalli-, phallo- [G. *phallos,* penis] Combining forms denoting the penis.

phal'lic [G. *phallos,* penis] Relating to or resembling the penis.

phal'loplasty [phallo- + G. *plassō,* to form] Reparative or plastic surgery of the penis.

phal'lus, pl. **phal'li** [L., G. *phallos*] Penis.

phan'tasm [G. *phantasma,* an appearance] The mental imagery produced by fantasy.

phan'tom [G. *phantasma,* an appearance] **1.** Phantasm. **2.** A model, especially a transparent one, of the human body or any of its parts.

pharmaceu'tic, pharmaceu'tical [G. *pharmakeutikos,* relating to drugs] Relating to pharmacy or to pharmaceutics.

pharmaceutics 1. Pharmacy. **2.** The science of pharmaceutical systems, *i.e.,* preparations, dosage forms, etc.

phar'macist [G. *pharmakon,* a drug] Chemist (2).

pharmaco- [G. *pharmakon,* drug, medicine] Combining form relating to drugs.

phar'macodynam'ics [pharmaco- + G. *dynamis,* force] The study of the actions of drugs on the living organism.

phar'macogenet'ics The study of genetically determined variations in responses to drugs.

phar'macokinet'ics [pharmaco- + G. *kinēsis,* movement] Movements of drugs within biological systems, as affected by uptake, distribution, elimination, and biotransformation.

pharmacol'ogy [pharmaco- + G. *logos,* study] The science concerned with drugs, their sources, appearance, chemistry, actions, and uses.

phar'macopoe'ia, [G. *pharmakopoiia,* fr. *pharmakon,* a medicine, + *poieo,* to make] A work containing monographs of therapeutic agents, standards for their strength and purity, and directions for making preparations.

pharmacopoe'ial Relating to a pharmacopoeia; denoting a drug in the list of a pharmacopoeia.

phar'macother'apy [pharmaco- + G. *therapeia,* therapy] Treatment of disease by means of drugs. See also chemotherapy.

phar'macy [G. *pharmakon,* drug] **1.** The practice of preparing and dispensing drugs. **2.** A place where drugs are prepared and dispensed.

pharyn'geal [Mod. L. *pharyngeus*] Relating to the pharynx.

pharyngec'tomy [pharyng- + G. *ektome,* excision] Excision of a part of the pharynx.

pharynges Plural of pharynx.

pharyngi'tis [pharyng- + G. *-itis,* inflammation] Inflammation of the mucous membrane and underlying parts of the pharynx.

pharyngo-, pharyng- [Mod. L. fr. G. *pharynx*] Combining forms denoting the pharynx.

pharyn'golaryng'eal Relating to both the pharynx and the larynx.

pharyn'golaryngi'tis Inflammation of both the pharynx and the larynx.

pharyn'goplasty [pharyngo- + G. *plasso,* to form] Plastic surgery of the pharynx.

pharyngot'omy [pharyngo- + G. *tome,* incision] Any cutting operation upon the pharynx either from without or from within.

phar'ynx, pl. **pharyn'ges** [Mod. L. fr. G. *pharynx* (pharyng-), the throat, the joint opening of the gullet and windpipe] [NA] The upper expanded portion of the digestive tube, between the oesophagus below and the mouth and nasal cavities above and in front.

phen-, pheno- [fr. G. *phaino,* to appear, show forth] Combining form denoting appearance; in chemistry, derivation from benzene.

phe'nobarbitone A long-acting oral or parenteral sedative and hypnotic.

phe'nol Carbolic acid; an antiseptic and disinfectant; locally and internally escharotic in concentrated form, and neurolytic in 3 to 4% solutions.

phenolphtha'lein A substance used as a hydrogen ion indicator and as a laxative.

phenom'enon, pl. **phenom'ena** [G. *phainomenon,* fr. *phaino,* to cause to appear] **1.** A symptom; an occurrence of any sort, whether ordinary or extraordinary, in relation to a disease. See also reaction; sign. **2.** Any unusual fact or occurrence.

    déjà vu p., the mental impression that a new experience (*e.g.,* a sight, sound, or action) has happened before; a common p. in normal persons that may occur more frequently or continuously in certain emotional or organic disorders.

    Raynaud's p., spasm of the digital arteries with blanching and numbness of the fingers.

phe'nothi'azine The parent compound for synthesis of a large number of antipsychotic compounds, such as chlorpromazine.

phe'notype [G. *phaino,* to display, show forth, + *typos,* model] In genetics, a category or group to which an individual may be assigned on the basis of one or more characteristics observable clinically or by laboratory means that reflect genetic variation or gene-environment interaction; may include more than one genotype.

phenox'yben'zamine hydrochloride An adrenergic (α-receptor) blocking agent that selectively blocks the excitatory response of smooth muscle and exocrine glands to adrenaline.

phenyl (Ph) The univalent radical, C_6H_5-, of phenol.

phenylal'anine (Phe) One of the common amino acids in proteins.

phenylalanine 4-monooxygenase An enzyme that catalyses the oxidation of phenylalanine to tyrosine.

phe'nylketonu'ria (PKU) [phenyl + ketone + G. *ouron,* urine] Congenital deficiency of phenylalanine 4-monooxygenase causing inadequate formation of tyrosine, elevation of serum phenylalanine, urinary excretion of phenylpyruvic acid, and accumulation of phenylalanine and its metabolites; produces brain damage resulting in severe mental retardation, often with seizures, other neurologic abnormalities such as retarded myelination, and deficient melanin formation that predisposes to eczema; autosomal recessive inheritance.

phere'sis A procedure in which blood is removed from a donor, separated, and a portion retained, with the remainder returned to the donor.

-phil, -phile, -philic, -philia [G. *philos*, fond, loving, *phileō*, to love] Suffix denoting affinity or craving for.

phil'trum, pl. **phil'tra** [L. from G. *philtron*, depression on upper lip, fr. *phileo*, to love] [NA] The infranasal depression; the indentation in the midline of the upper lip.

phimo'sis, pl. **phimo'ses** [G. a muzzling, fr. *phimos*, a muzzle] Narrowness of the opening of the prepuce, preventing its being drawn back over the glans.

phlebecta'sia [phlebo- + G. *ektasis*, a stretching] Vasodilation of the veins.

phlebec'tomy [phlebo- + G. *ektomē*, excision] Excision of a segment of a vein.

phlebi'tis [phlebo + G. *itis*, inflammation] Inflammation of a vein.

phlebo-, phleb- [G. *phleps*, vein] Combining forms denoting vein.

phleb'ogram [phlebo- + G. *gramma*, something written] A tracing of the jugular venous pulse.

phlebog'raphy [phlebo- + G. *graphē*, a writing] **1.** The recording of the venous pulse. **2.** Venography.

phleb'olith [phlebo- + G. *lithos*, stone] A calcareous deposit in a venous wall or thrombus.

Phlebot'omus [phlebo- + G. *tomos*, cutting] A genus of very small midges or blood-sucking sand flies (family Psychodidae), various species of which are vectors of kala azar, cutaneous leishmaniasis, and phlebotomus fever.

phlebot'omy [phlebo- + G. *tomē*, incision] Incision into a vein for the purpose of drawing blood.

phlegm [G. *phlegma*, inflammation] **1.** Mucus. **2.** One of the four humours of the body, according to the ancients.

phlegma'sia [G. fr. *phlegma*, inflammation] Inflammation, especially when acute and severe.

   p. al'ba do'lens, milk leg; an extreme oedematous swelling of the leg following childbirth, due to thrombosis of the veins that drain the part.

phlegmat'ic [G. *phlegmatikos*, relating to phlegm] Relating to the heavy one of the four

humours (phlegm), and therefore of a calm, apathetic, unexcitable temperament.

phlycte'na, pl. **phlycte'nae** [G. *phlyktaina*, a blister made by a burn] A small vesicle, especially one of a number of small blisters following a first degree burn.

phlycten'ula, pl. **phlycten'ulae** [Mod. L. dim. of G. *phlyktaina*, blister] A small red nodule of lymphoid cells, with ulcerated apex, occurring in the conjunctiva.

phlyc'tenule Phlyctenula.

pho'bia [G. *phobos*, fear] Any objectively unfounded morbid dread or fear; used as a termination in many terms expressing the object that inspires the fear, *e.g.*, agoraphobia.

pho'bic Pertaining to or characterized by phobia.

phocome'lia [G. *phokē*, a seal, + *melos*, extremity] Defective development of arms or legs, or both, so that the hands and feet are attached close to the body, resembling the flippers of a seal.

phona'tion [G. *phōnē*, voice] The utterance of sounds by means of vocal cords.

phono-, phon- [G. *phōnē*, sound, voice] Combining forms denoting sound, speech, or voice sounds.

phonocar'diogram A record of the heart sounds made by means of phonocardiograph.

phonocard'iograph An instrument for graphically recording the heart sounds, which are displayed on an oscilloscope or tracing.

phonocardiog'raphy [phono- + G. *kardia*, heart, | *graphō*, to record] **1.** Recording of the heart sounds with a phonocardiograph. **2.** The science of interpreting phonocardiograms.

pho'nocath'eter A cardiac catheter with diminutive microphone housed in its tip, for recording sounds and murmurs from within the heart and great vessels.

phos- [G. *phōs*, light] Combined form denoting light.

phosph-, phospho-, phosphor-, phosphoro- Prefixes indicating presence of phosphorus in a compound. See also phospho- (2).

phosphatae'mia [phosphate + G. *haima*, blood] An abnormally high concentration of inorganic phosphates in the blood.

phos'phatase Any of a group of enzymes that liberate inorganic phosphate from phosphoric esters.

phos'phate A salt or ester of phosphoric acid.

phosphatu'ria [phosphate + G. *ouron*, urine] Excessive excretion of phosphates in the urine.

phos'phene [G. *phōs*, light, + *phainō*, to show] Sensation of light produced by mechanical or electrical stimulation of the peripheral or central optic pathway of the nervous system.

phosphocre'atine A compound of creatine (through its NH₂ group) with phosphoric acid; a source of energy in the contraction of vertebrate muscle, its breakdown furnishing phosphate for the resynthesis of ATP from ADP by creating kinase.

phospholip'id A lipid containing phosphorus, thus including the lecithins and sphingomyelin.

pho'sphonecro'sis [phosphorus + G. *nekrōsis*, death] Necrosis of the osseous tissue of the jaw, as a result of poisoning with phosphorus.

phosphor-, phosphoro- See phosph-.

phospho'ric acid A solvent, dilute solutions of which have been used as urinary acidifiers and to remove necrotic debris.

phos'phorism Chronic poisoning with phosphorus.

phos'phorus [G. *phosphoros*, fr. *phōs*, light, + *phoros*, bearing] A nonmetallic chemical element, symbol P, atomic no. 15, atomic weight 30.975, occurring as the phosphate in essentially every living cell; its elemental form is extremely poisonous, causing intense inflammation, fatty degeneration, and necrosis of the jaw (phossy jaw).

photal'gia [photo- + G. *algos*, pain] Pain caused by light, an extreme degree of photophobia.

phot'ic Relating to light.

photo-, phot- [G. *phōs* (*phōt-*), light] Combining forms relating to light.

pho'tocoagula'tion [photo- + L. *coagulo*, pp. -*atus*, to curdle] Direction of an intense light beam to a desired area of the ocular fundus to produce localized coagulation by absorption of light energy and its conversion to heat; used for retinal detachment, peripheral degeneration, neovascularization, and angiomas.

pho'todermati'tis [photo- + G. *derma*, skin, + -*itis*, inflammation] Dermatitis caused or elicited by exposure to ultraviolet light.

photodyn'ia [photo- + G. *odynē*, pain] Photalgia.

pho'toinactiva'tion Inactivation by light; *e.g.*, as in the treatment of herpes simplex by local application of a photoactive dye followed by exposure to a fluorescent lamp.

photopho'bia [photo- + G. *phobos*, fear] **1.** Abnormal sensitiveness to light, especially of the eyes. **2.** Morbid dread and avoidance of light.

photopho'bic Relating to photophobia.

photophthal'mia [photo- + G. *ophthalmos*, eye] The inflammatory reaction caused by short-waved light on the external parts of the eye, as in snow blindness.

photop'sia [photo- + G. *opsis*, vision] A subjective sensation of lights, sparks, or colours due to retinal or cerebral disease.

photop'sin The protein moiety (opsin) of the pigment (iodopsin) in the cones of the retina.

photorecep'tor [photo- + L. *re-cipio*, pp. -*ceptus*, to receive] A receptor that is sensitive to light, *e.g.*, a retinal rod or cone.

pho'toradia'tion Therapeutic exposure to visible light; in cancer therapy, combined with intravenous injection of a photosensitizing agent and for deep-seated tumours by a fibre-optic system.

pho'toretinop'athy [photo- + retina, + G. *pathos*, suffering] A macular burn from excessive exposure to sunlight or other intense light, characterized subjectively by reduced visual acuity.

pho'tosensitiza'tion Sensitization of the skin to light, usually due to the action of certain drugs.

phototker'apy Treatment of disease by means of light rays.

phren'emphrax'is [phren- + G. *emphraxis*, a stoppage] Phreniclasia.

-phrenia [G. *phrēn*, the diaphragm, mind, heart (as seat of emotions)] Suffix denoting the diaphragm or the mind.

phren'ic **1.** Relating to the diaphragm. **2.** Relating to the mind.

phrenicec'tomy [phreni- + G. *ektomē*, excision] Exsection of a portion of the phrenic nerve, to prevent reunion such as may follow phrenicotomy.

phrenicla'sia [phreni- + G. *klasis*, a breaking away] Crushing of a section of the phrenic nerve as a substitute for phrenicotomy.

phrenicot'omy [phrenico- + G. *tomē*, incision] Sectioning of the phrenic nerve.

phreno-, phren-, phreni-, phrenico- [G. *phrēn*, diaphragm, mind, heart (as seat of emotions)] Combining forms denoting diaphragm, mind, or phrenic.

phrenople'gia [phreno- + G. *plēgē*, stroke] **1.** A psychosis of sudden onset. **2.** Paralysis of the diaphragm.

phthiri'asis [G. *phtheiriasis*, fr. *phtheir*, a louse] Infestation with the pubic or crab louse, *Pthirus pubis*.

Phthi'rus [L. *phthir*; G. *phtheir*, a louse] See *Pthirus*.

phthi'sis [G. a wasting] Obsolete term for: **(1)** a wasting or atrophy, local or general, and **(2)** consumption or, specifically, tuberculosis of the lungs.

phylax'is [G. a guarding, protection] Protection against infection.

phylo- [G. *phylon*, tribe] Combining form denoting tribe, race, or phylum.

phylogen'esis [phylo- + G. *genesis*, origin] The evolutionary development of any plant or animal species; ancestral history of the individual as opposed to ontogenesis, development of the individual.

phylog'eny Phylogenesis.

phy'lum, pl **phy'la** [Mod L fr G *phylon*, tribe] The taxanomic division below kingdom and above class.

physiat'rics [G. *physis*, nature, + *iatrikos*, healing] Physical *therapy*.

physi'atrist A physician who specializes in physical medicine.

physi'cian [Fr. *physicien*, a natural philosopher] A licensed practitioner of medicine; a doctor.

physio-, physi- [G. *physis*, nature] Combining forms denoting physical (physiologic) or natural (relating to physics).

physiolog'ic, physiolog'ical **1.** Relating to physiology. **2.** Normal as opposed to pathologic; denoting the various vital processes. **3.** Denoting the action of a drug when given to a healthy person, as distinguished from its therapeutic action.

physiol'ogy [L. or G. *physiologia*, fr. G. *physis*, nature, + *logos*, study] The science concerned with the normal vital processes of organisms.

physiother'apy [physio- + G. *therapeia*, treatment] Physical *therapy*.

physique' [Fr.] The physical or bodily structure; the "build."

physo- [G. *physao*, to inflate, distend] Combining form denoting **(1)** tendency to swell or inflate; **(2)** relation to air or gas.

phy'socele [physo- + G. *kelē*, tumour, hernia] **1.** A circumscribed swelling due to the presence of gas. **2.** A hernial sac distended with gas.

phyto-, phyt- [G. *phyton*, a plant] Combining form denoting plants

phytobe'zoar [phyto- + bezoar] A gastric concretion formed of vegetable fibres, with the seeds and skins of fruits, and sometimes starch granules and fat globules.

phytotox'in [phyto- + G. *toxikon*, poison] Any toxin elaborated by plants.

pi'a-arachni'tis Leptomeningitis.

pi'a ma'ter [L. tender, affectionate mother] A delicate vasculated fibrous membrane firmly adherent to the glial capsule of the brain and spinal cord; it and the arachnoid are collectively called leptomeninges.

pi'ca [L. *pica*, magpie] A depraved or perverted appetite; a hunger for substances not fit for food.

Picornavi'ridae [It. *piccolo*, very small, + RNA + -*viridae*] A family of very small nonenveloped viruses having a core of single-stranded RNA; includes the polioviruses, coxsackieviruses, and echoviruses.

picor'navirus A virus of the family Picornaviridae.

pie'dra [Sp. a stone] A fungus disease of hair characterized by the presence of numerous small black or white nodular masses.

pig'ment [L. *pigmentum*, paint] **1.** Any colouring matter, as that of the skin, hair, iris, etc., or the stains used in histologic or bacteriologic work, or that in paints. **2.** A medicinal preparation for external use, applied to the skin like paint.

   bile p.'s, colouring matter in the bile derived from porphyrins by rupture of a methane bridge; *e.g.*, bilirubin, biliverdin.

   respiratory p.'s, the oxygen-carrying (coloured) substances in blood and tissues; *e.g.*, haemoglobin, myoglobin.

visual p.'s, the photopigments in the retinal cones (photopsins) and rods (scotopsins) that absorb light and by photochemical processes initiate the phenomenon of vision.

pigmenta'tion Coloration, either normal or pathologic, of the skin or tissues resulting from a deposit of pigment.

pi'lar, pil'ary [L. *pilus,* a hair] Hairy; relating to pili.

pile [L. *pila,* ball] An individual haemorrhoidal tumour. See haemorrhoids.

piles [L. *pila,* a ball] Haemorrhoids.

pi'li [L.] [NA] Plural of pilus.

pill [L. *pilula;* dim of *pila,* ball] A small globular mass of some coherent but soluble substance, containing a medicinal substance to be swallowed.

pill'-rolling A circular movement of the opposed tips of the thumb and the index finger appearing as a form of tremor in paralysis agitans.

pilo- [L. *pilus,* hair] Combining form relating to hair.

pi'lomo'tor [pilo- + L. *motor,* mover] Moving the hair; denoting the arrectores pilorum muscles of the skin and the postganglionic sympathetic nerve fibres innervating them.

piloni'dal [pilo- + L. *nidus,* nest] Denoting a growth of hair in a dermoid cyst or in the deeper layers of the skin.

piloseba'ceous [pilo- + L. *sebum,* suet] Relating to the hair follicles and sebaceous glands.

pi'lus, pl. **pi'li** [L.] **1** [NA] Hair; one of the fine filamentous epidermal growths covering the body, except the palms, soles, and flexor surfaces of the joints, and composed of a bulbous root and cylindrical shaft slanting toward the follicular opening of invaginated epidermis at the skin surface. **2.** A fine filamentous appendage, somewhat analogous to the flagellum, that occurs on some bacteria.

pim'ple A papule or small pustule; usually meant to denote a lesion of acne.

pin'eal [L. *pineus,* relating to the pine, pinus] **1.** Shaped like a pine cone. **2.** Pertaining to the corpus pineale.

pinguec'ula, pinguic'ula [L. *pinguiculus,* fattish] A yellowish spot sometimes observed on either side of the cornea in the aged; a connective tissue thickening of the conjunctiva.

pink'eye Acute contagious or acute epidemic conjunctivitis.

pin'na, pl. **pin'nae** [L. *pinna* or *penna,* a feather; pl., a wing] **1.** Auricula. **2.** A feather, wing, or fin.

pi'nocyto'sis [pinocyte + G. *-osis,* condition] The cellular process of actively engulfing liquid, a phenomenon in which minute incuppings or invaginations are formed in the surface of the cell membrane and close to form fluid-filled vesicles; resembles phagocytosis.

pin'ta [Sp. spot, blemish] A disease caused by a spirochaete, endemic in Mexico and Central America, and characterized by an eruption of patches of varying colour that finally become white.

pin'worm A member of the genus *Enterobius* or related genera of nematodes in the family Oxyuridae, abundant in a large variety of vertebrates, including *Enterobius vermicularis* (the human p.).

piper'azine Formerly used in gout, based upon its property of dissolving uric acid *in vitro;* its compounds are now used as anthelmintics in oxyuriasis and ascariasis.

pir'iform [L. *pirum,* pear, + *forma,* form] Pear-shaped.

pi'siform [L. *pisum,* pea, + *forma,* appearance] Pea-shaped or pea-sized.

pit [L. *puteus*] **1.** Any natural depression on the surface of the body, such as the axilla. **2.** One of the pinhead-sized depressed scars following the pustule of acne, chickenpox, or smallpox (pockmark). **3.** A sharp-pointed depression in the enamel surface of a tooth, due to faulty or incomplete calcification or formed by the confluent point of two or more lobes of enamel. **4.** To become indented, said of the oedematous tissues when pressure is made with the fingertip.

pitu'itarism Pituitary dysfunction.

pitu'itary Relating to the pituitary gland (hypophysis).

pityri'asis [G. fr. *pityron,* bran, dandruff] A dermatosis marked by branny desquamation.

   p. al'ba, seborrhoeic *dermatitis.*

   p. ro'sea, a self-limited eruption of macules or papules involving principally the trunk and extremities; lesions are usually oval and follow the lines of cleavage of the skin.

Pityros'porum [G. *pityron,* bran, + *sporos,* seed] A genus of nonpathogenic fungi found in dandruff and seborrhoeic dermatitis.

place'bo [L. I will please, future of *placeo*]
1. An indifferent substance, in the form of a
medicine, given for the suggestive effect. **2.**
An inert compound, identical in appearance
with material being tested in experimental research, where the patient and the physician
may or may not know which is which.

placen'ta [L. a cake] [NA] The organ of
metabolic interchange between fetus and
mother, composed of a portion of embryonic
origin, derived from the outermost embryonic
membrane (chorion frondosum) and a maternal portion formed by a modification of the
part of the uterine mucosa (decidua basalis)
in which the chorionic vesicle is implanted.
There is no direct mixing of fetal and maternal
blood, but the intervening placental membrane is sufficiently thin to permit the absorption of nutritive materials, oxygen, and some
harmful substances, like viruses, into the fetal
blood and the release of carbon dioxide and
nitrogenous waste from it.

   p. pre'via, the condition in which the p. is
implanted in the lower segment of the uterus,
extending to the margin of the internal os of
the cervix or partially or completely obstructing the os.

placen'tal Relating to the placenta.

plagio- [G. *plagios*, oblique] Combining
form denoting oblique, slanting.

plagiocephal'ic Relating to or marked by
plagiocephaly.

plagioceph'aly [G. *plagios*, oblique, +
kephalē, head] An asymmetric craniosteno-
sis due to premature closure of the lambdoid
and coronal sutures on one side; characterized by an oblique deformity of the skull.

plague [L. *plaga*, a stroke, injury] **1.** Any
disease of wide prevalence or of excessive
mortality. **2.** Pest; an acute infectious disease
caused by *Pastuerella pestis* and marked clinically by high fever, toxaemia, prostration, a
petechial eruption, lymph node enlargement,
and pneumonia, or haemorrhage from the
mucous membranes; primarily a disease of
rodents and is transmitted to man by fleas that
have bitten infected animals.

   bubonic p., the usual form of p. marked
by inflammatory enlargement of the lymphatic glands in the groins, axillae, or other
parts.

   pneumonic p., a frequently fatal form
in which there are areas of pulmonary consol-

idation, with chill, pain in the side, bloody
expectoration, and high fever.

pla'na [L.] Plural of planum.

plane [L. *planus*, flat] **1.** A flat surface. **2.** An
imaginary surface formed by extension
through any axis or two definite points in
reference especially to craniometry and to
pelvimetry.

   coronal p., frontal p., a vertical p. at
right angles to a sagittal p., dividing the body
into anterior and posterior portions.

   horizontal p., transverse p., a p.
across the body at right angles to the coronal
and sagittal p.'s.

   median p., midsagittal p., a vertical p. through the midline of the body that
divides the body into right and left halves.

   sagittal p., the anteroposterior median
p., or any p. parallel to it.

plano-, plan-, plani- **1.** [l. *planum*,
plane; *planus*, flat] Combining forms relating
to a plane, or meaning flat or level. **2.** [G.
planos, roaming, wandering] Combining form
meaning wandering.

planog'raphy Tomography.

pla'noval'gus [plano- + L. *valgus*,
turned outward] A condition in which the longitudinal arch of the foot is flattened and
everted.

plan'ta, gen. and pl. **plan'tae** [L.] [NA] The
sole of the foot.

plan'tar [L. *plantaris*] Relating to the sole of
the foot.

plaque [Fr. a plate] **1.** Platelet. **2.** A patch or
small differentiated area on a surface. **3.** A
sharply defined zone of demyelination characteristic of multiple sclerosis.

   dental p., the noncalcified accumulation
of oral microorganisms and their products
that adheres to the teeth.

-plasia [G. *plassō*, to form] Suffix meaning
formation.

**plasma-, plasmat-, plasmato-,
plasmo-** [G. *plasma*, something formed]
Combining forms denoting plasma.

plas'ma [G. something formed] **1.** Blood p.;
the fluid (noncellular) portion of the circulating blood, distinguished from the serum obtained after coagulation. **2.** The fluid portion of
the lymph.

plas'macyte Plasma cell.

plas'macyto'ma [plasmacyte + G.
-oma, tumour] A discrete, presumably solitary mass of neoplastic plasma cells in bone

or in one of various extramedullary sites; probably the initial phase of developing plasma cell myeloma.

plas'maphere'sis [plasma + G. *aphairesis*, a withdrawal] Removal of whole blood from the body, separation of its cellular elements by centrifugation, and reinfusion of them suspended in saline or some other plasma substitute, thus depleting the body's own plasma protein without depleting its cells.

plasmat'ic, plas'mic Relating to plasma.

plas'min An enzyme hydrolysing peptides and esters of arginine and histidine, and converting fibrin to soluble products; occurs in plasma as plasminogen and is activated to plasmin by organic solvents.

plasmin'ogen See plasmin.

Plasmo'dium [Mid. L. from G. *plasma*, something formed, + *eidos*, appearance] A genus of the family Plasmodidae (order or suborder Haemosporidia) that are blood parasites of vertebrates; includes the causal agents of malaria in man and other animals, with an asexual cycle occurring in liver and red blood cells of vertebrates and a sexual cycle in mosquitoes.

P. falcip'arum, a species that is the causal agent of falciparum or malignant tertian malaria.

P. mala'riae, a species that is the causal agent of quartan malaria.

P. ova'le, a species that is the agent of the least common form of human malaria; resembles *P. vivax* in its earlier stages, but often modifies the cell membrane, causing it to form a fimbriated outline, and the cell often assumes an oval shape.

P. vi'vax, the species that is the most common malarial parasite of man.

plasmo'dium, pl. **plasmo'dia** [Mod. L. fr. G. *plasma*, something formed, + *eidos*, appearance] A protoplasmic mass containing several nuclei, resulting from multiplication of the nucleus without cell division.

plasmorrhex'is The splitting open of a cell from the pressure of the protoplasm.

plas'ter [L. *emplastrum*; G. *emplastron*, plaster or mould] **1.** A solid preparation which can be spread when heated, and which becomes adhesive at the temperature of the body; used to keep the edges of a wound in apposition, to protect raw surfaces, and, when

medicated, to redden or blister the skin or to apply drugs to the surface to obtain their systemic effects. **2.** See p. of Paris.

p. of Paris, exsiccated calcium sulphate from which the water of crystallization has been expelled by heat, but which, when mixed with water, will form a paste which subsequently sets; used for casts and making impressions.

plas'tic [G. *plastikos*, relating to moulding] **1.** Capable of being formed or moulded. **2.** A material that can be shaped by pressure or heat to the form of a cavity or mould.

-plasty [G. *plastos*, formed, shaped] Suffix meaning moulding or shaping or the result thereof, as of a surgical procedure.

plate [O.Fr. *plat*, a flat object] **1.** In anatomy, lamina; lamella; a thin, flat, differentiated structure. **2.** A metal bar applied to a fractured bone in order to maintain the ends in apposition. **3.** A denture. **4.** The agar layer within a Petri dish or similar vessel. **5.** To form a very thin layer of a bacterial culture by streaking it on the surface of agar to isolate individual organisms from which a colonial clone will develop.

   cutis p., dermatome (2).

   muscle p., myotome (2).

plate'let [see plate] An irregularly shaped disc found in blood, containing granules in the central part (granulomere) and, peripherally, clear protoplasm (hyalomere), but with no definite nucleus and no haemoglobin.

plateletphere'sis [platelet + G. *aphairesis*, a withdrawal] Removal of blood from a donor with replacement of all blood components except platelets.

platy- [G. *platys*, flat, broad] Combining form denoting width or flatness.

plat'ycephal'ic, platyceph'alous [platy- + G. *kephalē*, head] Having a flattened skull.

platyhel'minth [platy- + G. *helmins*, worm] Common name for any flatworm of the phylum Platyhelminthes; any cestode (tapeworm) or trematode (fluke).

Plat'yhelmin'thes [see platyhelminth] A phylum of flatworms that are bilaterally symmetric, flattened, and without a true body cavity; parasitic species of medical and veterinary importance are in the subclass Cestoda (the tapeworms) of the class Cestoidea, and in the subclass Digenea (the flukes) of the class Trematoda.

platypnoe'a [platy- + G. pnoē, a breathing] Difficulty in breathing when erect, relieved by recumbency.

platys'ma, pl. **platys'mas, platys'mata** [G. platysma, a flatplate] [NA] A muscle: origin, subcutaneous layer and fascia covering pectoralis major and deltoid at level of first or second rib; action, depresses lower lip, wrinkles skin of neck and upper chest.

-plegia [G. plēgē, stroke] Suffix denoting paralysis.

pleo- [G. plelōn, more] Combining form denoting more.

pleomorph'ism [pleo- + G. morphē, form] Polymorphism.

pless-, plessi- [G. plessō, to strike] Combining forms denoting a striking, especially percussion.

plessim'eter [G. plēssō, to strike, + metron, measure] A flexible oblong plate used in mediate percussion by being placed against the skin and struck with the plessor.

ples'sor [G. plēssō, to strike] A small hammer, usually with soft rubber head, used to tap the part directly, or with a plessimeter, in percussion of the chest or other part.

pleth'ora [G. plēthōrē, fullness] **1.** Hypervolaemia. **2.** An excess of any of the body fluids.

pletho'ric Relating to plethora.

plethys'mograph [G. plēthysmos, increase, + graphō, to write] A device for measuring and recording changes in volume of a part, organ, or whole body.

plethysmog'raphy [G. plēthysmos, increase, + graphē, a writing] Use of a plethysmograph

pleur-, pleura-, pleuro- [G. pleura, a rib, the side] Combining forms denoting rib, side, or pleura.

pleu'ra, gen. and pl. **pleu'rae** [G. pleura, a rib, pl. the side] [NA] The serous membrane enveloping the lungs (**pulmonary p.**) and lining the walls of the pleural cavity (**parietal p.**).

pleu'ral Relating to the pleura.

pleu'risy [L. pleurisis, fr. G. pleuritis] Inflammation of the pleura.

    serofibrinous p., the common form of p., characterized by a fibrinous exudate on the surface of the pleura and an extensive effusion of serous fluid into the pleural cavity.

pleurit'ic Pertaining to pleurisy.

pleurit'is [G. fr. pleura, side, + itis, inflammation] Pleurisy.

pleu'rocele [pleuro- + G. kēlē, hernia] Pneumonocele.

pleurod'esis [pleuro- + G. desis, a binding together] Surgical creation of a fibrous adhesion between the visceral and parietal layers of the pleura, thus obliterating the pleural cavity; a treatment in cases of recurrent spontaneous pneumothorax, malignant pleural effusion, and chylothorax.

pleurodyn'ia [pleuro- + G. odynē, pain] **1.** Pleuritic pain in the chest. **2.** A painful rheumatic affection of the tendinous attachments of the thoracic muscles, usually of one side only.

pleurol'ysis [pleuro- + lysis, dissolution] Surgical division of pleural adhesions.

pleu'ropericardi'tis [pleuro- + pericardium + G. -itis, inflammation] Combined inflammation of the pericardium and of the pleura.

pleuropul'monary Relating to the pleura and the lungs.

plex'iform [plexus + L. forma, form] Weblike, or resembling or forming a plexus.

plex'us, pl. **plex'uses, plex'us** [L. a braid] [NA] A network or interjoining of nerves and blood vessels or of lymphatic vessels.

    aortic p., **(1)** a p. of lymph nodes and connecting vessels lying along the lower portion of the abdominal aorta; **(2)** an autonomic p. surrounding the abdominal aorta, directly continuous with the thoracic aortic p.; **(3)** an autonomic p. surrounding the thoracic aorta and passing with it through the aortic opening in the diaphragm, to become continuous with the abdominal aortic p.

    p. autono'mici [NA], **autonomic p.'s,** p.'s of nerves in relation to blood vessels and viscera, the component fibres of which are sympathetic parasympathetic, and sensory.

    p. brachia'lis [NA], **brachial p.,** formed of the anterior branches of the fifth cervical to first thoracic nerves which converge in the posterior triangle of the neck between the scalenus anterior and medius muscles and pass down on the lateral side of the subclavian artery behind the clavicle into the axilla.

    p. celi'acus, coeliac p., [NA] solar p.; the largest of the autonomic p.'s, lying in front of the aorta at the level of origin of the coeliac artery and behind the stomach; through its connections with the other abdominal p.'s it sends branches to all the abdominal viscera.

p. choroi'deus [NA], **choroid p.,** a vascular proliferation of the cerebral ventricles that serves to regulate intraventricular pressure by secretion or absorption of cerebrospinal fluid.

p. coccyg'eus [NA], **coccygeal p.,** a small p. formed by the fifth sacral and the coccygeal nerves; gives origin to the anococcygeal nerves.

p. lymphat'icus [NA], **lymphatic p.,** a network of lymphatic capillaries, usually without valves, that opens into one or more larger lymphatic vessels.

solar p., p. celiacus.

pli'ca, pl. **pli'cae** [Mod. L. a plait or fold] [NA] An anatomical structure in which there is a folding over of the parts.

p. voca'lis [NA], vocal cord; the sharp edge of a fold of mucous membrane stretching along either wall of the larynx from the angle between the laminae of the thyroid cartilage to the vocal process of the arytenoid cartilage; vibration of the folds is used in voice production.

plica'tion [L. *plico,* to fold] An operation for reducing the size of a hollow viscus by taking folds or tucks in its walls.

plicot'omy [plica + G. *tomē,* incision] Division of the fold(s) of the tympanic membrane.

-ploid [G. *-plo-,* -fold, + *-ides,* in form; L. *-ploïdeus*] Adjectival suffix denoting multiple in form.

plug'ger An instrument used for condensing material in a cavity.

plum'bism [L. *plumbum,* lead] Lead poisoning.

pluri- [L. *plus, pluris,* more] Combining form denoting several or more. See also multi-, poly-.

plurip'otent, plu'ripoten'tial 1. Having the capacity to affect more than one organ or tissue. **2.** Not fixed as to potential development.

-pnoea [G. *pneō,* to breathe] Suffix denoting breath or respiration.

pneum-, pneuma-, pneumat-, pneumato- [G. *pneuma, pneumatos,* air, breath] Combining forms denoting presence of air or gas, the lungs, or breathing. See also pneumo-.

pneumat'ocele [G. *pneuma,* air, + *kēlē,* tumour, hernia] **1.** An emphysematous or gaseous swelling. **2.** Pneumonocele. **3.** A thin-walled cavity forming within the lung, characteristic of staphylococcus pneumonia.

pneumatu'ria [G. *pneuma,* air, + *ouron,* urine] Passage of gas or air from the urethra during or after urination.

pneumo-, pneumon-, pneumono- [G. *pneumōn, pneumonos,* lung] Combining forms denoting the lungs, air or gas, respiration, or pneumonia. See also pneum-.

pneu'moarthrog'raphy [G. *pneuma,* air, + *arthron,* joint, + *graphō,* to write] Radiographic study of a joint after injection of air.

pneumoceph'alus [G. *pneuma,* air, + *kephalē,* head] Presence of air or gas within the cranial cavity.

pneumococ'cal Pertaining to or containing the pneumococcus.

pneu'mococcosu'ria [pneumococcus + G. *ouron,* urine] Presence of pneumococci or their specific capsular substance in the urine.

pneumococ'cus, pl. **pneumococ'ci** [G. *pneumōn,* lung, + *kokkos,* berry (coccus)] *Streptococcus pneumoniae.*

pneu'moconio'sis, pl. **pneu'moconio'ses** [G. *pneumon,* lung, + *konis,* dust, + *-osis,* condition] Inflammation commonly leading to fibrosis of the lungs due to irritation caused by inhalation of dust incident to an occupation; the degree of disability depends on the particles inhaled, as well as the level of exposure to them.

pneumocra'nium [G. *pneuma,* air, + *kranion,* skull] Presence of air between the cranium and the dura mater.

Pneumocys'tis cari'nii [G. *pneuma,* air, breathing, + *kystis,* bladder, pouch] A parasite, transitional between fungi and protozoa, frequently occurring as aggregate forms within a rounded cystlike structure with a visible wall; the apparent cause of pneumocystosis.

pneu'mocystog'raphy [G. *pneuma,* air, + *kystis,* bladder, + *graphō,* to write] Radiography of the bladder following injection of air.

pneu'mocysto'sis Pneumonia resulting from infection with *Pneumocystis carinii,* particularly frequent among immunologically compromised or debilitated individuals, characterized by alveoli filled with a network of acidophilic material within which the organisms are enmeshed; throughout the alveolar walls and pulmonary sputa there is a diffuse infiltration of mononuclear inflammatory cells, chiefly plasma cells and macrophages.

pneu'moencephalog'raphy [G. pneuma, air, + enkephalos, brain, + graphō, to write] Radiographic visualization of cerebral ventricles and subarachnoid spaces by use of gas such as air.

pneumogas'tric [G. pneumōn, lung, + gastēr, stomach] Relating to the lungs and the stomach.

pneu'mogram [G. pneumōn, lung, + gramma, a drawing] 1. A record or tracing made by a pneumograph. 2. Radiograph following air injection as in encephalography.

pneu'mograph [G. pneumōn, lung, + graphō, to write] An instrument for recording the force and rapidity of the respiratory movements, usually by responding to changes in chest circumference.

pneumog'raphy [G. pneumōn, lung, + graphō, to write] Radiography of the lungs.

pneumon- See pneumo-.

pneumonec'tomy [G. pneumōn, lung, + ektomē, excision] Removal of all pulmonary lobes, in one operation, from a lung.

pneumo'nia [G. fr. pneumōn, lung, + -ia, condition] Inflammation of the lung parenchyma, excluding the bronchi, in which the affected part is consolidated, the alveolar air spaces being filled with blood cells and fibrin; distribution may be lobar, segmental, or lobular.

aspiration p., bronchopneumonia resulting from the entrance of foreign material, usually food particles or vomit into the bronchi.

bronchial p., bronchopneumonia.

double p., lobar p. involving both lungs.

lobar p., p. affecting a lobe, lobes, or part of a lobe where the consolidation is homogeneous; commonly due to infection by Streptococcus pneumoniae.

pneu'monitis [G. pneumōn, lung, + -itis, inflammation] Inflammation of the lungs.

pneumono- See pneumo-.

pneumon'ocele Protrusion of a portion of the lung through a defect in the chest wall.

pneu'mopericar'dium [G. pneuma, air, + pericardium] Presence of gas in the pericardial sac.

pneu'moperitone'um [G. pneuma, air, + peritoneum] Presence of air or gas in the peritoneal cavity as a result of disease or produced artificially for the treatment of certain conditions.

pneu'moradiog'raphy Radiographic study of a region after air has been injected into it.

pneumotho'rax [G. pneuma, air, + thorax] Presence of air or gas in the pleural cavity.

artificial p., p. produced by the injection of air or a gas into the pleural space to collapse the lung.

open p., a free communication between the atmosphere and the pleural space either via the lung or through the chest wall.

spontaneous p., p. occurring secondary to parenchymal lung disease.

pock'et [Fr. pochette] 1. A cul-de-sac or pouchlike cavity. 2. A diseased gingival attachment; a space between the inflammed gum and the surface of a tooth, limited apically by an epithelial attachment. 3. To enclose within a confined space. 4. A collection of pus in a nearly closed sac. 5. To approach the surface at a localized spot, as with the thinned out wall of an abscess which is about to rupture.

pod-, podo- [G. pous, podos, foot] Combining forms meaning foot or foot-shaped.

podag'ra [G. fr. pous, foot, + agra, a seizure] Typical gout in the great toe.

podal'gia [pod- + G. algos, pain] Pain in the foot.

podal'ic [G. pous (pod-), foot] Relating to the foot.

podarthri'tis [pod- + arthritis] Inflammation of any of the tarsal or metatarsal joints.

podi'atrist [pod- + G. iatros, physician] Chiropodist.

podi'atry [pod- + G. iatreia, medical treatment] Chiropody.

-poiesis [G. poiēsis, a making] Combining form denoting production.

poikilo- [G. poikilos, many coloured, varied] Combining form denoting irregular or varied.

poi'kilocyte [poikilo- + G. kytos, cell] A red blood cell of irregular shape.

poi'kilocythae'mia [poikilocyte + G. haima, blood] Poikilocytosis.

poi'kilocyto'sis [poikilocyte + G. -osis, condition] The presence of poikilocytes in the peripheral blood.

poikiloder'ma [poikilo- + G. derma, skin] A variegated hyperpigmentation and telangiectasia of the skin, followed by atrophy.

point [Fr.; L. punctum, fr. pungo, pp. punctus, to pierce] **1.** Punctum. **2.** A sharp end or apex. **3.** A slight projection. **4.** A stage or condition reached. **5.** To become ready to open, as an abscess or boil.

craniometric p.'s, fixed p.'s on the skull used as landmarks in craniometry.

McBurney's p., a p. between 1½ and 2 inches above the anterior superior spine of the ilium, on a straight line joining that process and the umbilicus, where pressure of the finger elicits tenderness in acute appendicitis.

pressure p., (1) any of the various locations on the body where pressure may be applied to control bleeding; **(2)** a p. of extreme sensitivity to pressure.

pointillage' [Fr. dotting, stippling] A massage manipulation with the tips of the fingers.

poi'son [Fr. from L. potio, potion, draught] Any substance (taken internally or applied externally) that is injurious to health or dangerous to life.

poi'soning 1. The administering of poison. **2.** The state of being poisoned.

bacterial food p., a term commonly used to refer to conditions limited to enteritis or gastroenteritis (excluding enteric or typhoid fevers and the dysenteries) caused by bacterial multiplication per se or a soluble exotoxin.

carbon monoxide p., intoxication caused by inhalation of carbon monoxide gas which competes favourably with oxygen for binding with haemoglobin and thus interferes with the transportation of oxygen and carbon dioxide by the blood.

lead p., intoxication by lead or any of its salts; symptoms of **acute l. p.** are usually those of acute gastroenteritis; **chronic l. p.** is manifested chiefly by anaemia, constipation, colicky abdominal pain, paralysis with wristdrop involving the extensor muscles of the forearm, bluish lead line of the gums, convulsions, and coma.

mercury p., a disease usually caused by the ingestion of mercury or mercury compounds: **acute m. p.** is associated with ulcerations of the stomach and intestine and nephrotoxic changes in the renal tubules; **chronic m. p.** may be related to metallic mercury and primarily involves the CNS, producing an intention tremor, increased tendon reflexes, and emotional instability.

poison ivy or **oak** See Rhus and Toxicodendron.

poi'sonous Toxic; pertaining to or caused by a poison.

po'lar [Mod. L. polaris, fr. polus, pole] **1.** Relating to a pole. **2.** Having poles, said of certain nerve cells having one or more processes.

polar'ity [Mod. L. polaris, polar] **1.** The property of having two opposite poles, as that possessed by a magnet, or opposite properties or characteristics. **2.** The direction or orientation of positivity relative to negativity.

polio- [G. polios, grey] Combining form denoting grey or the grey matter (substantia grisea).

po'lio Abbreviated term for poliomyelitis.

po'liodystro'phia Poliodystrophy.

p. cer'ebri progressi'va infanta'lis, Christensen-Krabbe disease; familial progressive spastic paresis of extremities with progressive mental deterioration, with development of seizures, blindness and deafness, beginning during the first year of life, and with destruction and disorganization of nerve cells of the cerebral cortex.

po'liodys'trophy [polio- + G. dys-, bad, + trophe, nourishment] Wasting of the grey matter of the nervous system.

po'lioencephali'tis [polio- + G. enkephalos, brain, + -itis, inflammation] An acute infectious inflammation of the grey matter of the brain, either of the cortex or of the central nuclei.

po'liomyeli'tis [polio- + G. myelos, marrow, + -itis, inflammation] Inflammation of the grey matter of the spinal cord.

acute anterior p., an acute infectious inflammation of the anterior cornua of the spinal cord caused by the poliomyelitis virus and marked by fever, pains, and gastroenteric disturbances, followed by flaccid paralysis of one or more muscular groups, and later by atrophy.

acute bulbar p., poliomyelitis virus infection affecting nerve cells in the medulla oblongata.

po′liomy′eloencephali′tis [polio- + G. *myelon*, marrow, + *enkephalos*, brain, + *-itis*, inflammation] Acute anterior poliomyelitis with pronounced cerebral signs.

po′liovi′rus hom′inis Poliomyelitis *virus*.

pol′itzeriza′tion Inflation of the auditory tube and middle ear with a Politzer bag.

pol′lex, pl. **pol′lices** [L.] [NA] The thumb.

pollino′sis [L. *pollen*, pollen, + G. *-osis*, condition] Hay fever excited by the pollen of various plants.

pollu′tion [L. *pollutio*, fr. *pol-luo*, pp. *-lutus*, to defile] Rendering unclean or unsuitable by contact or mixture with a dirty or toxic substance.

poly- [G. *polys*, much, many] **1.** Prefix denoting multiplicity; equivalent to *multi-*. See also pluri-. **2.** In chemistry, prefix meaning "polymer of," as in polypeptide.

polyadeni′tis Inflammation of many lymph nodes, especially with reference to the cervical group.

polyadenop′athy, polyadeno′sis A disorder affecting many lymph nodes.

polyangii′tis Inflammation of multiple blood vessels involving more than one type of vessel, *e.g.*, arteries and veins, or arterioles and capillaries.

polyarteri′tis Simultaneous inflammation of a number of arteries.

polyarthri′tis [poly- + G. *arthron*, joint, + *-itis*, inflammation] Simultaneous inflammation of several joints.

polyove′tis Composed of many cysts.

polycythae′mia [poly- + G. *kytos*, cell, + *haima*, blood] An increase above the normal in the number of red cells in the blood.

   p. ru′bra, p. ve′ra, erythraemia.

polydac′tyly, polydac′tylism [poly- + G. *daktylos*, finger] Presence of more than five digits on either hand or foot.

polydip′sia [poly- + G. *dipsa*, thirst] Frequent drinking because of extreme thirst.

pol′ygraph [poly- + G. *grapho*, to write] **1.** An instrument to obtain simultaneous tracings from several different pulsations. **2.** Lie detector; an instrument for recording physiological changes as indicators of emotional reactions, and thus whether a person is telling the truth.

pol′yhydram′nios [poly- + G. *hydor*, water, + *amnion*] An excess in the amount of amniotic fluid.

polymas′tia [poly- + G. *mastos*, breast] A condition in which, in the human, more than two breasts are present.

polyme′lia [poly- + G. *melos*, limb] Presence of supernumerary limbs or parts of limbs.

pol′ymenorrhoe′a [poly- + G. *men*, month, + *rhoia*, flow] The occurrence of menstrual cycles of greater than usual frequency.

pol′ymer [poly- + -mer] A substance of high molecular weight, made up of a chain of identical repeated "base units."

polym′eriza′tion A reaction in which a high molecular weight product is produced by successive additions to or condensations of a simpler compound.

polymor′phic [G. *polymorphos*, multiform] Occurring in more than one morphologic form.

polymor′phism Occurrence in more than one form; the existence in the same species or other natural group of more than one morphologic type.

pol′ymorphonu′clear [G. *polymorphos*, multiform, + L. *nucleus*, kernel] Having nuclei of varied forms; denoting a variety of leucocyte.

polymor′phous Polymorphic.

polymyal′gia [poly- + G. *mys*, muscle, + *algos*, pain] Pain in several muscle groups.

pol′ymyosi′tis [poly- + G. *mys*, muscle, + *-itis*, inflammation] Inflammation of a number of voluntary muscles simultaneously.

polymyx′in A mixture of antibiotic substances obtained from cultures of *Bacillus polymyxa* (*B. aerosporus*), of which there are five different types: A, B, C, D, and E, about equally effective against Gram-negative bacteria but differing in toxicity.

polyneuri′tis Simultaneous inflammation of a large number of the spinal nerves, marked by paralysis, pain, and wasting of muscles.

   acute idiopathic p., infectious p., Guillain-Barré syndrome; a neurologic syndrome, seemingly a sequela of certain virus infections, marked by paraesthesia of the limbs and muscular weakness or a flaccid paralysis; characteristic finding is increased protein in the cerebrospinal fluid without increase in cell count.

polyneurop′athy [poly- + G. *neuron*, nerve, + *pathos*, disease] A disease process involving a number of peripheral nerves.

polyo'pia [poly- + G. *ōps*, eye] Multiple vision; the perception of several images of the same object.

pol'yp [L. *polypus;* fr. G. *polys*, many, + *pous*, foot] Any mass of tissue that bulges or projects outward or upward from a surface by growing from a broad base (**sessile p.**) or a slender stalk (**pedunculated p.**).

polypec'tomy [polyp + G. *ektomē*, excision] Excision of a polyp.

polyphar'macy The mixing of many drugs in one prescription.

pol'yploidy [poly- + -ploid] The state of a cell nucleus containing three or a higher multiple of the haploid number of chromosomes.

polypo'sis [polyp + G. suffix *-osis*, condition] Presence of several polyps.

  familial or **multiple intestinal p., (1)** p. of the colon characterized by polyps only of the mucosa, with no associated lesions, which begin to form usually in late childhood, increase in numbers, and may carpet the mucosal surface; autosomal dominant inheritance; **(2)** p. of the small or large intestine as a feature of Zollinger-Ellison and other syndromes.

polypus, pl. **polypi** [L.] Polyp.

polyradic'uli'tis Inflammation of nerve roots.

polysac'charide A carbohydrate containing a large number of saccharide groups; *e.g.*, starch.

polyserosi'tis [poly- + L. *serum*, serum, + G. *-itis*, inflammation] Chronic inflammation with effusions in several serous cavities resulting in fibrous thickening of the serosa and constrictive pericarditis.

polysper'mia **1.** Polyspermy. **2.** An abnormally profuse spermatic secretion.

polysper'my The entrance of more than one spermatozoon into the ovum.

polysynap'tic Referring to neural conduction pathways formed by a chain of many synaptically connected nerve cells.

polyu'ria [poly- + G. *ouron*, urine] Excessive excretion of urine, or profuse micturition.

pom'pholyx [G. a bubble, fr. *pomphos*, a blister] Dyshidrosis.

pons, pl. **pon'tes** [L. bridge] **1.** [NA] That part of the brainstem intermediate between the medulla oblongata caudally and the mesencephalon rostrally, and composed of a ventral part and the tegmentum. **2.** Any bridgelike formation connecting two more or less disjoined parts of the same structure or organ.

pon'tile, pon'tine Relating to a pons.

pool [A.S. *pōl*] A collection of blood in any region of the body, due to a dilation and retardation of the circulation in the capillaries and veins of the part.

pop'les [L. the ham of the knee] [NA] The posterior region of the knee.

poplite'al Relating to the poples.

pore [G. *poros*, passageway] A hole, meatus, or foramen; one of the minute openings of the sweat glands of the skin.

porenceph'aly [G. *poros*, pore, + *enkephalos*, brain] The occurrence of cavities in the brain substance, communicating usually with the lateral ventricles.

por'phobilin'ogen (PBG) A porphyrin compound found in the urine in large quantities in cases of acute or congenital porphyria.

porphy'ria A disorder of prophyrin metabolism; may be a heritable disease, of which four types have been described, or may be acquired, as from the effects of certain chemical agents.

  acute intermittent p., p. caused by congenital hepatic overproduction of δ-aminolevulinic acid, with greatly increased urinary excretion of this compound and of porphobilinogen; characterized by intermittent hypertension, abdominal colic, psychosis, and neuropathy; autosomal dominant inheritance.

  congenital erythropoietic p., enhanced porphyrin formation by erythroid cells in bone marrow, leading to severe porphyrinuria, often in conjunction with haemolytic anaemia and persistent cutaneous photosensitivity; autosomal recessive inheritance.

porphy'rins Pigments widely distributed throughout nature (*e.g.*, haem, bile pigments, cytochromes), consisting of four pyrroles joined in a ring (porphin) structure; they combine with various metals (iron, copper, magnesium, etc.) to form metalloporphyrins, and with nitrogenous substances.

por'phyrinu'ria Excretion of porphyrins and related compounds in the urine.

porri'go [L. scurf, dandruff] Any disease of the scalp.

por'ta, pl. **por'tae** [L. gate] **1.** Hilum. **2.** *Foramen* interventriculare.

p. hep'atis [NA], a transverse fissure on the visceral surface of the liver between the caudate and quadrate lobes, lodging the portal vein, hepatic artery, hepatic nerve plexus, hepatic ducts, and lymphatic vessels.

portaca'val Concerning the portal vein and the inferior vena cava.

por'tal [L. *portalis*, pertaining to a porta (gate)] **1.** Relating to any porta. **2.** The point of entry into the body of a pathogenic microorganism.

porto- [L. *porta*, gate] Combining form meaning portal.

portog'raphy [porto- + G. *graphō*, to write] Radiographic delineation of the portal circulation using radiopaque material introduced into the spleen or into the portal vein.

po'rus, pl. **po'ri** [L. fr. G. *poros*, passageway] [NA] A pore, meatus, or foramen.

posi'tion [L. *positio*, a placing, position] **1.** An attitude, posture, or place occupied. **2.** In obstetrics, the relation of some arbitrarily chosen p. of the fetus to the right or left side of the mother.

flank p., a lateral recumbent p., but with the lower leg flexed, the upper leg extended, and convex extension of the upper side of the body; used for nephrectomy.

Fowler's p., an inclined p. obtained by raising the head of the bed to promote better dependent drainage after an abdominal operation.

knee-chest p., a prone posture resting on the knees and upper part of the chest, assumed for gynecologic or rectal examination.

knee-elbow p., a prone p. resting on the knees and elbows, assumed for rectal or vaginal examination or operation.

lithotomy p., a supine p. with buttocks at the end of the operating table, the hips and knees being fully flexed with feet strapped in p.

Mayo-Robson's p., a supine p. with a thick pad under the loins, causing a marked lordosis in this region; used in operations on the gallbladder.

Sims p., lateral recumbent p.; a p. to facilitate a vaginal examination; a semiprone p. with the under arm behind the back, the thighs flexed, the upper one more than the lower.

Trendelenburg p., a supine p. Inclined at an angle of 45°, so that the pelvis is higher than the head; used during and after operations in the pelvis or for shock.

pos'itive (+) [L. *positivus*, settled by arbitrary agreement] Affirmative; definite; not negative.

post- [L. *post*, after] Prefix denoting after, behind, or posterior; corresponding to *meta-*.

poste'rior [L. comparative of *posterus*, following] **1.** After, in relation to time or space. **2.** [NA] Dorsal; in human anatomy, denoting the back surface of the body or nearer the back of the body. **3.** Near the tail or caudal end of certain embryos.

postero- [L. *posterior*, q.v.] Combining form denoting posterior.

post'eroante'rior A term denoting the direction of view or progression, from posterior to anterior, through a part.

posterolat'eral Behind and to one side, specifically to the outer side.

postganglion'ic Distal to or beyond a ganglion; referring to the unmyelinated nerve fibres originating from cells in an autonomic ganglion.

posthi'tis [G. *posthē*, prepuce, + *-itis*] Inflammation of the prepuce.

posthypnot'ic Following hypnotism.

postic'tal Following a seizure.

postmature' Remaining in the uterus longer than the normal gestational period.

postmenopau'sal Relating to the period following the menopause.

postmor'tem **1.** Pertaining to or occurring during the period after death. **2.** Colloquialism for autopsy (1)

postna'sal **1.** Posterior to the nasal cavity **2.** Relating to the posterior portion of the nasal cavity.

postna'tal [L. *natus*, birth] Occurring after birth.

postop'erative Following an operation.

posto'ral [L. *os* (or-), mouth] In the posterior part of, or posterior to, the mouth.

post par'tum [L. *partus*, birth (noun), fr. *pario*, pp. *partus*, to bring forth] After childbirth; as an adjective, usually written postpartum.

postpran'dial [L. *prandium*, breakfast] Following a meal or the taking of food.

post-traumat'ic Temporally, and implied causally, related to a trauma.

pos'tural Relating to or effected by posture.

pos'ture [L. *positura*, fr. *pono*, pp. *positus*, to place] The position of the limbs or the carriage of the body as a whole.

potas'sium [Mod. L. fr. E. potash (fr. pot + ashes) + -*ium*] An alkaline metallic element, symbol K (*kalium*), atomic no 19, atomic weight 39.100, occurring always in combination; its salts are used medicinally.

po'tency [L. *potentia*, power] **1.** Power, force, or strength; the condition or quality of being potent. **2.** Specifically, **sexual p.**, the ability to carry out and consummate the sexual act; referring mainly to the male. **3.** In therapeutics, the pharmacological activity of a compound.

po'tion [L. *potio, potus*, fr. *poto*, to drink] A draught or large dose of liquid medicine.

pouch A pocket or cul-de-sac.

   Douglas p., *excavatio* rectouterina.

poul'tice [L. *puls* (*pult-*), a thick pap; G. *poltos*] A soft, moist mass prepared by wetting various powders or other absorbent substances with fluids, sometimes medicated, and usually applied hot to the surface; exerts an emollient, relaxing, stimulant, or counter-irritant effect upon the skin and underlying tissues.

pow'der [Fr. *poudre;* L. *pulvis*] **1.** A dry mass of minute separate particles. **2.** In pharmaceutics, a homogenous dispersion of finely divided, relatively dry, particulate matter consisting of one or more substances. **3.** A single dose of a powdered drug.

pox [variant of the pl. of pock] **1.** An eruptive disease, usually qualified by a descriptive term; *e.g.,* smallpox, chickenpox. **2.** An eruption, first papular then pustular, occurring in chronic antimony poisoning. **3.** Archaic term for syphilis.

Poxvi'ridae A family of large complex DNA viruses, with an affinity for skin tissue, that are pathogenic for man and other animals; replication occurs entirely in the cytoplasm of infected cells. Six genera are recognized: *Orthopoxvirus, Avipoxvirus, Capripoxvirus, Leporipoxvirus, Parapoxvirus,* and *Entomopoxvirus.*

pox'virus Any virus of the family Poxviridae.

prac'tice [Mediev. L. *practica*, business, G. *praktikos*, pertaining to action, fr. *prassō*, to do] The exercise of the profession of medicine or one of the associated health professions.

   family p., the medical specialty concerned with the delivery of comprehensive primary health care to members of the family on a continuing basis.

   general p., the provision of continuing comprehensive medical care regardless of the patient's age or of the disorder involved, even if it requires intervention by a specialist.

   group p., the p. of medicine by a group, each of whom usually confined to some special field, but shares a common facility.

practi'tioner One who practises medicine or an associated health care profession.

pre- [L. *prae*, before] Prefix denoting anterior or before in space or time. See also ante-, pro-.

precan'cer A lesion from which a malignant neoplasm is presumed to develop in a significant number of instances, and which may or may not be recognizable clinically or by microscopic changes in the affected tissue.

precan'cerous Pertaining to any lesion that is interpreted as a precancer.

precip'itant Anything causing a precipitation from a solution.

precip'itate [L. *praecipito*, pp. -*atus*, to cast headlong] **1.** To cause a substance in solution to separate as a solid. **2.** A solid separated out from a solution or suspension; a floc or clump, such as that resulting from the mixture of a specific antigen and its antibody. **3.** A punctate opacity on the posterior surface of the cornea, arising from inflammatory cells in the vitreous.

precipitin An antibody that under suitable conditions combines with and causes its specific and soluble antigen to precipitate from solution.

preclin'ical **1.** Before the onset of disease. **2.** A period in medical education before the student is involved with patients and clinical work.

preco'cious [L. *praecox*, premature] Developing unusually early.

precon'scious In psychoanalysis, one of the three divisions of the psyche according to Freud's topographical psychology; includes all ideas, thoughts, past experiences, and other memory impressions that with effort can be consciously recalled.

preconvul'sive Denoting the stage in an epileptic paroxysm preceding convulsions.

precor'dia [L. *praecordia*, the diaphragm, the entrails] The epigastrium and anterior surface of the lower part of the thorax.

precur'sor [L. *praecursor*, fr. *prae-*, pre- + *curro*, to run] Anything that precedes another or from which another is derived, applied especially to a physiologically inactive substance that is converted to an active enzyme, vitamin, hormone, etc., or to a chemical substance that is built into a larger structure in the course of synthesizing the latter.

prediabe'tes A state in which one or a few of the abnormalities typical of diabetes mellitus can be observed episodically or persistently, and are often mild in nature.

prediges'tion The artificial initiation of digestion of proteins (proteolysis) and starches (amylolysis) before they are eaten.

predisposi'tion A condition of special susceptibility to a disease.

prednis'olone A dehydrogenated analogue of cortisol with the same actions and uses as cortisol.

pred'nisone A dehydrogenated analogue of cortisone with the same actions and uses.

pre-eclamp'sia [pre- + G. *eklampsis*, a shining forth (eclampsia)] The development of hypertension with proteinuria or oedema, or both, due to pregnancy or the influence of a recent pregnancy.

pre'ganglion'ic Situated proximal to or preceding a ganglion; referring specifically to the preganglionic motor neurones of the autonomic nervous system (located in the spinal cord and brainstem) and the myelinated nerve fibres by which they are connected to the autonomic ganglia.

preg'nancy [L. *praegnans*, fr. *prae-*, before, + *gnascor*, pp. *natus*, to be born] Gestation; the state of a female after conception until the birth of the baby.

    ectopic p., extrauterine p., the development of an impregnated ovum outside the cavity of the uterus.

    false p., pseudocyesis.

preg'nant [see pregnancy] Gravid; denoting a female bearing within her the product of conception.

prehen'sile [L. *prehendo*, pp. *-hensus*, to lay hold of, seize] Adapted for taking hold of or grasping.

preic'tal [pre- + L. *ictus*, a stroke] Occurring before a convulsion or stroke.

premature' [L. *praematurus*, too early, fr. *prae-*, pre- + *maturus*, ripe (mature)] **1.** Occurring before the usual or expected time. **2.** Denoting an infant born after less than 37 weeks of gestation, birth weight no longer considered a critical criterion.

premedica'tion **1.** Administration of drugs prior to anaesthesia to allay apprehension, produce sedation, and facilitate the administration of anaesthesia to the patient. **2.** Drugs used for such purposes.

premen'strual Relating to the period preceding menstruation

premo'lar **1.** Anterior to a molar tooth. **2.** A bicuspid tooth

prena'tal [pre- + L. *natus*, born, pp. of *nascor*, to be born] Antenatal; preceding birth.

preop'erative Preceding an operation.

prepubes'cent Immediately prior to the commencement of puberty.

pre'puce [L. *praeputium*, foreskin] Preputium.

prepu'tium, pl. **prepu'tia** [L. *praeputium*] [NA] Prepuce; foreskin; the free fold of skin that covers the glans penis.

presby-, **presbyo-** [G. *presbys*, old man] Combining forms denoting old age. See also gero-.

presbyacu'sis,   **presbyacu'sia** [presby- + G. *akousis*, hearing] Loss of ability to perceive or discriminate sounds as a part of the aging process.

presbyophre'nia [presbyo- + G. *phrēn*, mind] One of the mental disorders of old age marked by loss of memory, disorientation, and confabulation, but with relative integrity of judgment.

presbyo'pia (Pr) [presby- + G. *ōps*, eye] The physiologic change in accommodation power in the eyes in advancing age, said to begin when the near point has receded beyond 22cm.

presbyop'ic Relating to or suffering from presbyopia.

prescrip'tion [L. *praescriptio*; see prescribe] **1.** A written formula for the preparation and administration of any remedy. **2.** A medicinal preparation compounded according to the directions formulated in a p., said to consist of four parts: *superscription*, consisting of the word *recipe*, take, or its sign; *inscription*, or main part of the p., containing the names and amounts of the drugs ordered;

subscription, directions for mixing the ingredients and designation of the form in which the drug is to be made (usually begins with *misce*, mix, M); and *signature*, directions to the patient regarding the dose and times of taking the remedy (preceded by *signa*, designate, or S).

prese'nile Displaying presenility.

presenil'ity [pre- + L. *senilis*, old] Premature old age; the condition of one, not old in years, who displays the physical and mental characteristics of old age.

present' [L. *praesens* (-*sent*-), pres. p. of *prae-sum*, to be before, be at hand] To precede or appear, as of the part of the fetus at the os uteri that is felt by the examining finger.

presenta'tion [see present] The part of the body of the fetus which is in advance during birth; the occiput, chin, and sacrum are the determining points in vertex, face, and breech p.'s, respectively.

pres'sor [L. *premo*, pp. *pressus*, to press] Exciting to vasomotor activity; producing increased blood pressure.

pres'sure [L. *pressura*, fr. *premo*, pp. *pressus*, to press] **1.** A stress or force acting in any direction against resistance. **2** (P, frequently followed by a subscript indicating location). In physics and physiology, the force per unit area exerted by a gas or liquid against the walls of its container.

   blood p., (BP), the p. or tension of the blood within the arteries, maintained by the contraction of the left ventricle, resistance of the arterioles and capillaries, elasticity of the arterial walls, as well as viscosity and volume of the blood; always expressed as relative to the ambient atmospheric p.

   diastolic p., the lowest blood p. reached during any given ventricular cycle.

   partial p., the p. exerted by a single component of a mixture of gases, commonly expressed in mm Hg or torr; for a gas dissolved in a liquid, the partial p. is that of a gas that would be in equilibrium with the dissolved gas. Symbol: P followed by subscripts denoting location and/or chemical species.

   systolic p., the highest blood pressure reached during any given ventricular cycle.

presynap'tic Pertaining to the area on the proximal side of a synaptic cleft.

presys'tole That part of diastole immediately preceeding systole.

presystol'ic Relating to the interval immediately preceding systole.

prev'alence The number of existing cases of a disease in a given population at a specific time.

pri'apism [L. *priapus* (*q.v.*), penis] Abnormal persistent erection of the penis.

prim'aquine phosphate An antimalarial agent especially effective against *Plasmodium vivax*, terminating relapsing vivax malaria; usually administered with chloroquine.

pri'mary [L. *primarius*, fr. *primus*, first] **1.** The first or foremost, as a disease or symptoms to which others may be secondary or occur as complications. **2.** Relating to the first stage of growth or development.

primigrav'ida [L. fr. *primus*, first, + *gravida*, a pregnant woman] A woman who is pregnant for the first time.

primip'ara [L. fr. *primus*, first, + *pario*, to bring forth] A woman who has given birth for the first time to an infant or infants, alive or dead, weighing 500 g or more and having a length of gestation of at least 20 weeks.

prin'ciple [L. *principium*, a beginning, fr. *princeps*, chief] **1.** A continuously acting power or force. **2.** The essential ingredient in a drug or chemical compound.

   active p., a constituent of a drug, usually an alkaloid or glycoside, upon the presence of which the characteristic therapeutic action of the substance largely depends.

pro- [L. and G. *pro*, before] **1.** Prefix denoting before or forward. See also ante-, pre-. **2.** In chemistry, prefix indicating precursor of. See also -gen.

proaccel'erin Factor V.

pro'bang A slender flexible rod, tipped with a globular piece of sponge or some other material, used chiefly for making applications or removing obstructions in the larynx or oesophagus.

probe [L. *probo*, to test] **1.** A slender rod with a blunt bulbous tip, used for exploring an open body part. **2.** To enter and explore a body part, as with a p.

pro'caine hydrochloride A local anaesthetic used for infiltration and spinal anaesthesia.

pro'cess [L. *processus*, an advance, progress] **1.** A method or mode of action used in the attainment of a certain result. **2.** An advance or progress, as of a disease. **3.** A projection or outgrowth. See processus.

mastoid p., *prooooouo* maotoidouo.

proces'sus, pl. **proces'sus** [L. see process] [NA] A projection or outgrowth.

p. mastoi'deus [NA], the nipple-like projection of the petrous part of the temporal bone.

proctal'gia [proct- + G. *algos*, pain] Pain at the anus, or in the rectum.

procti'tis [proct- + G. *-itis*, inflammation] Inflammation of the mucous membrane of the rectum

procto-, proct- [G. *prōktos*, anus] Combining forms signifying anus or, more frequently, rectum. See also recto-.

proctec'tomy [proct- + G. *ektomē*, excision] Surgical resection of the rectum.

proc'tocele [procto- + G. *kēlē*, tumour] Prolapse or herniation of the rectum.

proctoc'lysis [procto- + G. *klysis*, a washing out] Slow continuous administration of saline solution by instillation into the rectum and sigmoid colon.

proc'tocolec'tomy [procto- + G. *kolon*, colon, + *ektomē*, excision] Surgical removal of the rectum and part or all of the colon.

proc'tocystot'omy [procto- + G. *kystis*, bladder, + *tomē*, incision] incision into the bladder from the rectum.

proctodyn'ia [procto- + G. *odynē*, pain] Proctalgia.

proctol'ogy [procto- + G. *logos*, study] The surgical specialty concerned with the anus and rectum and their diseases.

proc'topexy [procto- + G. *pēxis*, fixation] Surgical fixation of a prolapsing rectum

proctople'gia [procto- + G. *plēge*, stroke] Paralysis of the anus and rectum occurring with paraplegia.

proctor'rhaphy [procto- + G. *rhaphe*, suture] Suturing of a lacerated rectum or anus.

proc'toscope [procto- + G. *skopeō*, to view] A rectal speculum.

proctos'copy Visual examination of the rectum and anus, as with a proctoscope.

proc'tosigmoidi'tis [procto- + sigmoid + G. *-itis*, inflammation] Inflammation of the sigmoid colon and rectum.

proctos'tomy [procto- + G. *stoma*, mouth] Formation of an artificial opening into the rectum.

proctot'omy [procto- + G. *tomē*, incision] An incision into the rectum.

procum'bent [L. *procumbens*, falling or leaning forward] In a prone position; lying face down

prodro'mal Relating to a prodrome.

pro'drome [G. *prodromos*, a running before] An early or premonitory symptom of a disease.

pro'drug A class of drugs the pharmacologic action of which results from conversion by metabolic processes within the body (biotransformation).

produc'tive [see product] Producing or capable of producing; denoting especially an inflammation leading to the production of new tissue with or without an exudate.

pro'file [It. *profilo*, fr. L. *pro*, forward, + *filum*, thread, line (contour)] **1.** An outline or contour, especially one representing a side view of the human head. **2.** A summary, brief account, or record.

test p., a combination of laboratory tests usually performed by automated methods and designed to evaluate organ systems of patients upon admission to a hospital or clinic.

proge'ria [pro- + G. *gēras*, old age] Premature senility syndrome, a condition in which normal development in the first year is followed by gross retardation of growth, with a senile appearance characterized by dry wrinkled skin, total alopecia, and bird-like facies.

proges'terone A progestin, an anti-oestrogenic steroid believed to be the active principle of the corpus luteum, isolated from the corpus luteum and placenta or synthetically prepared, and used to correct abnormalities of the menstrual cycle.

proges'tin 1. A hormone of the corpus luteum. **2.** Generic term for any substance, natural or synthetic, that effects some or all of the biological changes produced by progesterone.

proges'togen 1. Any agent capable of producing biological effects similar to those of progesterone. **2.** A synthetic derivative from testosterone or progesterone that has some of the physiologic activity and pharmacologic effects of progesterone.

proglos'sis [pro- + G. *glōssa*, tongue] Tip of the tongue.

proglot'tid, pl. **proglot'tids, proglot'tides** [pro- + G. *glóssa*, tongue] One of the segments of a tapeworm, containing the reproductive organs.

prognath'ic [pro- + G. *gnathos*, jaw] **1.** Having a projecting jaw; having a gnathic index above 103. **2.** Denoting a forward projection of either or both of the jaws relative to the craniofacial skeleton.

prog'nathism The condition of being prognathic.

prognath'ous Prognathic.

progno'sis [G. *prognósis*, fr. *pro*, before, + *gignóskó*, to know] **1.** The foretelling of the probable course of a disease. **2.** A forecast of the outcome of a disease.

prognos'tic [G. *prognóstikos*] **1.** Relating to a prognosis. **2.** A symptom upon which a prognosis is based.

progres'sive [L. *pro-gredior*, pp. *-gressus*, to go forth] Going forward; advancing; denoting the course of a disease, especially, when unqualified, an unfavourable course.

projec'tion [L. *projectio*; fr. *pro-jicio*, pp. *-jectus*, to throw before] **1.** A pushing out. **2.** A prominence. **3.** The referring of a sensation to the object producing it. **4.** A defence mechanism involving the referring to another of a repressed complex in the individual, as when one reprobates in others faults to the commission of which he himself has a constant inclination. **5.** Localization of visual impressions; straight ahead, right or left, above or below. **6.** In neuroanatomy, the system or systems of nerve fibres by which a group of nerve cells discharges its nerve impulses ("projects") to one or more other cell groups.

prokar'yote [pro- + G. *karyon*, kernel, nut] A unicellular microorganism whose cell does not contain a limiting membrane around the nuclear material.

prolac'tin (PRL) A hormone of the anterior lobe of the hypophysis cerebri that stimulates the secretion of milk and possibly during pregnancy, breast growth.

pro'lapse [L. *prolapsus*, a falling] **1.** To sink down, said of an organ or other part. **2.** A sinking of an organ or other part, especially its appearance at a natural or artificial orifice.

   p. of umbilical cord, presentation of part of the umbilical cord ahead of the fetus; it may cause fetal death due to compression of the cord between the presenting part of the fetus and the maternal pelvis.

   p. of uterus, falling of the uterus resulting from laxity and atony of the muscular and fascial structures of the pelvic floor, usually resulting from injuries of childbirth or advanced age.

prolif'erate [L. *proles*, offspring, + *fero*, to bear] To grow and increase in number by means of reproduction of similar forms.

prolif'erative, prolif'erous Increasing the numbers of similar forms.

pro'line (Pro) An amino acid found in proteins.

prom'inence [L. *prominentia*] A protuberance or projection.

   laryngeal p., Adam's apple; the projection on the anterior portion of the neck formed by the thyroid cartilage of the larynx.

   thenar p., thenar (1).

promy'elocyte [pro- + G. *myelos*, marrow, + *kytos*, cell] A large uninuclear cell occurring in the circulating blood in myelocytic leukaemia.

prona'tion The condition of being prone; the act of assuming or of being placed in a prone position; *e.g.*, eversion and abduction of foot, causing a lowering of the medial edge, or rotation of the forearm in such a way that the palm of the hand faces backward when the arm is in the anatomical position, or downward when the arm is extended at a right angle to the body.

prona'tor [L.] A muscle which turns a part into the prone position.

prone [L. *pronus*, bending down or forward] Denoting the hand or foot in pronation, or the body when lying face downward.

pronu'cleus In embryology, the nuclear material of the head of the spermatozoon (**male p.**) or of the ovum (**female p.**), after the ovum has been penetrated by the spermatozoon; each carries the haploid number of chromosomes.

pro'phase [G. *prophasis*, from *prophaino*, to foreshadow] The first stage of mitosis or meiosis, consisting of linear contraction and increase in thickness of the chromosomes (each composed of two chromatids) accompanied by division of the centriole and migration of the two daughter centrioles and their asters toward the poles of the cell.

prophylac'tic [G. *prophylaktikos*; see prophylaxis] **1.** Preventing disease; relating to prophylaxis. **2.** An agent that acts as a preventive against disease.

prophylax'is, pl. **prophylax'es** [Mod.L. fr. G. *pro-phy-lasso*, to take precaution] The prevention of disease.

propri'etary name [L. *proprietarius*] The patented brand name or trademark under which a manufacturer markets his product; written with a capital initial letter and is often further distinguished by a superscript R in a circle.

propriocep'tive [L. *proprius*, one's own, + *capio*, to take] Capable of receiving stimuli originating in muscles, tendons, and other internal tissues.

propriocep'tor One of a variety of sensory end organs in muscles, tendons, and joint capsules.

propto'sis [G. *proptōsis*, a falling forward] A forward displacement of any organ, as in exophthalmos.

propul'sion [G. *pro-pello*, pp. *-pulsus*, to drive forth] The tendency to fall forward that causes the festination in paralysis agitans.

pro'pyl The radical of propyl alcohol or propane; $CH_3CH_2CH_2-$.

 p. alcohol, a solvent; more toxic than ethyl alcohol.

prosenceph'alon [G. *prosō*, forward, + *enkephalos*, brain] [NA] Forebrain; the anterior primitive cerebral vesicle, which divides in further development into diencephalon and telencephalon.

prosopo-, prosop- [G. *prosōpon*, face, countenance] Combining forms denoting the face. See also facio-.

prostaglan'din [first found in genital fluids and accessory glands] Any of a class of physiologically active substances present in many tissues; among effects are those of vasodepressors, stimulation of intestinal smooth muscle, uterine stimulation, and antagonism to hormones influencing lipid metabolism.

pros'tata [Mod. L. from G. *prostatēs*, one standing before] [NA] Prostate gland; a chestnut-shaped body that surrounds the beginning of the urethra in the male, consisting of two lateral lobes connected anteriorly by an isthmus and posteriorly by a middle lobe lying above and between the ejaculatory ducts; its secretion is a milky fluid discharged by excretory ducts into the prostatic urethra at the time of the emission of semen.

pros'tate Prostata.

prostatec'tomy [prostat- + G. *ektomē*, excision] Removal of part or all of the prostate.

prostat'ic Relating to the prostate gland.

pros'tatism A clinical syndrome caused by enlargement of the prostate gland and characterized by significant obstruction to urinary flow and often a progressive increase in urgency and urinary frequency.

prostati'tis [prostat- + G. *-itis*, inflammation] Inflammation of the prostate.

prostato-, prostat- Combining forms denoting the prostate gland

pros'tatocysti'tis [prostato- + G. *kystis*, bladder, + *-itis*, inflammation] Inflammation of the prostate and the bladder; cystitis by extension of inflammation from the prostatic urethra.

pros'tatomeg'aly [prostato- + G. *megas*, large] Enlargement of the prostate gland.

pros'tatorrhoe'a [prostato- + G. *rhoia*, a flow] An abnormal discharge of prostatic fluid.

prostatot'omy [prostato- + G. *tomē*, incision] An incision into the prostate.

pros'thesis, pl. **pros'theses** [G. an addition] A fabricated substitute for a diseased or missing part of the body, as a limb, tooth, eye, or heart valve.

 surgical p., an appliance prepared as an aid or as a part of a surgical proceeding, such as a heart valve or cranial plate.

prosthet'ic Relating to a prosthesis or to an artificial part.

prostra'tion [L. *pro-sterno*, pp. *-stratus*, to strew before, overthrow] Marked loss of strength, as in exhaustion.

prot- See (1) proteo-; (2) proto-.

pro'tamine Any of a class of proteins, highly basic because rich in arginine and simpler in constitution than the albumins and globulins, etc., found in certain fish spermatozoa in combination with nucleic acid; neutralizes anticoagulant action of heparin.

protano'pia [G. *prōtos*, first, + a- priv. + *ōps (ōp-)* eye] A form of dichromatism characterized by absence of the red-sensitive pigment in cones, decreased luminosity for long wavelengths of light, and confusion in recognition of red and bluish-green.

pro'tease Descriptive term for proteolytic enzymes, both endopeptidases and exopeptidases.

pro'tein [G. *protein*, fr. *proteios*, primary] Macromolecules consisting of long sequences of α-amino acids, generally the 20 common ones. P. is three-fourths of the dry weight of most cell matter and is involved in structures, hormones, enzymes, muscle contraction, immunological response, and other essential life functions.

Bence Jones p., p. with unusual thermosolubility found in the urine of patients with multiple myeloma and occasional persons with other diseases of the reticuloendothelial system; similar in size and physical properties to the light chains of the myeloma p. synthesized by a given patient.

pro'teinases Enzymes hydrolysing native protein, or polypeptides, making internal cleavages.

protein hydrol'ysate A sterile solution of amino acids and soft chain peptides prepared from a suitable protein by acid or enzymic hydrolysis; used intravenously for the maintenance of positive nitrogen balance in severe illness, after surgery involving the alimentary tract, in the diets of infants allergic to milk, or as a supplement when high protein intake from ordinary foods cannot be accomplished.

proteino'sis [protein + G. *-osis*, condition] A state characterized by disordered protein formation and distribution, particularly as manifested by the deposition of abnormal proteins in tissues.

proteinu'ria [protein + G. *ouron*, urine] **1.** Presence of abnormal concentrations of urinary protein. **2.** Albuminuria.

proteo-, prot-, Combining forms indicating protein.

proteol'ysis [proteo- + G. *lysis*, dissolution] Protein hydrolysis; the decomposition of protein.

pro'teolyt'ic Relating to or effecting proteolysis.

pro'teose A descriptive term for protein derivatives resulting from further cleavage of metaprotein material; a mixture of intermediate products of proteolysis between protein and peptone.

Pro'teus [*Prōteus*, G. myth. char.] **1.** A former genus of the Sarcodina, now termed *Amoeba*. **2.** A genus of motile Gram-negative bacteria (family Enterobacteriaceae) occurring primarily in faecal matter and in putrefying materials. The type species is *P. vulgaris*.

P. morgan'ii, a species found in the intestinal canal and in normal and diarrhoeal stools.

P. vulgar'is, the type species of the genus *P.*, found in putrefying materials and in abscesses; certain strains are agglutinated by typhus serum and are therefore significant in the diagnosis of typhus.

prothrom'bin Factor II; a glycoprotein formed and stored in the parenchymal cells of the liver, and present in blood in a concentration of approximately 20 mg per 100 ml; in the presence of thromboplastin and calcium ion, p. is converted to thrombin, which in turn converts fibrinogen to fibrin, this process resulting in coagulation of the blood.

prothrom'binase Factor X; an enzyme hydrolysing prothrombin to thrombin.

proto- [G. *prōtos*, first] Prefix denoting the first in a series or the highest in rank.

pro'tocol A precise and detailed plan for the study of a biomedical problem or for a regimen of therapy.

pro'toplasm [proto- + G. *plasma*, thing formed] Living matter, the substance of which animal and vegetable cells are formed.

pro'toporphyr'ia Enhanced faecal excretion of protoporphyrin.

erythropoietic p., a benign disorder of porphyrin metabolism characterized by enhanced faecal excretion of protoporphyrin and elevated quantities of protoporphyrin in red blood cells, plasma, and faeces; acute solar urticaria or more chronic solar eczema develops quickly upon exposure to sunlight; autosomal dominant inheritance with variable penetrance.

protopor'phyrin The substituted porphin that, with iron, forms the haem of haemoglobin and the prosthetic groups of myoglobin, catalase, cytochromes, etc.

pro'totype [proto- + G. *typos*, type] The primitive form; the first form to which subsequent individuals of the class or species conform.

Protozo'a [proto- + G. *zōon*, animal] A phylum (sometimes regarded as a subkingdom) of the animal kingdom, including all of the so-called unicellular forms, consisting of a single functional cell unit or of an aggregation of nondifferentiated cells, loosely held together and not forming tissues.

protozo'an **1.** A member of the Protozoa. **2.** Relating to protozoa.

protozo'on, pl. **protozo'a** Protozoan (1).

protrac'tor [L. *pro-traho,* pp. *-tractus,* to draw forth] A muscle drawing a part forward, as antagonistic to a retractor.

protru'sion [L. *protrusio*] **1.** The state of being thrust forward or projected. **2.** In dentistry, a position of the mandible forward from centric relation.

protu'berance [Mod. L. *protuberantia*] A prominence, eminence, or projection.

provit'amin A substance that may be converted into a vitamin.

    p. A, a generic name for all carotenoids exhibiting qualitatively the biological activity of β-carotene, *i.e.,* vitamin A precursors (α-, β-, and γ-carotene and cryptoxanthin); they are contained in fish liver oils, spinach, carrots, egg yolk, milk products, and other green leaf or yellow vegetables and fruits.

    p. D_2, any substance that can give rise to ergocalciferol (vitamin D_2); in nature, the chief p. is ergosterol.

prox'imal [Mod. L. *proximalis,* fr. L. *proximus,* nearest, next] **1.** Nearest the trunk or the point of origin. **2.** Mesial. **3.** In dental anatomy, denoting the surface of a tooth in relation with its neighbour, nearer to or farther from the anteroposterior median plane.

prox'imate Immediate; next; proximal.

proximo-, prox-, proxi- Combining forms denoting proximal.

pruri'go [L. itch, fr. *prurio,* to itch] A chronic disease of the skin marked by a persistent eruption of papules that itch intensely.

prurit'ic Relating to pruritus.

pruri'tus [L. an itching, fr. *prurio,* to itch] **1.** Itching. **2.** Itch (3).

prus'sic acid Hydrocyanic acid.

psammo- [G. *psammos,* sand] Combining form denoting sand.

psammo'ma [psammo- + G. *-oma,* tumour] A firm cellular neoplasm derived from fibrous tissue of the meninges, choroid plexus, and certain other structures associated with the brain, characterized by the formation of multiple, discrete, concentrically laminated, calcareous bodies (psammoma bodies).

pseudae'sthesia [pseud- + G. *aisthēsis,* sensation] **1.** A subjective sensation not arising from an external stimulus. **2.** Phantom *limb.*

pseudarthro'sis [pseud- + G. *arthrōsis,* a jointing] A new, false joint arising at the site of an ununited fracture.

pseudo-, pseud- [G. *pseudēs,* false] Prefix denoting a resemblance, often deceptive.

pseudoan'eurysm False aneurysm; a dilation of an artery with actual disruption of one or more layers of its walls, rather than with expansion of all layers of the wall.

pseudoarthro'sis Pseudarthrosis.

pseudobul'bar Denoting a supranuclear paralysis of the bulbar nerves.

pseu'docoxal'gia [pseudo- + L. *coxa,* hip, + G. *algos,* pain] Legg-Calvé-Perthes *disease.*

pse'udocye'sis [pseudo- + G. *kyēsis,* pregnancy] False pregnancy; a condition in which some of the signs and symptoms suggest pregnancy although the woman is not pregnant.

pseu'dohaematu'ria A red pigmentation of urine caused by certain foods or drugs.

pseu'dohaemophil'ia A noninherited haemophilia-like syndrome due to some specific disorder or disorders.

    hereditary p., von Willebrand's *disease.*

pseu'dohermaph'roditism A state, somewhat resembling true hermaphroditism in which the individual is distinctly of one sex, possessing either testes (**male p.**) or ovaries (**female p.**), although having somatic characteristics of both sexes.

pseu'dohypoparathy'roidism A disorder resembling hypoparathyroidism, but with signs and symptoms unresponsive to treatment with parathyroid hormone, characterized by short stature, round face, achondroplasia, calcification of basal ganglia, true ectopic bone in fascial planes and skin, mental deficiency, hypocalcaemia, hyperphosphataemia, and parathyroid tissue that is hyperplastic; most commonly inherited as a sex-linked dominant trait.

pseudoic'terus Discoloration of the skin not due to bile pigments, as in Addison's disease.

pseu'doisochromat'ic Apparently of the same colour; denoting certain charts containing coloured spots mixed with figures printed in confusion colours; used in testing for colour blindness.

pseudojaun'dice Pseudoicterus.

Pseudomo'nas [pseudo- + G. *monas*, unit, monad] A genus of motile, Gram-negative, strictly aerobic bacteria (family Pseudomonadaceae) that occur commonly in soil and in fresh water and marine environments; some species are plant pathogens, others are occasionally pathogenic to animals. The type species is *P. aeruginosa*, the causative agent of blue pus.

pseu'doparal'ysis Apparent paralysis due to voluntary inhibition of motion because of pain, incoordination, or other cause, but without actual paralysis.

 arthritic general p., A disease, occurring in arthritic subjects, having symptoms resembling those of general paresis, the lesions of which consist of diffuse changes of a degenerative and noninflammatory character due to intracranial atheroma.

pseu'doparaple'gia Apparent paralysis in the lower extremities, in which the tendon and skin reflexes and the electrical reactions are normal.

pseudopare'sis 1. Pseudoparalysis. 2. A condition marked by the pupillary changes, tremors, and speech disturbances suggestive of early paresis, in which, however, the serologic tests are negative.

pseu'dopod Pseudopodium.

pseudopo'dium, pl. **pseudopo'dia** [pseudo- + G. *pous*, foot] A temporary protoplasmic process, put forth by an amoeboid organism for locomotion or for prehension of food.

pseu'dopolyp A projecting mass of granulation tissue, large numbers of which may develop in ulcerative colitis.

pseudopreg'nancy 1. Pseudocyesis. 2. A condition in which symptoms resembling those of pregnancy are present, but which is not pregnancy, occurring after sterile copulation in mammalian species in which copulation induces ovulation.

pseu'do-pseudohy'popara-thy'roidism A heritable disorder that closely simulates pseudohypoparathyroidism; manifestations of hypoparathyroidism are mild or absent and hypocalcaemia is not present, or the consequences thereof, such as tetanic convulsions.

pseudop'sia [pseudo- + G. *opsis*, vision] Visual hallucinations, illusions, or false perceptions.

pseudoscle'ro'sis [pseudo- + G. *sklērosis*, hardening] 1. Inflammatory induration or fatty or other infiltration simulating fibrous thickening. 2. The cerebral changes of hepatolenticular degeneration.

pseudos'mia [pseudo- + G. *osmē*, smell] Subjective sensation of an odour that is not present.

pseu'dotumour 1. An enlargement of non-neoplastic character which clinically resembles a true neoplasm. 2. A circumscribed fibrous exudate of inflammatory origin and temporary character. 3. A condition, commonly associated with obesity in young females, of cerebral oedema with narrowed small ventricles but with increased intracranial pressure and frequently papilloedema.

psittaco'sis [G. *psittakos*, a parrot, + *-osis*, condition] An infectious disease of birds, especially parrots, caused by *Chlamydia psittaci* and sometimes transmitted to man, in whom the symptoms are headache, nausea, epistaxis, constipation, and fever preceded by a chill, and usually with added symptoms of bronchopneumonia.

psori'asis [G. *psōriasis*, fr. *psōra*, the itch] A condition characterized by the eruption of circumscribed, discrete and confluent, reddish, silvery-scaled maculopapules pre-eminently on the elbows, knees, scalp, and trunk.

psy'che [G. mind, soul] Obsolete term for the subjective aspects of the mind and of the individual.

psychedel'ic [psyche- + G. *dēloun*, to manifest] 1. Pertaining to a category of drugs with mainly CNS action, and with effects said to be the expansion or heightening of consciousness. 2. A drug, visual display, music, or other sensory stimulus having such action.

psychiat'ric Relating to psychiatry.

psychi'atrist A specialist in psychiatry.

psychi'atry [psych- + G. *iatreia*, medical treatment] The medical specialty concerned with mental disorders and diseases.

psycho-, psych-, psyche- [G. *psychē*, soul, mind] Combining forms denoting the mind.

psychoac'tive Possessing the ability to alter mood, anxiety, behaviour, cognitive processes, or mental tension; usually applied to pharmacologic agents.

psy'choanal'ysis [psycho- + analysis, *q.v.*] 1. A method of psychotherapy, originated by Freud, designed to bring precon-scious and unconscious material to consciousness primarily through analysis of transference and resistance. **2.** A method of investigating the human mind and psychological functioning, especially through free association and dream analysis in the psychoanalytic situation. **3.** An integrated body of observations and theories on personality development, motivation, and behaviour. **4.** An institutionalized school of psychotherapy, as in jungian or freudian p.

psychoan'alyst A psychotherapist, usually a psychiatrist, trained in psychoanalysis and employing its methods in the treatment of emotional disorders.

psy'chodrama A method of psychotherapy in which patients act out their personal problems by taking roles in spontaneous dramatic performances.

psy'chodynam'ics [psycho- + G. dynamis, force] The systematized study and theory of human behaviour, emphasizing unconscious motivation and the functional significance of emotion.

psychogen'esis [psycho- + G. genesis, origin] The origin and development of the psychic processes including mental, behavioural, personality, and related psychological processes.

psychogen'ic 1. Of mental origin or causation. **2.** Relating to psychogenesis.

psycholog'ic, psycholog'ical Relating to psychology or to the mind and its processes.

psychol'ogist A specialist in psychology licensed to practise professional psychology, or certified to teach psychology as a scholarly discipline, or whose scientific specialty is a subfield of psychology.

psychol'ogy [psycho- + G. logos, study] The profession (o.g., clinical p.), scholarly discipline (academic p.), and science (research p.) concerned with the behaviour of man and animals, and related mental and physiological processes.

   behavioural p., behaviourism.

   developmental p., the study of the psychological changes which occur with aging.

   forensic p., the application of p. to legal matters in a court of law.

   gestalt p., see gestaltism.

psychomet'rics Psychometry.

psychom'etry [psycho- + G. metron, measure] The discipline pertaining to psychological and mental testing, and to any quantitative analysis of an individual's psychological traits or attitudes or mental processes.

psychomo'tor 1. Relating to the mental origin of muscular movement, to the production of voluntary movements. **2.** Relating to the combination of psychic and motor events, including disturbances.

psychoneuro'sis [psycho- + G. neuron, nerve, | osis, condition] **1.** A mental or behavioural disorder of mild or moderate severity. **2.** Formerly a classification of neurosis including hysteria, psychasthenia, and neurasthenia.

psy'chopath An obsolete and inexact term for an individual who engages in antisocial behaviour, shows no empathy or bonding with others, and manipulates others for his own ends. See sociopath.

psychopathol'ogy [psycho- + G. pathos, disease, + logos, study] **1.** The science concerned with the pathology of the psyche or mind. **2.** The science of mental and behavioural disorders, including psychiatry and abnormal psychology.

psychop'athy [psycho- + G. pathos, disease] An obsolete and inexact term referring to a pattern of antisocial or manipulative behaviour.

psy'chopharmacol'ogy [psycho- + G. pharmakon, drug, + logos, study] **1.** The use of drugs to influence affective and emotional states. **2.** The science of drug-behaviour relationships.

psychosex'ual Pertaining to the emotional or mental components of sex.

psycho'sis, pl. **psycho'ses** [G. an animating] **1.** A mental disorder causing gross distortion or disorganization of a person's mental capacity, affective response, and capacity to recognize reality, communicate, and relate to others to the degree of interfering with the capacity to cope with the ordinary demands of everyday life; divided into two major classifications according to their origins: those associated with organic brain syndromes and functional p.'s. **2.** Generic term for any of the insanities, the most common forms being the schizophrenias. **3.** A severe emotional illness.

manic-depressive p., a major mental disorder in which there are severe changes of mood and usually a tendency to remission and recurrence. In the manic state, the patient is over-elated and hyperactive; in the depressed state, he suffers from a depressed mood, anxiety, and possible physical slowing down that can lead to stupor. In the circular form of this disorder, at least one of each type of episode occurs.

postpartum p., an acute mental disorder in the mother following childbirth.

psychoso'cial Involving both psychological and social aspects.

psychosomat'ic [psycho- + G. *soma*, body] Pertaining to the influence of the mind or higher functions of the brain upon the functions of the body, especially in relation to bodily disorders or disease.

psychosur'gery The treatment of mental disorders by operation upon the brain, *e.g.*, lobotomy.

psychother'apist A person, usually a psychiatrist or clinical psychologist, professionally trained and engaged in psychotherapy.

psychother'apy [psycho- + G. *therapeia*, treatment] Treatment of emotional, behavioural, personality, and psychiatric disorders based primarily upon verbal or nonverbal communication with the patient, in contrast to utilizing chemical and physical measures.

psychot'ic Relating to or affected by psychosis.

psychot'omimet'ic 1. A drug or substance that produces psychological and behavioural changes resembling those of psychosis. 2. Denoting such a drug or substance.

psychotro'pic [psycho- + G. *tropē*, a turning] Affecting the mind, denoting drugs used in the treatment of mental illnesses.

psychro- [G. *psychros*, cold] Combining form relating to cold. See also cryo-, crymo-.

pteryg'ium [G. *pterygion*, anything like a wing] 1. A triangular patch of hypertrophied bulbar subconjunctival tissue, extending from the medial canthus to the border of the cornea or beyond, with apex pointing toward the pupil. 2. A forward growth of the eponychium with adherence to the proximal portion of the nail. 3. An abnormal skin web, as of the neck

extending from the acromion to the mastoid, usually bilateral.

pterygo- [G. *pteryx, pterygos,* wing] Combining form denoting wing-shaped.

pter'ygoid [G. *pteryx* (*pteryg-*), wing, + *eidos*, resemblance] Wing-shaped; resembling a wing; applied to various anatomical parts in the area of the sphenoid bone.

Pthi'rus [L. *phthir*; G. *phtheir*, a louse] A genus of lice (family Pediculidae) formerly grouped in the genus *Pediculus. P. pubis* (*Pediculus pubis*), the crab or pubic louse, is a parasite that infests the pubis and neighbouring hairy parts of the body.

-ptosis [G. *ptōsis*, a falling] Suffix denoting a falling or downward displacement of an organ.

pto'sis, pl. **pto'ses** [G. *ptōsis*, a falling] A sinking down or prolapse of an organ; specifically, a drooping of the upper eyelid.

ptyal-, ptyalo- [G. *ptyalon*, saliva] Combining forms denoting saliva, or the salivary glands. See also sialo-.

pty'alagogue Sialagogue.

pu'barche The onset of puberty, particularly as manifested by the appearance of pubic hair.

pu'berty [L. *pubertas,* fr. *puber,* grown up] The sequence of events by which a child is transformed into a young adult: gametogenesis begins, as well as secretion of gonadal hormones, growth of secondary sexual characters, and development reproductive functions; sexual dimorphism is accentuated.

precocious p., a state in which pubertal changes begin at an unexpectedly early age; often the result of a pathological process involving a gland capable of secreting oestrogens or androgens.

pu'bic Relating to the os pubis.

pubiot'omy [L. *pubis*, pubic bone, + G. *tomē*, incision] Severance of the pubic bone a few centimetres lateral to the symphysis, in order to increase the capacity of a contracted pelvis sufficiently to permit the passage of a living child.

pu'bis, pl. **pu'bes** [L. *pubes*, the hair on the genitals; the genitals] 1. *Os* pubis. 2. [NA] One of the pubic hairs; the hair of the pubic region just above the external genitals. 3. [NA] *Mons* pubis.

puden'dum, pl. **puden'da** [L. ntr. of *pudendus*, fr. *pudeo*, to feel ashamed] The external genitals, especially the female genitals (vulva).

puer'peral Relating to the puerperium, or period after childbirth.

puerpe'rium, pl. **puerpe'ria** [L. childbirth, fr. *puer*, child, + *pario*, to bring forth] The period from the termination of labour to complete involution of the uterus, usually defined as 42 days.

Pu'lex [L. flea] A genus of fleas (family Pulicidae), including *P. irritans*, the common human flea that infests man and many animals.

pulie'ioide, pu'lioide [L. *pulex* (*pulic-*), flea, + *caedo*, to kill] A chemical agent destructive to fleas.

pulmo-, pulmon-, pulmono- [L. *pulmo*, lung] Combining forms denoting the lungs. See also pneum-, pneumo-

pul'mo, gen. **pulmo'nis,** pl. **pulmo'nes** [L.] [NA] Lung.

pul'monary [L. *pulmonarius*, fr. *pulmo*, lung] Relating to the lungs, to the pulmonary artery, or to the aperture leading from the right ventricle into the pulmonary artery.

pulp [L. *pulpa*, flesh] A soft, moist, coherent solid.

dental p., the soft tissue within the pulp cavity, consisting of connective tissue containing blood vessels, nerves and lymphatics, and at the periphery a layer of odontoblasts capable of internal repair of the dentine.

pulpec'tomy [L. *pulpa*, pulp, + G. *ektome*, excision] Removal of the entire pulp structure of a tooth, including that in the roots.

pulsa'tion [L. *pulsatio*, a beating] A throbbing or rhythmical beating, as of the pulse or the heart.

pulse [L. *pulsus*] The rhythmical dilation of an artery, produced by the increased volume of blood thrown into the vessel by the contraction of the heart.

alternating p., pulsus alternans.

paradoxical p., an exaggeration of the normal variation in the p. volume with respiration, becoming weaker with inspiration and stronger with expiration; characteristic of constrictive pericarditis or pericardial effusion; so called because these changes are independent of changes in p. rate.

venous p., a pulsation occurring in the veins, especially the internal jugular vein.

pul'sion [L. *pulsio*] A pushing outward or swelling.

pul'sus [L. a stroke, pulse] Pulse.

p. alter'nans, a pulse regular in time but with alternate beats stronger and weaker, often detectable only with the sphygmomanometer and usually indicating serious myocardial disease.

pump-ox'ygena'tor A mechanical device that can substitute for both the heart (pump) and the lungs (oxygenator) during open heart surgery.

punc'tate [L. *punctum*, a point] Marked with points or dots differentiated from the surrounding surface by colour, elevation, or texture.

punc'tum, pl **punc'ta** [L. a prick, point] [NA] Point. **1.** The tip of a sharp process. **2.** A minute round spot differing in colour or otherwise in appearance from the surrounding tissues.

punc'ture [L. *punctura*, fr. *pungo*, pp. *punctus*, to prick] **1.** To make a hole with a small pointed object, such as a needle. **2.** A prick or small hole made with a pointed instrument.

lumbar p., spinal p., spinal tap; p. into the subarachnoid space of the lumbar region for diagnostic or therapeutic purposes.

sternal p., removal of bone marrow from the manubrium by needle.

pu'pil (p.) [L. *pupilla*, q.v.] Pupilla.

Argyll Robertson p., a form of reflex iridoplegia characterized by the loss of reflexes to light, direct and consensual, with normal pupillary contraction on accommodation and convergence, often present in tabes and general paresis.

pupil'la, pl. **pupil'lae** [L. dim. of *pupa*, a girl or doll] [NA] The circular orifice in the centre of the iris, through which the light rays enter the eye.

pu'pillary Relating to the pupil.

purga'tion [L. *purgatio*] Catharsis; evacuation of the bowels with the aid of a purgative or cathartic.

pur'gative [L. *purgativus*, purging] An agent used for purging the bowels.

purge [L. *purgo*, to cleanse] **1.** To cause a copious evacuation of the bowels. **2.** A cathartic remedy.

pu'rine The parent substance of naturally occurring purine bases, not known to exist as such in the body. There are three p. groups: oxypurines (hypoxanthine, xanthine, and uric acid), aminopurines (adenine and guanine), and methyl p.'s (caffeine, theophylline, and theobromine).

pur'pura [L. fr. G. *porphyra*, purple] A condition characterized by haemorrhage into the skin, the appearance of the lesions varying with the type of p., duration of the lesions, and acuteness of the onset; the colour is first red, gradually darkening to purple and then fading to a brownish yellow and usually disappearing; the colour of residual permanent pigmentation depends largely on the type of unabsorbed pigment of the extravasated blood; extravasations may occur also into the mucous membranes and internal organs.

   allergic p., nonthrombocytopenic p. due to foods, drugs, and insect bites.

   Henoch-Schönlein p., an eruption of nonthrombocytopenic purpuric lesions associated with joint pains or swelling, colic, vomiting of blood, passage of bloody stools, and sometimes glomerulonephritis, most commonly occurring in male children.

   idiopathic thrombocytopenic p. (ITP), a systemic illness characterized by extensive ecchymoses, haemorrhages from mucous membranes, deficiencies in platelet count, anaemia, and prostration.

   p. seni'lis, occurrence of petechiae and ecchymoses on the legs in aged and debilitated persons.

   thrombotic thrombocytopenic p., a rapidly fatal or occasionally protracted disease with varied symptoms in addition to p., including signs of CNS involvement, due to formation of fibrin or platelet thrombi in arterioles and capillaries in many organs.

pu'rulence [L. *purulentia*, a festering, fr. *pus* (*pur-*), pus] The condition of containing or forming pus.

pu'rulent Containing, consisting of, or forming pus.

pus [L.] A fluid product of inflammation, consisting of a liquid containing leucocytes and the debris of dead cells and tissue elements liquefied by proteolytic and histolytic enzymes elaborated by polymorphonuclear leucocytes.

   blue p., p. tinged with pyocyanin, a product of *Pseudomonas aeruginosa.*

pus'tular Relating to or marked by pustules.

pustula'tion The formation or presence of pustules.

pus'tule [L. *pustula*] A small circumscribed elevation of the skin, containing purulent material.

puta'men [L. that which falls off in pruning] [NA] The outer, larger, and darker grey of the three portions into which the nucleus lentiformis is divided by laminae of white fibres; its histological structure is similar to that of the caudate nucleus with which together it composes the striatum.

putrefac'tion [L. *putre-facio*, pp. *-factus*, to make rotten] Decay; decomposition or rotting, the breakdown of organic matter usually by bacterial action, resulting in the formation of other less complex substances with the evolution of ammonia or its derivatives and hydrogen sulphide; characterized usually by the presence of toxic or malodorous products.

pyae'mia [G. *pyon*, pus, + *haima*, blood] Septicaemia due to pyogenic organisms causing multiple abscesses.

pyarthro'sis [G. *pyon*, pus, + *arthrōsis*, a jointing] Suppurative *arthritis.*

pycno- See pykno-.

pyeli'tis [pyel- + G. *-itis*, inflammation] **1.** Inflammation of the renal pelvis. **2.** Obsolescent term for pyelonephritis.

pyelo-, pyel- [G. *pyelos*, trough, tub, vat (pelvis)] Combining forms denoting pelvis, usually the renal pelvis.

pyelog'raphy [pyelo- + G. *graphō*, to write] Radiologic study of the kidney and renal collecting system, usually with a contrast agent.

py'elolithot'omy [pyelo- + G. *lithos*, stone, + *tomē*, incision] Pelvilithotomy.

py'elonephri'tis [pyelo- + G. *nephros*, kidney, + *-itis*, inflammation] Inflammation of the renal parenchyma, calices, and pelvis, particularly due to local bacterial infection.

py'elonephro'sis [pyelo- + G. *nephros*, kidney, + *-osis*, condition] Any disease of the pelvis of the kidney.

py'eloplasty [pyelo- + G. *plassō*, to fashion] A plastic or reconstructive operation on the kidney pelvis to correct an obstruction.

pyk'nic [G. *pyknos*, thick] Denoting a constitutional body type characterized by well rounded external contours and ample body cavities.

pykno-, pyk- [G. *pyknos*, thick, dense] Combining forms meaning thick, dense, compact.

py'lephlebi'tis [G. *pylē*, a gate, + *phleps*, vein, + *-itis*, inflammation] Inflammation of the portal vein or any of its branches.

py'lethrombo'sis [G. *pylē*, gate, + *thrombos*, a clot, + *-osis*, condition] Thrombosis of the portal vein or its branches.

pylo'ric Relating to the pylorus.

pyloro-, pylor- [G. *pyloros*, gatekeeper] Combining forms denoting the pylorus.

pylo'romyot'omy [pyloro- + G. *mys*, muscle, + *tomē*, incision] Longitudinal incision through the anterior wall of the pyloric canal to the level of the submucosa, to treat hypertrophic pyloric stenosis.

pylo'roplasty [pyloro- + G. *plassō*, to form] An operation, commonly performed in conjunction with truncal vagectomy to treat peptic ulcer disease, in which an opening into pyloric canal is made in a longitudinal place and closed transversely; the latter destroys the normal closing mechanism at the gastric outlet and facilitates prompt emptying of gastric contents into the duodenum.

pylo'rospasm Spasmodic contraction of the pylorus.

pylo'rus, pl. **pylo'ri** [L. fr. G. *pylōros*, a gatekeeper] [NA] **1.** A muscular or myovascular device to open (dilator) and to close (sphincter) an orifice or the lumen of an organ. **2.** The muscular tissue surrounding and controlling the aboral outlet of the stomach.

pyo- [G. *pyon*, pus] Combining form denoting suppuration or an accumulation of pus.

pyocol'pos [pyo- + G. *kolpos*, bosom (vagina)] An accumulation of pus in the vagina.

pyoder'ma [pyo- + G. *derma*, skin] Any pyogenic infection of the skin.

   p. gangreno'sum, a chronic eruption of spreading, undermined ulcers showing central healing.

pyoge'nic Pus-forming; relating to pus formation.

py'ohaemotho'rax [pyo- + G. *haima*, blood, + thorax] Presence of pus and blood in the pleural cavity.

pyome'tra [pyo- + G. *mētra*, uterus] An accumulation of pus in the uterine cavity.

py'omyosi'tis [pyo- + G. *mys*, muscle, + *-itis*, inflammation] Abscesses, carbuncles, or infected sinuses lying deep in muscles.

pyonephri'tis [pyo- + G. *nephros*, kidney, + *itis*, inflammation] Suppurative inflammation of the kidney.

pyonephro'sis [pyo- + G. *nephros*, kidney, + *-osis*, condition] Distension of the pelvis and calices of the kidney with pus, usually associated with obstruction.

py'opericardi'tis Suppurative inflammation of the pericardium.

py'operitoni'tis Suppurative inflammation of the peritoneum.

py'opneumopericar'dium [pyo- + G. *pneuma*, air, + pericardium] Presence of pus and gas in the pericardial sac.

py'opneumotho'rax [pyo- + G. *pneuma*, air, + thorax] Presence of gas together with a purulent effusion in the pleural cavity.

pyorrhoe'a [pyo- + G. *rhoia*, a flow] A purulent discharge.

pyosal'pinx [pyo- + G. *salpinx*, trumpet (tube)] Distension of a fallopian tube with pus.

pyo'sis [G.] Suppuration.

pyotho'rax Empyema in a pleural cavity.

pyoure'ter Distension of a ureter with pus.

pyr'amid [G. *pyramis* (*pyramid-*), a pyramid] An anatomical structure having a pyramidal shape.

   renal p., *pyramis renalis.*

pyr'amis, pl. **pyram'ides** [Mod. L. fr. G. pyramid] [NA] Pyramid.

   p. rena'lis, pl. **pyram'ides rena'les** [NA], one of a number of pyramidal masses, seen on longitudinal section of the kidney, that contain part of the secreting tubules and the collecting tubules.

pyret'ic [G. *pyretikos*] Feverish; pertaining to fever.

pyrex'ia [G. *pyrexis*, feverishness] Fever.

pyrimeth'amine A potent folic acid antagonist used as an antimalarial agent effective against *Plasmodium falciparum;* also used in the treatment of toxoplasmosis.

pyrim'idine A heterocyclic substance, the formal parent of several "bases" present in nucleic acids (uracil, thymine, cytosine) as well as of the barbiturates.

pyro- [G. *pyr*, fire] **1.** Combining form denoting fire, heat, or fever. **2.** In chemistry, combining form denoting derivatives formed by removal of water (usually by heat) to form anhydrides.

pyrocat'echol A constituent of adrenaline and noradrenaline (both "catecholamines") and dopa; used externally as an antiseptic.

py'rogen [pyro- + -gen, producing] An agent that causes a rise in temperature.

pyro'sis [G. a burning] Heartburn; substernal pain or burning sensation, usually associated with regurgitation of acid-peptic gastric juice into the oesophagus.

pyu'ria [G. pyon, pus, + ouron, urine] Presence of pus in the urine. •

Q

quadri- [L. quattuor, four] Combining form denoting four.

quad'riceps [L. fr. quadri- + caput, head] Having four heads; denoting various muscles.

quadrigem'inal [quadri- + L. geminus, twin] Fourfold.

quadrigem'inum One of the corpora quadrigemina.

quadriple'gia [quadri- + G. plēgē, stroke] Paralysis of all four limbs.

quar'antine [It. quarantina fr. L. quadraginta, forty] **1.** A period (originally 40 days) of detention of vessels and their passengers coming from an area where an infectious disease prevails. **2.** To detain such vessels and their passengers until the incubation period of the disease has passed. **3.** A place where such vessels and their passengers are detained. **4.** The isolation of a person with a contagious disease.

quar'tan [L. quartanus, relating to a fourth (thing)] Recurring every fourth day.

quick'ening [A.S. cwic, living] The signs of life felt by the mother as a result of the fetal movements.

quies'cent At rest or inactive.

quin'idine One of the alkaloids of cinchona, a stereoisomer of quinine; used as an antimalarial and in the treatment of cardiac arrhythmias.

quin'ine An alkaloid derived from cinchona (family Rubiaceae), used as an antimalarial effective against the asexual and erythrocytic forms of the parasite, but having no effect on the exoerythrocytic (tissue) forms; also used as an antipyretic, analgesic, sclerosing agent, stomachic, and oxytocic (occasionally), and in the treatment of atrial fibrillation and certain myopathies.

quin'sy [M.E. quinsie (quinesie), a corruption of L. cynanche, sore throat] Peritonsillar abscess.

quin'tan [L. quintus, fifth] Recurring every fifth day.

quotid'ian [L. quotidianus, daily] Daily; occurring every day.

quo'tient [L. quoties, how often] The number of times one amount is contained in another.

   intelligence q. (IQ), an index of measured intelligence as one part of a two-part determination of intelligence (the other being an index of adaptive behaviour) used to denote a person's standing relative to his age peers on a test of general ability, ordinarily expressed as a ratio between the person's score on a given test and the score which the average individual his age attained on the same test.

   respiratory q., (R.Q.), the steady state ratio of carbon dioxide produced by tissue metabolism to oxygen consumed in the same metabolism; for the whole body, normally about 0.82 under basal conditions; in the steady state, equal to the respiratory exchange ratio.

R

rab'id [L. rabidus, raving, mad] Relating to or affected with rabies.

ra'bies [L. rage, fury, fr. rabio, to rave, to be mad] A highly fatal infectious disease transmitted by the bite of carnivorous animals and caused by a neurotropic lyssavirus that occurs in the CNS and the salivary glands; symptoms are those of a profound disturbance of the nervous system: excitement, aggressiveness, and dementia, followed by paralysis and death; cytoplasmic inclusion bodies (Negri bodies) found in many of the neurones are characteristic.

race'mic Denoting a mixture that is optically inactive, being composed of an equal number of dextro- and laevorotatory substances, which are separable; compounds internally compensated, and therefore not separable into D and L (or d and l) forms, are termed "meso."

ra'cemose [L. racemosus, full of clusters] Branching, with nodular terminations, resembling a bunch of grapes.

rachi-, rachio- [G. *rachis*, spine, backbone] Combining form denoting the spine.

ra'chicente'sis, ra'chiocente'sis [rachi- + G. *kentēsis*, puncture] Lumbar puncture.

rachid'ial, rachid'ian Spinal.

rachitogen'ic [rachitis + G. *genesis*, production] Producing or causing rickets.

ra'darkymog'raphy Video tracking of heart motion by means of image intensification and closed circuit television during fluoroscopy; enables cardiac motion to be measured by reproducible linear graphic tracing.

ra'dial [L. *radialis*, fr. *radius*, ray] **1.** Relating to the radius (bone of the forearm), to any structures named from it, or to the radial or lateral aspect of the upper limb as compared to the ulnar or medial aspect. **2.** Relating to any radius. **3.** Radiating; diverging in all directions from any given centre.

ra'diant 1. Giving out rays. **2.** A point from which light radiates to the eye.

ra'diate [L. *radio*, pp. *-atus*, to shine] **1.** To spread out in all directions from a centre. **2.** To emit radiation.

radia'tion [L. *radiatio*, fr. *radius*, ray, beam] **1.** The act or condition of diverging in all directions from a centre. **2.** The sending forth of light, short radio waves, ultraviolet or x-rays, or any other rays for treatment or diagnosis or for other purpose; *cf.* irradiation (2). **3.** Radiant energy or a radiant beam.

rad'ical [L. *radix* (*radic-*), root] **1.** In chemistry, a group of elements or atoms usually passing intact from one compound to another, but usually incapable of prolonged existence in a free state; in chemical formulas, often distinguished by being enclosed in parentheses or brackets. **2.** Thorough; relating or directed to the extirpation of the root or cause of a morbid process; *e.g.*, a r. operation. **3.** Denoting treatment by extreme, drastic, or innovative measures, as opposed to conservative.

radi'ces Plural of radix.

rad'icle [L. *radicula*, dim of *radix*, root] A rootlet or structure resembling one, as a minute veinlet joining with others to form a vein or a nerve fibre which joins others to form a nerve.

radic'ula [L. dim of *radix*, root] A spinal nerve root.

radio'uli'tis [radicul- + G. *itis*, inflammation] Inflammation of the intradural portion of a spinal nerve root prior to its entrance into the intervertebral foramen or of the portion between that foramen and the nerve plexus.

radiculo-, radicul- Combining forms denoting radicle, radicular.

radic'ulop'athy [radiculo- + G. *pathos*, suffering] Disease of the spinal nerve roots.

ra'dii [L.] Plural of radius.

radio- [L. *radius*, ray] Combining form denoting radiation, chiefly x-ray; the radioactive isotope of the element to which it is prefixed; radius.

ra'dioac'tive Possessing radioactivity.

ra'dioactiv'ity The property of some atomic nuclei of spontaneously emitting gamma rays or subatomic particles of matter.

     artificial r., induced r., the r. of isotopes that exist only because man-made through the bombardment of naturally occurring isotopes by subatomic particles, or high levels of x- or gamma radiation.

ra'diobiol'ogy The biologic study of the effects of ionizing radiation upon living things.

ra'diocar'diogram A graphic record of the concentration of injected radioisotope within the cardiac chambers.

ra'diocar'pal 1. Relating to the radius and the bones of the carpus. **2.** On the radial or lateral side of the carpus.

radiochem'istry The science that uses radionuclides and their properties to study chemical applications and problems.

ra'diodermati'tis Dermatitis due to exposure to ionizing radiation.

ra'diodiagno'sis Diagnosis by means of x-rays.

radiogold' col'loid A radioactive isotope of gold emitting negative beta particles and gamma radiation, with a half-life of 2.7 days; used for irradiation of closed serous cavities in the palliative treatment of ascites and pleural effusion due to metastatic malignancies, and for liver scans.

ra'diograph [radio- + G. *graphō*, write] The sensitized film or plate upon which a shadow image is produced by radiography.

     bitewing r., intraoral dental film adapted to show the coronal portion and cervical third of the root of the teeth in near occlusion.

     panoramic r., a radiographic view of the maxillae and mandible extending from the left to the right glenoid fossae.

radiog'raphy Examination of any part of the body for diagnostic purposes by means of x-rays, the record of the findings being impressed upon a photographic plate or film.

electron r., a radiographic imaging process in which the incident x-radiation is converted to a latent charge image subsequently developed by a special printing process; it improves detail enhancement by the virtual absence of background fog and image noise.

serial r., several x-ray exposures, over a period of time, of a region under study.

ra'dioimmu'nity Lessened sensitivity to radiation.

radioim'munoas'say An immunological procedure in which radioisotope-labeled antigen is reacted with specific antiserum and an aliquant part of the same antiserum previously treated with test fluid; any specific substance in the test fluid sample would have reacted with antibody and, accordingly, a greater quantity of free, labeled antigen in the test fluid, with reference to the specific antiserum, would be a measure of the substance in the test fluid sample.

radioi'sotope An unstable isotope that decays to a stable state by emitting radiation.

radiolog'ic, radiolog'ical Pertaining to radiology.

radiol'ogist A specialist in the diagnostic and/or therapeutic use of x-rays and other forms of radiant energy.

radiol'ogy [radio- + G. *logos,* study] Science concerned with radiant energy, with the chemical and other actions of rays proceeding from luminous bodies, and with the sources of these rays.

radiom'eter [radio- + G. *metron,* measure] A device for determining the penetrative power of x-rays.

ra'diomimet'ic [radio- + G. *mimētikos,* imitative] Imitating the action of radiation, as in the case of chemicals such as nitrogen mustards which affect cells as high-energy radiation does.

ra'dionecro'sis Necrosis due to excessive exposure to radiation.

radionu'clide A nuclide of artificial or natural origin that exhibits radioactivity.

radiopaque' [radio- + Fr. opaque fr. L. *opacus,* shady] Exhibiting relative impenetrability by x-rays or any other form of radiation.

ra'diopharmaceu'ticals Radioactive chemical or pharmaceutical preparations, used as diagnostic or therapeutic agents.

radios'copy [radio- + G. *skopeō,* to view] Fluoroscopy.

radiosens'itive Affected by radiation.

ra'diosensitiv'ity The condition of being readily acted upon by radioactive forces.

ra'diotherapeu'tic Relating to radiotherapy or to radiotherapeutics.

ra'diotherapeu'tics The study and use of radiotherapeutic agents.

ra'diother'apist One who practises radiotherapy or is knowledgeable in radiotherapeutics.

ra'diother'apy The medical specialty concerned with the use of electromagnetic or particulate radiations in the treatment of disease.

ra'diotoxae'mia [radio- + G. *toxikon,* poison, + *haima,* blood] Radiation sickness caused by the products of disintegration produced by the action of x-rays or other forms of activity and by the depletion of certain cells and enzyme systems.

ra'dium [L. *radius,* ray] A metallic element, symbol Ra, atomic no. 88, atomic weight 226.05, extracted from pitchblende; its therapeutic action is similar to that of x-rays and is applied as one of its salts: the bromide, carbonate, chloride, and sulphate.

ra'dius, pl. **ra'dii** [L. spoke of a wheel, rod, ray] **1.** A straight line passing from the centre to the periphery of a circle. **2.** [NA] The lateral and shorter of the two bones of the forearm.

ra'dix, pl. **ra'dices** [L.] [NA] Root; the primary or beginning portion of a part or organ buried in a tissue or by which it arises from another structure.

rale [Fr. rattle] Ambiguous term for an added sound heard on auscultation of the chest; used by some to denote rhonchus and by others for crepitation.

ra'mus, pl. **ra'mi** [L.] [NA] **1.** A branch. **2.** One of the primary divisions of a nerve or blood vessel. **3.** A part of an irregularly shaped bone (less slender than a "process") that forms an angle with the main body. **4.** One of the primary divisions of a cerebral sulcus.

ran'ula [L. tadpole, dim. of *rana,* frog] **1.** Hypoglottis. **2.** A cystic tumour of the undersurface of the tongue, or floor of the mouth due to obstruction of the duct of the sublingual glands.

rape [L. *rapio*, to seize, to drag away] **1.** Sexual intercourse with a woman by force or without her legal consent. **2.** To perform such an act.

raphe [G. *rhaphē*, suture seam] [NA] The line of union of two contiguous, bilaterally symmetrical structures.

rarefac'tion [L. *rarus*, thin, + *facio*, to make] Expansion; the condition of becoming or being light or less dense.

rash [O. Fr. *rasche*, skin eruption, fr. L. *rado*, pp. *rasus*, to scratch, scrape] A cutaneous eruption.

  butterfly r., a scaling lesion on each cheek, joined by a narrow band across the nose; seen in lupus erythematosus and seborrhoeic dermatitis.

  drug r., drug *eruption*.

  heat r., *miliaria* rubra.

  napkin r., napkin *dermatitis*.

rate [L. *ratum*, a reckoning] A record of the measurement of an event or process in terms of its relation to some fixed standard; measurement expressed as the ratio of one quantity to another.

  birth r., the precise number of births for a year related to an exact population and place.

  mortality r., death r.; the ratio of the total number of deaths to the total population of a given community, usually expressed as deaths per 1000, 10,000, or 100,000 population.

  neonatal mortality r., the number of deaths in the first 28 days of life divided by the number of live births occurring in the same population during the same period of time.

  pulse r., r. of the pulse as observed in an artery; invariably recorded as beats per minute.

  sedimentation r., the sinking velocity of blood cells, *i.e.,* the degree of rapidity with which the red cells sink in a mass of drawn blood.

ray [L. *radius*] **1.** A line of light, heat, or other form of radiation. **2.** A part or line that extends radially from a structure.

  gamma r.'s, electromagnetic radiation emitted from radioactive substances; analogous to the x-rays but originating from the nucleus rather than the orbital shell and not deflected by a magnet.

  x-r., see under x.

reac'tant A substance taking part in a chemical reaction.

reac'tion **1.** The response of living tissue or an organism to a stimulus. **2.** The colour change effected in litmus and certain other organic pigments by contact with various substances (acids or alkalies); also the property that such substances possess of producing this change. **3.** In chemistry, the intermolecular action of two or more substances upon each other, whereby these substances are caused to disappear, new ones being formed in their place. **4.** In immunology, *in vivo* or *in vitro* action of antibody on specific antigen, with or without involvement of complement or other components of the immunological system. See also response; test.

  adverse r., a result of drug therapy which is neither intended nor expected in normal therapeutic use and which causes significant, sometimes life-threatening morbidity.

  allergic r., a local or general r. of an organism to internal or external contact with a specific allergen to which the organism has been previously sensitized.

reac'tivate To render active again; said of an inactivated immune serum to which normal serum (complement) is added.

rea'gent [Mod. L. *reagens*] Any substance added to a solution of another substance to participate in a chemical reaction.

real'ity testing In psychiatry, the ego function by which the objective or real world and one's relationship to it are evaluated and appreciated.

rebreath'ing Inhalation of part or all of gases previously exhaled.

re'call The process of remembering thoughts, words, and actions of a past event in an attempt to recapture actual happenings.

recan'aliza'tion **1.** Restoration of a lumen in a blood vessel following thrombotic occlusion, by organization of the thrombus with formation of new channels. **2.** Spontaneous restoration of the continuity of the lumen of any occluded duct or tube.

receptac'ulum, pl. **receptac'ula** [L. fr. *re-cipio*, pp. *-ceptus*, to receive] Reservoir; a receptacle.

recep'tor [L. receiver, fr. *recipio*, to receive] **1.** In Ehrlich's theory of immunity, one of the side chains of the cell which combine with foreign substances, conceived as being of three orders; although much of his theory is now obsolete, the concept of specific sites (*i.e.*, molecular configurations) of attachment continues to play a major role in immunology and pharmacology. **2.** Any one of the various sensory nerve endings in the skin, deep tissues, viscera, and special sense organs.

reces'sion [L. *recessio* (see recessus)] A withdrawal or retreating of tissue. See also retraction.

reces'sive 1. Drawing away; receding. **2.** In genetics, denoting an allele possessed by one parent of a hybrid which is not expressed in the latter because of suppression by a contrasting allele (dominant) from the other parent.

recidiva'tion [L. *recidivus*, falling back, recurring, fr. *recido*, to fall back, fr. *cado*, to fall] Relapse of a disease, symptom or behavioural pattern such as an illegal activity for which one was previously hospitalized or imprisoned.

recid'ivism [L. *recidivus*, recurring] The tendency of an individual toward recidivation.

rec'ipe [L. imperative *recipio*, to receive] **1.** Take; the superscription of a prescription, usually indicated by the sign ℞. **2.** A prescription or formula.

recom'binant DNA DNA resulting from the insertion into the chain, by chemical or biological means, of a sequence (a whole or partial chain of DNA) not originally (biologically) present in that chain.

rec'rement [L. *recrementum*, refuse, filth, fr. re- + *cerno*, to separate] A secretion, like saliva, that is reabsorbed after having performed its function.

recrudes'cence [L. *re-crudesco*, to become raw again, break out afresh] A recurrence of a morbid process or its symptoms after a period of improvement.

recrudes'cent Becoming active again, relating to a recrudescence.

recruit'ment [Fr. *recrutement*, fr. L. *recresco*, pp. -*cretus*, to grow again] **1.** The unequal reaction of the ear to equal steps of increasing intensity, measured in decibels, when such inequality of response results in a greater than normal increment of loudness. **2.** The bringing into activity of additional motor neurones and thus causing greater activity in response to increased duration of the stimulus applied to a given receptor or afferent nerve.

rec'tal Relating to the rectum.

recto-, rect- Combining forms denoting the rectum. See also procto-.

rec'tocele [recto- + G. *kēlē*, tumour, hernia] Proctocele.

rectosig'moid The rectum and sigmoid colon considered as a unit; also applied to the junction of the sigmoid colon and rectum.

rec'tum, pl. **rec'tums, rec'ta** [L. *rectus*, straight, pp. of *rego*, to make straight] [NA] The terminal portion of the digestive tube, extending from the sigmoid colon to the anal canal.

recum'bent [L. *recumbo*, to lie back, recline, fr. re-, back, + *cubo*, to lie] Leaning; reclining; lying down.

recu'perate [L. *recupero* (or recip-), pp. -*atus*, to take again, recover] To recover; to regain health and strength.

recur'rence [L. *re-curro*, to run back, recur] **1.** A return of the symptoms, occurring as a phenomenon in the natural history of the disease, as seen in recurrent fever. **2.** Relapse.

recur'rent 1. In anatomy, turning back on itself. **2.** Returned; denoting symptoms or lesions reappearing after an intermission or remission.

recurva'tion [L. *re-curvus*, bent back] A backward bending or flexure.

reduce' [L. *re-duco*, pp. -*ductus*, to lead back, restore, reduce] **1.** To perform reduction (1). **2.** In chemistry, to initiate a reaction involving a gain of electrons by the substance in question; the substance supplying the electrons or the hydrogen, or removing the oxygen, is itself oxidized in so doing.

reduc'tion [L. *reductio*, see reduce] **1.** Repositioning; restoration, by surgical or manipulative procedures, of a part to its normal anatomical relation. **2.** In chemistry, the gain of one or more electrons by an ion or compound.

re'flex [L. *reflexus*, pp. of *re-flecto*, to bend back] An involuntary reaction in response to a stimulus applied to the periphery and transmitted to the nervous centres in the brain or spinal cord.

accommodation r., constriction of the pupil, convergence of the eyes, and increased convexity of the lens when the eyes view a near object.

conditioned r. (CR), a r. gradually developed by training and association through frequent repetition of a definite stimulus.

deep r., an involuntary muscular contraction following percussion of a tendon or bone.

patellar r., knee or knee-jerk r.; a sudden contraction of the anterior muscles of the thigh, caused by a smart tap on the patellar tendon while the leg hangs loosely at a right angle with the thigh.

pilomotor r., contraction of the smooth muscle of the skin resulting in "gooseflesh" caused by mild application of a tactile stimulus or by local cooling.

plantar r., the response to tactile stimulation of the ball of the foot, normally plantar flexion of the toes; the pathologic response is Babinski's *sign* (1).

pupillary r., change in diameter of the pupil as a reflex response to light or to any type of stimulus.

re'flux [L. *re-,* back, + *fluxus,* a flow] A backward flow. See also regurgitation.

refract' [L. *refringo,* pp. *-fractus,* to break up] **1.** To bend a ray of light. **2.** To detect an error of refraction in the media of the eye and to correct it by means of lenses.

refrac'tion [L. *refractio* (see refract)] **1.** Deflection of a ray of light when it passes from one medium into another of different optical density. **2.** The act of determining the nature and degree of the refractive errors in the eye and correction of the same by lenses.

refractiv'ity Ability of a substance to refract rays of light.

refrac'tory [L. *refractarius,* fr. *refringo,* pp. *-fractus,* to break in pieces] **1.** Intractable; resistant to treatment, as of a disease. **2.** Obstinate (1).

refrac'ture [re- + fracture] The breaking again of a bone that has united, after a previous fracture.

refrigera'tion [L. *refrigeratio*] The act of cooling or reducing fever.

refrin'gence Refraction.

regenera'tion [L. *re-genero,* pp. *-atus,* to reproduce] **1.** Reproduction or reconstitution of a lost or injured part. **2.** A form of asexual reproduction, as when a worm is divided into two or more parts, each segment is regenerated into a new individual.

reg'imen [L. direction, rule] A regulation of the mode of living, diet, sleep, exercise, etc., for a hygienic or therapeutic purpose.

re'gion [L. *regio*] **1.** An arbitrarily defined portion of the body's surface. **2.** A portion of the body having a special nervous or vascular supply, or a part of an organ having a special function.

abdominal r.'s, topographical subdivisions of the abdomen: right and left hypochondriac, right and left lateral, right and left inguinal, and the unpaired epigastric, umbilical and pubic regions.

regres'sion [L. *re-gredior,* pp. *-gressus,* to go back] **1.** A subsidence of symptoms. **2.** A relapse; return of symptoms. **3.** Any retrograde movement or action. **4.** Return to a more primitive mode of behaviour due to an inability to function adequately at a more adult level. **5.** An unconscious defence mechanism by which there occurs a return to earlier patterns of adaptation.

regres'sive Relating to or characterized by regression.

regur'gitate [L. *re-,* back, + *gurgito,* pp. *-atus,* to flood] **1.** To flow backward. **2.** To expel the contents of the stomach in small amounts, short of vomiting.

regurgita'tion [L. *regurgitatio* (see regurgitate)] **1.** A backward flow, as of blood through an incompetent heart valve. **2.** The return of contents in small amounts from the stomach.

re'habilita'tion [L. *rehabilitare,* pp. *-tatus,* to make fit] Restoration, following disease, illness, or injury, of ability to function in a normal or near normal manner.

rehydra'tion The return of water to a system after its loss.

re'implanta'tion Replantation.

reinfec'tion A second infection by the same microorganism, after recovery from or during the course of a primary infection.

reinforce'ment **1.** An increase of force or strength. **2.** In conditioning, the totality of the process in which the conditioned stimulus is followed by presentation of the unconditioned stimulus which, itself, elicits the response to be conditioned.

re'innerva'tion Restoration of nerve control of a paralysed muscle or organ by means of regrowth of nerve fibres, either spontaneously or after anastomosis.

re'integra'tion In psychiatry, the return to well adjusted functioning following disturbances due to mental illness.

rejec'tion [L. *rejectio*, a throwing back] **1.** The immunological response to incompatibility in a transplanted organ. **2.** A refusal to accept, recognize, or grant; a denial. **3.** Elimination of small ultrasonic echoes from display.

relapse' [L. *re-labor*, pp. *-lapsus*, to slide back] The return of the symptoms of a disease after convalescence has begun.

relax'ant **1.** Relaxing; causing relaxation; reducing tension, especially muscular tension. **2.** An agent that so acts.

relaxa'tion [L. *relaxatio*, fr. *re-laxo*, to loosen] Dilation; loosening; lengthening or lessening of tension, as in a muscle.

rem'edy [L. *remedium*, fr. *re-*, again, + *medeor*, cure] An agent that cures disease or alleviates its symptoms.

remin'eraliza'tion The return to the body of necessary mineral constituents lost through disease or dietary deficiencies; commonly referring to the content of calcium salts in bone.

remis'sion [L. *re-mitto*, pp. *-missus*, to send back, slacken, relax] **1.** Abatement or lessening in severity of the symptoms of a disease. **2.** The period during which such abatement occurs.

remit'tence A temporary amelioration, without actual cessation, of symptoms.

remit'tent Characterized by temporary remissions or periods of abatement of the symptoms.

ren, pl. **re'nes** [L.] [NA] Kidney.

re'nal Nephric.

re'nin An enzyme that converts angiotensinogen to angiotensin.

ren'ipor'tal [reni- + L. *porta*, gate] **1.** Relating to the hilum of the kidney. **2.** Relating to the portal, or venous capillary circulation in the kidney.

ren'nin Chymosin.

reno-, reni- [L. *ren*, kidney] Combining forms denoting the kidney. See also nephro-.

renog'raphy Radiography of the kidney.

renopri'val [reno- + L. *privus*, deprived of] Relating to, characterized by, or resulting from total loss of kidney function or from removal of all functioning renal tissue.

renovas'cular Pertaining to the blood vessels of the kidney, denoting especially disease of these vessels.

Reovi'ridae [Respiratory *E* nteric Orphan + -viridae] A family of double stranded ether-resistant RNA viruses comprising six genera: *Reovirus, Orbivirus*, rotavirus group, cytoplasmic polyhedrosis virus group, and two plant reovirus groups.

Re'ovirus A genus of viruses (family Reoviridae) of three antigenically distinct human types related by a common complement-fixing antigen; recovered from children with mild fever and sometimes diarrhoea, and from children with no apparent infection; hosts are vertebrates, but the virus does not multiply in vertebrates.

repair' Restoration of diseases or damaged tissues naturally by healing processes or artificially, as by surgical means.

replanta'tion [G. *re-*, again, + *planto*, pp. *-atus*, to plant] Replacement of an organ or part back in its original site and reestablishing of its circulation.

rep'licate **1.** One of several identical processes or observations. **2.** To repeat; to produce an exact copy.

replica'tion [L. *replicatio*, a reply, fr. *replico*, pp. *-atus*, to fold back] **1.** Repeating a process or observation, commonly used in describing experimental work. **2.** Autoreproduction.

repres'sion [L. *re-primo*, pp. *-pressus*, to press back] In psychoanalysis, the defence mechanism by which ideas, impulses, and affects once available to conscious thought are removed from consciousness.

resec'tion **1.** Removal of articular ends of one or both bones forming a joint. **2.** Excision of a segment of a part.

  transurethral r., endoscopic removal of the prostate gland or bladder lesions, usually for relief of prostatic obstruction or treatment of bladder malignancies.

  wedge r., removal of a wedge-shaped portion of tissue, as of the ovary.

resec'toscope A special endoscopic instrument for the transurethral electrosurgical removal of lesions involving the bladder, prostate gland, or urethra.

res'erpine An ester alkaloid isolated from certain species of *Rauwolfia* which decreases the 5-hydroxytryptamine and catecholamine concentrations in the CNS and in peripheral tissues; used in conjunction with other hypotensive agents in the management of essential hypertension and as a tranquilizer in psychotic states.

res'ervoir [Fr.] Receptaculum.

r. of infection, living or nonliving material in or on which an infectious agent multiplies and/or develops and is dependent for its survival in nature.

resid'ual Relating to or of the nature of a residue.

res'idue [L. *residuum*] That which remains after removal of substances.

resis'tance [L. *re-sisto*, to stand back, withstand] **1.** The natural ability of an organism to remain unaffected by pathogenic or toxic agents. **2.** The opposition in a conductor to the passage of a current of electricity, whereby there is a loss of energy and a production of heat; specifically, the potential difference in volts across the conductor per ampere of current flow; unit: ohm. **3.** The opposition to flow through one or more passageways. **4.** In psychoanalysis, opposition to the uncovering of the unconscious. **5.** The power residing in the red blood cells to resist haemolysis and to preserve their shape under varying degrees of osmotic pressure.

resolu'tion [L. *resolutio*, a slackening] **1.** The arrest of an inflammatory process without suppuration; the absorption or breaking down and removal of the products of inflammation or of a new growth. **2.** The ability optically to distinguish detail such as the separation of closely approximated objects.

res'onance [L. *resonantia*, echo] **1.** Sympathetic or forced vibration of air in body cavities above, below, in front of, or behind a source of sound. **2.** The sound obtained on percussing a part that can vibrate freely **3.** The intensification and hollow character of the voice sound obtained on auscultating over a cavity.

nuclear magnetic r. (NMR), a method for defining the character of covalent bonds by measuring the magnetic moment of the atomic nuclei involved.

resorb' [L. *re-sorbeo*, to suck back] To reabsorb; to absorb what has been excreted, as an exudate or pus.

resor'cinol *m*-Dihydroxybenzene; used internally for the relief of nausea, asthma, whooping cough, and diarrhoea, but chiefly as an external antiseptic in psoriasis, eczema, seborrhoea, and ringworm.

resorp'tion **1.** The act of resorbing; removal of an exudate, a blood clot, pus, etc., by absorption. **2.** A loss of substance by physiologic or pathologic means.

respira'tion (R) [L. *respiratio*, fr. *respiro*, pp. *-atus*, to exhale, breathe] **1.** A fundamental process of life in which oxygen is used to oxidize organic fuel molecules, providing a source of energy as well as carbon dioxide and water. **2.** Ventilation (2).

artificial r., artificial *ventilation*.

assisted r., assisted *ventilation*.

Biot's r., abrupt and irregular alternating periods of apnoea and constant rate and depth of breathing, as that resulting from lesions due to increased intracranial pressure.

Cheyne-Stokes r., the pattern of breathing with gradual increase in depth and sometimes in rate to a maximum, followed by a decrease resulting in apnoea; characteristically seen in coma from affection of the nervous centres of respiration.

Kussmaul r., deep rapid r. characteristic of diabetic acidosis or coma.

mouth-to-mouth r., a method of artificial ventilation involving an overlap of the patient's mouth (and nose in small children) with the operator's mouth, to inflate the patient's lungs by blowing, followed by an unassisted expiratory phase brought about by elastic recoil of the patient's chest and lungs.

res'pirator **1.** An appliance fitting over the mouth and nose, used for the purpose of excluding dust, smoke, or other irritants, or of otherwise altering the air before it enters the respiratory passages. **2.** An apparatus for administering artificial respiration, especially for a prolonged period, in cases of paralysis of inadequate spontaneous ventilation.

Drinker r., iron lung; a mechanical r. in which the whole body except the head is encased within a metal tank, which is sealed at the neck with an airtight gasket; artificial respiration is induced by making the air pressure inside alternately negative and positive.

respi'ratory Relating to respiration.

respirom'eter [L. *respiro*, to breathe, + G. *metron*, measure] **1.** An instrument for measuring the extent of the respiratory movements. **2.** An instrument for measuring oxygen consumption or carbon dioxide production, usually of an isolated tissue.

response' [L. *responsus* (noun), an answer] **1.** The reaction of a muscle or other part to any stimulus. **2.** Any act or behaviour, or its constitutents, that an organism is capable of emitting.

conditioned r., a r. already in an individual's repertoire but which, through repeated pairings with its natural stimulus, has been acquired or conditioned anew to a previously neutral or conditioned stimulus.

evoked r., an alteration in the electrical activity of a particular part of the nervous system produced by an incoming sensory stimulus.

re'steno'sis [re- + G. *stenōsis*, a narrowing] Recurrence of stenosis after corrective surgery on the heart valve.

res'tiform [L. *restis*, rope, + *forma*, form] Ropelike; rope-shaped.

restora'tion [L. *restauro*, pp. *-atus*, to restore, to repair] **1.** Any inlay, crown, bridge, partial denture, or complete denture which restores or replaces lost tooth structure, teeth, or oral tissues. **2.** Any substance used for restoring the missing portion of a tooth.

resuscita'tion [L. *resuscitatio*] Restoration to life after apparent death. See also artificial *ventilation*.

cardiopulmonary r. (CPR), restoration of cardiac output and pulmonary ventilation following cardiac arrest and apnoea, using artificial respiration and closed chest massage.

resus'citator An apparatus that forces gas (usually O_2) into lungs to produce artificial respiration.

retain'er Any type of clasp, attachment, or device used for the fixation or stabilization of a prosthesis; an appliance used to prevent the shifting of teeth following orthodontic treatment.

continuous bar r., a metal bar, usually resting on lingual surfaces of teeth, to aid in their stabilization and to act as indirect r.'s.

retarda'tion A slowness or limitation of development.

mental r., subaverage general intellectual functioning that originates during the developmental period and is associated with impairment in adaptive behaviour.

retch [A.S. *hraecan*, to hawk] To make an involuntary effort to vomit.

retch'ing Dry vomiting; movements of vomiting without effect.

rete, pl. **re'tia** [L. net] [NA] **1.** A network of nerve fibres or small vessels. **2.** A structure composed of a fibrous network or mesh.

reten'tion [L. *retentio*, a holding back, see retain] **1.** The keeping in the body of what normally belongs there, especially the retaining of food and drink in the stomach, or of what normally should be discharged, as urine or faeces. **2.** Retaining that which has been learned so that it can be utilized later as in recall, recognition, or, if r. is partial, relearning.

retic'ular, retic'ulated Relating to a reticulum.

reticulo-, reticul- Combining forms denoting reticulum or reticular.

retic'ulocyte [reticulo- + G. *kytos*, cell] A young red blood cell with a network of precipitated basophilic substance, occurring during the process of active blood regeneration.

retic'ulocytope'nia [reticulocyte + G. *penia*, poverty] Paucity of reticulocytes in the blood.

retic'ulocyto'sis [reticulocyte + G. *-osis*, condition] An increase in the number of circulating reticulocytes above the normal (less than 1% of the total number of red blood cells).

retic'uloendothe'lial Denoting or referring to reticuloendothelium.

retic'uloendothe'lium [reticulo- + endothelium] The cells making up the reticuloendothelial system.

reticulo'sis [reticulo- + G. *-osis*, condition] An increase in histiocytes, monocytes, or other reticuloendothelial elements.

retic'ulum, pl. **retic'ula** [L. dim of *rete*, a net] **1.** [NA] A fine network formed by cells, or formed of certain structures within cells or of connective tissue fibres between cells. **2.** Neuroglia. **3.** The second compartment of the stomach of a ruminant.

endoplasmic r., (ER), the network of tubules or flattened sacs (cisternae) with or without ribosomes on the surface of their membranes.

ret'ina [Mediev. L. prob. fr. L. *rete*, a net] [NA] The innermost tunic of the eyeball, consisting of three parts: optic, ciliary, and iridial. The optic part, the physiologic portion that receives the visual light rays, is further divided into two parts, pigmented and nervous, which are arranged in the following layers: pigment layer, layer of rods and cones, external limiting membrane, outer nuclear layer, outer plexiform layer, inner nuclear layer, inner plexiform layer, layer of ganglion cells, layer of nerve fibres, and internal limiting membrane. The ciliary and iridial parts are forward prolongations of the pigmented layer and a layer of supporting columnar or epithelial cells over the ciliary body and the posterior surface of the iris, respectively.

retinac'ulum, pl. **retinac'ula** [L. a band, a halter, fr. *retineo*, to hold back] [NA] A frenum, or a retaining band or ligament.

ret'inal Relating to the retina.

retini'tis [retina + G. -*itis*, inflammation] Inflammation of the retina.

exudative r., a chronic inflammatory condition characterized by the appearance of white or yellowish raised areas encircling the optic disc due to the accumulation of oedematous fluid beneath the retina.

r. pigmento'sa, a progressive abiotrophy of the neuroepithelium, with atrophy and pigmentary infiltration of the inner layers.

retino-, retin- Combining forms denoting the retina.

ret'inoblasto'ma [retino- + G. *blastos*, germ, + -*oma*, tumour] A malignant neoplasm composed of primitive retinal cells, occurring sporadically (mainly uniocularly) and as an autosomal dominant trait (mainly binocularly).

ret'inol Vitamin A (2); **r. dehydrogenase** is an oxidoreductase catalysing interconversion of retinaldehyde and retinol, a reaction of importance in the chemistry of rod vision.

retinop'athy [retino- + G. *pathos*, suffering] Noninflammatory degenerative disease of the retina, as distinguished from retinitis.

diabetic r., retinal changes occurring in diabetes of long standing, marked by punctate haemorrhages, microaneurysms, and sharply defined waxy exudates.

ret'inopexy [retino- + G. *pexis*, fixation] Formation of chorioretinal adhesions surrounding a retinal tear for correction of retinal detachment.

ret'inoscope [retino- + G. *skopeō*, to view] An optical device used in retinoscopy.

retinos'copy [retino- + G. *skopeō*, to view] A method of detecting errors of refraction by illuminating the retina and noting the direction of movement of the light when the mirror is rotated.

retrac'tile Retractable; capable of being drawn back.

retrac'tion [L. *retractio*, a drawing back] **1.** A shrinking, drawing back, or pulling apart.

2. Posterior movement of teeth, usually with the aid of an orthodontic appliance.

retrac'tor **1.** An instrument for drawing aside the edges of a wound or for holding back structures adjacent to the operative field. **2.** A muscle that draws a part backward.

retro- [L. back, backward] Prefix, to words formed from Latin roots, denoting backward or behind.

retroces'sion [L. *retro- cedo*, pp. -*cessus*, to go back, retire] **1.** A going back; a relapse. **2.** Cessation of the external symptoms of a disease followed by signs of involvement of some internal organ or part. **3.** Denoting a position of the uterus or other organ further back than is normal.

retroflex'ion [retro- + L. *flecto*, pp. *flexus*, to bend] Backward bending, as of the uterus when the corpus is bent back, forming an angle with the cervix.

retrognath'ic Denoting retrognathism.

retrognath'ism [retro- + G. *gnathos*, jaw] A condition of facial disharmony in which one or both jaws are posterior to normal in their craniofacial relationships.

ret'rograde [L. *retrogradus*, fr. retro- + *gradior*, to go] **1.** Moving backward. **2.** Degenerating; reversing the normal order of growth and development.

retrogres'sion [L. *retrogressus*, fr. *retrogradior*, to go backwards] Degeneration, deterioration, or return to a previous, less complex condition.

ret'roperitoni'tis Inflammation of the cellular tissue behind the peritoneum.

ret'rophar'ynx The posterior part of the pharynx.

retropul'sion [retro- + L. *pulsio*, a pushing] An involuntary backward walking or running, occurring in patients with the parkinsonian syndrome. **2.** A pushing back of any part.

retrover'sion [retro- + L. *verto*, pp. *versus*, to turn] **1.** A turning backward, as of the uterus. **2.** A condition in which the teeth are located in a more posterior position than is normal.

Retrovi'ridae A family of viruses resembling the orthomyxoviruses in size and shape, but structurally more complex; they possess RNA-dependent DNA polymerases (reverse transcriptases) and are grouped in three subfamilies: Oncovirinae (RNA tumor viruses), Spumavirinae (foamy viruses), and Lentivirinae (visna and related agents).

ret'rovirus Any virus of the family Retroviridae.

revas'culariza'tion Re-establishment of blood supply to a part.

rever'sal [L. *re-verto*, pp. *-versus*, to turn back or about] **1.** A turning in the opposite direction, as of a disease, symptom, or a state. **2.** Denoting the difficulty of some persons in distinguishing the lower case printed or written letter *p* from *q* or *g*, *b* from *d*, or *s* from *z*. **3.** In psychoanalysis, the change of an instinct of affect into its opposite, as from love into hate.

reviv'ifica'tion [L. *re-*, again, + *vivo*, to live, + *facio*, to make] Refreshening the edges of a wound by paring or scraping to promote healing.

rhabdo-, rhabd- [G. *rhabdos*, rod] Combining forms denoting rod, rod-shaped.

rhab'domyol'ysis [rhabdo- + G. *mys*, muscle, + *lysis*, loosening] An acute, fulminating, potentially fatal disease of skeletal muscle which entails destruction of skeletal muscle as evidenced by myoglobinaemia and myoglobinuria.

rhabdomyo'ma [rhabdo- + G. *mys*, muscle, + *-oma*, tumour] A benign neoplasm derived from striated muscle.

rhab'domyosarco'ma [rhabdo- + G. *mys*, muscle, + *sarkōma*, sarcoma] A malignant neoplasm derived from skeletal (striated) muscle; characterized in adults by poorly differentiated oblong, as well as rounded and bizarre, cells with large hyperchromatic nuclei.

Rhabdovi'ridae A family of rod- or bullet-shaped RNA viruses of vertebrates, insects, and plants, including rabies virus; two genera have been assigned: *Vesiculovirus* and *Lyssavirus*.

rhab'dovirus Any virus of the family Rhabdoviridae.

rhag'ades [G. *rhagas*, pl. *rhagades*, a crack] Chaps, cracks, or fissures occurring at mucocutaneous junctions; seen in vitamin deficiency diseases and in congenital syphilis.

rheum [G. *rheuma*, a flux] A mucous or watery discharge.

rheumat'ic [G. *rheumatikos*, subject to flux] Relating to or characterized by rheumatism.

rheu'matism [G. *rheumatismos*, rheuma, a flux] Indefinite term applied to various conditions with pain or other symptoms which are of articular origin or related to other elements of the musculoskeletal system.

rheu'matoid [G. *rheuma*, flux, + *eidos*, resemblance] Resembling rheumatism in one or more features.

rheumatol'ogist A specialist in the diagnosis and treatment of rheumatic conditions.

rhex'is [G. *rhexis*, rupture] Bursting or rupture of an organ or vessel.

rhin-, rhino- [G. *rhis*, nose] Combining form denoting the nose.

rhinenceph'alon [rhin- + G. *enkephalos*, brain] Collective term denoting the parts of the cerebral hemisphere directly related to the sense of smell: the olfactory bulb, olfactory peduncle, olfactory tubercle, and olfactory or piriform cortex including the cortical nucleus of the amygdala.

rhini'tis [rhin- + G. *-itis*, inflammation] Inflammation of the nasal mucous membrane.

   acute r., an acute catarrhal inflammation of the mucous membrane of the nose, marked by sneezing, lacrimation, and a profuse secretion of watery mucus; usually associated with infection by one of the common cold viruses.

   allergic r., r. associated with hay fever.

rhi'nolith [rhino- + G. *lithos*, stone] A calcareous concretion in the nasal cavity.

rhinol'ogy [rhino- + G. *logos*, study] The branch of medical science concerned with the nose and its diseases.

rhinop'athy [rhino- + G. *pathos*, suffering] Disease of the nose.

rhinophy'ma [rhino- + G. *phyma*, tumour, growth] Hypertrophy of the nose with follicular dilation, resulting from hyperplasia of sebaceous glands with fibrosis and increased vascularity.

rhi'noplasty [rhino- + G. *plassō*, to form] **1.** Repair of a partial or complete defect of the nose with tissue taken from elsewhere. **2.** A plastic operation to change the shape or size of the nose.

rhinorrha'gia [rhino- + G. *rhēgnymi*, to burst forth] Epistaxis or nosebleed, especially if profuse.

rhinorrhoe'a [rhino- + G. *rhoia*, flow] A discharge from the nasal mucous membrane.

rhi'noscope A small mirror with an angled handle, used in posterior rhinoscopy.

rhinos'copy [rhino- + G. *skopeō*, to view] Inspection of the nasal cavity.

rhi'nosporidio'sis Invasion of the nasal cavity by *Rhinosporidium seeberi*, a yeastlike organism, resulting in a chronic granulomatous disease producing polyps or other forms of hyperplasia on mucous membranes.

Rhi'novirus A proposed genus of acid-labile viruses (family Picornaviridae) associated with the common cold in man and foot-and-mouth disease in cattle; there are 100 or more antigenic types classified as M strains (culturable in rhesus monkey kidney cells) and H strains (growing only in cultures of human cells).

Rhipiceph'alus [G. *rhipis*, fan, + *kephalē*, head] A genus of inornate hard ticks (family Ixodidae) that includes vectors of diseases in man and domestic animals.

rhizo- [G. *rhiza*, root] Combining form denoting root.

rhizot'omy [G. *rhiza*, root, + *tomē*, section] Section of the spinal nerve roots for the relief of pain or spastic paralysis.

rhodo-, rhod- [G. *rhodon*, rose] Combining forms denoting rose or red colour.

rhodogen'esis [rhodopsin + G. *genesis*, production] The production of rhodopsin by the combination of 11- *cis*-retinal and opsin in the dark.

rhodop'sin A red thermolabile protein found in the external segments of the rods of the retina; bleached by the action of light, which converts it to opsin and all- *trans*-retinal, and restored in the dark (see rhodogenesis).

rhombenceph'alon [rhombo + G. *enkephalos*, brain] [NA] Hindbrain; that part of the brain developed from the posterior of the three vesicles of the embryonic neural tube; it includes the pons, cerebellum, and medulla oblongata.

rhon'chus, pl. **rhon'chi** [L. fr. G. *rhenchos*, a snoring] An added sound with musical pitch occurring during inspiration or expiration, heard on auscultation of the chest, caused by air passing through bronchi that are narrowed by inflammation, spasm of smooth muscle, or by the presence of mucus in the lumen. A similar sound, produced in like manner, heard by air conduction from the mouth, is called a wheeze.

rhyth'm [G. *rhythmos*] Measured time or motion; the regular alternation of two different or opposite states; especially applied to the pattern of the heart's beat.

rhytidec'tomy [G. *rhytis* (*rhytid*-), a wrinkle] Elimination of wrinkles from, or reshaping of, the face by excising any excess skin and tightening the remainder; the so-called "face-lift."

rib [A.S. *ribb*] Costa (1).

ribofla'vin(e) One of the heat-stable factors of the vitamin B complex; dietary sources include green vegetables, liver, kidneys, wheat germ, milk, eggs, and cheese; used as replacement therapy in general vitamin B complex deficiencies.

ribonu'clease (RNase) An enzyme that catalyses the hydrolysis of ribonucleic acid.

ribonucle'ic acid (RNA) A macromolecule consisting of ribonucleoside residues connected by phosphate from the 3′ hydroxyl of one to the 5′ hydroxyl of the next nucleoside; found in all cells, in both nuclei and cytoplasm and in particulate and nonparticulate form, and also in many viruses.

   messenger RNA (mRNA), RNA reflecting the exact nucleoside sequence of the genetically active DNA and carrying the "message" of the latter, coded in its sequence, to the cytoplasmic areas where protein is made in amino-acid sequences specified by the mRNA, and hence primarily by the DNA.

   transfer RNA (tRNA), short chain RNA molecules present in cells in at least 20 varieties, each variety capable of combining with a specific amino acid. By joining (through their anticodons) with particular spots (codons) along the messenger RNA molecule and carrying their amino acids along, they lead to the formation of protein molecules with a specific amino-acid arrangement — the one ultimately dictated by a segment of DNA in the chromosomes.

ri'bonucleopro'tein (RNP) A combination of protein and ribonucleic acid.

ri'bonu'cleoside A nucleoside in which the sugar component is ribose.

ri'bonu'cleotide A nucleotide in which the sugar component is ribose.

ri'bose (Rib) The pentose present in ribonucleic acid.

ri'bosome A granule of ribonucleoprotein that is the site of protein synthesis from aminoacyl-tRNA's as directed by mRNA's.

ribosu'ria [ribose + G. *ouron*, urine] Enhanced urinary excretion of D-ribose; a common manifestation of muscular dystrophy.

ri'cin A phytotoxic protein occurring in the seeds of the castor oil plant, *Ricinus sanguineus;* a violent irritant that may be fatal.

rick'ets [E. *wrick*, to twist] A vitamin-D deficiency disease characterized by overproduction and deficient calcification of osteoid tissue, with associated skeletal deformities, enlargement of the liver and spleen, profuse sweating, and general tenderness of the body when touched.

    adult r., a disease resembling r. in many of its features, occurring in adult life.

    vitamin D-resistant r., a heritable form of r., characterized by hypophosphataemia due to defective renal tubular reabsorption of phosphate and subnormal absorption of dietary calcium; X-linked recessive inheritance.

Rickett'sia A genus of Gram-negative bacteria (order Rickettsiales) that usually occur intracytoplasmically in lice, fleas, ticks, and mites; pathogenic species are parasitic on man and other animals. The type species is *R. prowazekii.*

    R. ak'ari, a species that causes human rickettsialpox.

    R. austral'is, a species causing a spotted fever in which the patient's serum contains a different antibody from that reacting with *R. ricketsii, R. prowazekii,* and others.

    R. conor'ii, R. conori, a species causing boutonneuse fever in man.

    R. prowazek'ii, a species causing epidemic typhus fever; the type species of the genus *R.*

    R. ricketts'ii, a species causing Rocky Mountain spotted fever, South African tick-bite fever, São Paulo exanthematic typhus of Brazil, Tobia fever of Colombia, and spotted fevers of Minas Gerais and Mexico.

    R. tsutsugam'ushi, a species causing scrub typhus.

rickett'sialpox An acute disease caused by *Rickettsia akari* and transmitted by the mite *Liponnysoides sanguineus;* a papule in the skin of a covered part of the body develops into a deep-seated vesicle and then shrinks to form a black eschar; symptoms develop about a week after the appearance of the papule and consist of fever, chills, headache, backache, sweating, and local adenitis.

rifam'picin An antibacterial agent used in the treatment of tuberculosis.

rigid'ity [L. *rigidus*, rigid, inflexible] **1.** Stiffness or inflexibility. **2.** In psychiatry and clinical psychology, an aspect of personality characterized by resistance to change.

rig'or [L. stiffness] Rigidity (1).

    r. mor'tis, stiffening of the body after death, from hardening of the muscular tissues as a result of coagulation of myosinogen and paramyosinogen; disappears when decomposition begins.

ri'ma, pl. **ri'mae** [L. a slit] [NA] A slit or fissure, or narrow elongated opening between two symmetrical parts.

    r. glot'tidis [NA], the interval between the true vocal cords.

ri'mose [L. *rimosus*, fr. *rima*, a fissure] Fissured; marked by cracks in various directions.

ring'worm Tinea.

ri'sus sardon'icus The semblance of a grin caused by a facial spasm, especially in tetanus.

RNA Ribonucleic acid.

rod [A.S. *rōd*] **1.** A straight slender cylindrical formation. **2.** Rod cell of retina; the photosensitive, outward-directed process of a rhodopsin-containing rod cell in the external granular layer of the retina.

roent'genogram Radiograph.

roentgenog'raphy Radiography.

role [Fr.] The pattern of behaviour that one exhibits in relationship to significant persons in one's life.

    gender r., the sex of a child assigned by a parent or significant other.

    sex r., a stereotyped masculine or feminine pattern in everyday behaviour.

    sick r., the individual regarded, by himself or others, as a patient; may be assumed voluntarily or it may be imposed.

role'-playing A psychotherapeutic method used in psychodrama to understand and treat emotional conflicts through the enactment or re-enactment of stressful interpersonal events.

rom'bergism Romberg's *sign.*

rosa'cea [L. *rosaceus*, rosy] Vascular and follicular dilation involving the nose and contiguous portions of the cheeks; may vary from very mild but persistent erythema to extensive hyperplasia of the sebaceous glands with deep-seated papules and pustules and accompanied by telangiectasia at the affected erythematous sites.

roseo'la [Mod. L. dim. of L. *roseus*, rosy] A symmetrical eruption of small, closely aggregated patches of rose-red colour.

   epidemic r., rubella.

   r. infan'tilis, r. infan'tum, *exanthema* subitum.

   syphilitic r., usually the first eruption of syphilis, occurring 6 to 12 weeks after the initial lesion.

rosette' [Fr. a little rose] **1.** The quartan malarial parasite of *Plasmodium malariae* in its segmented or mature phase. **2.** A grouping of cells, characteristic of neoplasms of neuroblastic or neuroectodermal origin, in which a number of nuclei form a ring from which neurofibrils extend to interlace in the centre.

rota'tion [L. *roto*, pp. *rotatus*, to revolve, rotate] **1.** Turning or movement of a body round its axis. **2.** A recurrence in regular order of certain events, such as the symptoms of a periodical disease.

   optical r., the change in the plane of polarization of polarized light upon passing through optically active substances.

ro'tator [L. See rotation] A muscle by which a part can be turned circularly.

ro'tavirus A group of viruses (family Reoviridae) which probably form a separate genus that includes the infantile gastroenteritis viruses of man.

rough'age 1. Anything in the diet, *e.g.*, fibre, serving as a stimulant of intestinal peristalsis **2.** Hay or other coarse feed fed to cattle and other herbivores.

round'worm A nematode member of the phylum Nemathelminthes; commonly restricted to the parasitic forms.

-rrhagia [G. *rhēgnymi*, to burst forth] Suffix denoting excessive or unusual discharge.

-rrhaphy [G. *rhaphē*, suture] Suffix denoting surgical suturing.

-rrhoea [G. *rhoia*, a flow] Suffix denoting a flowing or flux.

rubefa'cient [L. *rubi-facio*, fr. *ruber*, red, + *facio*, to make] **1.** Causing a reddening of the skin. **2.** A counterirritant that produces erythema when applied to the skin surface.

rubel'la [L. *rubellus*, fem. *-a*, reddish] German measles; an acute exanthematous disease caused by rubella virus (*Rubivirus*) and marked by enlargement of lymph nodes, usually with little fever or constitutional reaction;

of importance because of the high incidence of abnormalities in children from infection during the first several months of fetal life.

rubeo'la [Mod. L. dim. of *ruber*, red, reddish] Used as a synonym for two different virus diseases of man: measles and rubella.

ru'bor [L.]. Redness, as one of the four signs of inflammation (r., calor, dolor, tumor) enunciated by Celsus.

ru'ga, pl. **ru'gae** [L. a wrinkle] [NA] A fold, ridge, or crease; a wrinkle.

ru'gose, ru'gous [L. *rugosus*] Marked by rugae; wrinkled.

rup'ture [L. *ruptura*, a break, fracture] **1.** Hernia. **2.** A tear of solution of continuity; a break of any organ or other of the soft parts.

S

sac [L. *saccus*, a bag] **1.** A pouch or bursa. **2.** An encysted abscess at the root of a tooth. **3.** The capsule of a tumour, or envelope of a cyst.

   amniotic s., amnion.

saccad'ic [Fr. *saccade*, sudden check of a horse] Jerky.

sac'charides Carbohydrates; classified as mono-, di-, tri-, and polysaccharides according to the number of monosaccharide groups composing them.

sac'charin A sugar substitute; in dilute aqueous solution, 300 to 500 times sweeter than sucrose.

sac'charine Relating to sugar; sweet.

saccharo-, acchar-, acchari- [G. *sakcharon*, sugar] Combining forms denoting sugar.

saccula'tion 1. A structure formed by a group of sacs. **2.** Formation of a sac or pouch.

sac'cule Sacculus.

   s. of larynx, *sacculus* laryngis.

sac'culus, pl. **sac'culi** [L. dim. of *saccus*, sac] [NA] The smaller of the two membranous sacs in the vestibule of the labyrinth.

   s. laryn'gis [NA], a small diverticulum extending upward from the ventricle of the larynx between the vestibular fold and the lamina of the thyroid cartilage.

sac'cus, pl. **sac'ci** [L. a bag, sack] [NA] A sac.

   s. lacrima'lis [NA], the upper portion of the nasolacrimal duct into which empty the two lacrimal canaliculi.

sa'cral Relating to or in the neighbourhood of the sacrum.

sacro-, sacr- [L. *sacrum, q.v.*] Combining forms denoting the sacrum.

sa'crococcyg'eal Relating to both sacrum and coccyx.

sacroil'iac Relating to the sacrum and the ilium.

sacrover'tebral Relating to the sacrum and the vertebrae above.

sa'crum, pl. **sa'cra** [L. sacred bone, fr. *sacer,* sacred] *Os* sacrum.

sad'dle Sella; a structure shaped like, or suggestive of, a seat or saddle.

sa'dism [Marquis de *Sade*] A form of sexual perversion in which the subject finds pleasure in inflicting pain.

sadomas'ochism [sadism + masochism] A form of sexual perversion marked by love of cruelty in its active and/or passive form.

sag'ittal [L. *sagitta,* an arrow] **1.** Resembling an arrow. **2.** In the line of an arrow shot from a bow, *i.e.,* in an anteroposterior direction.

salicyl'amide The amide of salicylic acid, an analgesic, antipyretic and antiarthritic, similar in action to aspirin.

salic'ylate A salt or ester of salicylic acid.

salicyl'ic acid A component of aspirin; also used externally as a keratolytic agent, antiseptic, and fungicide.

sa'line 1. Relating to, of the nature of, or containing salt; salty. **2.** A salt solution.

   physiological s., an isotonic aqueous solution of salts in which cells will remain alive for a time; contains 0.9% sodium chloride.

sali'va [L. akin to G. *sialon*] Spittle; a slightly acid viscid fluid, consisting of the secretion from the parotid, sublingual, and submaxillary salivary glands and the mucous glands of the oral cavity; keeps the mucous membrane of the mouth moist, lubricates food during mastication, and converts starch into maltose.

sal'ivary [L. *salivarius*] Relating to saliva.

saliva'tion Sialism.

Salmonel'la [D. E. *Salmon*] A genus of aerobic to facultatively anaerobic Gram-negative bacteria (family Enterobacteriaceae) that are pathogenic for man and other animals. The type species is *S. cholerae-suis.*

   S. chol'erae-su'is, a species which occurs in pigs, and occasionally causes acute gastroenteritis and enteric fever in humans; the type species of the genus *S.*

   S. enterit'idis, a species that causes gastroenteritis in humans.

   S. hirschfeld'ii, a species causing enteric fever in man.

   S. paraty'phi, a species causing enteric fever in man.

   S. schottmül'leri, a species causing enteric fever in man.

   S. ty'phi, typhoid bacillus; a species found in cases of typhoid fever and in contaminated water and food.

   S. typhimu'rium, a species causing food poisoning in humans.

   S. typho'sa, *S. typhi.*

sal'monello'sis [*Salmonella* + G. *-osis,* condition] Infection with organisms of the genus *Salmonella.*

salping- See salpingo-.

salpingec'tomy [salping- + G. *ektomē,* excision] Removal of the fallopian tube.

sal'pingemphrax'is [salping- + G. *emphraxis,* a stopping] Obstruction of the eustachian or fallopian tube.

salpingi'tis [salping- + G. *-itis,* inflammation] Inflammation of the fallopian or the eustachian tube.

salpingo-, salping- [G. *salpinx,* trumpet (tube)] Combining forms denoting a tube, usually the fallopian or eustachian tubes, See also tubo-.

salpin'gocele [salpingo- + G. *kēle,* hernia] Hernia of a fallopian tube.

salpingog'raphy [salpingo- + G. *graphō,* to write] Radiographic imaging of the uterine tubes after the injection of a radiopaque substance.

salpingol'ysis [salpingo- + G. *lysis,* loosening] Freeing the fallopian tube from adhesions.

salpin'go-oophorec'tomy Removal of the ovary and its fallopian tube.

salpin'go-oophori'tis Inflammation of both fallopian tube and ovary.

salpin'goplasty [salpingo- + G. *plassō,* to fashion] Plastic operation upon the uterine tubes.

salpingos'tomy [salpingo- + G. *stoma,* mouth] Establishment of an artificial opening in a fallopian tube in which the fimbriated extremity has been closed by inflammation.

salpingot'omy [salpingo- + G. *tomē,* incision] Incision into a fallopian tube.

sal'pinx, pl. **salpin'ges** [G. a trumpet (tube)] **1.** Uterine *tube.* **2.** Auditory *tube.*

salt 1. A compound formed by the interaction of an acid and a base, the hydrogen atoms of the acid being replaced by the positive ion of the base. **2.** Sodium chloride, the prototypical salt. **3.** A saline cathartic (magnesium sulphate, sodium sulphate, or potassium sodium tartrate); often called salts.

    Epsom s.'s, *magnesium* sulphate.

    smelling s.'s, ammonium carbonate, scented with aromatic oils and sniffed as a general stimulant.

salve [A.S. *sealf*] Ointment.

sanato'rium [Mod. L. neuter of *sanatorius,* curative] An institution for the treatment of chronic diseases and for recuperation under medical supervision; often improperly called sanitarium.

sangui-, sanguin-, sanguino- [G. *sanguis,* blood] Combining forms meaning blood, bloody.

sanguifa'cient [sangui- + L. *facio,* to make] Haemopoietic.

sanguif'erous [sangui- + L. *fero,* to carry] Conveying blood.

sanguin'eous [L. *sanguineus*] Relating to blood; bloody.

sanitar'ium [L. *sanitas,* health] A health resort, as contrasted with sanatorium.

san'itary [L. *sanitus,* health] Healthful; conducive to health; usually in reference to a clean environment.

sanita'tion [L. *sanitas,* health] The establishment and use of measures designed to promote health and prevent disease.

saphe'nous [G. *saphēnēs,* clearly visible] Relating to or associated with a saphenous vein; denoting a number of structures in the leg.

sapo-, sapon- [L. *sapo,* soap] Combining forms relating to soap.

sapona'ceous Soapy; relating to or resembling soap.

sapon'ifica'tion [L. *sapo,* soap, + *facio,* to make] Conversion into soap; denoting the hydrolytic action of an alkali upon fat.

sapro-, sapr- [G. *sapros,* rotten] Combining forms denoting rotten, putrid, decayed.

sap'robe [sapro- + G. *bios,* life] An organism that lives upon dead organic material. This term is preferable to saprophyte, since bacteria and fungi are no longer regarded as plants.

saprogen'ic, saprog'enous Causing or resulting from decay.

sap'rophyte [sapro- + G. *phyton,* plant] See saprobe.

sarco- [G. *sarx* (sark-), flesh] Combining form denoting muscular substance or a resemblance to flesh.

sar'cocele [sarco- + G. *kēlē,* tumour] A fleshy tumour or sarcoma of the testis.

sar'coid [sarco- + G. *eidos,* resemblance] **1.** Sarcoidosis. **2.** A tumour resembling a sarcoma.

    Boeck's s., sarcoidosis.

sarcoido'sis [sarcoid + G. *-osis,* condition] A systemic granulomatous disease of unknown cause, especially involving the lungs with resulting fibrosis, but also involving lymph nodes, skin, liver, spleen, eyes, phalangeal bones, and parotid glands; granulomas are composed of epithelioid and multinucleated giant cells with little or no necrosis.

sarcolem'ma [sarco- + G. *lemma,* husk] The plasma membrane of a muscle fibre.

sarco'ma [G. *sarkōma,* a fleshy excrescence, fr. *sarx,* flesh, + *-oma,* tumour] A connective tissue neoplasm, usually highly malignant, formed by proliferation of mesodermal cells.

    Kaposi's s., a multifocal malignant or benign neoplasm of primitive vasoformative tissue, occurring in the skin and sometimes in lymph nodes or viscera; consists of spindle cells and small vascular spaces frequently infiltrated by haemosiderin-pigmented macrophages

    osteogenic s., the most common and malignant of bone s.'s, which arises from bone-forming cells and affects chiefly the ends of long bones.

sar'comato'sis [sarcoma + G. *-osis,* condition] Occurrence of several sarcomatous growths on different parts of the body.

sarcom'atous Relating to or of the nature of sarcoma.

Sarcop'tes scabie'i [sarco- + G. *koptō,* to cut; L. *scabies,* scurf] The itch mite, varieties of which affect man and various domestic and wild animals, and cause scabies and mange.

sarco'sis [G. *sarkōsis,* the growth of flesh] **1.** An abnormal increase of flesh. **2.** A multiple growth of fleshy tumours. **3.** A diffuse sarcoma involving the whole of an organ.

sardon'ic grin [G. *sardanios, sardonios,* an epithet of bitter, scornful laughter] *Risus sardonicus.*

sat'urnine [L. *saturnus,* lead, fr. *saturnis,* the god and planet Saturn] **1.** Relating to lead. **2.** Due to or symptomatic of lead poisoning.

satyri'asis [G. *satyros,* a satyr] Excessive sexual excitement and behaviour in the male.

sau'ceriza'tion Excavation of tissue to form a shallow depression, performed in wound treatment to facilitate drainage from infected areas.

saxitox'in A potent neurotoxin found in shellfish, such as the mussel or the clam, produced by the dinoflagellate *Gonyaulax catenella,* which is ingested by the shellfish.

scab [A.S. *scaeb*] A crust formed by coagulation of blood, pus, serum, or a combination of these, on the surface of an ulcer, erosion, or other type of wound.

sca'bicide An agent lethal to itch mites.

sca'bies [L. fr. *scabo,* to scratch] A skin eruption due to the female *Sarcoptes scabiei* var. *hominis,* which burrows into the skin, producing a vesicular eruption with intense pruritus between the fingers, on the male genitalia, buttocks, and elsewhere on the trunk and extremities.

sca'la, pl. **sca'lae** [L. a stairway] [NA] One of the cavities of the cochlea winding spirally around the modiolus.

     s. tym'pani [NA], the division of the spiral canal of the cochlea lying below the lamina spiralis.

     s. vestib'uli [NA], vestibular canal; the division of the spiral canal of the cochlea lying above the lamina spiralis and vestibular membrane.

scald [L. *excaldo,* to wash in hot water] **1.** To burn by contact with a hot liquid or steam. **2.** The lesion resulting from such contact.

scale [L. *scala,* a stairway] **1.** A strip of metal, glass, or other substance, marked off in lines, for measuring. **2.** A standardized test for measuring psychological, personality, or behavioural characteristics. [O.E. *scealu,* fr. O.Fr. *escale,* shell, husk] **3.** Squama. **4.** A small thin plate of horny epithelium, resembling a fish s., cast off from the skin. **5.** To desquamate. **6.** To remove tartar from the teeth.

     Celsius s., centigrade s., the temperature s. in which there are 100 degrees between the freezing point (0°C) and boiling point (100°C) of water at sea level.

     Fahrenheit s., a thermometer s., in which the freezing point of water is 32°F and the boiling point of water 212°F.

     Kelvin s., a s. in which temperature is measured in degrees Celsius from absolute zero ($-273.16°C$).

scalp [M. E. fr. Scand. *skalpr,* sheath] The skin covering the cranium.

scal'pel [L. *scalpellum;* dim. of *scalprum,* a knife] A knife used in surgical dissection.

scan **1.** To move a beam in search of a structure; *e.g.,* to move an ultrasonic beam to make a trace follow in synchronism. **2.** In computed tomography, the mechanical motion of the CT machine required to produce the image(s).

scan'ning [L. *scando,* to climb] Determination of the distribution of a specific radioactive element or compound or an internally administered radiopharmaceutical in the body by recording the emitted ray on a photographic film.

scaph'a [L. fr. G. *skaphē,* skiff] [NA] **1.** A boat-shaped structure. **2.** The longitudinal furrow between the helix and the antihelix of the auricle.

scapho- [G. *skaphē,* skiff, boat] Combining form denoting scapha or scaphoid.

scaphocephal'ic, scapho-
ceph'alous [scapho- + G. *kephalē,* head] Denoting a long narrow skull with a ridge along the prematurely ossified sagittal suture.

scaph'oid [scapho- + G. *eidos,* resemblance] Boat-shaped; hollowed.

scap'ula, pl. **scap'ulae** [L.] [NA] The shoulder blade; a large triangular flattened bone lying over the ribs, posteriorly on either side, articulating laterally with the clavicle and the humerus.

scapulo- [L. *scapulae,* shoulder blades] Combining form denoting scapula or scapular.

scapulohu'meral Relating to both scapula and humerus.

scar [G. *eschara,* scab] The fibrous tissue replacing normal tissues destroyed by injury or disease.

scar'ifica'tion [L. *scarifico,* to scratch] The making of a number of superficial incisions in the skin.

scarlati'na [through It. fr. Med. L. *scarlatum*, scarlet, a scarlet cloth] Scarlet fever; an acute exanthematous disease caused by streptococcal erythrogenic toxin and marked by fever and other constitutional disturbances, and a generalized eruption of closely aggregated points or small macules of a bright red colour, followed by desquamation.

scato- [G. *skōr* (*skat-*), faeces, excrement] Combining forms denoting faeces. See also copro-, sterco-.

scatol'ogy [scato- + G. *logos*, study] **1.** The study and analysis of the faeces for physiologic and diagnostic purposes. **2.** The study relating to the psychiatric aspects of excrement or the oxeromental (anal) function.

schisto- [G. *schistos*, split] Combining form denoting split or cleft. See also schizo.

Schistoso'ma [schisto- + G. *sōma*, body] A genus of trematodes, including the important blood flukes of man and domestic animals, that cause schistosomiasis.

 S. haemato'bium, the vesical blood fluke, a species with terminally spined eggs that occurs as a parasite in the portal system and mesenteric veins of the bladder (causing human schistosomiasis haematobium) and rectum; found along waterways, irrigation ditches, or streams throughout Africa and in parts of the Middle East; intermediate hosts are snails of the subfamily Bulininae (*Bulinus, Physopsis, Pyrgophysa*).

 S. japon'icum, the Oriental or Japanese blood fluke, a species having eggs with small lateral spines, causes schistosomiasis japonicum, with extensive pathology from on capsulation of the eggs, particularly in the liver; intermediate hosts are amphibious snails (species of *Oncomelania,* family Amnicolidae); many domestic animals serve as reservoir hosts.

 S. manso'ni, a common species in Africa, parts of the Middle East, the West Indies, South America, and certain Caribbean islands and the cause of human schistosomiasis mansoni; characterized by large eggs with a strong lateral spine and transmitted by snails of the genus *Biomphalaria.*

schis'tosome Common name for a member of the genus *Schistosoma.*

schis'tosomi'asis Infection with a species of *Schistosoma;* manifestations of which vary with the infecting species but depend in large measure upon tissue reaction (granula-tion and fibrosis) to the eggs deposited in venules and in the hepatic portals, the latter resulting in portal hypertension and oesophageal varices, as well as liver damage leading to cirrhosis.

schizo-, schiz- [G. *schizō*, to split or cleave] Combining forms denoting split, cleft, or division. See also schisto-.

schiz'oid [schizo(phrenia), + G. *eidos*, resemblance] **1.** Schizophrenia-like; resembling the personality characteristic of schizophrenia, but in milder form. **2.** Also used to describe the withdrawal or "shut-in-ness" of the introverted personality.

schizophre'nia [schizo- + G. *phrēn*, mind] A term synonymous with and replacing dementia praecox; the most common type of psychosis, characterized by a disorder in the thinking processes, such as delusions and hallucinations, and extensive withdrawal of the individual's interest from other people and the outside world, and the investment of it in one's own; now considered a group of mental disorders rather than as a single entity.

 catatonic s., s. characterized by marked disturbances in activity, with either generalized inhibition or excessive activity.

 paranoid s., s. characterized predominantly by delusions of persecution and megalomania.

schizophren'ic Relating to or suffering from one of the schizophrenias.

sciat'ic [Med. L. *sciaticus*, fr. G. *ischion*, the hip joint] **1.** Relating to or situated in the neighbourhood of the ischium or hip. **2.** Relating to sciatica.

sciat'ica [see sciatic] Pain in the lower back and hip radiating down the back of the thigh into the leg, usually due to herniated lumbar disc.

scin'tigram [fr. L. *scintilla*, spark, + G. *gramma*, something written] Scintiscan.

scintig'raphy Scintiphotography.

scintilla'tion [L. *scintilla*, a spark] **1.** A flashing or sparkling; a subjective sensation of sparks or flashes of light. **2.** In nuclear medicine, the light emitted when an x- or gamma ray is absorbed by a crystal or liquid radiation detector.

scin'tiphotog'raphy The process of obtaining a photographic recording of the distribution of an internally administered radiopharmaceutical with the use of a stationary scintillation detector device, a gamma camera.

scin'tiscan The record obtained by scanning; the photographic display of the distribution of an internally administered radiopharmaceutical.

scir'rhous Hard; indurated.

scissu'ra, pl. **scissu'rae** [L.] **1.** A cleft or fissure. **2.** A splitting.

scle'ra, pl. **scle'ras, scle'rae** [Mod. L. fr. G. *sklēros,* hard] [NA] White of the eye; a fibrous tunic forming the outer envelope of the eye, except for its anterior sixth occupied by the cornea.

scle'ral Sclerotic; relating to the sclera.

sclerec'tomy [scler- + G. *ektomē,* excision] **1.** Excision of a portion of the sclera. **2.** Removal of the fibrous adhesions formed in chronic otitis media.

sclere'ma [scler- + oedema] Induration of the subcutaneous fat.

scleri'tis Inflammation of the sclera.

sclero-, scler- [G. *sklēros,* hard] Combining forms denoting hardness (induration), sclerosis, or relationship to the sclera.

sclerocor'nea 1. The cornea and sclera regarded as forming together the hard outer coat of the eye. **2.** A congenital anomaly in which the whole or part of the cornea is opaque and resembles the sclera; other ocular abnormalities are frequently present.

scleroder'ma [sclero- + G. *derma,* skin] Thickening of the skin caused by swelling and thickening of fibrous tissue, with eventual atrophy of the epidermis; a manifestation of progressive systemic sclerosis and used synonymously for that disease.

    circumscribed s., morphoea.

sclero'ma [G. *sklērōma,* an induration] A circumscribed indurated focus of granulation tissue in the skin or mucous membrane.

sclerose' To harden; to undergo sclerosis.

sclero'sis [G. *sklērōsis,* hardness] **1.** Induration of chronic inflammatory origin. **2.** In neuropathy, induration of nervous and other structures by a hyperplasia of the interstitial fibrous or glial connective tissue.

    amyotrophic lateral s., Charcot's disease; a disease of the motor tracts of the lateral columns and anterior horns of the spinal cord, causing progressive muscular atrophy, increased reflexes, fibrillary twitching, and spastic irritability of muscles.

    arterial s., arteriosclerosis.

    multiple s. (MS), the occurrence of patches of s. (plaques) in the brain and spinal cord, causing some degree of paralysis, tremor, nystagmus, and disturbances of speech, the various symptoms depending upon the seat of the lesions; occurs chiefly in early adult life, with characteristic exacerbations and remissions.

    progressive systemic s., a systemic disease characterized by formation of hyalinized and thickened collagenous fibrous tissue, with thickening of the skin and adhesion to underlying tissues, especially of the hands and face.

scleros'tomy [sclero- + G. *stoma,* mouth] Surgical perforation of the sclera, as for the relief of glaucoma.

sclerother'apy Treatment involving the injection of a sclerosing solution into vessels or tissues.

sclerot'ic 1. Relating to or characterized by sclerosis. **2.** Scleral.

sclerot'omy [sclero- + G. *tomē,* incision] An incision through the sclerotic coat of the eye.

sco'lex, pl. **sco'leces, sco'lices** [G. *skōlēx,* a worm] The head or anterior end of a tapeworm; attached by suckers and, frequently, by rostellar hooks to the wall of the intestine, the wide variety of the form of the s. characterizes the orders of cestodes.

scolio'sis [G. *skoliōsis,* a crookedness] A lateral curvature of the spine; depending on aetiology, there may be just one curve, or primary and secondary compensatory curves, which may be fixed as a result of muscle and/or bone deformity, or mobile as a result of unequal muscle contraction.

-scope [G. *skopeō,* to view] Suffix usually denoting an instrument for viewing but extended to include other methods of examination.

scopol'amine Hyoscine; an alkaloid found in the leaves and seeds of solanaceous plants; the 6,7-epoxide of atropine.

-scopy [G. *skopeō,* to view] Suffix denoting an action or activity involving the use of an instrument for viewing.

scorbu'tic [Med. L. *scorbutus,* fr. Teutonic *schorbuych,* scurvy] Relating to scurvy.

scoto- [G. *skotos,* darkness] Combining form denoting darkness.

scoto'ma [G. *skotōma,* vertigo, fr. *skotos,* darkness] **1.** An isolated area of varying size and shape, within the visual field, in which vision is absent or depressed. **2.** A blind spot in psychological awareness.

mental s., absence of insight into, or inability to grasp, a mental problem.

physiological s., blind spot (1); a negative scotoma in the visual field, corresponding to the optic disc.

scoto'pic Referring to low illumination to which the eye is dark-adapted.

scotop'sin The protein moiety of the pigment in the rods of the retina.

screen'ing 1. Examination of a group of usually asymptomatic individuals to detect those with a high probability of having a given disease, typically by means of an inexpensive diagnostic test. **2.** In psychiatry, initial patient evaluation that includes medical and psychiatric history, mental status evaluation, and diagnostic formulation to determine the patient's suitability or a particular treatment modality.

screw-worm The larve of the botfly, *Cochliomyia hominivorax,* and other similar forms that cause human and animal myiasis.

scro'tum, pl. **scro'ta, scro'tums** [L.] [NA] The musculocutaneous sac containing the testes, formed of skin, a network of nonstriated muscular fibres (dartos), cremasteric fascia, cremaster muscle, and the serous coverings of the testes and epididymides.

scurf [A.S.] Dandruff.

scur'vy [fr. A.S. scurf] A disease marked by inanition, debility, anaemia, oedema of the dependent parts, a spongy condition, sometimes with ulceration, of the gums, and haemorrhages into the skin and from the mucous membranes; due to a deficiency of sources of vitamin C in the diet.

scy'balum, pl. **scy'bala** [G. *skybalon,* excrement] A hard round mass of inspissated faeces.

sea'sickness Mal de mer; a form of motion sickness caused by the motion of a floating platform or vessel.

seba'ceous [L. *sebaceus*] Relating to sebum; oily; fatty.

sebo-, seb-, sebi- [L. *sebum,* suet, tallow] Combining forms denoting sebum, sebaceous.

seborrhoe'a [sebo- + G. *rhoia,* a flow] Overactivity of the sebaceous glands, resulting in an excessive amount of sebum.

seborrhoe'ic Relating to seborrhoea.

se'bum [L. tallow] Secretions of the sebaceous glands.

secre'ta [L. *secretus,* pp. of *se-cerno,* to separate] Secretions.

secre'tin A hormone, formed by the epithelial cells of the duodenum under the stimulus of acid contents from the stomach, that incites secretion of pancreatic juice.

gastric s., gastrin.

secre'tion [see secreta] **1.** Production by a cell or gland of some substance differing in chemical and physical properties from the body from which or by which it is produced. **2.** The product, solid, liquid, or gaseous, of cellular or glandular activity that is stored in or utilized by the organism in which it is produced.

secre'toinhib'itory Restraining or curbing secretion.

secre'tomo'tor, secre'tomo'tory Stimulating secretion.

sec'tion [L. *sectio,* a cutting] **1.** The act of cutting. **2.** A cut or division. **3.** A segment or part of any organ or structure delimited from the remainder. **4.** A cut surface. **5.** A thin slice of tissue, cells, microorganisms, or any material for examination under the microscope.

caesarean s. [so called not because performed at the birth of Julius Caesar, but because included under *lex cesarea,* Roman law], incision through the abdominal wall and the uterus (abdominohysterotomy) for extraction of the fetus.

seda'tion [L. *sedatio,* to calm, allay] The act of calming, especially by the administration of a sedative, or the state of being calm.

sed'ative [see sedation] **1.** Calming; quieting. **2.** An agent that quiets nervous excitement, designated according to the part or the organ upon which their specific action is exerted.

sed'iment [L. *sedimentum* a settling] **1.** An insoluble material that sinks to the bottom of a liquid. **2.** To cause, or effect, the formation of a sediment or deposit.

seg'ment [L. *segmentum,* fr. *seco,* to cut] **1.** A section; a part of an organ or other structure delimited naturally, artificially, or in the imagination from the remainder. **2.** A territory of an organ having independent function, supply, or drainage.

segrega'tion [L. *segrego,* pp. *-atus,* to set apart, separate] **1.** Separation; removal of certain parts from a mass. **2.** Separation of contrasting characters in the offspring of heterozygotes. **3.** Separation of the paired state of genes which occurs at the reduction division of meiosis.

sei'zure [O. Fr. *seisir*, to grasp, take possession of] An attack; the sudden onset of a disease or of certain symptoms, such as convulsions.

self 1. A sum of the attitudes and behavioural predispositions that make up the personality. **2.** The individual as represented in his own awareness and in his environment.

self-lim'ited Denoting a disease that tends to cease after a definite period, as a result of its own processes.

sel'la [L. saddle] Saddle.

s. tur'cica, [Turkish saddle] [NA], a saddle-like prominence on the upper surface of the sphenoid bone, situated in the middle cranial fossa and dividing it into two halves.

se'men, pl. **semi'na, se'mens** [L. *semen*, seed] **1.** [NA] Seminal fluid; the penile ejaculate, containing spermatozoa; a mixture of the secretions of the testes, seminal vesicles, prostate, and bulbourethral glands. **2.** A seed.

semi- [L. *semis*, half] Prefix denoting one-half or partly, corresponding to *hemi-*.

semico'ma A mild degree of coma from which it is possible to arouse the patient.

semico'matose Denoting semicoma.

semilu'nar [semi- + L. *luna*, moon] Lunar (2).

sem'inal Relating to the semen.

seminif'erous [L. *semen*, seed, + *fero*, to carry] Carrying or conducting the semen; denoting the tubules of the testis.

semino'ma [L. *semen*, seed, + G. *-oma*, tumour] A malignant testicular neoplasm, arising from the sex cells in young male adults, which metastasizes to the paraortic lymph nodes.

semiper'meable Permeable to water and small ions or molecules, but not to larger molecules or colloidal matter.

senes'cence [L. *senesco*, to grow old, fr. *senex*, old] The state or process of growing old.

senil'ity Old age; the sum of the physical and mental changes occurring in advanced life.

seno'pia [L. *senilis*, senile, + G. *ōps*, eye] An improvement in near vision in the aged caused by the myopia of increasing lenticular

nuclear sclerosis, a precursor of eventual nuclear cataract.

sensa'tion [L. *sensatio*, perception, feeling] A feeling; the translation into consciousness of the effects of a stimulus exciting any of the organs of sense.

sense [L. *sentio*, pp. *sensus*, to feel, to perceive] Feeling; sensation; consciousness; the faculty of perceiving any stimulus.

pressure s., the faculty of discriminating various degrees of pressure on the body's surface.

special s., one of the five senses related to the organs of sight, hearing, smell, taste, and touch.

visceral s., the perception of the existence of the internal organs.

sen'sible [L. *sensibilis*, fr. *sentio*, to feel, perceive] **1.** Perceptible to the senses. **2.** Capable of sensation.

sen'sitive 1. Capable of perceiving sensations. **2.** Responding to a stimulus. **3.** Acutely perceptive of interpersonal situations **4.** In immunology, denoting 1) a sensitized antigen; 2) one who has been rendered susceptible to immunological reactions by previous exposure of the immunological system to the antigen concerned.

sensitiv'ity [L. *sentio*, pp. *sensus*, to feel] **1.** The state of being sensitive. **2.** The proportion of individuals with a positive test result for the disease that the test is intended to reveal, *i.e.,* true positive results as a proportion of the total of true positive and false negative results.

sen'sitiza'tion Immunization, especially with reference to antigens (immunogens) not associated with infection; the induction of acquired sensitivity or allergy.

sensori- [L. *sensorius*, sensory] Combining form denoting sensory.

sen'sorimo'tor Both sensory and motor, denoting a mixed nerve with afferent and efferent fibres.

sen'sory [L. *sensorius*, fr. *sensus*, sense] Relating to sensation.

sep'sis, pl. **sep'ses** [G. *sēpsis*, putrefaction] Presence of various pus-forming and other pathogenic organisms, or their toxins, in the blood or tissues.

sep'tal Relating to a septum.

sep'tate [L. *saeptum*, septum] Having a septum; divided into compartments.

septi-, sept- [L. *septem*, seven] Combining forms meaning seven.

sep'tic Relating to or caused by sepsis.

septicae'mia [G. *sēpsis*, putrefaction, + *haima*, blood] Systemic disease caused by the multiplication of microorganisms in the circulating blood.

sep'tum, pl. **sep'ta** [L. *saeptum*, a partition] [NA] A thin wall dividing two cavities or masses of softer tissue.

 s. interatria'le [NA], **interatrial s.,** the wall between the atria of the heart.

 s. interventriculа're [NA], **interventricular s.,** the wall between the ventricles of the heart.

 s. na'si [NA], **nasal s.,** the wall dividing the nasal cavity into halves, composed of a central supporting skeleton covered by a mucous membrane.

seque'la, pl **seque'lae** [L. a sequel, fr. *sequor*, to follow] A morbid condition following as a consequence of a disease.

sequestra'tion [L. *sequestratio*, fr. *sequestro*, pp. -*atus*, to lay aside] **1.** Formation of a sequestrum. **2.** Loss of blood or of its fluid content into spaces within the body so that it is withdrawn from the circulating volume.

seques'trum, pl. **seques'tra** [Med. L. *sequestrum*, something laid aside] A piece of necrosed tissue, usually bone, that has become separated from the surrounding healthy tissue.

se'ra Plural of serum.

ser'ine (Ser) One of the amino acids occurring in proteins.

sero- [L. *serum*, whey] Combining form denoting serum or serous.

serolog'ic Relating to serology.

serol'ogy [sero- + G. *logos*, study] The branch of science concerned with serum, especially with specific immune or lytic serums.

seromu'cous Pertaining to a mixture of watery and mucinous material such as that of certain glands.

sero'sa, pl. **sero'sae** [fem. of Mod. L. *serosus*, serous] **1.** *Tunica serosa.* **2.** The outermost of the extraembryonic membranes that encloses the embryo and all its other membranes.

se'rosanguin'eous Composed of or containing serum and blood.

serosi'tis Inflammation of a serous membrane.

seroto'nin A vasoconstrictor, liberated by the blood platelets, that inhibits gastric secretion and stimulates smooth muscle; present in relatively high concentrations in some areas of the CNS, and occurs in many peripheral tissues and cells and in carcinoid tumours.

se'rous Relating to, containing, or producing serum or a substance having a watery consistency.

serpig'inous [Med. L. *serpigo* (-gin), ringworm] Creeping; denoting an ulcer or other cutaneous lesion that extends with an arciform border and has a wavy margin.

se'rum, pl. **se'rums** or **se'ra** [L. whey] **1.** A clear watery fluid, especially that moistening surface of serous membranes, or exuded in inflammation of any of those membranes. **2.** The fluid portion of the blood obtained after removal of the fibrin clot and blood cells; sometimes used as a synonym for antiserum or antitoxin.

ses'sile [L. *sessilis*, low-growing, fr. *sedeo*, pp. *sessus*, to sit] Having a broad base of attachment; not pedunculated.

set 1. A readiness to perceive or to respond in some way; an attitude which facilitates or predetermines an outcome. **2.** To reduce a fracture; to bring the bones back into a normal position or alinement.

sex [L. *sexus*] **1.** The character or quality that distinguishes between male and female as expressed in the nature of the sex chromosomes, the gonads, and the accessory sexual organs, as contrasted with gender role. **2.** The physiological and psychological processes within an individual which prompt behaviour related to procreation and/or erotic pleasure.

sex'ual [L. *sexualis*, fr. *sexus*, sex] **1.** Relating to sex; erotic; genital. **2.** Denoting a person considered in his or her s. relation or tendencies.

sexual'ity The sum of a person's sexual behaviours and tendencies, and the latter's strength; the quality of having sexual functions or implications.

shaft [A.S. *sceaft*] An elongated rodlike structure, as the part of a long bone between the epiphyseal extremities.

shank [A.S. *sceanca*] The tibia; the shin; the leg or a leglike part.

sheath [A.S. *scaeth*] **1.** Any enveloping structure. **2.** Vagina (1).

myelin s., medullary s., the lipopro-teinaceous envelope in vertebrates sur-rounding most axons of more than 0.5-μm diameter; consists of a double plasma mem-brane wound tightly around the axon and sup-plied by oligodendroglia cells (in the brain and spinal cord) or Schwann cells (in periph-eral nerves).

Shigel'la [K. *Shiga*] A genus of Gram-nega-tive bacteria (family Enterobacteriaceae) whose normal habitat is the intestinal tract and which produce dysentery. The type spe-cies is *S. dysenteriae*.

S. boy'dii, a species that occurs in a low proportion of cases of bacillary dysentery.

S. dysenter'iae, a species causing dysentery.

S. flexne'ri, a species that is the most common cause of dysentery epidemics and sometimes of infantile gastroenteritis.

S. son'nei, a species causing mild dys-entery and also summer diarrhoea in chil-dren.

shigello'sis Bacillary dysentery caused by bacteria of the genus *Shigella*, often occur-ring in epidemic patterns.

shin [A.S. *scina*] The anterior portion of the leg.

shin'gles [L. *cingulum*, girdle] *Herpes zoster.*

shin-splints Tenderness and pain with induration and swelling of pretibial muscles, following athletic overexertion by the un-trained.

shock 1. A sudden physical or mental dis-turbance. **2.** A state of profound mental and physical depression consequent upon severe physical injury or an emotional disturbance. **3.** The abnormally palpable impact, appreci-ated by a hand on the chest wall, of an accen-tuated heart sound.

anaphylactic s., a severe, often fatal form of s. characterized by smooth muscle contraction and capillary dilation initiated by cytotropic (IgE class) antibodies.

cardiogenic s., s. resulting from de-cline in cardiac output secondary to serious heart disease, usually myocardial infarction.

haemorrhagic s., hypovolaemic s. re-sulting from acute haemorrhage, character-ized by hypotension, tachycardia, pale, cold, and clammy skin, and oliguria.

hypovolaemic s., s. caused by a re-duction in volume of blood, as from haemor-rhage or dehydration.

insulin s., s. produced by overdosage of insulin, characterized by sweating, tremor, anxiety, vertigo, and diplopia, followed by de-lirium, convulsions, and collapse.

short-sight'edness Myopia.

shoul'der [A.S. *sculder*] The lateral por-tion of the scapular region, where the scapula joins with the clavicle and humerus and is covered by the rounded mass of the deltoid muscle.

frozen s., adhesive *capsulitis*.

shoulder blade Scapula.

show [A.S. *sceáwe*] An appearance; specifi-cally: **(1)** the first appearance of blood in beginning menstruation; **(2)** a sign of impend-ing labour, characterized by the discharge from the vagina of a small amount of blood-tinged mucus which represents the extrusion of the mucous plug that has filled the cervical canal during pregnancy.

shunt A bypass or diversion of accumula-tions of fluid to an absorbing or excreting system by fistulation or a mechanical device; nomenclature commonly includes origin and terminus of structures involved.

sial'agogue [sial- + G. *agōgos*, drawing forth] Promoting the flow of saliva.

si'alism, sialis'mus [G. *sialismos*] Hy-persalivation; an excess secretion of saliva.

sialo-, sial- [G. *sialon*, saliva] Combining forms denoting saliva or the salivary glands. See also ptyal-.

sial'ogogue Sialagogue.

sialog'raphy [sialo- + G. *graphō*, to write] Radiographic examination of the sali-vary glands and ducts after the introduction of a radiopaque material into the ducts.

si'alolith [sialo- + G. *lithos*, stone] A sali-vary calculus.

sib'ling, sib [A. S. *sib*, relation] One of two or more children of the same parents.

sicklae'mia Presence of sickle- or cres-cent-shaped erythrocytes in peripheral blood; seen in sickle cell anaemia and sickle cell trait.

sick'ling Production of sickle-shaped erythrocytes in the circulation.

sick'ness Disease (1).

altitude s., a syndrome caused by low inspired oxygen pressure and characterized by nausea, headache, dyspnoea, malaise, and insomnia.

decompression s., bends; a symptom complex caused by the escape from solution In body fluids of nitrogen bubbles absorbed originally at high atmospheric pressure, as a result of abrupt reduction in atmospheric pressure; characterized by headache, pain in the arms, legs, joints, and epigastrium, itching of the skin, vertigo, dyspnoea, coughing, choking, vomiting, weakness and sometimes paralysis, and severe peripheral circulatory collapse.

morning s., the nausea and vomiting of early pregnancy.

motion s., the syndrome of pallor, nausea, weakness, and malaise which may progress to vomiting and incapacitation, caused by the stimulation of the semicircular canals during travel or motion.

radiation s., the condition that follows x-radiation at levels in excess of about 100 rem; severity of the effect in dose dependent. In mild forms there are anorexia, nausea, vomiting, malaise, and leucopenia; In more severe forms there are reduction or disappearance of platelets with bleeding, reduction or disappearance of leucocytes with risk of infection, and reduction of new red cells leading to anaemia.

side effect A result of drug or other therapy In addition to or in extension of the desired therapeutic effect; usually connotes an undesirable effect.

sidero- [G. *sideros*, iron] Combining form denoting iron.

sidero'sis [sidero + G. *osis*, condition] **1.** Pneumoconiosis due to the presence of iron dust. **2.** Discoloration of any part by an iron pigment. **3.** An excess of iron in the circulating blood.

sig'moid [G. *sigma*, S, + *eidos*, resemblance] Resembling in outline the letter S or one of the forms of the Greek sigma.

sigmoidi'tis [sigmoid- + G. -*itis*, inflammation] Inflammation of the sigmoid colon.

sigmoido-, sigmoid- [G. *sigma*, S, + *eidos*, resemblance] Combining forms denoting sigmoid, usually the sigmoid colon.

sigmoi'dopexy [sigmoido- + G. *pēxis*, fixation] Operative attachment of the sigmoid colon to a firm structure to correct rectal prolapse.

sigmoi'doscope [sigmoido- + G. *skopeō*, to view] A speculum for viewing the cavity of the sigmoid colon.

sigmoidos'tomy [sigmoido- + G. *stoma*, mouth] Establishment of an artificial anus by opening into the sigmoid colon.

sign [L. *signum*, mark] **1.** Any abnormality indicative of disease, discoverable by examination; an objective symptom of disease. **2.** In psychology, any object or artefact that represents a specific thing or conveys a specific idea to the person who perceives it.

Babinski's s., (1) extension of the great toe and abduction of the other toes instead of the normal flexion reflex to plantar stimulation, considered indicative of pyramidal tract involvement; **(2)** in hemiplegia, weakness of the platysma muscle on the affected side, evident in such actions as blowing or opening the mouth; **(3)** when the patient is lying upon his back with arms crossed on the front of his chest, and attempts to assume the sitting posture, the thigh on the side of an *organic* paralysis is flexed and the heel raised, whereas the limb on the sound side remains flat; **(4)** in hemiplegia, the forearm on the affected side when placed in a position of supination turns into the pronated position.

Braxton Hicks s., irregular uterine contractions occurring after the third month of pregnancy.

Brudzinski's s., (1) in meningitis, on passive flexion of the leg on one side, a similar movement occurs in the opposite leg; **(2)** in meningitis, if the neck is passively flexed, flexion of the legs occurs.

Chaddock s., when the external malleolar skin area is irritated extension of the great toe occurs In cases of organic disease of the corticospinal reflex paths.

Chvostek's s., facial irritability In tetany, unilateral spasm being excited by a slight tap over the facial nerve.

clenched fist s., the gesture of the patient with angina pectoris by pressing a clenched fist against the chest to indicate the constricting, pressing quality of the pain.

doll's eye s., dissociation between the movements of the eyes and those of the head, the eyes being lowered as the head is raised, and the reverse; also characterized by protrusion of the eyeballs and sluggish movements of the eyes and lids; both s.'s may occur in diphtheria.

Erb-Westphal s., abolition of the patellar tendon reflex, in tabes and certain other diseases of the spinal cord, and occasionally also in brain disease.

Homans s., slight pain at the back of the knee or calf when the ankle is slowly and gently dorsiflexed (with the knee bent), indicative of incipient or established thrombosis in the veins of the leg.

Kernig's s., when the subject lies upon the back and the thigh is flexed to a right angle with the axis of the trunk, complete extension of the leg on the thigh is impossible; present in various forms of meningitis.

Leri's s., voluntary flexion of the elbow is impossible in a case of hemiplegia when the wrist on that side is passively flexed.

Lhermitte's s., sudden electric-like shocks extending down the spine when the patient flexes his head; seen in multiple sclerosis and in compression and other cervical cord disorders.

Remak's s., dissociation of the sensations of touch and of pain in tabes dorsalis and polyneuritis.

Romberg's s., if a patient standing is more unsteady with the eyes closed it indicates a loss of proprioceptive control.

Stewart-Holmes s., rebound phenomenon; the inability to check a movement when passive resistance is suddenly released, present in cerebellar deficit.

Tinel's s., a sensation of tingling, or "pins and needles," felt in the distal extremity of a limb when percussion is made over the site of an injured nerve, indicating a partial lesion or early regeneration in the nerve; sometimes called "distal tingling on percussion" (DTP).

Trendelenburg's s., in congenital dislocation of the hip, or in hip abductor weakness, if the patient stands on the dislocated leg and flexes the hip and knee on the other side the pelvis on this side will sag, whereas if normal, it will be raised on the side of the flexed hip and knee.

Trousseau's s., in latent tetany, the occurrence of carpal spasm or accoucheur's hand, elicited when the upper arm is compressed, as by a tourniquet or a blood pressure cuff.

vital s.'s, manifestation of breathing, heart beat, and sustained blood pressure.

sig'nature [L. *signum*, a sign, mark] The part of a prescription containing the directions to the patient.

sil'ica [Mod. L. fr. L. *silex*, flint] Silicon dioxide; SiO_2; the chief constituent of sand, hence of glass.

sil'icon A nonmetallic element, symbol Si, atomic no. 14, atomic weight 28.086.

sil'icone A plastic compound of silicon oxides which may be a liquid, gel, or solid, depending on the extent of polymerization.

silico'sis [L. *silex*, flint, + -*osis*, condition] A form of pneumoconiosis due to the inhalation of dust containing silica; a slowly progressive fibrosis of the lungs is a predominant feature, which may result in restrictive and obstructive impairment of lung function.

sil'ver [A.S. *seolfor*] A metallic element with a specific gravity of 10.4 to 10.7, symbol Ag, atomic no. 47, atomic weight 107.873.

s. nitrate, an antiseptic and astringent; used externally, in solution, in the prevention of ophthalmia neonatorum; also used in the special staining of the nervous system, spirochaetes, reticular fibres, Golgi apparatus, and calcium.

simula'tion [L. *simulatio*, fr. *simulo*, pp. -*atus*, to imitate] Imitation; said of a disease or symptom that resembles another, or of the feigning of illness, as by a malingerer.

sin'ciput, pl. **sincip'ita, sin'ciputs** [L. half of the head] [NA] The anterior part of the head just above and including the forehead.

sin'ew [A.S. *sinu*] A tendon.

sinis'ter (S) [L.] [NA] Left.

sinistro- [L. *sinister*, left] Combining form denoting left, or toward the left.

sin'istrotor'sion [sinistro- + L. *torsio*, a twisting (torsion)] A turning or twisting to the left.

sin'istrocar'dia [sinistro- + G. *kardia*, heart] Displacement of the heart beyond the normal position on the left side.

sinoa'trial Relating to the sinus venosus and the right atrium of the heart.

si'nus, pl. **si'nus, si'nuses** [L. *sinus*, cavity, channel, hollow] **1.** [NA] A channel for the passage of blood or lymph, which does not have the coats of an ordinary vessel, as in the gravid uterus or the cerebral meninges. **2.** [NA] A hollow in bone or other tissue. **3.** A fistula or tract leading to a suppurating cavity.

s. carot'icus [NA], **carotid s.,** a dilation of the common carotid artery at its bifurcation into external and internal carotids; contains baroreceptors which, when stimulated, cause slowing of the heart, vasodilation, and a fall in blood pressure.

s. corona'rius [NA], **coronary s.,** a short trunk receiving most of the veins of the heart, running in the posterior part of the coronary sulcus and emptying into the right atrium between the inferior vena cava and the atrioventricular orifice.

s. ethmoida'les [NA], **ethmoidal s.'s,** evaginations of the mucous membrane of the middle and superior meatuses of the nasal cavity; subdivided into s. anterior middle, and posterior s.'s.

s. fronta'lis [NA], **frontal s.,** a hollow formed on either side in the lower part of the squama of the frontal bone; communicates by the ethmoidal infundibulum with the middle meatus of the nasal cavity of the same side.

mastoid s.'s, numerous small intercommunicating cavities in the mastoid process of the temporal bone that empty into the mastoid or tympanic antrum.

s. maxilla'ris [NA], **maxillary s.,** an air cavity in the body of the maxilla, communicating with the middle meatus of the nose.

s. paranasa'les [NA], **paranasal s.'s,** paired cavities (frontal, sphenoidal, maxillary, ethmoidal) in the bones of the face lined by mucous membrane continuous with that of the nasal cavity.

s. sphenoida'lis [NA], **sphenoidal s.,** one of a pair of cavities in the body of the sphenoid bone communicating with the nasal cavity.

s. vena'rum cava'rum [NA], **s. of venae cavae,** the portion of the cavity of the right atrium of the heart that receives the blood from the venae cavae and is separated from the rest of the atrium by the crista terminalis.

s. veno'sus [NA], a cavity at the caudal end of the embryonic cardiac tube in which the veins from the intra- and extraembryonic circulatory arcs unite; in the course of development it forms the portion of the right atrium known in adult anatomy as the s. venarum cavarum.

s. veno'sus scle'rae [NA], **venous s. of the sclera,** Schlemm's canal; a ringlike vein in the sclera, near its anterior edge, encircling the cornea.

sinusi'tis [sinus + G. -*itis,* inflammation] Inflammation of the lining membrane of any sinus, especially of one of the paranasal sinuses.

si'nusoid [sinus + G. *eidos,* resemblance] **1.** Resembling a sinus. **2.** A terminal blood vessel having an irregular and larger calibre than an ordinary capillary.

si'tus inver'sus, A transposition of the viscera, the liver being on the left side, the heart on the right, etc.

skel'etal Relating to the skeleton.

skel'eton [G. *skeletos,* dried, ntr. *skeleton,* a mummy] **1.** The bony framework of the body in vertebrates (endoskeleton) or the hard outer envelope of insects (exoskeleton or dermoskeleton). **2.** All the dry parts (ligaments, cartilages, bones) remaining after the destruction and removal of the soft parts. **3.** All the bones of the body taken collectively.

skin [A.S. *scinn*] Cutis.

skull [Early Eng. *skulle,* a bowl] Cranium.

sleep [A.S. *slaep*] A physiologic state of relative unconsciousness and inaction of the voluntary muscles, the need for which recurs periodically.

paradoxical s., a deep s., with a brain wave pattern more like that of waking states than of other states of sleep, which occurs during the rapid eye movement state of s.

rapid eye movement (REM) s., that state of deep s. in which rapid eye movements, alert EEG pattern, and dreaming occur.

twilight s., **(1)** a stage of anaesthesia between s. and wakefulness in which the person is analgesic and amnestic; **(2)** formerly, a popular method of producing s. for delivery by a combination of morphine and scopolamine.

slough **1.** Necrosed tissue separated from the living structure. **2.** To separate from the living tissue, said of a dead or necrosed part.

small'pox [E. *small pocks,* or pustules] Variola; an acute eruptive contagious disease caused by a poxvirus (*Orthopoxvirus*) and marked at the onset by chills, high fever, backache, and headache, followed by papules which become umbilicated vesicles and develop into pustules; the pustules dry and form scabs which on falling off leave a permanent marking of the skin (pock marks).

smear A thin specimen for examination, usually prepared by spreading material uniformly onto a glass slide, fixing it, and staining it before examination.

Pap s., Papanicolaou s., a s. of vaginal mucosa obtained for a Pap test.

smeg'ma [G. unguent] Sebum; especially the whitish secretion that collects under the prepuce of the foreskin of the penis or of the clitoris, composed chiefly of desquamating epithelial cells.

snare [A.S. *snear*, a cord] A wire loop passed around the base of a polyp or other projection and gradually tightened to remove it.

snuf'fles Obstructed nasal respiration, especially in the newborn infant, sometimes due to congenital syphilis.

soap [A.S. *sape*, L. *sapo*, G. *sapōn*] The sodium or potassium salts of long chain fatty acids; used for cleansing purposes and as an excipient in the making of pills and suppositories.

socializa'tion [L. *socia*, partner, companion] The process of learning interpersonal and interactional skills which are in conformity with the values of one's society.

socio- [L. *socius*, companion] Combining form denoting social, society.

so'ciopath A person with antisocial personality disorder.

sock'et [thr. O. Fr. fr. L. *soccus*, a shoe, a sock] **1.** The hollow part of a joint; the excavation in one bone of a joint which receives the articular end of the other bone. **2.** Any hollow or concavity into which another part fits, as the eye or tooth s.

so'da [It., possibly fr. Mediev. L. barilla plant] See bicarbonate, *sodium* carbonate, and *sodium* hydroxide.

s. lime, a mixture of calcium and sodium hydroxides used to absorb carbon dioxide in rebreathing apparatus and circuits.

so'dium [Mod. L. fr. *soda*] Natrium; a caustic alkaline metallic element, symbol Na, atomic no. 11, atomic weight 22.99; its salts are extensively used in medicine.

s. ben'zoate, C_6H_5COONa; used in chronic and acute rheumatism and as a liver function test.

s. bicarbonate, baking soda; $NaHCO_3$; used as a gastric and systemic antacid, to alkalize urine, and for washes of body cavities.

s. carbonate, washing soda; Na_2CO_3 $10H_2O$; used in the treatment of scaly skin

diseases; otherwise rarely used in medicine because of its irritant action.

s. chloride, common or table salt; NaCl; used as in making isotonic and physiological salt solutions, as an emetic, and in treatment of salt depletion.

s. fluoride, used as a dental prophylactic in drinking water, and topically as a 2% solution applied on the teeth.

s. hydroxide, caustic soda; NaOH; used externally as a caustic.

s. nitrite, $NaNO_2$; used to lower systemic blood pressure, to relieve local vasomotor spasms, especially in angina pectoris and Raynaud's disease, to relax bronchial and intestinal spasms, and as an antidote for cyanide poisoning.

s. sulphate, $Na_2SO_4 \cdot 10H_2O$; an ingredient of many of the natural laxative waters, also used as a hydragogue cathartic.

s. thiosul'phate, $Na_2S_2O_3 \cdot 5H_2O$; used as an antidote in cyanide poisoning in conjunction with s. nitrite, as a prophylactic agent against ringworm infections in swimming pools and baths, and to measure the extracellular fluid volume of the body.

sod'omist, sod'omite [G. *sodomitēs*, inhabitant of biblical city of Sodom] One who practises sodomy.

sod'omy [see sodomist] A term denoting a variety of sexual practices considered abnormal, especially copulation of man and animal (bestiality), fellatio, and anal intercourse.

sol'ute [L. *solutus*, dissolved] The dissolved substance in a solution.

solu'tion (sol.) [L. *solutio*] **1.** Incorporation of a solid, a liquid, or a gas in a liquid or noncrystalline solid resulting in a homogeneous single phase. **2.** Generally, an aqueous s. of a nonvolatile substance. **3.** Termination of a disease by crisis. **4.** A break, cut, or laceration of the solid tissues.

sol'vent [L. *solvens*, pres. p. of *solvo*, to dissolve] **1.** Capable of dissolving a substance. **2.** A liquid that holds another substance in solution, *i.e.*, dissolves it.

so'ma [G. *sōma*, body] **1.** The axial part of a body: head, neck, trunk, and tail. **2.** All of an organism with the exception of the germ cells.

so'matagno'sia [somat- + G. a- priv. + gnōsis, recognition] Inability to identify parts of one's own body and parts of another's body.

somat'ic [G. *sōmatikos*, bodily] **1.** Relating to the soma or trunk, the wall of the body cavity, or the body in general. **2.** Relating to the vegetative, as distinguished from the generative, functions.

somato-, somat-, somatico- [G. *sōma*, body] Combining forms denoting the body, bodily.

so'matogen'ic [somato- + G. *genesis*, origin] **1.** Originating in the body under the influence of external forces. **2.** Having origin in body cells.

so'matother'apy 1. Therapy directed at bodily or physical disorders. **2.** In psychiatry, a variety of therapeutic interventions employing chemical or physical, as opposed to psychological, methods.

so'matotro'pin, so'matotro'phin Growth hormone, a protein hormone of the anterior lobe of the pituitary, produced by the acidophil cells; promotes body growth, fat mobilization, and inhibition of glucose utilization.

so'matotype The constitutional or body type of an individual, especially that associated with a particular personality type.

somnam'bulism [L. *somnus*, sleep, + *ambulo*, to walk] **1.** Sleepwalking; a disorder of sleep, involving complex motor acts, that occurs primarily during the first third of the night but not during rapid eye movement sleep. **2.** A form of hysteria in which purposeful behaviour is forgotten.

son'ogram [L. *sonus*, sound, + G. *gramma*, a drawing] The image obtained by ultrasonography.

sonog'raphy [L. *sonus*, sound + G. *graphō*, to write] Ultrasonography.

sor'des [L. fifth fr *sordeo*, to be foul] A dark brown or blackish crustlike collection on the lips, teeth, and gums of a person with dehydration in chronic debilitating disease.

sore [A.S. *sār*] **1.** A wound, ulcer, or any open skin lesion. **2.** Painful.

 bed s., decubitus *ulcer*.

 canker s.'s, ulcerative *stomatitis*.

 cold s., colloquialism for *herpes* simplex.

 pressure s., decubitus *ulcer*.

sorp'tion Adsorption or absorption.

souf'fle [Fr. *souffler*, to blow] A soft blowing sound heard on auscultation.

 cardiac s., a soft puffing heart murmur.

 fetal s., funic s., funicular s., a blowing murmur, synchronous with the fetal heart beat, sometimes only systolic and sometimes continuous, heard on auscultation over the pregnant uterus.

 uterine s., placental s., a blowing sound, synchronous with the cardiac systole of the mother, heard on auscultation of the pregnant uterus.

sound 1. Noise; the vibrations produced by a sounding body, transmitted by the air or other medium, and perceived by the internal ear. **2.** An elongated cylindrical, usually curved, instrument used for exploring the bladder or other cavities of the body, dilating strictures of the urethra, oesophagus, or other canal, calibrating the lumen of a body cavity, or detecting the presence of a foreign body in a body cavity. **3.** Whole; healthy; not diseased or injured.

 heart s., one of the s.'s heard on auscultation over the heart **first h. s.,** occurs with ventricular systole and is mainly produced by closure of the atrioventricular valves; **second h. s.,** signifies the beginning of diastole, due to closure of the semilunar valves; **third h. s.,** occurs in early diastole and corresponds with the first phase of rapid ventricular filling; **fourth h. s.,** occurs in late diastole and corresponds with atrial contraction.

spas'm [G. *spasmos*] **1.** An involuntary muscular contraction; if painful, usually referred to as a cramp; if violent, a convulsion. **2.** Muscle s.; increased muscular tension and shortness which cannot be released voluntarily and which prevent lengthening of the muscles involved.

 carpopedal s., s. of the feet and hands observed in hyperventilation, calcium deprivation, and tetany; flexion of the hands at the wrists and of the fingers at the metacarpophalangeal joints and extension of the fingers at the phalangeal joints; feet are dorsiflexed at the ankles and toes plantar flexed.

 clonic s., alternate involuntary contraction and relaxation of a muscle.

 habit s., tic.

 intention s., a spasmodic contraction of the muscles occurring when a voluntary movement is attempted.

 nodding s., spasmus nutans **(1)** in infants, a drop of the head on the chest due to loss of tone in the neck muscles as in epilepsy or to tonic spasm of anterior neck muscles. **(2)** in adults, a psychogenic nodding of the head from clonic s.'s of the sternomastoid muscles.

saltatory s., a spasmodic affection of the muscles of the lower extremities.

tonic s., a continuous involuntary muscular contraction.

torsion s., a spasmodic twisting of the body and pelvis.

spasmo- [G. *spasmos*, spasm] Combining form denoting spasm.

spasmod'ic [G. *spasmōdes*, convulsive] Relating to or marked by spasm.

spasmol'ysis [spasmo- + G. *lysis*, dissolution] Arrest of a spasm or convulsion.

spasmolyt'ic 1. Relating to spasmolysis. **2.** Denoting a chemical agent that relieves smooth muscle spasms.

spas'mus [L. fr. G. *spasmos*, spasm] Spasm.

s. nu'tans, (1) nodding *spasm;* **(2)** nystagmus associated with head-nodding movements.

spas'tic [L. *spasticus*, fr. G. *spastikos*, drawing in] **1.** Hypertonic (1). **2.** Relating to spasm or to spasticity.

spastic'ity A state of increased muscular tone with exaggeration of the tendon reflexes.

spe'cies, pl. **spe'cies** [L. appearance, form, kind, fr. *specio*, to look at] **1.** A biological division between the genus and variety or the individual; a group of organisms which generally bear a close resemblance to one another in the more essential features of their organization, and with sexual forms which produce fertile progeny. **2.** A class of pharmaceutical preparations consisting of a mixture of dried plants in sufficiently fine division to be used in making extemporaneous decoctions or infusions.

spec'imen [L. fr. *specio*, to look at] A small part, or sample, of any substance or material obtained for testing.

spec'tacles [L. *specto*, pp. *-atus*, to watch, observe] Eyeglasses; lenses set in a frame which holds them in front of the eyes, used to correct errors of vision or to protect the eyes.

spectro- Combining form denoting a spectrum.

spectrom'etry [spectro- + G. *metron*, measure] The procedure of observing and measuring the wavelengths of light and other electromagnetic rays.

spec'trophotom'eter [spectro- + photometer] An instrument for measuring the intensity of light of a definite wavelength transmitted by a substance or a solution, giving a quantitative measure of the amount of material in the solution absorbing the light.

spec'troscope [spectro- + G. *skopeō*, to view] An instrument for resolving light from any luminous body into its spectrum, and for the observation of the spectrum so formed.

spec'trum, pl. **spec'tra, spec'trums** [L. an image] **1.** The colour image presented when white light is resolved into its constituent colours by being passed through a prism or through a diffraction grating; arranged according to the increasing frequency of vibration or decreasing wavelength: red, orange, yellow, green, blue, indigo, violet. **2.** Figuratively, the pathogenic microorganisms against which an antibiotic or other antibacterial agent is active. **3.** The plot of intensity vs. wavelength of light emitted or absorbed by a substance, usually characteristic of the substance and used in qualitative and quantitative analysis.

spec'ulum, pl. **spec'ula** [L. a mirror, fr. *specio*, to look at] An instrument for enlarging the opening of any canal or cavity in order to facilitate inspection of its interior.

speech [A.S. *spaec*] Speaking; talk; the use of the voice in conveying ideas.

oesophageal s., a technique for speaking following total laryngectomy; the swallowing of air and regurgitating of it to produce a vibration in the hypopharynx.

subvocal s., slight movements of the muscles of s. related to thinking but producing no sound.

sperm [G. *sperma*, seed] [NA] **1.** Spermatozoon. **2.** Semen.

sperma-, spermato-, spermo- [G. *sperma*, seed] Combining forms denoting semen or spermatozoa.

spermat'ic Relating to sperm or semen.

sper'matocele [spermato- + G. *kēlē*, tumour] A cyst of the epididymis containing spermatozoa.

sper'matocide [spermato- + L. *caedo*, to kill] An agent destructive to spermatozoa.

sper'matogen'esis [spermato- + G. *genesis*, production] Formation and development of the spermatozoon.

sper'matorrhoe'a [spermato- + G. *rhoia*, a flow] An involuntary discharge of semen, without orgasm.

sper'matozo'on, pl. **sper'matozo'a** [G. *sperma*, seed, + *zoōn*, animal] The male gamete or sex cell, composed of a head and a tail, which contains genetic information to be transmitted by the male, exhibits autokinesis, and is able to effect zygosis with an ovum.

sper'micide Spermatocyte.

spheno- [G. *sphēn*, wedge] Combining form denoting wedge or wedge-shaped, or the sphenoid bone.

sphe'noid, **sphenoi'dal** [G. *sphēnoeidēs*, fr. *sphēn*, wedge, + *eidos*, resemblance] **1.** Relating to the sphenoid bone. **2.** Wedge-shaped.

sphero- Combining form denoting spherical or a sphere.

sphe'rocyte [sphero- + G. *kytos*, cell] A small spherical red blood cell.

spherocyto'sis [spherocyte + G. *-osis*, condition] The presence of sphere-shaped red blood cells in the blood.

   hereditary s., a congenital defect of the erythrocyte cell membrane, which is abnormally permeable to sodium, resulting in thickened and almost spherical erythrocytes that are fragile and susceptible to spontaneous haemolysis, with decreased survival in the circulation; results in chronic anaemia with reticulocytosis, episodes of mild jaundice due to haemolysis, and acute crises with fever and abdominal pain; autosomal dominant inheritance.

sphinc'ter [G. *sphinktēr*, a band or lace] A muscle that encircles an organ or orifice in such a way that its contraction constricts or closes the lumen or orifice; the closing component of a pylorus.

sphincterec'tomy [sphincter + G. *ektomē*, excision] **1.** Excision of a portion of the pupillary border of the iris. **2.** Dissecting away any sphincter muscle.

sphincterot'omy [sphincter + G. *tomē*, incision] Incision or division of a sphincter muscle.

sphingolip'id Any lipid containing a long chain base; a constituent of nerve tissue.

sphin'golipido'sis Collective designation for a variety of diseases characterized by abnormal sphingolipid metabolism.

   cerebral s., any one of a group of inherited diseases characterized by failure to thrive, hypertonicity, progressive spastic paralysis, loss of vision and occurrence of blindness, usually with macular degeneration and optic atrophy, convulsions, and mental deterioration.

sphingomy'elins A group of phospholipids found in the brain, spinal cord, kidney, and egg yolk, containing 1-phosphocholine combined with a ceramide.

sphyg'mic Relating to the pulse.

sphygmo-, sphygm- [G. *sphygmos*, pulse] Combining forms denoting pulse.

sphyg'mograph [sphygmo- + G. *graphō*, to write] An instrument that graphically records the excursions of the radial artery pulse.

sphyg'momanom'eter [sphygmo- + G. *manos*, thin, scanty, + *metron*, measure] An instrument for measuring the blood pressure.

spic'ule [L. *spiculum*, dim. of *spicum*, a point] A small, needle-shaped body.

spi'der [O. E. *spinnan*, to spin] **1.** An arthropod (subclass Arachnida) characterized by four pairs of legs, a cephalothorax, a globose smooth abdomen, and a complex of webspinning spinnerets. *Many species are venomous.* **2.** Arterial s.

   arterial s., vascular s., spider naevus; a telangiectatic arteriole in the skin with radiating capillary branches simulating the legs of a s.

spi'na, pl. **spi'nae** [L. a thorn, the backbone, spine] [NA] Any spine or sharp thornlike process.

   s. bif'ida, a limited defect in the spinal column, consisting in absence of the vertebral arches, through which the spinal membranes, with or without spinal cord tissue, may protrude.

   s. bif'ida occul'ta, s. bifida with no protrusion of the cord or its membrane.

spi'nal [L. *spinalis*] **1.** Relating to any spine or spinous process. **2.** Relating to the vertebral column.

spine [L. *spina*] **1.** A short sharp process of bone; a spinous process. **2.** *Columna* vertebralis.

spinn'barkheit [Ger. "spinnability"] The stringy, elastic character of cervical mucus during the ovulatory period.

spino- Combining form denoting the spine; spinous.

spi'nocerebel'lar Relating to the spine and cerebellum.

spi'nous Relating to, shaped like, or having a spine or spines.

spiril'lar S-shaped; referring to a bacterial cell with an S shape.

spir'it [L. *spiritus*, a breathing, life, soul] **1.** An alcoholic liquor stronger than wine, obtained by distillation. **2.** Any distilled liquid. **3.** An alcoholic or hydroalcoholic solution of volatile substances.

spiro-, spir- 1 [G. *speira*, a coil] Combining forms denoting coil or coil-shaped. **2** [L. *spiro*, to breathe] Combining forms denoting breathing.

Spirochae'ta [Mod. L. fr. G. *speira*, a coil, + *chaitē*, hair] A genus of motile bacteria containing presumably Gram-negative, flexible, undulating, spiral-shaped rods which may or may not possess flagelliform, tapering ends. They are not parasitic but are found free-living in fresh or sea water slime; they are commonly found in sewage and foul waters. At present the genus contains five species.

spirochae'tal Relating to spirochaetes, especially to infection with such organisms.

spi'rochaete A vernacular term used to refer to any member of the genus *Spirochaeta*.

spi'rograph [L. *spiro*, to breathe, + G. *graphō*, to write] A device for representing graphically the depth and rapidity of respiratory movements.

spirom'eter [L. *spiro*, to breathe, + G. *metron*, measure] A device used for measuring respiratory gases.

Spirom'etra [G. *speira*, coil, + *metra*, womb (uterus)] A genus of tapeworms, the larval form of which (sparganum) may survive in human tissues via active migration from skin infections or from eating any vertebrate harbouring these tapeworms.

spirom'etry Making pulmonary measurements with a spirometer.

spis'sated [L. *spisso*, pp. *spissatus*, to thicken] Inspissated; thickened.

splanch'nic Visceral.

splanchnicec'tomy [splanchni- + G. *ektomē*, excision] Resection of the splanchnic nerves and, usually, of the coeliac ganglion.

splanchno-, splanchn-,
splanchni- [G. *splanchnon*, viscus] Combining forms denoting the viscera. See also viscero-

splanch'nocele [G. *kēlē*, hernia] Hernia of any of the abdominal viscera.

splay'foot *Talipes* planus.

spleen [G. *splēn*] Lien; a large vascular lymphatic organ between the stomach and diaphragm that acts as a blood-forming organ in early life, a storage organ for red corpuscles, and, because of the large number of macrophages, as a blood filter.

splenec'tomy [splen- + G. *ektomē*, excision] Removal of the spleen.

splen'ic Relating to the spleen.

spleni'tis [splen- + G. *-itis*, inflammation] Inflammation of the spleen.

spleno-, splen- [G. *splēn*, spleen] Combining forms denoting the spleen.

splenog'raphy [spleno- + G. *graphō*, to write] Radiography of the spleen after injection of contrast material into it.

splenomeg'aly [spleno- + G. *megas* (*megal-*), large] Enlargement of the spleen.

splen'oportog'raphy [spleno- + portography] The introduction of radiopaque material into the spleen to obtain radiographic delineation of the portal vessel of the portal circulation.

splint [Middle Dutch *splinte*] An appliance for preventing movement of a joint or for the fixation of displaced or movable parts.

spondyli'tis [spondyl- + G. *-itis*, inflammation] Inflammation of one or more of the vertebrae.

    ankylosing s., arthritis of the spine, resembling rheumatoid arthritis, that may progress to bony ankylosis with lipping of vertebral margins.

    s. defor'mans, arthritis and osteitis deformans involving the spinal column; marked by nodular deposits at the edges of the intervertebral discs, with ossification of the ligaments and bony ankylosis of the intervertebral articulations; results in a rounded kyphosis with rigidity.

    tuberculous s., tuberculous infection of the spine associated with a sharp angulation of the spine at the point of disease.

spondylo-, spondyl- [G. *spondylos*, vertebra] Combining forms denoting the vertebrae.

spon'dylolisthe'sis [spondylo- + G. *olisthēsis*, a slipping and falling] Forward movement of the body of one of the lower lumbar vertebrae on the vertebra below it, or upon the sacrum.

spondylos'chisis [spondylo- + G. *schisis*, fissure] Congenital fissure of one or more of the vertebral arches.

spondylo'sis [G. *spondylos*, vertebra] Vertebral ankylosis; also applied nonspecifically to any degenerative lesion of the spine.

spongio- [G. *spongia*, sponge] Combining form denoting sponge-like, spongy.

spon'giocyte [spongio- + G. *kytos*, cell] A neuroglial cell.

sporad'ic [G. *sporadikos*, scattered] Occurring singly, not grouped; neither epidemic nor endemic.

spore [G. *sporos*, seed] **1.** The asexual reproductive body of sporozoan protozoa or of Cryptogamia. **2.** A cell of a plant lower in organization than the seed-bearing spermatophytic plants. **3.** A resistant form of certain species of bacteria.

sporici'dal [spori- + L. *caedo*, to kill] Lethal to spores.

sporo-, spori-, spor- [G. *sporos*, seed] Combining forms denoting seed or spore.

Spo'rothrix [Mod. L. fr. G. *sporos*, seed, + *thrix*, hair] A genus of dimorphic imperfect fungi, including the species *S. schenckii*, the causative agent of sporotrichosis.

spo'rotricho'sis A chronic subcutaneous mycosis spread by way of the lymphatics and caused by *Sporothrix schenckii*; may remain localized or become generalized, involving bones, joints, lungs, and the CNS; lesions may be granulomatous or suppurative, ulcerative or draining.

Sporozo'a [Mod. L. fr. G. *sporos*, seed, + *zoön*, animal] A large class of protozoans consisting of obligatory parasites that includes the gregarines and coccidia.

sporozo'an **1.** An individual organism of the class Sporozoa. **2.** Relating to the Sporozoa.

spot **1.** Macula. **2.** To lose a slight amount of blood through the vagina.

Bitot's s.'s, small greyish foamy triangular deposits on the bulbar conjunctiva adjacent to the cornea in the area of the palpebral fissure, associated with vitamin A deficiency.

blind s., (1) physiological *scotoma*; (2) mental *scotoma*; (3) *discus* nervi optici.

café au lait s.'s, uniformly light brown, sharply defined, and usually oval-shaped patches of the skin characteristic of neurofibromatosis, but also found in normal individuals.

liver s., senile *lentigo*.

sprain **1.** An injury to a ligament when the joint is carried through a range of motion greater than normal, but without dislocation or fracture. **2.** To cause a s. of a joint.

sprue [D. *spruw*] **1.** Primary intestinal malabsorption with steatorrhoea. **2.** In dentistry, wax or metal used to form the aperture or apertures for molten metal to flow into a mould to make a casting.

nontropical s., s. occurring in persons away from the tropics; usually called coeliac disease.

tropical s., tropical diarrhoea; s. occurring in the tropics, often associated with enteric infection and nutritional deficiency, and frequently complicated by folate deficiency with macrocytic anaemia.

spur [A.S. *spora*] Calcar.

spu'rious [L. *spurius*] False; not genuine.

spu'tum, pl. **spu'ta** [L. *spuo*, pp. *sputus*, to spit] **1.** Expectorated matter, especially mucus or mucopurulent matter expectorated in diseases of the air passages. **2.** An individual mass of such matter.

squa'ma, pl. **squa'mae** [L. a scale] **1.** [NA] A thin plate of bone. **2.** An epidermic scale.

squamo'sa, pl. **squamo'sae** [L. *squamosus*, scaly, fr. *squama*, scale] The squama of the frontal, occipital, or temporal bone, especially the latter.

squa'mous [L. *squamosus*] Squamate; scaly; relating to or covered with scales.

squint Strabismus.

sta'bile [L. *stabilis*] Stable; steady; resistant to change.

stage [M.E. thr. O. Fr. *estage*, standing place] **1.** A period in the course of a disease; the distribution and extent of dissemination of a malignant neoplastic disease. **2.** The part of a microscope on which the microslide bears the object to be examined. **3.** A particular step, phase, or position in a developmental process.

sta'ging Classification of neoplasms according to the extent of the tumour.

stain [M.E. *steinen*] **1.** A dye used in histologic and bacteriologic technique. **2.** A procedure in which a dye or combination of dyes and reagents is used to colour the constituents of cells and tissues.

Gram's s., a method for differential staining of bacteria in which Gram-positive organisms stain purple black and Gram-negative organisms stain pink; useful in bacterial taxonomy and identification, and also in indicating fundamental differences in cell wall structure.

stam'mering A speech disorder characterized by hesitation and repetition of sounds, or by mispronunciation or transposition of certain consonants, especially *l*, *r*, and *s*.

stan'nous [L. *stannum*, tin] Relating to tin, especially denoting compounds containing tin in its lower valency.

stannous fluoride A preparation containing not less than 71.2% of stannous tin and not less than 22.3% and not more than 25.5% of fluoride; used as a dental prophylactic.

stapedec'tomy [stapes + G. *ektomē*, excision] Removal of the stapes in whole or part and replacement with various prostheses and tissues.

stape'dial Relating to the stapes.

sta'pes, pl. **sta'pes, stape'des** [Mod. L. stirrup] [NA] Stirrup; smallest of the three auditory ossicles; its base, or footpiece, fits into the vestibular (oval) window, while its head is articulated with the lenticular process of the long limb of the incus.

staphylec'tomy [staphyl- + G. *ektomē*, excision] Uvulectomy.

staphylo-, staphyl- [G. *staphylē*, a bunch of grapes] Combining forms denoting resemblance to a grape or a bunch of grapes, hence relating usually to staphylococci. See also uvulo-.

staph'ylococ'cal,

staph'ylococ'cic Relating to or caused by any species of *Staphylococcus*.

Staph'ylococ'cus [staphylo- + G. *kokkos*, a berry] A genus of Gram-positive bacteria (family Micrococcaceae) that form irregular clusters; found on the skin, in skin glands, on the nasal and other mucous membranes of warm-blooded animals, and in a variety of food products. The type species is *S. aureus.*

S. au'reus, a common species that causes furunculosis, pyaemia, osteomyelitis, suppuration of wounds, and food poisoning.

S. pyog'enes al'bus, mutants of *S. aureus* which form white colonies.

staphylo'ma [G.] A bulging of the cornea or sclera due to inflammatory softening, usually containing adherent uveal tissue.

starch [A.S. *stearc*, strong] A polysaccharide that exists in most plant tissues; converted into dextrin when subjected to the action of dry heat, and into dextrin and glu-cose by amylases and glucoamylases in saliva and pancreatic juice.

sta'sis, pl. **sta'ses** [G. a standing still] Stagnation of the blood or other fluids.

-stat [G. *statēs*, stationary] Suffix indicating an agent intended to keep something from changing or moving.

statoco'nia, sing. **statoco'nium** [L. fr. G. *statos*, standing, *konis*, dust] [NA] Otoliths; crystalline particles of calcium carbonate and a protein adhering to the gelatinous membrane of the maculae of the utricle and saccule.

sta'tus [L. a way of standing] State; condition.

  s. asthmat'icus, a condition of severe, prolonged asthma.

  s. epilep'ticus, a condition in which one major attack of epilepsy succeeds another with little or no intermission.

steal Diversion of blood via alternate routes or reversed flow, from a vascularized tissue to one deprived by proximal arterial obstruction.

steap'sin Triacylglycerol lipase.

stear'ic acid One of the most abundant fatty acids found in animal lipids; used in pharmaceutical preparations, ointments, soaps, and suppositories.

stearo-, stear- [G. *stear*, tallow] Combining forms denoting fat. See also steato-.

steati'tis [G. *stear* (*steat-*), tallow, + *-itis*, inflammation] Inflammation of adipose tissue.

steato- [G. *stear* (*steat-*), tallow] Combining form denoting fat. See also stearo-.

steatol'ysis [steato- + G. *lysis*, dissolution] Hydrolysis or emulsion of fat in the digestive process.

ste'atopyg'ia [steato- + G. *pygē*, buttocks] An excessive accumulation of fat on the buttocks.

ste'atorrhoe'a [steato- + G. *rhoia*, a flow] Passage of fat in large amounts in the faeces, as noted in pancreatic disease and the malabsorption syndromes.

steato'sis [steato- + G. *-osis*, condition] Fatty *degeneration*.

stel'late [L. *stella*, a star] Star-shaped.

steno- [G. *stenos*, narrow] Combining form denoting narrowness or constriction.

stenosed' Narrowed; contracted: strictured.

steno'sis, pl. **steno'ses** [G. *stenōsis*, a narrowing] A stricture of any canal; especially of one of the cardiac valves.

    aortic s., pathologic narrowing of the aortic valve orifice.

    mitral s., pathologic narrowing of the orifice of the mitral valve.

    pyloric s., narrowing of the gastric pylorus, especially by congenital muscular hypertrophy or scarring resulting from a peptic ulcer.

stent [C. *Stent*] **1.** A device used to maintain a bodily orifice or cavity during skin grafting, or to immobilize a skin graft after placement. **2.** A slender thread, rod, or catheter placed within the lumen of tubular structures to provide support during or after their anastomosis, or to assure patency of an intact but contracted lumen.

step'page [Fr.] The peculiar gait seen in neuritis of the peroneal nerve and from tabes dorsalis; in consequence of this, dorsal flexion of the foot is impossible, and in walking the foot must be raised very high in order to clear the ground with the drooping toes.

sterco- [L. *stercus*, faeces, excrement] Combining form denoting faeces. See also copro-; scato-.

stercobi'lin A brown degradation product of haemoglobin present in the faeces.

ster'colith [sterco- + G. *lithos*, stone] Coprolith.

stercora'ceous, ster'coral Relating to or containing faeces.

stereo- [G *stereos*, solid] **1.** Combining form denoting a solid, or a solid condition or state. **2.** Prefix denoting spatial qualities, three-dimensionality.

ste'reochem'istry The branch of chemistry concerned with atoms in their spatial three-dimensional relations, the positions the atoms in a compound bear in relation to one another in space.

stereog'nosis [stereo- + G. *gnōsis*, knowledge] The appreciation of the form of an object by means of touch.

stereoi'somer [stereo- + G. *isos*, equal, + *meros*, part] A molecule containing the same number and kind of atom groupings as another but in a different arrangement in space, by virtue of which it exhibits different properties.

ste'reotaxy Stereotactic surgery; a precise method of destroying deep-seated brain structures located by use of three-dimensional coordinates.

ste'reotypy [stereo- + G. *typos*, impression, type] **1.** Maintenance of one attitude for a long period. **2.** Constant repetition of certain meaningless gestures or movements.

ster'ile [L. *sterilis*, barren] Relating to or characterized by sterility.

steril'ity [L. *sterilitas*] **1.** In general, the incapability of fertilization or reproduction. **2.** The state of being aseptic, or free from all living microorganisms and their spores.

steriliza'tion **1.** The act or process by which an individual is rendered incapable of fertilization or reproduction. **2.** Destruction of all microorganisms in or about an object, as by steam, chemical agents, high-velocity electron bombardment, ultraviolet light radiation.

ster'nal Relating to the sternum.

sterno-, stern- Combining form denoting the sternum.

ster'noclavic'ular Relating to the sternum and the clavicle.

ster'nocleidomas'toid Relating to sternum, clavicle, and mastoid process.

sternocos'tal [L. *costa*, rib] Relating to the sternum and the ribs.

sternot'omy [sterno- + G. *tomē*, incision] Incision into or through the sternum

ster'nover'tebral Relating to the sternum and the vertebrae; denoting the true ribs (seven upper ribs) that articulate with the vertebrae and the sternum.

ster'num, pl. **ster'na** [Mod. L. fr. G. *sternon*, the chest] [NA] The breast bone; a long flat bone, articulating with the cartilages of the first seven ribs and with the clavicle, forming the middle part of the anterior wall of the thorax; consists of three portions: corpus, manubrium, and xiphoid process.

ste'roid **1.** Pertaining to the steroids. **2.** One of the steroids. **3.** Generic designation for compounds closely related in structure to steroids, such as sterols, bile acids, cardiac glycosides, and precursors of vitamin D. **4.** Jargon for a compound having biological actions similar to a steroid hormone, of semisynthetic or synthetic origin, and whose structure may or may not resemble that of a steroid.

ste'roids A large family of chemical substances, comprising many hormones, vitamins, body constituents, and drugs, each containing tetracyclic cyclopenta[α]phenanthrene skeleton.

ster'tor [L. *sterto*, to snore] A noisy inspiration occurring in coma or deep sleep, sometimes due to obstruction of the larynx or upper airways.

ster'torous Relating to or characterized by stertor or snoring.

stetho-, steth- [G. *stēthos*, chest] Combining forms denoting the chest.

steth'oscope [stetho- + G. *skopeō*, to view] An instrument used in auscultation of sounds in the body.

stethos'copy 1. Examination of the chest by means of auscultation, either mediate or immediate, and percussion. 2. Mediate auscultation with the stethoscope.

stig'ma, pl. **stig'mas** or **stigma'ta** [G. a mark, fr. *stizō*, to prick] 1. Visible evidence of a disease. 2. Any spot or blemish on the skin. 3. A bleeding spot on the skin which is considered a manifestation of conversion hysteria.

stigmat'ic Relating to or marked by a stigma.

stil'bene An unsaturated hydrocarbon, the nucleus of stilboestrol and other synthetic oestrogenic compounds.

stilboes'trol A synthetic crystalline compound, not a steroid, possessing oestrogenic activity when given orally or by injection.

still'birth The birth of an infant who shows no evidence of life.

stim'ulant [L. *stimulans*, pres. p. of *stimulo*, pp. *-atus*, to goad, incite] 1. Stimulating; exciting to action. 2. Stimulator; an agent that arouses organic activity, increases vitality, and promotes a sense of well-being; classified, according to the parts upon which they chiefly act.

stim'ulus, pl. **stim'uli** [L. a goad] 1. A stimulant. 2. That which can elicit or evoke action (response) in an excitable tissue, or cause an augmenting action upon any function or metabolic process.

sting 1. Sharp momentary pain produced by the puncture of the skin by many species of arthropods, or by contact with venomous species of aquatic life forms. 2. The venom apparatus of a stinging organism. 3. To introduce (or the process of introducing) a venom by stinging.

stitch [A.S. *stice*, a pricking] 1. A sharp sticking pain of momentary duration. 2. A single suture. 3. Suture (2).

sto'ma, pl. **sto'mas** or **sto'mata** [G. a mouth] 1. [NA] A minute opening or pore. 2. The mouth. 3. An artificial opening between two cavities or canals, or between such and the surface of the body.

stom'ach [G. *stomachos*, L. *stomachus*] Ventriculus; gaster; that part of the digestive tract between the oesophagus and the small intestine, lying just beneath the diaphragm.

  hourglass s., a condition in which there is an abnormal constriction of the wall of the s. dividing it into two cavities, cardiac and pyloric.

stomach'ic An agent that improves appetite and digestion.

stomati'tis [stomat- + G. *-itis*, inflammation] Inflammation of the mucous membrane of the mouth.

  angular s., inflammation at the corners of the mouth usually associated with a wrinkled or fissured epithelium, stopping at the mucocutaneous junction and not involving the mucosa.

  ulcerative s., canker sores; destructive ulceration of the mucous membrane of the mouth.

stomato-, stom-, stomat- [G. *stoma*, mouth] Combining forms denoting mouth.

sto'matomyco'sis [stomato- + G. *mykēs*, fungus, + *-osis*, condition] A fungal disease of the mouth.

stomatop'athy [stomato- + G. *pathos*, suffering] Any disease of the mouth.

sto'matoplasty [stomato- + G. *plassō*, to form] Reconstructive or plastic surgery of the mouth.

-stomy [G. *stoma*, mouth] Combining form denoting an artificial or surgical opening.

stone [A.S. *stān*] Calculus.

stool [A.S. *stōl*, seat] 1. A discharging of the bowels. 2. Evacuation; the matter discharged at one movement of the bowels.

strabis'mus [Mod. L. fr. G. *strabismos*, a squinting] Heterotropia; squint; a manifest lack of parallelism of the visual axes of the eyes.

  convergent s., esotropia.

  divergent s., exotropia.

strain [A.S. *stryand; streōnan*, to beget] 1. A race or stock; in bacteriology, the set of descendants that originates from a common ancestor and retains the characteristics of the ancestor. 2. An hereditary tendency. 3. [L.

stringere, to bind] To make an effort to the limit of one's strength. **4.** To injure by overuse or improper use. **5.** Injury resulting from improper use or overuse. **6.** To filter; to percolate.

stran'gle [G. *strangaloō*, to choke, fr. *strangalē*, a halter] To suffocate; to choke; to compress the trachea so as to prevent sufficient passage of air.

stran'gulated [L. *strangulo*, pp. *-atus*, to choke] Constricted so as to prevent sufficient passage of air, as through the trachea, or to cut off venous return, as in the case a hernia.

stran'gury [G. *stranx*, something squeezed out, + *ouron*, urine] Difficulty in micturition, the urine being passed drop by drop with pain and tenesmus.

strat'ifica'tion [L. *stratum*, layer, + *facio*, to make] An arrangement in layers or strata.

strat'ified Arranged in the form of layers or strata.

stra'tum, pl. **stra'ta** [L. *sterno*, pp. *stratus*, to spread out, strew] [NA] One of the layers of differentiated tissue, the aggregate of which forms any given structure. See also lamina.

strepto- [G. *streptos*, twisted] Combining form denoting curved or twisted.

Strep'tobacil'lus [strepto- + *bacillus*] A genus of Gram-negative bacteria (family Bacteroidaceae) that are parasitic to pathogenic for rats, mice, and other mammals. Type species is *S. moniliformis*.

streptococ'cal Relating to or caused by any organism of the genus *Streptococcus*.

Streptococ'cus [strepto- + G. *kokkus*, berry (coccus)] A genus of Gram-positive bacteria (family Lactobacillaceae) containing spherical or ovoid cells which occur in pairs or short or long chains; some species are pathogenic. Type species is *S. pyogenes*.

  S. mu'tans, a species associated with the production of dental caries.

  S. pneumo'niae, *Diplococcus pneumoniae;* pneumococcus; a species of Gram-positive diplococci that is the common causative agent of lobar pneumonia, meningitis, sinusitis, and other infections. Type species of the genus *Diplococcus*.

  S. pyog'enes, a species that causes formation of pus and septicaemias.

streptococ'cus, pl. **streptococci** Any member of the genus *Streptococcus*.

streptodor'nase (SD) A deoxyribonuclease obtained from streptococci; used with streptokinase to facilitate drainage in septic surgical conditions.

streptoki'nase (SK) *Streptomyces griseus* neutral proteinase, an extracellular enzyme that cleaves plasminogen, producing plasmin, which causes the liquefaction of fibrin; used usually in conjunction with streptodornase.

streptoly'sin A haemolysin produced by streptococci.

Streptomy'ces [strepto- + G. *mykēs*, fungus] A genus of Gram-positive bacteria (family Streptomycetaceae) that are predominantly saprophytic soil forms; some are parasitic and many produce antibiotics. Type species is *S. albus*.

streptomy'cin An antibiotic agent obtained from *Streptomyces griseus* that is active against the tubercle bacillus and a large number of Gram-positive and -negative bacteria.

stress [L. *strictus*, tight] **1.** Reactions of the animal body to forces of a deleterious nature, infections, and various abnormal states that tend to disturb homeostasis. **2.** The resisting force set up in a body as a result of an externally applied force. **3.** In psychology, a physical or psychological stimulus which, when impinging upon an individual, produces strain or disequilibrium.

stri'a, pl. **stri'ae** [L. channel, furrow] **1.** [NA] A stripe, band, streak, or line, distinguished from the tissue in which it is found. **2.** *Striae cutis distensae*.

  striae cu'tis disten'sae, striae gravida'rum, bands of thin wrinkled skin, initially red but becoming purple and white, which occur commonly on the abdomen, buttocks, and thighs during and following pregnancy, and result from atrophy of the dermis and overextension of the skin; also associated with ascites and Cushing's syndrome.

stri'ate, stri'ated [L. *striatus*, furrowed] Striped; marked by striae.

stria'tion 1. Stria (1). **2.** A striate appearance. 3. The act of streaking or making striae.

stria'tum [L. neut. of *striatus*, furrowed] Collective name for the caudate nucleus and putamen which together with the globus pallidus form the corpus striatum.

stric'ture [L. *strictura* drawn tight] A circumscribed narrowing of a hollow structure.

stri'dor [L. a harsh, creaking sound] A high-pitched noisy respiration; a sign of respiratory obstruction.

strid'ulous [L. *stridulus*, fr. *strideo*, to creak, to hiss] Having a shrill or creaking sound.

strip [A.S. *strypan*, to rob] **1.** To express the contents from a tube or canal by running the finger along it. **2.** Subcutaneous excision of a vein in its longitudinal axis.

stro'bila, pl. **stro'bilae** [G. *stobilē*, a twist of lint] A chain of segments, less the scolex and unsegmented neck portion, of a tapeworm.

stroke [A.S. *strāc*] A sudden neurological affliction usually related to the cerebral blood supply; more accurately, a thrombosis, haemorrhage, or embolism.

    heat s., see heatstroke.

    sun s., see sunstroke.

stro'ma, pl. **stro'mata** [G. *strōma*, bed] [NA] The framework, usually of connective tissue, of an organ, gland, or other structure.

stro'mal, stromat'ic. Relating to the stroma.

Strongyloi'des [G. *strongylos*, round, + *eidos*, resemblance] The threadworm, a genus of small nematode intestinal parasites (superfamily Rhabditoidea) characterized by a life cycle that involves a generation of free-living adult worms; species include *S. stercoralis*, which causes strongyloidiasis in man.

stron'tium [*Strontian*, Scotland] A metallic element, symbol Sr, atomic no. 38, atomic weight 87.62; one of the alkaline earth series and similar to calcium in chemical and biological properties.

stroph'ulus [L. fr. G. *strophus*, colic] *Miliaria* rubra.

stru'ma, pl. **stru'mae** [L. fr. *struo*, to pile up] **1.** Goitre. **2.** Formerly, any enlargement.

strumec'tomy [struma + G. *ektomē*, excision] Surgical removal of all or a portion of a goitrous tumour.

stru'miform [struma + L. *forma*, form] Resembling a goitre.

strych'nine A poisonous alkaloid from *Strychnos nux-vomica*.

strych'ninism Chronic strychnine poisoning, the symptoms being those that arise from CNS stimulation: tremors and twitching, progressing to severe convulsions and respiratory arrest.

stu'por [L. fr. *stupeo*, to be stunned] A state of impaired consciousness in which the individual shows a marked diminution in his reactivity to environmental stimuli.

stu'porous Relating to or marked by stupor.

stut'tering A phonatory or articulatory disorder, characteristically beginning in childhood with intense anxiety about the efficiency of oral communications; characterized by difficult enunciation of words with frequent halting and repetition of the initial consonant or syllable.

    urinary s., frequent involuntary interruption occurring during the act of urination.

sty, stye, pl. **sties, styes** Hordeolum.

sty'let, stylette' [It. *stilletto*, a dagger] **1.** A flexible metallic rod inserted in the lumen of a flexible catheter to stiffen it and give it form during its passage. **2.** A slender probe.

stylo- [G. *stylos*, pillar, post] Prefix denoting styloid; specifically, the styloid process of the temporal bone.

stylohy'al, stylohy'oid Relating to the styloid process of the temporal bone and to the hyoid bone.

sty'loid [stylo- + G. *eidos*, resemblance] Denoting a slender bony process, found on the temporal bone, ulna, radius, and third metacarpal bone.

sty'lus [L. *stilus* or *stylus*, a stake or pen] **1.** Any pencil-shaped structure. **2.** A pencil-shaped medicinal preparation for external application. **3.** Stylet.

styp'tic [G. *styptikos*] Having an astringent or haemostatic effect.

sub- [L. *sub*, under] Prefix denoting beneath, less than the normal or typical, inferior.

subacute' Between acute and chronic; denoting the course of a disease.

subap'ical Below the apex of any part.

subclin'ical Denoting a period prior to the appearance of manifest symptoms in the evolution of a disease.

subcon'scious 1. Not wholly conscious. **2.** Denoting an idea or impression which is present in the mind, but of which there is at the time no conscious perception.

subcor'tex Any part of the brain lying below the cerebral cortex, and not itself organized as cortex.

subcor'tical Relating to the subcortex; beneath the cerebral cortex.

subcuta'neous (s.c.) [sub- + L. *cutis*, skin] Beneath the skin.

subduce', subduct' [L. *sub-duco*, pp. -*ductus*, to lead away] To pull or draw downward.

subglos'sal Below or beneath the tongue.

subinfec'tion A secondary infection occurring in one exposed to and successfully resisting an epidemic of another infectious disease.

subinvolu'tion An arrest in the normal involution of the uterus following childbirth, the organ remaining abnormally large.

subja'cent [L. *sub-jaceo*, to lie under] Below or beneath another part.

subject'ive [L. *subjectivus*, fr. *subjicio*, to throw under] Perceived by the individual only and not evident to the examiner.

sub'limate [L. *sublimo*, pp. -*atus*, to raise on high] 1. Any substance that has been submitted to sublimation. 2. To accomplish sublimation.

sublima'tion 1. The process of vaporizing a solid substance without passing through a liquid state. 2. In psychoanalysis, an unconscious defence mechanism in which unacceptable instinctual drives and wishes are modified into more personally and socially acceptable channels.

sublim'inal [sub- + L. *limen* (*limin*-), threshold] Below the limit of sensory perception or threshold of consciousness.

sublin'gual Subglossal.

subluxa'tion [sub- + L. *locatio*, dislocation] An incomplete dislocation, though a relationship is altered, contact between joint surfaces remains.

submax'illari'tis [sub- + maxilla + G. -*itis*, inflammation] Inflammation, usually due to mumps virus, affecting the submandibular salivary gland.

submax'illary Mandibular.

submicroscop'ic Too minute to be visible under the most powerful light microscope.

submuco'sa A layer of tissue beneath a mucous membrane.

subpap'ular Denoting the eruption of few and scattered papules, in which the lesions are very slightly elevated, being scarcely more than macules.

subscrip'tion [L. *subscriptio*, to write under] The part of a prescription preceding the signature, in which are the directions for compounding.

sub'stance [L. *substantia*, essence, material] Matter; stuff; material. See also substantia.

Nissl s., Nissl bodies or granules; material consisting of granular endoplasmic reticulum and ribosomes which occurs in nerve cell bodies and dendrites.

substan'tia, pl. **substan'tiae** [L.] [NA] Substance.

s. al'ba [NA], white matter; those regions of the brain and spinal cord largely or entirely composed of nerve fibres and containing few or no neuronal cell bodies or dendrites.

s. gris'ea [NA], grey matter; those regions of the brain and spinal cord made up primarily of the cell bodies and dendrites of nerve cells rather than myelinated axons.

substitu'tion [L. *substitutio*] 1. In chemistry, the replacement of an atom or group in a compound by another. 2. In psychiatry, an unconscious defence mechanism by which the unacceptable or unattainable is replaced by one that which is more acceptable or attainable.

sub'strate [L. *sub-sterno*, pp. -*stratus*, to spread under] The substance acted upon and changed by an enzyme.

subun'gual, subun'guial [L. *unguis*, nail] Beneath the finger or toe nail.

subvolu'tion [L. *sub*, under, + *volvo*, pp. *volutus*, to turn] Turning over a flap of mucous membrane to prevent adhesion.

suc'cus, pl. **suc'ci** [L.] 1. The fluid constituents of the body tissues. 2. A fluid secretion, especially the digestive juices. 3. Formerly, a pharmacopoeial preparation obtained by expressing the juice of a plant and adding to it sufficient alcohol to preserve it.

su'crose A nonreducing disaccharide made up of glucose and fructose, obtained from sugar cane, several species of sorghum, and the sugar beet.

sucrosu'ria [sucrose + G. *ouron*, urine] Excretion of sucrose in the urine.

sucto'rial Relating to or adapted for sucking.

suda'men, pl. **sudam'ina** [Mod. L. fr. *sudo*, to sweat] A minute vesicle due to retention of fluid in a sweat follicle or in the epidermis.

sudomo'tor [L. *sudor*, sweat, + *motor*, mover] Denoting the nerves that stimulate the sweat glands to activity.

sudor- [L. *sudor*, sweat] Combining form denoting sweat, perspiration.

su'dor [L.] Perspiration (3).

sudorif'erous [sudor- L. *fero*, to bear] Carrying or producing sweat.

sudorif'ic [sudor- + L. *facio*, to make] Causing sweat.

suf'focate [L. *suffoco*, pp. -*atus*, to choke, strangle] **1.** To impede respiration; to asphyxiate. **2.** To suffer from lack of oxygen; to be unable to breathe.

suffu'sion [L. *suffusio*, to pour out] **1.** The act of pouring a fluid over the body. **2.** Reddening of the surface. **3.** The condition of being wet with a fluid. **4.** Extravasate (2).

sug'ar [G. *sakcharon*; L. *saccharum*] One of the sugars.

  blood s., glucose.

  fruit s., fructose.

  invert s., a mixture of equal parts of glucose and fructose.

sug'ars Saccharides; those carbohydrates having the general composition $(CH_2O)_n$ and simple derivatives thereof; generally identifiable by the ending -ose or, if in combination with a nonsugar, -oside or -osyl. S.'s, especially glucose, are the chief source of energy and in polymeric form are major constituents of mucoproteins, bacterial cell walls, and plant structural material.

sugges'tible Susceptible to suggestion.

sugges'tion [L. *sug-gero*, pp. -*gestus*, to bring under] Implanting of an idea in the mind of another by some word or act, the subject being influenced in his conduct or physical condition.

  posthypnotic s., s. given to a subject who is under hypnosis for certain actions to be performed after removal from the hypnotic trance.

suggilla'tion [L. *suggillo*, pp. -*atus*, to beat black and blue] **1.** Ecchymosis; a black and blue mark. **2.** Livedo.

sul'cus, gen. and pl. **sul'ci** [L. a furrow or ditch] **1.** [NA] One of the grooves or furrows on the surface of the brain, bounding the several convolutions or gyri; a fissure. See also fissura. **2** [NA] Any long narrow groove, furrow, or slight depression.

sulph-, sulpho- Prefix denoting sulphur, sulphonic acid, or sulphonate.

sul'pha The sulpha drugs, or sulphonamides.

sulphae'moglobin Sulphmethaemoglobin.

sulphae'moglobinae'mia. Presence of sulphaemoglobin in the blood, marked by persistent cyanosis, but the blood count does not reveal any special abnormality in that fluid.

sul'phate A salt or ester of sulphuric acid (H_2SO_4).

sul'phide A compound of sulphur in which sulphur has a valency of -2.

sul'phite A salt of sulphurous acid (H_2SO_3).

  s. oxidase, a liver oxidoreductase (a haemoprotein) catalysing the oxidation of inorganic sulphate ion with O_2, producing H_2O_2.

sulphmethae'moglobin The complex formed by H_2S (or sulphides) and ferric ion in methaemoglobin.

sul'phobro'mophtha'lein sodium A triphenylmethane derivative excreted by the liver; used in testing hepatic function, particularly of the reticuloendothelial cells.

sulphon'amides The sulpha drugs; a group of bacteriostatic drugs containing the sulphanilamide group (sulphanilamide, sulphapyridine, sulphathiazole, sulphadiazine, and other derivatives).

sulphon'ic acid Any compound in which a hydrogen atom of a CH group is replaced by the sulphonic acid group, $-SO_3H$.

sul'phonylu'reas Hypoglycaemic agents that are chemically related to the sulphonamides.

sul'phur [L. *sulfur*, sulphur, brimstone] An element, symbol S, atomic no. 16, atomic weight 32.066, that combines with oxygen to form s. dioxide and s. trioxide, and with many of the metals and nonmetallic elements to form sulphides.

sulphu'ric acid H_2SO_4; a colourless, nearly odourless, corrosive liquid containing 96% of the absolute acid; used occasionally as a caustic.

sun'burn Erythema caused by exposure to critical amounts of ultraviolet light, usually within the range of 2600 to 3200 Å.

sun'stroke A form of heatstroke resulting from undue exposure to the sun's rays; symptoms are those of heatstroke, often without fever, but with prostration and collapse.

super- [L. *super*, above, beyond] Prefix denoting in excess, above, superior, or in the upper part of. See also hyper-, supra-.

supercil'ium, pl. **supercil'ia** [L. *super*, above, + *cilium*, eyelid] [NA] **1.** Eyebrow; the line of hairs at the superior edge of the orbit. **2.** An individual hair of the eyebrow.

supere'go In psychoanalytic theory, an outgrowth of the ego that has identified itself unconsciously with important persons from early life, and which results from incorporating the values and wishes of these persons as part of one's own standards to form the "conscience."

superfi'cial [L. *superficialis*, fr. *superficies*, surface] **1.** Cursory; not thorough. **2.** Situated nearer the surface of the body in relation to a specific reference point.

su'perinfec'tion A fresh infection added to one of the same nature already present.

su'perinvolu'tion An extreme reduction in size of the uterus, after childbirth, below the normal size of the nongravid organ.

supe'rior [L. comparative of *superus*, above] **1.** Situated above or directed upward. **2.** [NA] In human anatomy, situated nearer the vertex of the head in relation to a specific reference point.

supernu'merary [super- + L. *numerus*, number] Exceeding the normal number.

superscrip'tion [L. *super-scribo*, pp. *-sciptus*, to write upon or over] The beginning of a prescription, consisting of the injunction, *recipe*, take, usually denoted by the sign ℞.

su'pinate [L. *supino*, pp. *-atus*, to bend backwards, place on back] **1.** To assume, or to be placed in, a supine position. **2.** To perform supination.

supina'tion The condition or act of assuming or of being placed in a supine position, as inversion and abduction of the foot, causing an elevation of the medial edge, rotation of the forearm in such a way that the palm of the hand faces foreward when the arm is in the anatomical position, or upward when the arm is extended at a right angle to the body.

supine' [L. *supinus*] Denoting the hand or foot in supination, or the body when lying face upward.

suppos'itory [L. *suppositorius*, placed underneath] A medicated mass shaped for introduction into one of the orifices of the body other than the oral cavity, solid at ordinary temperatures, and dissolving at body temperature.

suppres'sion [L. *sub-primo*, pp. *-pressus*, to press down] **1.** Deliberately excluding from conscious thought, as distinguished from repression. **2.** Arrest of the secretion of a fluid, as distinguished from retention. **3.** Checking of an abnormal flow or discharge. **4.** The effect of a second mutation which cancels a phenotypic change caused by a previous mutation at a different point on the chromosome.

sup'purant [L. *suppurans*, causing suppuration] Causing or inducing suppuration.

sup'purate [L. *sup-puro*, pp. *-atus*] To form pus.

suppura'tion [L. *suppuratio* (see suppurate)] The formation of pus.

supra- [L. above] Prefix denoting a position above. See also super-.

supracos'tal Above the ribs.

suprascle'ral On the outer side of the sclera, denoting the space between the sclera and the fascia bulbi.

su'praventric'ular Above the ventricles; especially applied to rhythms originating from centres proximal to the ventricles, in the atrium or A-V node.

su'ra [L.] [NA] Calf, the muscular swelling of the back of the leg below the knee, formed chiefly by the bellies of the gastrocnemius and soleus muscles.

surface-active Indicating the property of certain agents of altering the physicochemical nature of surfaces and interfaces, bringing about lowering of interfacial tension.

surfac'tant 1. A surface-active agent; includes substances commonly referred to as wetting agents, surface tension depressants, detergents, dispersing agents, emulsifiers. **2.** Term in current use to describe those surface-active agents forming a monomolecular layer over pulmonary alveolar surfaces and stablizing alveolar volume by reducing surface tension and altering the relationship between surface tension and surface area.

sur'geon [G. *cheirourgos*; L. *chirurgus*] A physician who treats disease, injury, and deformity by operation or manipulation.

sur'gery [L. *chirurgia*; G. *cheir*, hand, + *ergon*, work] **1.** The branch of medicine concerned with the treatment of disease, injury, and deformity by operation or manipulation. **2.** The performance or procedures of an operation.

   oral s., the branch of dentistry concerned with the diagnosis and surgical and adjunctive treatment of diseases, injuries, and deformities of the oral and maxillofacial region.

plastic s., the surgical specialty or procedure concerned with the restoration, construction, reconstruction, or improvement in the shape and appearance of body structures that are missing, defective, damaged, or misshapened.

sur'gical Relating to surgery.

sur'rogate [L. *surrogare,* to put in another's place] **1.** A person who functions in another's life as a substitute for some third person. **2.** A person who reminds one of another person so that one uses the first as an emotional substitute for the second.

suspen'sion [L. *suspensio,* fr. *sus-pendo,* pp. *-pensus,* to hang up, suspend] **1.** Fixation of an organ to other tissue for support. **2.** Dispersion through a liquid of a solid in finely divided particles of a size large enough to be detected by purely optical means. **3.** A class of pharmacopoeial preparations of finely divided, undissolved drugs dispersed in liquid vehicles for oral or parenteral use.

suspen'sory **1.** Suspending; supporting; denoting a ligament, a muscle, or other structure that keeps an organ or other part in place. **2.** A supporter applied to uplift a dependent part, such as the scrotum or a pendulous breast.

sustentac'ular Relating to a sustentaculum; supporting.

sustentac'ulum, pl. **sustentac'ula** [L. a prop] [NA] A structure that serves as a stay or support to another.

sutu'ra, pl. **sutu'rae** [L. a sewing, a suture] [NA] A form of fibrous joint in which two bones formed in membrane are united by a fibrous membrane continuous with the periosteum.

su'ture [L. *sutura,* a seam] **1.** Sutura. **2.** Stitch; to unite two surfaces by sewing. **3.** The surgical material so used. **4.** The seam so formed.

swab A wad of cotton, gauze, or other absorbent material used for applying or removing a substance from a surface.

swal'low [A.S. *swelgan*] To pass anything through the fauces, pharynx, and oesophagus into the stomach; to perform deglutition.

somatic s., an adult or mature swallowing pattern with muscular contractions which appear to be under control at a subconscious level.

visceral s., the immature swallowing pattern of an infant or a person with tongue thrust, resembling peristaltic wavelike muscular contractions observed in the gut.

sweat [A.S. *swāt*] **1.** Perspiration; especially sensible perspiration. **2.** To perspire.

sweat'ing Perspiration (1).

syco'sis [G. *sykōn,* fig, + *-osis,* condition] A pustular folliculitis, particularly of the bearded area.

sym- See syn-.

symbio'sis [G. *symbiōsis,* state of living together] **1.** Any intimate association between two species; *e.g.,* mutualism, commensalism, parasitism. **2.** In psychiatry, the mutual cooperation or interdependence of two persons; sometimes denoting excessive or pathological interdependence.

symbiot'ic Relating to symbiosis.

symbleph'aron [sym- + G. *blepharon,* eyelid] Adhesion of one or both lids to the eyeball.

sympath-, sympatheto-, sympathico-, sympatho- Combining forms relating to the sympathetic part of the autonomic nervous system.

sympathec'tomy [sympath- + G. *ektomē,* excision] Excision of a segment of a sympathetic nerve or of one or more sympathetic ganglia.

sympathet'ic [G. *syn,* with, + *pathos,* suffering] **1.** Relating to or exhibiting sympathy. **2.** Denoting the sympathetic part of the autonomic nervous system.

sympatholyt'ic [sympatho- + G. *lysis,* a loosening] Denoting antagonism to or inhibition of adrenergic nerve activity.

sym'pathomimet'ic [sympatho- + G. *mimikos,* imitating] Denoting mimicking of action of the sympathetic system.

symphys'eal Relating to a symphysis; grown together; fused.

symphysiot'omy [symphysis + G. *tomē,* incision] Division of the pubic symphysis to increase the capacity of a contracted pelvis sufficiently to permit the passage of a living child.

sym'physis, pl. **sym'physes** [G. a growing together] **1.** [NA] A form of cartilaginous joint in which union between two bones is effected by means of fibrocartilage. **2.** A union, meeting point, or commissure of any two structures. **3.** A pathologic adhesion or growing together.

s. pu'bica [NA], **pubic s.,** the firm fibro-cartilaginous joint between the two pubic bones.

symp'tom [G. *symptōma*] Any morbid phenomenon or departure from the normal in function, appearance, or sensation which is experienced by the patient and indicative of disease. See also sign.

   objective s., a s. evident to the observer; a sign.

   pathognomonic s., a s. that, when present, points unmistakably to a certain definite disease.

   withdrawal s.'s, a group of morbid s 's, predominantly erethistic, occurring in an addict deprived of the accustomed dose of the addicting agent.

symptomat'io Indicative; relating to or constituting the semiology of symptoms of a disease.

symp'tomatol'ogy [symptom + G. *logos*, study] **1.** The science of the symptoms of disease, their production, and the indications they furnish. **2.** The aggregate of symptoms of a disease.

syn- [G. *syn*, with, together] Prefix indicating together; *sym-* before b, p, ph, or m.

syn'apse, pl. **synap'ses** [syn- + G. *haptein*, to clasp] The functional membrane-to-membrane contact of a nerve cell with another nerve cell, an effector (muscle, gland) cell, or a sensory receptor cell which subserves the transmission of nerve impulses from an axon terminal (presynaptic element) to the receiving cell's axon, dendrite, or plasma membrane (postsynaptic element); in most cases the impulse is transmitted by a chemical transmitter substance released into a synaptic cleft separating the presynaptic from the postsynaptic membrane; in others, transmission takes place by direct propagation of the bioelectrical potential from the presynaptic to the postsynaptic membrane.

synap'sis [G. a connection, junction] The point-for-point pairing of homologous chromosomes during the prophase of meiosis.

synap'tic Relating to synapse or synapsis.

synchondro'sis, pl. **synchondro'ses** [G. *syn*, together, + *chondros*, cartilage, + *-osis*, condition] [NA] A union between two bones formed either by hyaline cartilage or fibrocartilage.

syn'chronous [G. *synchronos*] Occurring simultaneously.

syn'chysis [G. a mixing together, fr. syn- + *chysis*, a pouring] Collapse of the collagenous framework of the vitreous humour with liquefaction of the vitreous body.

syn'clitism [G. *syn-klinō*, to incline together] A condition of parallelism between the planes of the fetal head and of the pelvis, respectively.

syn'cope [G. *synkopē*, a cutting short, a swoon] A fainting or swooning; a sudden fall of blood pressure or failure of the cardiac systole, resulting in cerebral anaemia and subsequent loss of consciousness.

syndac'tyly, syndac'tylism [syn- + G. *daktylos*, finger or toe] Any degree of webbing or fusion of the digits, involving soft parts only or including bone structure; usually autosomal dominant inheritance.

syndesmec'tomy [syndesm- + G. *ektomē*, excision] Cutting away a section of a ligament.

syndesmo-, syndesm- [G. *syndesmos*, a fastening] Combining forms denoting a ligament or ligamentous.

syndesmor'rhaphy [syndesmo- + G. *rhaphē*, suture] Suture of ligaments.

syndesmo'sis, pl. **syndesmo'ses** [syndesmo- + G. *-osis*, condition] [NA] A form of fibrous joint in which opposing surfaces that are relatively far apart are united by ligaments.

syn'drome [G. *syn*, together, + *dromos*, a running] The aggregate of signs and symptoms associated with any morbid process and constituting together the picture of the disease.

   acquired immunodeficiency s., AIDS.

   adult respiratory distress s. (ARDS), interstitial and/or alveolar oedema and haemorrhage as well as perivascular lung oedema associated with hyaline membrane, proliferation of collagen fibres, and swollen epithelium with increased pinocytosis.

   amnestic s., an organic brain s. with short term (but not immediate) memory disturbance, regardless of the aetiology.

   anterior tibial compartment s., ischaemic necrosis of the muscles of the anterior tibial compartment of the leg, presumed due to compression of arteries by swollen muscles following unaccustomed exertion.

Apert's s., type I *acrocephalosyndactyly.*

Apert-Crouzon s., type II *acrocephalosyndactyly.*

Banti's s., chronic congestive splenomegaly that occurs as a sequel to hypertension in the portal or splenic veins; characterized by anaemia, splenomegaly, and irregular episodes of gastrointestinal bleeding variously with ascites, jaundice, leucopenia, and thrombocytopenia.

Bassen-Kornzweig s., abetalipoproteinaemia.

battered baby s., the clinical presentation of child abuse: multiple traumatic lesions of the bones and/or soft tissues wilfully inflicted by an adult.

Brown-Séquard's s., hemiparaplegia and hyperaesthesia, but with loss of joint and muscle sense on the side of the lesion, and hemianaesthesia of the opposite side, in case of a unilateral involvement of the spinal cord.

Budd-Chiari s., Chiari's s.

carpal tunnel s., pain and paraesthesia in the hand in the area of distribution of the median nerve, caused by compression of the median nerve by fibres of the flexor retinaculum.

Carpenter's s. [G. Carpenter], acrocephalopolysyndactyly.

cervical rib s., symptoms due to pressure upon nerves of the brachial plexus by a supernumerary rib which arises from the seventh cervical vertebra: pain and tingling along the forearm and hand over the distribution of the first thoracic nerve root; later, anaesthesia with cyanosis and coldness over the ulnar area of the hand.

Charcot's s., intermittent *claudication.*

Chiari's s., Chiari-Budd s., thrombosis of the hepatic vein with great enlargement of the liver and extensive development of collateral vessels, intractable ascites, and great portal hypertension.

Chinese restaurant s., development of chest pain, feelings of facial pressure, and sensation of burning over variable portions of the body surface after ingestion of monosodium glutamate.

Conn's s., primary *aldosteronism.*

Costen's s., temporomandibular joint s.

cri-du-chat s., cat-cry s., a disorder due to partial deletion of chromosome 5: microcephaly, antimongoloid palpebral fissures, epicanthal folds, micrognathia, strabismus, mental and physical retardation, and a characteristic high-pitched catlike whine.

crush s., (1) the shocklike state that follows release of a body part after a prolonged period of compression, as by a heavy weight; characterized by suppression of urine, probably the result of damage to the renal tubules by myoglobin from the damaged muscles; **(2)** compression fracture of a vertebra as a rare delayed complication of electric shock therapy.

Cushing's s., a disorder resulting from increased adrenocortical secretion of cortisol, caused by adrenocortical hyperplasia or tumour; characterized by centripetal obesity, moon face, acne, abdominal striae, hypertension, decreased carbohydrate tolerance, protein catabolism, psychiatric disturbances, and amenorrhoea and hirsutism in females; when associated with a pituitary adenoma, sometimes called Cushing's disease.

Down's s., mongolism; trisomy 21 s.; a syndrome of mental retardation associated with a variable constellation of abnormalities caused by representation of at least a critical portion of chromosome 21 three times instead of twice in some or all cells; abnormalities include retarded growth, flat hypoplastic face with short nose, prominent epicanthic skin folds, small rounded ears with prominent antihelix, broad hands and feet, and transverse palmar crease.

Fanconi's s., (1) Fanconi's *anaemia:* **(2)** a group of conditions with characteristic disorders of renal tubular function classified as 1) *cystinosis,* a recessive hereditary disease of early childhood; 2) *adult Fanconi s.,* a rare hereditary form, characterized by the tubular malfunction seen in cystinosis and by osteomalacia, but without cystine deposit in tissues; and 3) *acquired Fanconi s.,* which may be associated with multiple myeloma or may result from damage of proximal tubular epithelium due to various causes, leading to multiple defects of tubular function.

fetal alcohol s., a specific pattern of fetal malformation with growth deficiency, craniofacial anomalies, and limb defects, found among offspring of mothers who are chronic alcoholics; mental retardation is often demonstrated later.

Ganser's s., a psychotic-like condition, without the symptoms and signs of a traditional psychosis, occurring typically in in those who feign insanity; *e.g.*, when asked to multiply 6 by 4, will answer 23, or will call a key a lock.

Gilles de la Tourette's s., Gilles de la Tourette's *disease*.

Guillain-Barré s., acute idiopathic *polyneuritis*.

Horner's s., ptosis, miosis, anhidrosis, and enophthalmos due to a lesion of the cervical sympathetic chain or its central pathways.

Hunt's s., Ramsay Hunt's s.; **(1)** an intention tremor beginning in one extremity, gradually increasing in intensity, and subsequently involving other parts of the body; **(2)** facial paralysis, otalgia, and herpes zoster resulting from viral infection of the seventh cranial nerve and geniculate ganglion; **(3)** a form of juvenile paralysis agitans associated with primary atrophy of the pallidal system.

Hunter's s., type II mucopolysaccharidosis; gargoylism (X-linked recessive type); an error of mucopolysaccharide metabolism clinically similar to Hurler's s. but distinguished by less severe skeletal changes and no corneal clouding; X-linked recessive inheritance.

Hurler's s., type I mucopolysaccharidosis; gargoylism (autosomal recessive type); an error of mucopolysaccharide metabolism characterized by severe abnormality in development of skeletal cartilage and bone, corneal clouding, hepatosplenomegaly, mental retardation and gargoyle-like facies; autosomal recessive inheritance.

Klinefelter's s., a chromosomal anomaly with chromosome count 47, XXY sex chromosome constitution; patients are male in development, but with seminiferous tubule dysgenesis, elevated urinary gonadotropins, variable gynaecomastia, and eunuchoid habitus; some patients are chromosomal mosaics, with two or more cell lines of different chromosome constitution.

Klippel-Feil s., a congenital defect manifest as a short neck, extensive fusion of the cervical vertebrae, and abnormalities of the brain stem and cerebellum.

Korsakoff's s., an alcohol amnestic s. characterized by confusion and severe im-

pairment of memory for which the patient compensates by confabulation; delirium tremens may precede the s., and Wernicke's s. often coexists.

Lesch-Nyhan s., a heritable disorder, associated with failure to form hypoxanthine-guanine phosphoribosyl transferase, that occurs only in males and is characterized by hyperuricaemia and uric acid urolithiasis, choreoathetosis, mental retardation, spastic cerebral palsy, and self-mutilation of fingers and lips by biting; X-linked recessive inheritance.

malabsorption s., a state characterized by diverse features such as diarrhoea, weakness, oedema, lassitude, weight loss, poor appetite, protuberant abdomen, pallor, bleeding tendencies, paraesthesias, muscle cramps, etc., caused by any of several disorders in which there is ineffective absorption of nutrients.

Marfan's s., congenital changes in the mesodermal and ectodermal tissues, skeletal changes (arachnodactyly, excessive length of extremities, laxness of joints), bilateral ectopia lentis, and vascular defects (particularly aneurysm of the aorta); autosomal dominant inheritance.

Morquio's s., type IV mucopolysaccharidosis; an error of mucopolysaccharide metabolism with excretion of keratosulphate in urine; characterized by severe skeletal defects with short urine, severe deformity of spine and thorax, long bones with irregular epiphyses but with shafts of normal length, enlarged joints, flaccid ligaments, and waddling gait; autosomal recessive inheritance.

Morton's s., congenital shortening of the first metatarsal with pain between the heads of two or more of the metatarsals, usually caused by irritation of the nerve between the heads of the metatarsals.

Munchausen s., habitual fabrication of a clinically convincing simulation of disease to seek and maintain hospital treatment.

Nelson s., a s. of hyperpigmentation, third nerve damage, and enlarging sella turcica caused by development of a pituitary tumour after adrenalectomy for Cushing's s.

nephrotic s., a clinical state characterized by oedema, albuminuria, decreased plasma albumin, doubly refractile bodies in the urine, and usually increased blood cholesterol; lipid droplets may be present in the cells of the renal tubules, but the basic lesion is increased permeability of the glomerular capillary basement membranes.

Pancoast s., pain and tingling of the arm over the area of distribution of the ulnar nerve, constriction of the pupil, and paralysis of the levator palpebrae superioris muscle, due to pressure on the brachial plexus by a malignant tumour in the region of the superior pulmonary sulcus.

pickwick'ian s., [after the "fat boy" in Dickens' *Pickwick Papers*], grotesque and deforming obesity, hypoventilation, and general debility, theoretically resulting from disability induced by extreme fatness.

Pierre Robin s., micrognathia and abnormal smallness of the tongue, often with cleft palate and bilateral eye defects including high myopia, congenital glaucoma, and retinal detachment.

Plummer-Vinson s., dysphagia due to degeneration of the muscle of the oesophagus, atrophy of the papillae of the tongue, and hypochromic anaemia.

polycystic ovary s., a condition commonly characterized by hirsutism, obesity, menstrual abnormalities, infertility, and enlarged ovaries.

premenstrual s. (PMS), the regular monthly experience of physiological and emotional distress, usually during the several days preceding menses, typically involving fatigue, oedema, irritability, tension, anxiety, and depression.

pseudo-Turner's s., a s. characterized by short stature and a webbed neck; unlike Turner's s., patients with this disorder may be of either sex, have normal chromosomes, have no renal abnormalities, are often mentally retarded, and have various forms of congenital heart disease.

punchdrunk s., a condition seen in boxers and alcoholics, presumably caused by repeated cerebral concussions: weakness in lower limbs, unsteadiness of gait, slowness of muscular movements, tremors of hands, hesitancy of speech, and slow cerebration.

Ramsay Hunt's s., Hunt's s.

Reiter's s., a triad of urethritis, iridocyclitis, and arthritis which appear in that order; one or more of these conditions may recur.

respiratory distress s. of newborn, hyaline membrane *disease*.

Reye's s., sudden loss of consciousness in children following a prodromal infection, usually resulting in death with cerebral oedema and marked fatty change in the liver and renal tubules.

Sheehan's s., hypopituitarism arising from a severe circulatory collapse post partum, with resultant pituitary necrosis.

Sjögren's s., sicca s., keratoconjunctivitis sicca, dryness of mucous membranes, telangiectasias or purpuric spots on the face, and bilateral parotid enlargement, seen in menopausal women, and often associated with rheumatoid arthritis, Raynaud's phenomenon, and dental caries.

Stein-Leventhal s., polycystic ovary s.

Stevens-Johnson s., a bullous form of erythema multiforme which may be extensive, involving the mucous membranes and large areas of the body.

Stokes-Adams s., Adams-Stokes s.

Sturge-Weber s., congenital cutaneous angioma in the distribution of the trigeminal nerve, homolateral meningeal angioma with intracranial calcification and neurologic signs, and angioma of choroid, often with secondary glaucoma; incomplete forms of the s. may exhibit any two of the major features in variable degree, occasionally with angiomas elsewhere.

sudden infant death s. (SIDS), cot death; abrupt and inexplicable death of an apparently healthy infant; various theories have been advanced to explain such deaths, but none has been generally accepted or demonstrated at autopsy.

temporomandibular joint s., various symptoms of discomfort, pain, or pathosis caused by loss of vertical dimension, lack of posterior occlusion, or other malocclusion, trismus, muscle tremor, arthritis, or direct trauma to the temporomandibular joint.

toxic shock s., a staphylococcal endotoxic infection, mostly of the vagina in menstruating women using superabsorbent tampons, characterized by high fever, vomiting, diarrhoea, a scarlatinaform rash followed by desquamation, and decreasing blood pressure and shock which can result in death.

trisomy 21 s., Down's s.

Turner's s., a chromosomal anomaly with chromosome count 45, including only a single X chromosome; buccal and other cells are usually sex chromatin-negative; anomalies include dwarfism, webbed neck, valgus of elbows, shield-shaped chest, infantile sexual development, and amenorrhoea; the ovary has no primordial follicles and may be represented only by a fibrous streak; some patients are chromosomal mosaic, with two or more cell lines of different chromosome constitution.

Waterhouse-Friderichsen s., acute fulminating meningococcal septicaemia characterized by vomiting, diarrhoea, extensive purpura, cyanosis, toniclonic convulsions and circulatory collapse, and usually haemorrhage into the adrenal glands.

Werner's s., scleroderma-like skin changes, bilateral juvenile cataracts, progeria, hypogonadism, and diabetes mellitus; autosomal recessive inheritance.

Wernicke's s., Wernicke's encephalopathy, a condition frequently encountered in chronic alcoholics, largely due to thiamine deficiency and characterized by disturbances in ocular motility, pupillary alterations, nystagmus, and ataxia with tremors; an organic-toxic psychosis is often associated and Korsakoff's s. often coexists.

Wernicke-Korsakoff s., coexistence of Wernicke's and Korsakoff's s.'s.

XO s., Turner's s.

XXY s., Klinefelter's s.

XYY s., a chromosomal anomaly with chromosome count 47, XYY sex chromosome constitution, and sex chromatin-negative buccal and other cells; males are likely to be tall and thin, with less than normal intelligence, and are said to be more likely to commit minor nonagressive crimes than the general population.

Zollinger-Ellison s., peptic ulceration with gastric hypersecretion and non-beta cell tumour of the pancreatic islets, sometimes associated with familial polyendocrine adenomatosis.

syne′chia, pl. **syne′chiae** [G. *syn*, together, + *echo*, to have, hold] Any adhesion; specifically of the iris to the cornea (anterior) or to the capsule of the lens (posterior).

syn′ergist A structure or drug that aids the action of another.

syn′ergy, syn′ergism [G. *synergia*, fr. *syn*, together, + *ergon*, work] Coordinated or correlated action by two or more structures or drugs.

syn′gamy [syn- + G. *gamos*, marriage] Conjugation of gametes in fertilization.

synkine′sis [syn- + G. *kinesis*, movement] Involuntary movement accompanying a voluntary one.

synosto′sis [syn- + G. *osteon*, bone, + *-osis*, condition] Osseous union between the bones forming a joint.

synovec′tomy [synovial membrane + G. *ektome*, excision] Exsection of a portion or all of the synovial membrane of a joint.

syno′via [L. fr. G. *syn*, together, + *oon*, egg] [NA] A clear thixotropic fluid, the function of which is to serve as a lubricant in a joint, tendon sheath, or bursa.

syno′vial 1. Relating to, containing, or consisting of synovia. **2.** Relating to a synovial membrane.

synovi′tis [synovial membrane + G. *-itis*, inflammation] Inflammation of a synovial membrane, especially that of a joint; generally, when unqualified, the same as arthritis.

syno′vium *Membrana* synovialis.

syn′thesis, pl. **syn′theses** [G. fr. *syn*, together, + *thesis*, a placing, arranging] **1.** A building up, putting together, composition. **2.** Formation of compounds by the union of simpler compounds or elements. **3.** A period in the cell cycle.

syph′ilid Any of the several kinds of cutaneous and mucous membrane lesions of secondary and tertiary syphilis.

syph′ilis [?] An acute and chronic infectious venereal disease caused by *Treponema pallidum* (*Spirochaeta pallida*) and transmitted by direct contact, usually through sexual intercourse.

congenital s., s. acquired by the fetus *in utero*, thus present at birth.

primary s., the first stage of the disease with the development of the chancre.

secondary s., the second stage of the disease, beginning with the appearance of the dermatologic eruption, slight fever, and various constitutional symptoms.

tertiary s., the final stage of the disease, marked by the formation of gummas, cellular infiltration, and cardiovascular and CNS lesions.

syphilit′ic Relating to, caused by, or suffering from syphilis.

syringe [G. *syrinx*, pipe or tube] An instrument used for injecting or withdrawing fluids.

hypodermic s., a small s. with a calibrated barrel, plunger, and tip used with a hollow needle for subcutaneous injections and for aspiration.

syringi'tis [syring- + G. *-itis,* inflammation] Inflammation of the eustachian tube.

syringo-, syring- Combining forms relating to a syrinx.

syrin'gomye'lia [syringo- + G. *myelos,* marrow] Presence in the spinal cord of fluid-filled longitudinal cavities lined by dense gliogenous tissue not caused by vascular insufficiency; marked clinically by pain and paraesthesia followed by muscular atrophy of the hands, analgesia with thermoanaesthesia of the hands and arms with the tactile sense preserved, spastic paralysis in the lower extremities, and scoliosis of the lumbar spine.

syringomy'elocele [syringo- + myelocele] Spina bifida, consisting of a protrusion of the membranes and spinal cord through a dorsal defect in the vertebral column, the fluid of the syrinx of the cord being increased and expanding the cord tissue into a thin-walled sac which then expands through the vertebral defect.

syr'inx, pl. **syrin'ges** [G. a tube, pipe] **1.** Rarely used synonym for fistula. **2.** A pathologic tube-shaped cavity in the brain or spinal cord.

sys'tem [G. *systēma,* an organized whole] A consistent and complex whole made up of correlated and semi-independent parts, as an entire organism; any complex of structures anatomically or functionally related.

autonomic nervous s., that part of the nervous s. which represents motor innervation of the internal organs' smooth muscle, cardiac muscle (heart), and gland cells. It consists of two physiologically and anatomically distinct, mutually antagonistic components: the sympathetic and parasympathetic s.'s whose pathway of innervation consists of a synaptic sequence of two motor neurones, a preganglionic neurone in the spinal cord or brainstem, the myelinated axon of which emerges with a spinal or cranial nerve and synapses with one or more ganglionic neurones composing the autonomic ganglia, whose unmyelinated fibres innervate the internal organs.

cardiovascular s., the heart and blood vessels considered as a whole.

central nervous s. (CNS), the brain and spinal cord considered as a whole.

circulatory s., vascular s.

digestive s., the digestive tract from mouth to anus with associated organs and glands concerned with the ingestion, digestion, and absorption of foodstuffs and nutrients.

endocrine s., collective designation for those tissues capable of secreting hormones.

extrapyramidal motor s., literally, all of the brain structures affecting bodily (somatic) movement, excluding the motor neurones, the motor cortex, and the pyramidal (corticobulbar and corticospinal) tract; commonly used to denote in particular the corpus striatum (basal ganglia), its associated structures (substantia nigra; subthalamic nucleus), and its descending connections with the midbrain and, indirectly, with the rhombencephalic and spinal motor neurones.

limbic s., collective term denoting a heterogeneous array of brain structures at or near the edge (limbus) of the medial wall of the cerebral hemisphere (hippocampus, amygdala, and gyrus fornicatus) also used to include the interconnections of these structures, as well as their connections with the septal area, the hypothalamus, and a medial zone of mesencephalic tegmentum; the s. influences the endocrine and autonomic motor s.'s and appears to affect motivational and mood states.

lymphatic s., the lymphatic vessels, lymph nodes, and lymphoid tissue.

nervous s., the entire neural apparatus: brain, spinal cord, nerves, and ganglia.

neuromuscular s., the muscles of the body collectively and the nerves supplying them.

parasympathetic nervous s., that part of the autonomic nervous s. whose preganglionic motor neurones compose the visceral motor nuclei of the brainstem and the lateral column of the second to fourth sacral segments of the spinal cord.

peripheral nervous s., that part of the nervous s. other than the central nervous s.

portal s., a s. of vessels in which blood, after passing through one capillary bed, is conveyed through a second capillary network.

reticuloendothelial s., collectively, the cells in different organs chiefly concerned with macrophagocytosis: in connective tissue and lymphatic structures, Kupffer cells; in connective tissue, histiocytes; in the lung, alveolar phagocytes; in nervous tissue, microglia.

sympathetic nervous s., that part of the autonomic nervous s. whose preganglionic motor neurones lie in the lateral column of the thoracic and upper two lumbar segments of the spinal cord.

urinary s., the kidneys, ureters, bladder, and urethra.

vascular s., circulatory s.; the cardiovascular and lymphatic s.'s collectively.

systematic name As applied to chemical substances, a name composed of specially coined or selected words or syllables, each of which has a precisely defined chemical structural meaning, so that the structure may be derived from the name.

system'ic Relating to a system; specifically somatic, relating to the entire organism as distinguished from any of its individual parts.

sys'tole [G. *systolē̄*, a contracting] Contraction of the heart, especially of the ventricles, by which the blood is driven through the aorta and pulmonary artery to traverse the systemic and pulmonary circulations, respectively.

systol'ic Relating to, or occurring during cardiac systole.

T

ta'bes [L. a wasting away] Progressive wasting or emaciation.

t. dorsa'lis, spinal atrophy; a chronic inflammation and progressive sclerosis of the posterior proximal spinal roots, the posterior columns of the spinal cord, and the peripheral nerves; symptoms include muscular incoordination and atrophy, anaesthesia, neuralgia, lancinating pains, visceral crises, and trophic disorders of the joints; a tertiary form of syphilis.

tabet'ic Relating to tabes.

tab'let [Fr. *tablette*, L. *tabula*] A solid dosage form containing medicinal substances with or without suitable diluents; classed according to the method of manufacture as moulded and compressed.

enteric coated t., a t. coated with a substance that delays release of the medication until the t. has passed into the intestine.

sustained action or **release t.,** a drug product formulation that provides the required dosage initially and then maintains or repeats it at desired intervals.

tabopare'sis A condition in which the symptoms of tabes dorsalis and general paresis are associated.

tache [Fr. spot] A circumscribed discoloration of the skin or mucous membrane, as a macule or freckle.

tachy- [G. *tachys*, quick, rapid] Combining form denoting rapid.

tachyoar'dia [tachy- + G. *kardia*, heart] Rapid beating of the heart, usually applied to rates over 100 per minute.

tachycrot'ic [tachy- + G. *krotos*, a striking] Relating to, causing, or characterized by a rapid pulse.

tachypnoe'a [tachy- + G. *pnoē̄(pnoiē)*, breathing] Rapid breathing.

tachyrhyth'mia [tachy- + G. *rhythmos*, rhythm] Tachycardia.

tac'tile [L. *tactilis*] Relating to touch or to the sense of touch.

Tae'nia [see taenia] A genus of cestodes that formerly included most of the tapeworms, but is now restricted to those species infecting carnivores with a cysticercus.

T. sagina'ta, the beef, hookless, or unarmed tapeworm of man, acquired by eating insufficiently cooked flesh of cattle infected with *Cysticercus bovis.*

T. so'lium, the pork, armed, or solitary tapeworm of man, acquired by eating insufficiently cooked pork infected with *Cysticercus cellulosae.*

tae'nia [L. fr. G. *tainia*, band, tape, a tapeworm] Common name for a tapeworm, especially of the genus *Taenia.*

tae'niacide [L. taenia, tapeworm, + caedo, to kill] An agent destructive to tapeworms.

tae'niafuge [L. taenia, tapeworm, + fugo, to put to flight] An agent that causes expulsion of tapeworms.

taeni'asis Presence of a tapeworm in the intestine.

tag 1. To incorporate into a compound an element or other substance that is more readily detected, whereby the compound can be detected and its metabolic or chemical history followed. **2.** A small outgrowth or polyp.

ta'lar Relating to the talus.

talc [Ar. *talq*] Native hydrous magnesium silicate, sometimes containing small proportions of aluminum silicate, purified by boiling powdered t. with hydrochloric acid in water; used as a dusting powder and in cosmetics.

talco'sis A pneumoconiosis related to silicosis, caused by inhalation of talc mixed with silicates.

tal'cum [L.] Talc.

tal'ipes [L. *talus*, heel, ankle, + *pes*, foot] Any deformity of the foot involving the talus.

  t. calca'neus, a deformity, due to weakness or absence of the calf muscles, in which the axis of the calcaneus becomes vertically oriented.

  t. ca'vus, an exaggeration of the normal arch of the foot.

  t. equi'nus, permanent extension of the foot so that only the ball rests on the ground.

  t. pla'nus, flatfoot; splayfoot; a deformity in which the arch of the foot is broken down, the entire sole touching the ground.

  t. val'gus, permanent eversion of the foot, the inner side alone of the sole resting on the ground.

  t. va'rus, inversion of the foot, with only outer side of the sole touching the ground.

talipoman'us [*talipes* + L. *manus*, hand] A fixed deformity of the hand, either congenital or acquired.

talo- [L. *talus*, ankle, ankle bone] Combining form denoting the talus.

ta'lus, pl. **ta'li** [L. ankle bone, heel] [NA] Ankle bone; the bone of the foot that articulates with the tibia and fibula to form the ankle joint.

tam'pon [O. Fr.] **1.** A cylinder or ball of cotton-wool, gauze, or other loose substance; used as a plug or pack in a canal or cavity to restrain haemorrhage, absorb secretions, or maintain a displaced organ in position. **2.** To insert such a plug or pack.

tamponade', tam'ponage The insertion of a tampon.

  cardiac t., compression of venous return to the heart due to increased volume of fluid in the pericardium.

tan'nic acid $C_{76}H_{52}O_{46}$, occurring in many plants, used as a styptic, astringent, and in the treatment of diarrhoea.

tap **1.** To withdraw fluid from a cavity by means of a trocar and cannula, hollow needle, or catheter. **2.** To strike lightly with the finger or a hammer-like instrument in percussion or to elicit a tendon reflex. **3.** A light blow.

  spinal t., lumbar *puncture*.

tape'toretinop'athy [tapetum + retinopathy] Hereditary degeneration of the retina and pigmentary epithelium and of the retinal neurepithelium.

tape'tum, pl. **tape'ta** [L. *tapēte*, a carpet] **1.** Any membranous layer or covering. **2.** A thin sheet of fibres in the lateral wall of the temporal horn of the lateral ventricle, continuous with the fasciculus subcallosus, and largely composed of fibres passing from the temporal cortex to the caudate nucleus.

tape'worm An intestinal parasitic worm, commonly restricted to members of the class Cestoidea, consisting of a scolex, variously equipped with spined or sucking structures by which the worm is attached to the intestinal wall of the host, and strobila having several to many proglottids that lack a digestive tract at any stage of development.

tapotement' [Fr. fr. *tapoter*, to tap] A massage movement consisting in striking with the side of the hand, usually with partly flexed fingers.

tar'dive Late; tardy.

tarsadeni'tis [tarsus + G. *adēn*, gland, + *-itis*, inflammation] Inflammation of the tarsal borders of the eyelids and of the meibomian glands.

tar'sal Relating to a tarsus in any sense.

tarsal'gia [tarsus + G. *algos*, pain] Podalgia.

tarsec'tomy [tarsus + G. *ektomē*, excision] Excision of the tarsus of the foot or of a segment of the tarsus of an eyelid.

tarsi'tis **1.** Inflammation of the tarsus of the foot. **2.** Inflammation of the tarsal border of an eyelid.

tarso-, tars- Combining forms relating to a tarsus.

tar'somet'atar'sal Relating to the tarsal and metatarsal bones.

tar'soplasty Blepharoplasty.

tarsor'rhaphy [tarso- + G. *rhaphē*, suture] Suturing together of the eyelid margins, partially or completely, to shorten the palpebral fissure or to protect the cornea in case of chronic ulcer or paralysis of the orbicularis muscle.

tar'sus, pl. **tar'si** [G. *tarsos*, a flat surface] [NA] **1.** Instep; the seven bones of the instep: talus, calcaneus, navicular, three cuneiform, and cuboid. **2.** The fibrous plates giving solidity and form to the edges of the eyelids.

tar'tar [Mediev. L. *tartarum*, ult. etym. unknown] Dental calculus; a white or brownish deposit at or below the gingival margin of teeth, chiefly hydroxyapatite in an organic matrix.

taste [It. *tastare*; L. *tango*, to touch] **1.** To perceive through the medium of the gustatory nerves. **2.** The sensation produced by a suitable stimulus applied to the gustatory nerve endings in the tongue.

tax'is [G. orderly arrangement] **1.** Reduction of a hernia or of a dislocation of any part by means of manipulation. **2.** Systematic classification or orderly arrangement. **3.** The reaction of protoplasm to a stimulus, leading an organism to move or act in certain definite ways in relation to its environment.

taxonom'ic Relating to taxonomy.

taxon'omy [G. *taxis*, orderly arrangement, + *nomos*, law] The classification of various living things or organisms, divided into groups to show degrees of similarity or presumed evolutionary relationships (higher categories being more inclusive and broad, lower categories being more restricted); in descending order: Phylum, Class, Order, Family, Genus, Species, Subspecies (Variety).

tear [A.S. *tēar*] A drop of the fluid secreted by the lacrimal glands by means of which the conjunctiva is kept moist.

teat [A.S. *tit*] **1.** *Papilla mammae.* **2.** Breast; mamma. **3.** Papilla.

techne'tium [G. *technetos*, artificial] An artificial radioactive element, symbol Tc, atomic no. 43.

technetium-99m (⁹⁹ᵐ Tc) A radioisotope of technetium with a physical half-life of 6 hr; used to prepare radiopharmaceuticals for scanning.

teeth Dentes. See tooth.

teg'men, pl. **teg'mina** [L. a covering, fr. *tego*, to cover] [NA] A structure that covers or roofs over a part.

tegmen'tal Relating to, characteristic of, or placed or oriented toward a tegmentum or tegmen.

tegmen'tum, pl. **tegmen'ta** [L. covering structure, fr. *tego*, to cover] [NA] A covering structure.

teg'ument [L. fr. *tegmentum*] Integument

teichop'sia [G. *teichos*, wall, + *opsis*, vision] A transient visual sensation of bright shimmering colours, such as that which precedes scintillating scotoma in migraine.

tel-, tele-, telo- [G. *tēle*, distant; *telos*, end] Combining forms denoting distance, end, or other end.

te'la, pl. **te'lae** [L. a web] [NA] **1.** Any thin weblike structure. **2.** A tissue; especially one of delicate formation.

telan'giecta'sia, telan'giec'tasis [G. *telos*, end, + *angeion*, vessel, + *ektasis*, a stretching out] Dilation of the previously existing small or terminal vessels of a part.

telan'giectat'ic Relating to or marked by telangiectasia.

tel'ediagno'sis Detection of a disease by evaluation of data transmitted from patient-monitoring instruments and a transfer link to a diagnostic centre.

telem'etry [G. *tēle*, distant, + *metron*, measure] The science of measuring a quantity, transmitting the results to a distant station, and there interpreting, indicating, and/or recording the results.

telenceph'alon [G. *telos*, end, + *enkephalos*, brain] [NA] Endbrain; the anterior division of the prosencephalon corresponding to the cerebral hemispheres; together with the diencephalon it composes the prosencephalon.

telep'athy [G. *tēle*, distant, + *pathos*, feeling] The transmittal and reception of thoughts by means other than through the normal senses; a form of extrasensory perception.

teleradiog'raphy [G. *tēle*, distant, + radiography] Radiography with the tube held about 2 m from the body, thereby securing practical parallelism of the rays.

telether'apy [G. *tēle*, distant, + *therapeia*, treatment] Radiation therapy administered at a distance from the body.

tel'ophase [G. *telos*, end, + *phasis*, appearance]. The final stage of mitosis or meiosis beginning when migration of chromosomes to the poles of the cell is complete.

tem'perament [L. *temperamentum*, disposition] The psychophysical organization peculiar to the individual, including his character or personality predispositions, which influence his manner of thought and action, and general views of life.

tem'perature [L. *temperatura*, due measure] The sensible intensity of heat of any substance; the measure of the average kinetic energy of the molecules making up a substance. See also entries under scale.

tem'ple [L. *tempus*, time, the temple] The area of the temporal fossa on the side of the head above the zygomatic arch.

tem'poral [L. *temporalis*, fr. *tempus*, time, temple] **1.** Relating to time; limited in time; temporary. **2.** Relating to the temple.

temporo- [L. *temporalis*, temporal] Combining form denoting the temple.

tem'poromandib'ular Relating to the temporal bone and the mandible; denoting the articulation of the lower jaw.

tena'cious [L. *tenax*, fr. *teneo*, to hold] Sticky; glutinous; viscid; not easily diverted.

tenac'ulum, pl. **tenac'ula** [L. a holder, fr. *teneo*, to hold] A surgical clamp designed to hold or grasp tissue during dissection.

ten'der [L. *tener*, soft, delicate] Sensitive; painful on pressure or contact.

ten'derness The condition of being tender.

   rebound t., t. felt when pressure, particularly abdominal pressure, is suddenly released.

tendini'tis Tendonitis.

ten'dinous Relating to, composed of, or resembling a tendon.

ten'do, pl. **ten'dines** [L. *tendo*, to stretch out, extend] [NA] Tendon.

   t. calca'neus [NA], **t. achil'lis** [NA], Achilles tendon; the tendon of insertion of the triceps surae muscle into the tuberosity of the calcaneus.

tendo- Combining form denoting a tendon. See also teno-.

tendol'ysis [tendo- + G. *lysis*, dissolution] Release of a tendon from adhesions.

ten'don [L. *tendo*] A fibrous cord or band that connects a muscle with its bony attachment; consists of fascicles of very densely arranged, almost parallel collagenous fibres, rows of elongated tendon cells, and a minimum of ground substance.

   Achilles t., *tendo* calcaneus.

   hamstring t., see hamstring.

   heel t., *tendo* calcaneus.

tendoni'tis Inflammation of a tendon.

tenes'mus [G. *teinesmos*, ineffectual effort to defaecate] A painful spasm of the anal sphincter with an urgent desire to evacuate the bowel or bladder, involuntary straining, and passage of little matter.

teno-, tenon-, tenonto- [G. *tenōn*, tendon] Combining forms meaning tendon. See also tendo-.

tenontomy'oplasty [tenonto- + G. *mys*, muscle, + *plassō*, to form] Combined tenontoplasty and myoplasty, used in the radical correction of hernia.

tenon'toplasty,   **ten'oplasty** [tenonto- + G. *plassō*, to form] Reparative or plastic surgery of the tendons.

tenor'rhaphy [teno- + G. *raphē*, suture] Suture of the divided ends of a tendon.

ten'osynovi'tis [teno- + synovia + G. *-itis*, inflammation] Inflammation of a tendon and its enveloping sheath.

tenot'omy [teno- + G. *tomē*, incision] Surgical division of a tendon to correct a deformity caused by congenital or acquired shortening of a muscle.

ten'sion [L. *tensio*, to stretch] **1.** The act or condition of being stretched or tense, or a stretching or pulling force. **2.** The partial pressure of a gas, especially that of a gas dissolved in a liquid such as blood. **3.** Mental, emotional, or nervous strain; strained relations or barely controlled hostility between persons or groups.

   arterial t., the blood pressure within an artery.

   intraocular t. (Tn), the resistance of the tunics of the eye to indentation.

   premenstrual t., premenstrual *syndrome*.

   surface t., the expression of intermolecular attraction at the surface of a liquid, in contact with air or another gas, a solid, or another immiscible liquid, tending to pull the molecules of the liquid inward from the surface.

ten'sor, pl. **tenso'res** [L. *tendo*, pp. *tensus*, to stretch] A muscle the function of which is to render a part firm and tense.

tent 1. A canopy used in various types of inhalation therapy to control humidity and concentration of oxygen in inspired air. **2.** A cylinder of some material, usually absorbent, introduced into a canal or sinus to maintain its patency or to dilate it. **3.** To elevate or pick up a segment of skin, fascia, or tissue at a given point, giving it the appearance of a t.

ter'as, pl. **ter'ata** [G.] A malformed fetus with deficient, redundant, misplaced, or grossly misshapen parts.

terato- [G. *teras*, monster] Combining form denoting a teras.

ter'atogen [terato- + G. *-gen*, producing] An agent that causes abnormal development.

teratogen'esis [terato- + G. *genesis*, origin] The origin or mode of production of a malformed fetus.

teratogen'ic, ter'atogenet'ic 1. Relating to teratogenesis. **2.** Causing abnormal development.

terato'ma [terato- + G. *-oma*, tumour] A neoplasm composed of multiple tissues, including tissues not normally found in the organ in which it arises.

ter'es, pl. **ter'etes** [L. round, smooth, fr. *tero*, to rub] Round and long; denoting certain muscles and ligaments.

ter'minal [L. *terminus*, a boundary, limit] **1.** Pertaining to the end; final. **2.** Relating to an extremity or end. **3.** A termination, extremity, end, or ending.

   axon t.'s, the somewhat enlarged, often club-shaped endings by which axons make synaptic contacts with other nerve cells or with effector cells.

ter'tian [L. *tertianus*, fr. *tertius*, third] Occurring every third day (by inclusive reckoning); actually, occurring every 48 hours or every other day.

test [L. *testum*, an earthen vessel] **1.** A trial, examination, or experiment. **2.** To perform such. See also reaction; sign. **3.** A reagent used in making a t.

   Coombs t., antiglobulin t., a t. for antibodies: **(1) direct:** for detecting sensitized erythrocytes in erythroblastosis fetalis and in acquired haemolytic anaemia, indicated by presence of incomplete or univalent antibodies on erythrocytes; **(2) indirect:** in cross matching blood or investigating transfusion reactions, for presence of specific antibodies attached to the antigen of donor erythrocytes.

   galactose tolerance t., a liver function t., based on the ability of the liver to convert galactose to glycogen, measured by the rate of excretion of galactose following ingestion or intravenous injection of a known amount.

   glucose tolerance t., a t. for diabetes, based upon the ability of the normal liver to absorb and store excessive amounts of glucose as glycogen: following ingestion of 100 g of glucose, the fasting blood sugar promptly rises, then falls to normal within 2 hours; in a diabetic patient, the increase is greater and the return to normal unusually prolonged.

   Guthrie t., bacterial inhibition assay for direct measurement of serum phenylalanine, to detect phenylketonuria in the newborn.

   histamine t., for maximal production of gastric acidity or anacidity: after preliminary administration of an antihistamine, histamine acid phosphate is injected subcutaneously in a dose of 0.04 mg/kg of body weight, followed by analysis of gastric contents.

   Ishihara's t., a t. for colour blindness which utilizes a series of pseudoisochromatic cards; all of the figures or letters are easily read by the normal person but not by one with defective colour vision.

   Pap t., Papanicolaou smear t., microscopic examination of cells exfoliated or scraped from a mucosal surface after staining with Papanicolaou's stain; used especially for detection of cervical cancer.

   patch t., a t. of skin sensitiveness. a small piece of blotting paper or cloth, wet with the t. fluid, is applied to the skin, and on removal of the patch the area previously covered is compared with the uncovered surface.

   plasmacrit t., a serologic screening method used as an aid in the diagnosis of syphilis: heparinized blood (obtained from a pricked finger) is centrifuged to collect plasma, mixed with antigen, agitated, and the presence or absence of flocculation observed; a positive result is not conclusively diagnostic, but a negative result is exclusive.

   precipitin t., an *in vitro* t. in which antigen is in soluble form and precipitates when it combines with added specific antibody in the presence of an electrolyte.

   prothrombin t., Quick's t., for prothrombin in blood, based on the clotting time of oxalated blood plasma in the presence of thromboplastin and calcium chloride.

   pulp t., vitality t.

   Queckenstedt-Stookey t., compression of the jugular vein in a healthy person causes a rapid increase in the pressure of the spinal fluid and an equally rapid fall to normal on release of the pressure; when there is a block of subarachnoid channels, compression of the vein causes little or no increase of pressure in the cerebrospinal fluid.

Rinne's t., (1) positive t.: a vibrating tuning fork is held in contact with the skull (usually the mastoid process) until the sound is lost, its prongs are then brought close to the auditory orifice when, if the hearing is normal, a faint sound will again be heard; **(2) negative t.:** a vibrating tuning fork is heard longer and louder when in contact with the skull than when held near the auditory orifice, indicating a disorder of the sound conducting apparatus.

Schick t., an intracutaneous t. for susceptibility to *Corynebacterium diphtheriae* toxin.

scratch t., a form of skin t. in which antigen is applied through a scratch.

screening t., any testing procedure designed to separate people or objects according to a fixed characteristic or property.

sex t., a method to determine genetic sex by examination of stained smears of buccal mucosal squamous epithelial cells for the presence and number, or absence, of sex chromatin bodies; normal males have none, normal females have one per cell nucleus.

skin t., a method for determining induced sensitivity (allergy) by applying an antigen (allergen) to, or inoculating it into, the skin.

tuberculin t., application of the skin t. to the diagnosis of infection by *Mycobacterium tuberculosis* in which tuberculin or its "purified" protein derivative serves as an antigen (allergen): injection of graduated doses of tuberculin or of purified protein derivative into the skin, most often by means of a needle and syringe (Mantoux t.) or by means of tines (tine t.); the t. is read on the basis of induration and erythema, the former being considered more diagnostic of infection.

vitality t., a group of thermal and electrical t.'s used to aid in assessment of dental pulp health.

Wassermann t., a complement-fixation t. used in the diagnosis of syphilis.

Weber's t., application of a vibrating tuning fork to one of several points in the midline of the head or face, to ascertain in which ear the sound is heard best by bone conduction, that ear being the affected one if the middle ear apparatus is at fault (positive

t.), but probably the normal one if the sensori-neural apparatus is diseased (negative t.).

tes'ticle [L. *testiculus,* dim. of *testis*] Testis.

testic'ular Relating to the testes.

tes'tis, pl. **tes'tes** [L.] [NA] Testicle; one of the two male reproductive glands, located in the cavity of the scrotum.

testos'terone The male hormone, most potent naturally occurring androgen, formed by the interstitial cells of the testes, possibly secreted also by the ovary and adrenal cortex, and may be produced in nonglandular tissues from precursors such as androstenedione; used in the treatment of hypogonadism, cryptorchism, certain carcinomas, and menorrhagia.

tetan'ic [G. *tetanikos*] **1.** Relating to or marked by tetanus. **2.** An agent that in poisonous doses produces tonic muscular spasm.

tetano-, tetan- Combining forms denoting tetanus or tetany.

tet'anus [L. fr. G. *tetanos,* convulsive tension] **1.** A disease marked by painful tonic muscular contractions, caused by the neurotropic toxin (tetanospasmin) of *Clostridium tetani* acting upon the CNS. **2.** A sustained muscular contraction caused by a series of stimuli repeated so rapidly that the individual muscular responses are fused.

tet'any [G. *tetanos,* tetanus] A disorder marked by intermittent tonic muscular contractions, accompanied by fibrillary tremors, paraesthesias, muscular pains, and increased irritability of the motor and sensory nerves to electrical and mechanical stimuli; occurs with gastric and intestinal disorders, alkalosis, or a deficiency of calcium salts.

tetra- [G. four] Prefix meaning four.

tet'racaine hydrochloride A local anaesthetic used for spinal, nerve block, and topical anaesthesia.

tetracy'cline A broad spectrum antibiotic, parent of oxytetracycline, prepared from chlortetracycline and also obtained from the culture filtrate of several species of *Streptomyces;* available as t. hydrochloride and t. phosphate complex.

tetradac'tylous [tetra- + G. *daktylos,* finger or toe] Having only four fingers or toes on a hand or foot.

tetral'ogy [G. *tetralogia*] A collection of four things having something in common.

Fallot's t., The most common form of cyanotic congenital heart disease: high pulmonic stenosis, ventricular septal defect, dextroposition of the aorta, and right ventricular hypertrophy.

tet'rodotox'in A potent neurotoxin found in the liver and ovaries of the Japanese pufferfish, *Sphoeroides rubripes*, other species of pufferfish, and certain newts; produces axonal blocks of the preganglionic cholinergic fibres and the somatic motor nerves.

thalam'ic Relating to the thalamus.

thalamo-, thalam- Combining forms relating to the thalamus.

thalamot'omy [thalamus + G. *tomē*, incision] Destruction of a selected portion of the thalamus by stereotaxy for the relief of pain, involuntary movements, epilepsy, and, rarely, emotional disturbances.

thal'amus, pl. **thal'ami** [G. *thalamos*, a bed, a bedroom] [NA] The large ovoid mass of grey matter that forms the larger dorsal subdivision of the diencephalon, located medial to the internal capsule and the body and tail of the caudate nucleus, and is composed of a large number of anatomically and functionally distinct cell groups or nuclei: 1) sensory relay nuclei, each receiving a modally specific sensory conduction system and in turn projecting each to the corresponding primary sensory area of the cortex; 2) secondary relay nuclei receiving fibres from the medial segment of the globus pallidus as well as cerebellothalamic fibres and projecting to the precentral motor cortex; 3) a nucleus associated with the limbic system; 4) association nuclei, each projecting to a large expanse to association cortex; 5) the midline and intralaminar nuclei; and 6) the habenula.

thalassae'mia [G. *thalassa*, the sea, + *haima*, blood] Any of a group of inherited disorders of haemoglobin metabolism in which there is a decrease in net synthesis of a particular globin chain without change in the structure of that chain; several genetic types exist, and the corresponding clinical picture may vary from barely detectable haematologic abnormality to severe and fatal anaemia.

    t. ma'jor, Cooley's anaemia; the syndrome of severe anaemia resulting from the homozygous state of one of the t. genes or one of the haemoglobin Lepore genes with onset, in infancy or childhood, of pallor, icterus, weakness, splenomegaly, cardiac enlargement, thinning of inner and outer tables of skull, microcytic hypochromic anaemia with poikilocytosis, anisocytosis, stippled cells, target cells, and nucleated erythrocytes; types of haemoglobin are variable and depend on the gene involved.

    t. mi'nor, the heterozygous state of a t. gene or a haemoglobin Lepore gene; usually asymptomatic, with leptocytosis, mild hypochromic microcytosis, and often slightly reduced haemoglobin level with slightly increased erythrocyte count; types of haemoglobin are variable and depend on the gene involved.

thalid'omide A hypnotic drug which, if taken in early pregnancy, may cause the birth of infants with phocomelia and other defects.

thanato- [G. *thanatos*, death] Combining form denoting death.

thanatol'ogy [thanato- + G. *logos*, study] The branch of science concerned with the study of death.

the'ca, pl. **the'cae** [G. *thēkē*, a box] A sheath or capsule.

the'cal [see theca] Relating to a sheath, especially a tendon sheath

theco'ma [G. *thēkē*, box (theca), + *-oma*, tumour] A neoplasm derived from ovarian mesenchyme, consisting chiefly of spindle-shaped cells that frequently contain small droplets of fat; generally resembles a granulosa cell tumour and may form considerable quantities of oestrogens, thereby resulting in precocious development of secondary sexual features in prepubertal girls, or hyperplasia of the endometrium in older patients.

the'larche [thel- + G. *arche*, beginning] The beginning of development of the breasts in the female

thelo-, thel- [G. *thēlē*, nipple] Combining form denoting the nipples.

the'nar [G. the palm of the hand] **1.** [NA] The fleshy mass on the lateral side of the palm; the ball of the thumb. **2.** Pertaining to any structure in relation with this part.

theoph'ylline An alkaloid found with caffeine in tea leaves; a smooth muscle relaxant, diuretic, cardiac stimulant, and vasodilator.

the'orem A proposition that can be proved, and so is established as a law or principle. See also law.

the'ory [G. *theōria*, a beholding, speculation] **1.** A reasoned explanation of the manner in which something occurs, lacking absolute proof, but more nearly established than hypothesis, which is closer to speculation. **2.** The underlying science, as distinguished from the art or practice, of a profession.

therapeu'tic [G. *therapeutikos*] Relating to therapeutics, or to the treatment of disease.

therapeu'tics [G. *therapeutikē*, medical practice] The practical branch of medicine concerned with the treatment of disease.

ther'apist One skilled in the practice of some type of therapy.

ther'apy [G. *therapeia*, medical treatment] Treatment of disease by various methods.

   behaviour t., an offshoot of psychotherapy involving the use of procedures and techniques associated with conditioning and learning for treatment of a variety of psychological conditions; systematic desensitization, flooding, counter-conditioning, and biofeedback are some techniques employed; distinguished from psychotherapy because specific symptoms are selected as the target for change, planned interventions or remedial steps to extinguish or modify these symptoms are then employed, and the progress of changes is continuously and quantitatively monitored.

   client-centred t., a system of nondirective psychotherapy based on the assumption that the client (patient) both has the internal resources to improve and is in the best position to resolve his own personality dysfunction.

   electroconvulsive t. (ECT), electroshock t., a treatment of mental disorders in which convulsions are produced by the passage of an electric current through the brain.

   group t., psychotherapy involving two or more patients participating together with one or more therapists to effect behavioural changes through interpersonal exchanges.

   occupational t. (OT), use of avocational or vocational tasks as a form of t., or the training in such as a means of rehabilitation.

   physical t. (PT), treatment of disease by use of natural forces, massage, and therapeutic exercises.

   play t., t. used with children in which the young patient reveals his problems and fantasies by playing with dolls, clay, or other toys.

   radiation t., use of radiant energy in the treatment of disease.

   replacement t., t. designed to compensate for a lack or deficiency arising from inadequate nutrition, from certain dysfunctions, or from losses; replacement may be physiological or may entail administration of a substitute substance.

therm- See thermo-.

ther'macogen'esis [G. *thermē*, heat, + *pharmakon*, drug, + *genesis*, production] Elevation of body temperature by drug action.

ther'mal Pertaining to heat.

thermalge'sia [therm- + G. *algēsis*, sense of pain] Excessive sensibility to heat; pain caused by a slight degree of heat.

thermo-, therm- [G. *thermē*, heat; *thermos*, warm or hot] Combining forms denoting heat.

ther'moanaesthe'sia [thermo- + G. *an-* priv. + *aisthēsis*, sensation] Loss of the temperature sense or of the ability to distinguish between heat and cold.

thermocau'tery [thermo- + G. *kautērion*, branding iron] Use of an actual cautery, such as an electrocautery.

thermogen'esis [thermo- + G. *genesis*, production] The physiologic process of heat production in the body.

ther'mogram [thermo- + G. *gramma*, a writing] **1.** A regional temperature map of a body or organ obtained, without direct contact, by infrared sensing devices; measures radiant heat, and thus blood flow. **2.** The record made by a thermograph.

ther'mograph [thermo- + G. *graphō*, to write] A registering thermometer, one form of which records every variation of temperature.

thermog'raphy A process for measuring temperature by means of a thermograph.

thermola'bile [thermo- + L. *labilis*, perishable] Subject to alteration or destruction by heat.

thermol'ysis [thermo- + G. *lysis*, dissolution] **1.** Loss of body heat by evaporation, radiation, etc. **2.** Chemical decomposition by heat.

thermom'eter [thermo- + G. *metron*, measure] An instrument for indicating the temperature of any substance. See also entries under scale.

   clinical t., a small, self-registering t., consisting of a simple glass tube with etched scale, used for taking the temperature of the body.

   self-registering t., a t. in which the maximum or minimum temperature, during the period of observation, is registered by means of a special appliance.

thermom'etry [thermo- + G. *metron*, measure] Measurement of temperature.

ther'mophile, ther'mophil [thermo- + G. *phileō*, to love] An organism which grows best at a temperature of 50°C or higher.

ther'morecep'tor A nerve ending sensitive to heat.

thermosta'bile, thermosta'ble [thermo- + L. *stabilis*, stable] Not subject to alteration or destruction by heat.

thermotac'tic, thermotax'ic Relating to thermotaxis.

thermotax'is [thermo- + G. *taxis*, orderly arrangement] **1.** Reaction of living protoplasm to the stimulus of heat. **2.** Regulation of the temperature of the body.

thermother'apy [thermo- + G. *therapeia*, treatment] Treatment of disease by application of heat.

thia- Prefix indicating the replacement of carbon by sulphur in a compound. Cf. thio-.

thi'amine Vitamin B_1; a heat-labile vitamin contained in milk, yeast, grains, and also artificially synthesized; essential for growth.

thieth'ylper'azine maleate An antiemetic agent used to control nausea and vomiting.

thigh Femur; the part of the leg between the hip and the knee.

thio- Prefix denoting the replacement of oxygen by sulphur in a compound. Cf. thia-.

thiopen'tone sodium An ultra-short-acting barbiturate administered intravenously or rectally for induction of anaesthesia or for general anaesthesia.

thixotrop'ic Pertaining to, or characterized by, thixotropy.

thix'otropy [G. *thixis*, a touching, + *tropē*, turning] The property of certain gels of becoming less viscous when shaken or subjected to shearing forces and returning to the original viscosity upon standing.

tho'racente'sis [thoraco- + G. *kentēsis*, puncture] Paracentesis of the pleural cavity.

thorac'ic Relating to the thorax.

thoracic cage The skeleton enclosing the thorax, consisting of the thoracic vertebrae, ribs, costal cartilages, and sternum.

thoraco-, thorac-, thoracico- [G. *thōrax*, chest] Combining forms denoting the chest (thorax).

tho'racocente'sis Thoracentesis.

thoracos'copy [thoraco- + G. *skopeō*, to view] Endoscopic examination of the pleural cavity.

thoracos'tomy [thoraco- + *stoma*, mouth] Establishment of an opening into the chest cavity, as for drainage.

thoracot'omy [thoraco- + G. *tomē*, incision] Incision into the chest wall.

tho'rax, pl. **tho'races** [L. fr. G. *thōrax*, breastplate, the chest] [NA] The chest; the upper part of the trunk between the neck and the abdomen, encased by the ribs.

thread'worm Common name for species of the genus *Strongyloides;* sometimes applied to any of the smaller parasitic nematodes.

thre'onine (Thr) One of the naturally occurring amino acids, included in the structure of most proteins, and essential to the diet of man and other mammals.

thresh'old [A.S. *therxold*] **1.** The point where a stimulus begins to produce a sensation, the lower limit of perception of a stimulus. **2.** The minimal stimulus that produces excitation of any structure, eliciting a motor response. **3.** Limen.

thrill The vibration accompanying a cardiac or vascular murmur, which can be felt on palpation.

throat [A.S. *throtu*] **1.** Gullet; the fauces and pharynx. **2.** The anterior aspect of the neck.

sore t., angina; a condition characterized by pain or discomfort on swallowing; may be due to any of a variety of inflammations.

thrombec'tomy [thromb- + G. *ektomē*, excision] Excision of a thrombus.

throm'bi Plural of thrombus.

throm'bin 1. An enzyme, formed in shed blood from prothrombin by the action of prothrombinase, that converts fibrinogen into fibrin. **2.** Sterile protein substance prepared from prothrombin through interaction with thromboplastin in the presence of calcium; causes clotting of whole blood, plasma, or a fibrinogen solution.

thrombo-, thromb- [G. *thrombos*, clot (thrombus)] Combining forms denoting blood clot or relation thereto.

throm'boangii'tis [thrombo- + G. *angeion*, vessel, + *-itis*, inflammation] Inflammation of the intima of a blood vessel, with thrombosis.

t. oblit'erans, inflammation of the entire wall and connective tissue surrounding medium-sized arteries and veins, especially of the legs, associated with thrombotic occlusion and commonly resulting in gangrene.

throm'boarteri'tis Arterial inflammation with thrombus formation.

throm'bocyte [thrombo- + G. *kytos*, cell] Platelet.

throm'bocytope'nia [thrombocyte + G. *penia*, poverty] An abnormally small number of platelets in the circulating blood.

   essential t., a primary form of t., in contrast to secondary forms that are associated with metastatic neoplasms, tuberculosis, and leukaemia involving the bone marrow, or with direct suppression of bone marrow by the use of chemical agents, or with other conditions.

throm'bocytopoie'sis [thrombocyte + G. *poiēsis*, a making] The process of formation of thrombocytes or platelets.

thrombocyto'sis [thrombocyte + G. *-osis*, condition] An increase in the number of platelets in the circulating blood.

thromboem'bolism Embolism from a thrombus.

throm'boendar'terec'tomy Surgical opening of an artery, removing an occluding thrombus along with the intima and atheromatous material, and leaving a clean fresh plane internal to the adventitia.

thromboki'nase Thromboplastin.

thrombol'ysis [thrombo- + G. *lysis*, a dissolving] Fluidifying or dissolving . of a thrombus.

thrombolyt'ic Breaking up or dissolving a thrombus.

thrombope'nia. Thrombocytopenia.

thrombophil'ia [thrombo- + G. *philos*, fond] A disorder of the haemopoietic system in which there is a tendency to the occurrence of thrombosis.

throm'bophlebi'tis [thrombo- + G. *phleps*, vein, + *-itis*, inflammation] Venous inflammation with thrombus formation.

thromboplas'tin Thrombokinase; a substance present in tissues, platelets, and leucocytes necessary for the coagulation of blood; in the presence of calcium ions, it is necessary for the conversion of prothrombin to thrombin.

throm'bopoie'sis [thrombo- + G. *poiēsis*, a making] The process of a clot forming in blood; generally referring to formation of blood platelets (thrombocytes).

thrombo'sis, pl. **thrombo'ses** [G. *thrombōsis*, a clotting, fr. *thrombos*, clot] Formation or presence of a thrombus; clotting within a blood vessel which may cause infarction of tissues supplied by the vessel.

   coronary t., coronary occlusion by thrombus formation, usually the result of atheromatous changes in the arterial wall and leading to myocardial infarction.

   mural t., formation of a thrombus in contact with the endocardial lining of a cardiac chamber, or a large blood vessel, if not occlusive.

thrombot'ic Relating to, caused by, or characterized by thrombosis.

throm'bus, pl. **throm'bi** [L. fr. G. *thrombos*, a clot] A clot in the cardiovascular systems formed from constituents of blood; may be occlusive or attached to the vessel or heart wall without obstructing the lumen.

thrush [fr. thrush fungus, *Candida albicans*] Infection of the oral tissues with *Candida albicans.*

thymec'tomy [thymus + G. *ektomē*, excision] Removal of the thymus gland.

-thymia [G. *thymos*, the mind or heart as the seat of strong feelings or passion] Suffix denoting relation to the mind, soul, or emotions. See also thymo-.

thy'mic Relating to the thymus gland.

thy'midine (dThd, dT) Thymine deoxyribonucleoside; one of the four major nucleosides in DNA.

thymidyl'ic acid Thymidine 5'-phosphate; a hydrolysis product of DNA.

thy'mine A constituent of thymidylic acid and DNA.

thymo-, thym-, thymi- 1 [G. *thymos*, thymus] Combining forms denoting the thymus. **2.** [G. *thymos*, the mind or heart as the seat of strong feelings or passions] Combining forms denoting relation to the mind, soul, or emotions.

thy'mocyte [thymo- (1) + G. *kytos*, cell] A cell that develops in the thymus as the precursor of the thymus-derived lymphocyte (T lymphocyte) that effects cell-mediated (delayed type) sensitivity.

thymo'ma [thymo- (1) + G. *-oma*, tumour] A usually benign neoplasm in the anterior mediastinum, originating from thymic tissue and frequently encapsulated.

thy'mus, pl. **thy'muses, thy'mi** [G. *thymos*, thymus, sweetbread] [NA] Thymus gland; a lymphoid organ, located in the superior mediastinum and lower part of the neck, that is necessary in early life for the normal development of immunological function; at puberty, it begins to involute and much of the lymphoid tissue is replaced by fat.

thyro-, thyr- Combining forms denoting the thyroid gland.

thy′rocalcito′nin A hypocalcaemic polypeptide hormone secreted by the parafollicular cells of the thyroid gland; believed to inhibit the resorption of bone and used in the treatment of Paget's disease.

thyrogen′ic, thyrog′enous [thyro- + G. -gen, producing] Of thyroid gland origin.

thyroglob′ulin 1. A thyroid hormone-containing protein, usually stored in the colloid within the thyroid follicles; biosynthesis entails iodination of its tyrosine moieties and the combination of two iodotyrosines to form thyroxine, the fully iodinated thyronine; secretion of thyroid hormone requires proteolytic degradation of t., with the attendant release of free hormone. **2.** A substance obtained by the fractionation of thyroid glands from the hog, used as a thyroid hormone in the treatment of hypothyroidism.

thyroglos′sal Relating to the thyroid gland and the tongue.

thy′roid [G. thyreos, an oblong shield, + eidos, form] **1.** Resembling a shield, scutiform; denoting the t. gland or the t. cartilage. **2.** A pharmaceutical preparation of cleaned, dried, and powdered t. gland obtained from a domesticated food animal. It contains 0.17 to 0.23% of iodine; used in the treatment of cretinism and myxoedema, in certain cases of obesity, and in skin disorders.

thyroideo′tomy [thyroid + G. ektomē, excision] Removal of the thyroid gland.

thyroidi′tis Inflammation of the thyroid gland.

　chronic atrophic t., replacement of the thyroid gland by fibrous tissue.

　Hashimoto's t., Hashimoto's disease.

thyromeg′aly [thyro- + G. megas, large] Enlargement of the thyroid gland.

thy′ropar′athyroidec′tomy Excision of thyroid and parathyroid glands.

thyropri′val, thyropriv′ic [thyro- + L. privus, deprived of] Denoting hypothyroidism produced by disease or thyroidectomy.

thyrot′omy [thyro- + G. tomē, a cutting] **1.** Any cutting operation on the thyroid gland. **2.** Laryngofissure.

thyrotox′ic Designating the state produced by excessive quantities of endogenous or exogenous thyroid hormone.

thy′rotoxico′sis [thyro- + G. toxikon, poison, + -osis, condition] The state produced by excessive quantities of endogenous or exogenous thyroid hormone.

thyrotro′phic [thyro- + G. tropē, a turning] Stimulating or nurturing the thyroid gland.

thyrotro′phin, thyrotro′pin Thyroid-stimulating hormone; a glycoprotein hormone produced by the anterior pituitary gland which stimulates the growth and function of the thyroid gland, and is used as a diagnostic test to differentiate primary and secondary hypothyroidism.

thyrotro′phic [thyro- + G. trophē, nourishment] Thyrotropic.

thyrox′ine, thyrox′in (T$_4$) The active iodine compound existing normally in the thyroid gland and extracted therefrom in crystalline form for therapeutic use; also prepared synthetically.

tib′ia, pl. **tib′iae** [L.] [NA] Shin bone; the medial and larger of the two bones of the leg, articulating with the femur, fibula, and talus.

tibio- [L. tibia, the large shinbone] Combining form denoting the tibia.

tic [Fr.] Habit spasm; an involuntary repeated contraction of a certain group of associated muscles; a habitual spasmodic movement or contraction of any part. See also spasm.

　t. douloureux′ [Fr. painful], trigeminal neuralgia.

　facial t., involuntary twitching of the facial muscles, sometimes unilateral.

tick An acarine of the families Ixodidae (hard t.'s) or Argasidae (soft t.'s), which contain many bloodsucking species that are important pests and vectors of a variety of disease agents; differentiated from the much smaller true mites by possession of an armed hypostome and a pair of tracheal spiracular openings located behind the basal segment of the third or fourth pair of walking legs.

ti′dal Relating to or resembling the tides, alternately rising and falling.

time [A.S. tima] A certain period during which something definite or determined is done.

coagulation t., clotting t., the t. required for blood to coagulate.

prothrombin t., the t. required for clotting after thromboplastin and calcium are added in optimal amounts to blood of normal fibrinogen content; if prothrombin is diminished, the clotting t. increases.

reaction t., the interval between the presentation of a stimulus and the response to it.

tinc′ture (tinct., tr.) [L. *tinctura*, a dyeing] An alcoholic or hydroalcoholic solution prepared from vegetable materials or from chemical substances. T.'s of potent drugs essentially represent the activity of 10 g of the drug in each 100 ml of t.; most other t.'s represent 20 g of drug in each 100 ml of t.

tin′ea [L. worm, moth] Ringworm; a fungus infection of the hair, skin, or nails.

t. bar′bae, t. sycosis.

t. cap′itis, ringworm of the scalp; a fungus infection of the scalp caused by various species of *Microsporn* and *Trichophyton*, characterized by patches of apparent baldness, scaling, block dots, and occasionally erythema and pyoderma.

t. circina′ta, t. cor′poris, ringworm of the body; a scaling macular eruption that frequently forms annular lesions on any part of the body.

t. cru′ris, jock itch; ringworm of the genitocrural region, including the inner side of the thighs, perineum, and groin.

t. pe′dis, athlete's foot; ringworm of the foot, especially of the skin between the toes, caused by a species of *Trichophyton* or *Epidermophyton*; consists of small vesicles, fissures, scaling, maceration, and eroded areas between toes and on the plantar surfaces of the feet.

t. syco′sis, ringworm of the beard, occurring as a follicular infection or as a granulomatous lesion; primary lesions are papules and pustules.

t. un′guium, onychomycosis.

t. versic′olor, pityriasis versicolor; an eruption of tan or brown branny patches on the skin of the trunk, often appearing white in contrast with hyperpigmented skin after exposure to the summer sun; caused by *Malassezia furfur*.

tinni′tus [L. *tinnio*, pp. *tinnitus*, to jingle, clink] The sensation of noises in one or both ears; associated with disease in the middle ear, the inner ear, or the central auditory apparatus.

tis′sue [Fr. *tissu*, woven, fr. L. *texo*, to weave] A collection of similar cells and the intercellular substances surrounding them, of four basic types: epithelium, connective tissue, muscle tissue, nerve tissue.

connective t., interstitial t., the supporting or framework t. of the animal body, formed of fibrous and ground substance; varieties are: areolar, adipose; fibrous, elastic, mucous, lymphatic, cartilage, and bone; blood and lymph may be regarded as connective t.'s, the ground substance of which is liquid.

muscular t., flesh; t. characterized by the ability to contract upon stimulation, of three varieties: skeletal, cardiac, and smooth. See under muscle.

nerve t., a highly differentiated t. composed of nerve cells, nerve fibres, dendrites, and neuroglia.

titra′tion [Fr. *titre*, standard] Volumetric analysis by means of the addition of definite amounts of a test solution to a solution of the substance being assayed.

toco- [G. *tokos*, birth] Combining form denoting childbirth.

to′codynamom′eter [toco- + G. *dynamis*, force, + *metron*, measure] An instrument for measuring the force of uterine contractions.

tocog′raphy [toco- + G. *graphō*, to write] The process of recording uterine contractions.

tocoph′erol (T) Generic term for vitamin E and compounds chemically related to it, with or without biological activity.

α-tocopherol (α-T). Vitamin E; obtained from wheat germ oil or by synthesis, and biologically exhibiting the most vitamin E activity of the t.'s.

toe [A.S. *ta*] Digitus pedis; one of the digits of the feet.

hammer t., permanent flexion at the midphalangeal joint of one or more of the t.'s.

toe-drop A drooping of the anterior portion of the foot, due to paralysis of the muscles that dorsally flex the foot.

toe′nail See unguis.

ingrown t., ingrown *nail*.

Togavi′ridae The family of viruses that includes the antigenic groups A and B arboviruses, which constitute the genera *Alphavirus* and *Flavivirus*, respectively, rubella virus (*Rubivirus*), and *Pestivirus*.

to'gavirus Any virus of the family Togaviridae.

tolbu'tamide An orally active hypoglycaemic agent that appears to stimulate the synthesis and release of endogenous insulin from functional islets; available as t. sodium for injection.

tol'erance [L. *tolero*, pp. -*atus*, to endure] **1.** The ability to endure or be less responsive to a stimulus, especially over a period of continued exposure. **2.** The power of resisting the action of a poison, or of taking a drug continuously or in large doses without injurious effects.

  cross t., the resistance to one or several effects of a compound as a result of t. developed to a pharmacologically similar compound.

  immunological t., acquired specific failure of the immunological mechanism to respond, induced by exposure to the given antigen.

-tome [G. *tomos*, cutting, sharp] Termination denoting a cutting instrument; a segment, part, or section.

tomog'raphy [G. *tomos*, a cutting (section), + *graphō*, to write] The taking of sectional radiographs in which the image of the selected plane remains clear while the images of all other planes are blurred or obliterated.

  computed t. (CT), computerized axial t. (CAT), the gathering of anatomical information from a cross-sectional plane of the body, presented as an image generated by a computer synthesis of x-ray transmission data obtained in many different directions through the given plane.

  positron emission t. (PET), tomographic imaging of local metabolic and physiological functions in tissues, as an indicator of the presence or absence of disease, the image being formed by computer synthesis of data transmitted by positron-emitting radionuclides that have been incorporated into natural biochemical substances administered to the patient.

-tomy [G. *tomē*, incision] Termination denoting a cutting operation. See also -ectomy.

tone [G. *tonos*, tone, or a tone] **1.** A musical sound. **2.** The character of the voice expressing an emotion. **3.** The tension present in resting muscles. **4.** Firmness of the tissues; normal functioning of all the organs.

tongue [A.S. *tunge*] Lingua (1).

  black t., the presence of a blackish to yellowish brown patch or patches on the t., accompanied by elongation of the papillae; *Candida albicans*, flourishes in this environment, especially after the use of antibiotics.

  coated t., a t. with a whitish layer on its upper surface, composed of epithelial debris, food particles, and bacteria.

  geographical t., occurrence on the dorsum of the t. of peripherally spreading patches of temporary papillary atrophy or transitory benign migrating plaques.

  hairy t., a t. with black hairlike elongations of the papillae.

ton'ic [G. *tonikos*, fr. *tonos*, tone] **1.** In a state of continuous unremitting action; denoting especially a muscular contraction. **2.** Invigorating; increasing physical or mental tone or vigour. **3.** A remedy that restores enfeebled function and promotes vigour and a sense of well being, qualified according to the organ or system on which they act; *e.g.*, cardiotonic.

tonic'ity [G. *tonos*, tone] **1.** Tonus; a state of normal tension of the tissues by virtue of which the parts are ready to function in response to a suitable stimulus. **2.** The osmotic pressure or tension of a solution, usually relative to that of blood.

ton'icoclon'ic Both tonic and clonic, referring to muscular spasms.

tono- [G. *tonos*, tone, tension] Combining form relating to tone, tension, pressure.

tonofi'bril One of a system of fibres, found in the cytoplasm of epithelial cells.

tonog'raphy Continuous measurement of intraocular pressure by means of a recording tonometer, for determining the facility of aqueous outflow.

tonom'eter [tono- + G. *metron*, measure] An instrument for determining pressure or tension, especially intraocular tension.

tonom'etry **1.** Measurement of the tension of a part. **2.** Measurement of intraocular tension.

ton'sil [L. *tonsilla*, a stake; pl, tonsils] **1.** Tonsilla. **2.** *Tonsilla* palatina.

  palatine t., *tonsilla* palatina.

  pharyngeal t., *tonsilla* pharyngea.

tonsil'la, pl. **tonsil'lae** [L.] [NA] Tonsil; any collection of lymphoid tissue.

t. palati'na [NA], a large oval mass of lymphoid tissue embedded in the lateral walls of the oral pharynx between the pillars of the fauces.

t. pharyn'gea [NA], a collection of aggregated lymphoid nodules on the posterior wall of the nasopharynx, hypertrophy of which constitutes adenoids.

ton'sillar, ton'sillary Relating to a tonsil, especially the palatine tonsil.

tonsillec'tomy [tonsil + G. *ektomē*, excision] Surgical removal of the entire tonsil.

tonsilli'tis [tonsil + G. *-itis*, inflammation] Inflammation of a tonsil, especially the palatine tonsil.

to'nus [L. fr. G. *tonos*] Tonicity (1).

tooth, pl. **teeth** [A.S. *tōth*] Dens; one of the hard conical structures set in the alveoli of the upper and lower jaws, used in mastication and assisting also in articulation, composed of dentine encased in cement on the covered portion and enamel on its exposed portion.

buck t., an anterior t. in labioversion.
baby t., *dens* deciduus.
bicuspid t., *dens* premolaris.
canine t., cuspid t., *dens* caninus.
deciduous t., *dens* deciduus.
Hutchinson's teeth, the teeth of congenital syphilis in which the incisal edge is notched and narrower than the cervical area.
impacted t., a t. whose normal eruption is prevented by adjacent teeth or bone.
incisor t., *dens* incisivus.
molar t., *dens* molaris.
permanent t., *dens* permanens.
premolar t., *dens* premolaris.
wisdom t., *dens* serotinus.

topagno'sis [top- + G. a- priv. + *gnosis*, recognition] Inability to localize tactile sensations.

to'phus, pl. **to'phi** [L. calcareous deposit from springs] **1.** A deposit of the uric acid and urates in gout. **2.** A salivary calculus, or tartar.

top'ical [G. *topikos*, fr. *topos*, place] Local; relating to a definite place or locality.

topo-, top- [G. *topos*, place] Combining forms denoting place, topical.

topog'raphy [topo- + G. *graphē*, a writing] In anatomy, the description of any part of the body, especially in relation to a definite and limited area of the surface.

tor'pid [L. *torpidus*, fr. *torpeo*, to be sluggish] Inactive; sluggish.

tor'por [L. sluggishness, numbness] Inactivity, sluggishness.

tor'sion [L. *torsio*, fr. *torqueo*, to twist] **1.** A twisting or rotation of a part upon its long axis. **2.** Twisting of the cut end of an artery to arrest haemorrhage. **3.** Rotation of the eye around its anteroposterior axis.

tor'so [It.] The trunk; the body without relation to head or extremities.

torticol'lis [L. *tortus*, twisted, + *collum*, neck] A contraction, often spasmodic, of the muscles of the neck, chiefly those supplied by the spinal accessory nerve; the head is drawn to one side and usually rotated.

tor'ulus, pl. **tor'uli** [L. dim. of *torus*, a protuberance, swelling] A minute elevation in the skin.

tour'niquet [Fr. fr. *tourner*, to turn] An instrument for temporarily arresting the flow of blood to or from a distal part by pressure applied with an encircling device.

toxae'mia [G. *toxikon*, arrow poison, + *haima*, blood] **1.** Clinical manifestations observed during certain infectious diseases, assumed to be caused by toxins and other noxious substances elaborated by the infectious agent. **2.** The clinical syndrome caused by toxic substances in the blood.

tox'ic [G. *toxikon*, arrow poison] **1.** Poisonous. **2.** Pertaining to a toxin.

tox'icant **1.** Poisonous. **2.** Any poisonous agent, specifically an alcoholic poison.

toxic'ity The state of being poisonous.
oxygen t., a condition resulting from breathing high partial pressures of oxygen; characterized by visual and hearing abnormalities, unusual fatigue, muscular twitching, anxiety, confusion, incoordination, and convulsions.

toxico-, tox-, toxi-, toxo- Combining form denoting a toxin or poison.

Toxicoden'dron [toxico- + G. *dendron*, tree] A genus of poisonous plants (family Anacardiaceae) comprising members of the genus *Rhus* such as poison ivy and poison oak.

toxicol'ogy [toxico- + G. *logos*, study] The science of poisons: their source, chemical composition, action, tests, and antidotes.

toxico'sis [toxico- + G. *-osis*, condition] Systemic poisoning; any disease of toxic origin.

tox'in [G. *toxikon*, arrow poison] A noxious or poisonous substance formed or elaborated either as an integral part of the cell (endotoxin) or tissue, as an extracellular product (exotoxin), or as a combination of two, during the metabolism and growth of an organism.

botulinum t., a potent neurotoxin from *Clostridium botulinum.*

Schick test t., diagnostic diphtheria t.; the inoculated dose of *Corynebacterium diptheriae* t. used in the Schick test.

tetanus t., the neurotropic heat-labile exotoxin of *Clostridium tetani* that causes tetanus.

toxocari'asis Infection with nematodes of the genus *Toxocara;* parenterally migrating larvae, chiefly of *T. canis* from dogs, may cause visceral larva migrans in man.

Toxoplas'ma gondii [G. *toxon,* bow, + *plasma,* anything formed] A sporozoan species that is an intracellular, non-host-specific parasite in a great variety of vertebrates but develops its sexual cycle, leading to oocyst production, exclusively in cats and other felids; proliferative stages and tissue cysts develop in other animals that acquire the infection from ingestion of oocysts from cats, tissue cysts from infected meat, or by transplacental migration leading to infection *in utero.*

tox'oplasmo'sis Disease caused by presence of or reaction to *Toxoplasma gondii.* Manifestations vary widely but chorioretinitis and uveitis are common; in prenatal infections, death or severe brain and eye damage usually occur; acute disease may develop, especially in immunologically compromised individuals, leading to generalized infection.

acquired t. in adults, a form of t. that may result in fever, encephalomyelitis, chorioretinopathy, maculopapular rash, arthralgia, myalgia, myocarditis, and pneumonitis; a lymphadenopathic form is manifested by fever, lymphadenopathy, malaise, and headache.

congenital t., t. apparently resulting from parasites in an infected mother being transmitted *in utero* to the fetus; may be observed as three syndromes: **1)** *acute,* most of the organs containing foci of necrosis in association with fever, jaundice, encephelomyelitis, pneumonitis, cutaneous rash, ophthalmic lesions, hepatomegaly, and splenomegaly; **2)** *subacute,* most of the lesions are partly healed or calcified, but those in the brain and eye seem to remain active; **3)** *chronic,* usually

not recognized during the newborn period, but chorioretinitis and cerebral lesions are detected later.

trabec'ula, pl. **trabec'ulae** [L. dim. of *trabs,* a beam] [NA] **1.** One of the supporting bundles of fibres traversing the substance of a structure, usually derived from the capsule or one of the fibrous septa. **2.** A small piece of the spongy substance of bone usually interconnected with other similar pieces.

trabec'ular, trabec'ulate Relating to or containing trabeculae.

tra'cer 1. An element or compound containing atoms that can be distinguished from their normal counterparts and that can thus be used to trace the course of the normal substances in metabolism or similar chemical changes. **2.** An instrument used in dissecting out nerves and blood vessels.

tra'chea, pl. **tra'cheae** [G. *tracheia artēria,* rough artery] [NA] Windpipe; the airway extending from the larynx into the thorax, where it divides into the right and left main bronchi; composed of rings of hyaline cartilage connected by a membrane, the annular ligament.

tra'cheal Relating to the trachea.

trachei'tis [trachea + G. *-itis,* inflammation] Inflammation of the lining membrane of the trachea.

trach'elism, trachelis'mus [G. *trachēlismos,* a seizing by the throat] A spasmodic bending backward of the neck, such as sometimes precedes an epileptic attack.

trachelo-, trachel- [G. *trachēlos,* neck] Combining forms denoting neck.

trach'eloplasty [trachelo- + G. *plastos,* formed] Surgical repair of the uterine cervix.

trachelor'rhaphy [trachelo- + G. *rhaphē,* suture] Suture of a laceration of the uterine cervix.

tracheo-, trache- Combining form denoting the trachea.

tra'cheobronchi'tis Inflammation of the mucous membrane of the trachea and bronchi.

tra'cheosteno'sis [tracheo- + G. *stenōsis,* constriction] Narrowing of the lumen of the trachea.

tracheos'tomy [tracheo- + G. *stoma,* mouth] Surgical creation of an opening into the trachea, or that opening.

tracheot'omy [tracheo- + G. *tomē*, incision] Incision into the trachea through the neck.

tracho'ma [G. *trachōma*, fr. *trachys*, rough, harsh] Chronic contagious microbial inflammation, with hypertrophy, of the conjunctiva caused by *Chlamydia trachomatis*.

tract [L. *tractus*, a drawing out, extent] An elongated assembly of tissue or organs having a common origin, function, and termination, or a serial arrangement serving a common function.

digestive t., alimentary t., the passage leading from the mouth to the anus through the pharynx, oesophagus, stomach, and intestine.

gastrointestinal t., the stomach, small intestine, and large intestine.

genital t., the genital passages of the urogenital system.

optic t., *tractus* opticus.

pyramidal t., *tractus* pyramidalis.

respiratory t., the air passages from the nose to the pulmonary alveoli, through the pharynx, larynx, trachea, and bronchi.

urinary t., the passage from the pelvis of the kidney to the urinary meatus through the ureters, bladder, and urethra.

trac'tion [L. *traho*, pp. *tractus*, to draw] **1.** The act of drawing or pulling. **2.** A pulling force.

axis t., t. upon the fetal head in the line of the birth canal by means of forceps.

skeletal t., t. pull on a bone structure mediated through a pin or wire inserted into the bone to reduce a fracture of long bones.

trac'tus, pl. **trac'tus** [L.] [NA] Tract.

t. op'ticus [NA], continuation of the optic nerve beyond its hemidecussation in the optic chiasm; each of the two tracts is composed of fibres originating from the temporal half of the retina of the ipsilateral eye and a nearly equal number of fibres from the nasal half of the contralateral retina.

t. pyramida'lis [NA], a massive bundle of fibres originating from the precentral motor cortex, to a lesser extent also in the postcentral gyrus, and emerge on the ventral surface of the medulla oblongata as the pyramis. Most of the fibres cross to the opposite side in the pyramidal decussation to descend throughout the length of the spinal cord to innervate distal extremity muscles subserving in particular hand-and-finger or foot-and-toe movements.

tra'gus, pl. **tra'gi** [G. *tragos*, goat, fr. hairs growing on the part] **1.** [NA] A tongue-like projection of the cartilage of the auricle in front of the opening of the external acoustic meatus and continuous with the cartilage of this canal. **2.** [NA] Plural, the hairs at the entrance to the external acoustic meatus.

trait [Fr. from L. *tratus*, a drawing out, extension] A characteristic, especially one that distinguishes an individual from others.

sickle cell t., the heterozygous state of the gene for haemoglobin S; heterozygotes produce both Hb S and Hb A, a portion of their erythrocytes assume sickle shape on reduction of oxygen tension.

trance [L. *trans-eo*, to go across] An altered state of consciousness as in hypnosis, catalepsy, or ecstasy.

tran'quilizer A drug that brings tranquility by calming, soothing, quieting, or pacifying without depression.

trans- [L. *trans*, through, across] **1.** Prefix meaning across, through, beyond; opposite of cis-. **2.** In genetics, denoting the location of two genes on opposite chromosomes of a homologous pair. **3.** In organic chemistry, denoting a form of isomerism in which the atoms attached to two carbon atoms, joined by double bonds, are located on opposite sides of the molecule. **4.** In biochemistry, prefix to group name in an enzyme name or a reaction denoting transfer of that group from one compound to another.

transam'inases Aminotransferases.

transam'ina'tion The reaction between an α-amino acid and an α-keto acid through which the amino group is transferred from the former to the latter.

transcor'tical 1. Across or through the cortex of an organ. **2.** From one part of the cerebral cortex to another; denoting the various association tracts.

transec'tion [trans- + L. *seco*, pp. *sectus*, to cut] **1.** A cross section. **2.** Cutting across.

trans'ference 1. The shifting of symptoms from one part of the body to another, as in certain cases of conversion hysteria. **2.** Displacement of affect from one person or one idea to another.

transfu'sion [L. *trans-fundo*, pp. *-fusus*, to pour from one vessel to another] **1.** Transfer of blood from one individual to another. **2.**

Intravascular injection of physiologic saline solution.

direct t., t. of blood from the donor directly to the receptor.

exchange t., removal of most of a patient's blood followed by introduction of an equal amount from donors.

indirect t., introduction into a patient of blood previously obtained from a donor and stored in a suitable container.

transloca'tion Transposition of two segments between nonhomologous chromosomes as a result of abnormal breakage and refusion of reciprocal segments.

transmigra'tion [L. *trans migro,* pp. *-atus,* to remove from one place to another] Movement from one site to another; may entail the crossing of some usually limiting barrier, as in diapedesis.

transmis'sible Capable of being conveyed from one person to another, as a t. disease.

transmis'sion [L. *transmissio,* a sending across] Transfer, as in the conveyance of disease from one person to another, or the passage of a nerve impulse across synapses or at myoneural junctions.

transpira'tion [trans- + L. *spiro* pp. *-atus,* to breathe] Passage of watery vapour through the skin or any membrane.

trans'plant [trans- + L. *planto,* to plant] **1.** To transfer from one part to another, as in grafting and transplantation **2.** The tissue or organ so used. See also graft.

transplanta'tion [L *trans-planto,* pp. *-atus,* to transplant] Implanting in one part a tissue or organ taken from another part or from another person.

trans'port [L. *transporto,* to carry over] Movement or transference of biochemical substances in biologic systems.

transposi'tion 1. Removal from one place to another. **2.** The state of being transposed or of being on the wrong side of the body, as of the viscera.

t. of the great vessels, a cyanotic form of congenital cardiovascular malformation in which the aorta arises from the right ventricle while the pulmonary artery arises from the left ventricle; life requires an associated septal defect or patent ductus arteriosus to permit crossflow between the two circulations.

transsex'ual 1. A person with the external genitalia and secondary sexual characteristics of one sex, but whose personal identification and psychosocial configuration is that of the opposite sex. **2.** Denoting or relating to such a person. **3.** Relating to medical and surgical procedures designed to alter a patient's external sexual characteristics so that they resemble those of the opposite sex.

transsex'ualism 1. The state of being a transsexual. **2.** An overwhelming desire to change one's anatomic sexual characteristics, stemming from the conviction that one is a member of the opposite sex.

trans'udate [trans- + L. *sudo,* pp. *-atus,* to sweat] Any fluid (solvent and solute) that has passed through a normal membrane as a result of imbalanced hydrostatic and osmotic forces.

trans'verse [L. *transversus*] Crosswise; lying across the long axis of the body or of a part.

transves'tism [trans- + L. *vestio,* to dress] Dressing or masquerading in the clothes of the opposite sex, especially adoption of feminine mannerisms and costume by a male.

transves'tite One who practises transvestism.

trau'ma, pl. **trau'mata, trau'mas** [G. wound] A wound or injury, accidental or inflicted.

birth t., (1) physical injury to an infant during its delivery; **(2)** the supposed emotional injury, inflicted by the events incident to birth, upon the psyche of the infant.

psychic t., an upsetting experience precipitating or aggravating an emotional or mental disorder.

traumat'ic [G. *traumatikos*] Relating to or caused by a wound or injury.

traumato-, traumat-, traum- [G. *trauma,* wound] Combining forms denoting a wound or injury.

treat [Fr. *traiter,* fr. L. *tracto,* to drag, handle, perform] To manage a disease or to care for a patient.

treat'ment [Fr. *traitment* (see treat)] Medical, surgical, or other management of a patient. See also therapy; therapeutics.

palliative t., t. to alleviate symptoms without curing the disease.

prophylactic t., preventive t., institution of measures designed to protect a person from a disease to which he has been, or is liable to be exposed.

Tremato'da [G. *trēmatōdēs*, full of holes] The flukes; a class of parasites in the phylum Platyhelminthes (flatworms), having a leaf-shaped body and two muscular suckers; flukes of medical interest belong to the subclass Digenea.

trem'atode Any fluke of the class Trematoda.

trem'or [L. a shaking] **1.** An involuntary trembling movement. **2.** Minute ocular movement occurring during fixation of an object.

trephina'tion Removal of a circular piece of cranium by a trephine.

trephine' [fr. L. *tres fines*, three ends] **1.** A cylindrical or crown saw for the removal of a disc of bone, especially from the skull, or of other firm tissue as that of the cornea. **2.** To remove a disc of bone or other tissue by means of a t.

Trepone'ma [G. *trepō*, to turn, + *nēma*, thread] A genus of anaerobic bacteria (order Spirochaetales) consisting of cells with acute, regular, or irregular spirals and no obvious protoplasmic structure; some species are pathogenic and parasitic for man and other animals. Type species is *T. pallidum*.

T. pal'lidum, a species that causes syphilis in man; the type species of the genus *T*.

T. perten'ue, a species that causes yaws.

trep'oneme Any member of the genus *Treponema*.

treponemi'asis Infection caused by *Treponema*.

trep'onemici'dal [*Treponema* + L. *caedo*, to kill] Destructive to any species of Treponema.

tri- [L. and G.] Prefix denoting three.

triacylglyc'erol Triglyceride; glycerol esterified at each of its three hydroxyl groups by a fatty (aliphatic) acid.

t. lipase, sometimes called simply lipase; the fat-splitting enzyme in pancreatic juice.

triage' [Fr. sorting] Medical screening of large numbers of patients, to determine priority for treatment, into three groups: those who cannot be expected to survive even with treatment; those who will recover without treatment; and the priority group of those who need treatment in order to survive.

tri'ceps [L. fr. *tri-*, three, + *caput*, head] Three-headed, denoting musculus t. brachii and t. surae.

trich-, trichi- See tricho-.

-trichia [G. *thrix* (*trich-*), hair, + *-ia*, condition] Combining form denoting condition or type of hair.

trichi'asis [trich- + G. *-iasis*, condition] A condition in which hairs around a natural orifice, or eyelashes, turn in and cause irritation.

trichi'na, pl. **trichi'nae** A larval worm of the genus *Trichinella*, infective form in pork.

Trichinel'la A parasitic nematode genus in the aphasmid group; *T. spiralis*, the pork or trichina worm, that causes trichinosis.

trichino'sis The disease resulting from ingestion of raw or inadequately cooked meat of carnivores, especially pork, that contains encysted viable larvae of *Trichinella spiralis*. Signs and symptoms may be related to the following: 1) intestinal phase: abdominal discomfort, nausea, and loose stools, associated with inflammation caused by adult worms in the jejunum and ileum; 2) dissemination phase: fever, leucocytosis and eosinophilia, and exaggeration of previous symptoms, associated with circulation of large numbers of larvae in the blood; 3) inflammation phase: intense inflammatory reactions in sites where the larvae degenerate and die; 4) phase of recession: decreasing manifestation of previous signs and symptoms, but larvae coiled within oval cysts may be found in biopsies of skeletal muscle.

trichlo'roeth'ylene An analgesic and inhalation anaesthetic used in minor surgical operations and in obstetrics.

tricho-, trich-, trichi- [G. *thrix* (*trich-*), hair] Combining form denoting the hair or a hairlike structure.

trichobe'zoar Hairball; a hair cast in the stomach or intestinal tract.

trichomo'nad Any member of the family Trichomonadidae (*e.g.*, *Trichomonas*).

Trichomo'nas [tricho- + G. *monas*, single (unit)] A genus of parasitic protozoan flagellates (family Trichomonadidae) that cause trichomoniasis.

T. te'nax, a species that lives as a commensal in the mouth, especially in tartar around the teeth or in defects of carious teeth.

T. vagina'lis, a species found in the vagina and urethra of women and in the urethra and prostate gland of men (only natural hosts), in whom it causes trichomoniasis vaginitis.

trich'omoni'asis Disease caused by infection with a species of *Trichomonas* or related genera.

t. vagini'tis, acute or subacute vaginitis or urethritis caused by infection with *Trichomonas vaginalis;* infection is venereal or by other forms of contact.

trich'omyco'sis [tricho- + G. *mykēs,* fungus, + *-osis,* condition] Formerly, any disease of the hair caused by a fungus; presently synonymous with trichonocardiosis or t. axillaris.

t. axilla'ris, infection of axillary and pubic hairs with development of yellow (flava), black (nigra), or red (rubra) concretions around the hair shafts.

trich'onocardio'sis [tricho- + *Nocardia* + G. *-osis,* condition] An infection of hair shafts, especially of the axillary and pubic regions, with nocardiae; yellow, red, or black concretions develop around the infected hair shafts. See also *trichomycosis axillaris.*

Trichophy'ton [tricho- + G. *phyton,* plant] A genus of pathogenic fungi causing dermatophytosis in man and animals. Species may be anthropophilic, zoophilic, or geophilic, and attack hair, skin, and nails. Many of the 20 to 30 species which have been listed are now known to be variants. The three groups of species are characterized by their growth in hair: endothrix species grow from the skin into the hair follicle, penetrate the shaft, and grow into it, producing rows of arthrospores as the hyphae septate; there is no growth on the external surface of the shaft. Ectothrix species are of two kinds, large spored and small spored. In both, the fungus grows into the hair follicle, surrounds the hair shaft, and penetrates it, but continues to grow both within and outside the hair shaft.

T. concen'tricum, an anthropophilic species that causes tinea imbricata.

T. mentagrophy'tes, a zoophilic small-spored ectothrix species that causes infection of hair, skin, and nails.

T. ru'brum, an anthropophilic endoectothrix species that causes persistent infections in the nails that are unusually resistant to therapy.

T. schoenlei'nii, an anthropophilic endothrix species that causes favus.

T. ton'surans, an anthropophilic endothrix species that causes epidemic dermatophytosis.

T. viola'ceum, an anthropophilic endothrix species that causes black-dot ringworm or favus infection of the scalp.

trichophyto'sis [tricho- + G. *phyton,* plant, + *-osis,* condition] Superficial fungus infection caused by species of *Trichophyton.*

trichorrhex'is [tricho- + G. *thōxio,* a breaking] A condition in which the hairs readily break or split.

trichuri'asis Infection with a species of *Trichuris;* usually asymptomatic and not associated with peripheral eosinophilia, but in massive infections it frequently induces diarrhoea or rectal prolapse.

Trichu'ris [tricho- + G. *oura,* tail] Whipworm; a genus of aphasmid nematodes related to the trichina worm, *Trichinella spiralis. T. trichiura* causes trichuriasis in man.

tricus'pid, tricus'pidal, tricus'pidate Having three points, prongs, or cusps.

tri'fid [l. *trifidus,* three-cleft] Split into three.

triglyc'eride Triacylglycerol.

tri'gone [L. *trigonum,* fr. G. *trigōnon,* triangle] **1.** A triangle or trigonum. **2.** The first three dominant cusps of an upper molar tooth.

t. of the bladder, *trigonum* vesicae. **inguinal t.,** *trigonum* inguinale.

trigoni'tis [trigone + G. *-itis,* inflammation] Inflammation of the urinary bladder, localized in the mucous membrane at the trigonum vesicae.

trigo'num, pl. **trigo'na** [L. from G. *trigōnon,* a triangle] [NA] Any triangular area.

t. inguina'le [NA], the triangular area in the lower abdominal wall bounded by the inguinal ligament below, the rectus abdominis muscle medially, and the inferior epigastric vessels laterally; the site of direct inguinal hernia.

t. lumba'le [NA], an area in the posterior abdominal wall bounded by the edges of the latissimus dorsi and external oblique muscles and the iliac crest; herniations occasionally occur here.

t. vesi'cae [NA], a triangular smooth area at the base of the bladder between the openings of the two ureters and that of the urethra.

3,5,3'-tri-iodothy'ronine (TITh, T₃) A thyroid hormone normally synthesized in smaller quantities than thyroxine; present in blood and in thyroid gland and exerts the same biological effects as thyroxine but, on a molecular basis, is more potent and the onset of its effect more rapid.

tri'labe [tri- + G. *labē*, a handle, hold] A three-pronged forceps for removal of foreign bodies from the bladder.

trilo'bate, tri'lobed Having three lobes.

triloc'ular Having three cavities or cells.

trimes'ter [L. *trimestris*, of three-month duration] A period of 3 months; one-third of the length of a pregnancy.

tri'ose A three-carbon monosaccharide.

triplo'pia [G. *triploos*, triple, + *opsis*, sight] A visual defect in which three images are seen of the same object.

-tripsy [G. *tripsis*, a rubbing] Suffix denoting a surgical procedure in which a structure is crushed, as a calculus.

tris'mus [L. fr. G. *trismos*, a creaking, rasping] Lockjaw; a firm closing of the jaw due to tonic spasm of the muscles of mastication from disease of the motor branch of the trigeminal nerve; usually associated with and due to general tetanus.

tri'somy [tri- + (chromo)some] State of an individual or cell with an extra chromosome; instead of the normal pair of homologous chromosomes there are three of a particular chromosome.

triv'ial name A name of a chemical that gives no clue as to chemical structure; commonly used for drugs, hormones, proteins, and other biologicals, but not officially sanctioned; *e.g.*, aspirin, chlorophyll, caffeine.

tro'car [Fr. *trocart*] An instrument for withdrawing fluid from a cavity, or for use in paracentesis, consisting of a metal tube (cannula) into which fits an obturator with a sharp three-cornered tip, which is withdrawn after the instrument has been pushed into the cavity; usually applied to the obturator alone, the entire instrument being designated t. and cannula.

trochan'ter [G. *trochantēr*, a runner, fr. *trechō*, to run] One of the bony prominences developed from independent osseous centres near the upper extremity of the femur.

t. ma'jor [NA], **greater t.,** a strong process overhanging the root of the neck of the femur.

t. mi'nor [NA], **lesser t.,** a pyramidal process projecting from the shaft of the femur at the junction of the shaft and the neck.

tro'che [L. *trochiscus*, small wheel] Lozenge; a small disc-shaped or rhombic body containing a drug, used for local treatment of the mouth or throat, being held in the mouth until dissolved.

troch'lea, pl. **troch'leae** [L. pulley] [NA] **1.** A structure serving as a pulley. **2.** A smooth articular surface of bone upon which another glides. **3.** A fibrous loop in the orbit, near the nasal process of the frontal bone, through which passes the tendon of the superior oblique muscle of the eye.

Trombic'ula The chigger mite, a genus of mites (family Trombiculidae) whose larvae (chiggers, red bugs) include pests of man and other animals.

-trophic [G. *trophē*, nourishment] Suffix denoting nutrition.

troph'ic [G. *trophē*, nourishment] **1.** Relating to or dependent upon nutrition. **2.** Resulting from interruption of nerve supply.

tropho-, troph- [G. *trophē*, nourishment] Combining forms denoting food or nutrition.

tro'phoblast [tropho- + G. *blastos*, germ] The mesectodermal cell layer covering the blastocyst which erodes the uterine mucosa and through which the embryo receives nourishment from the mother; it contributes to the formation of the placenta.

trophoblas'tic Relating to the trophoblast.

tro'phoneuro'sis [tropho- + G. *neuron*, nerve, + *-osis*, condition] A trophic disorder occurring as a consequence of disease or injury of the nerves of the part.

-trophy [G. *trophē*, nourishment] Suffix meaning food, nutrition.

-tropic [G. *tropē*, a turning] Suffix denoting a turning toward, having an affinity for.

trun'cal Relating to the trunk of the body or to any arterial or nerve trunk, etc.

trun'cus, pl. **trun'ci** [L. stem, trunk] [NA] **1.** Trunk; the body, excluding the head and extremities. **2.** A primary nerve or vessel before its division. **3.** A large collecting lymphatic vessel.

t. a'trioventricula'ris [NA], His bundle; the bundle of modified cardiac muscle fibres that begins at the atrioventricular node and passes through the right atrioventricular fibrous ring to the membranous part of the interventricular septum where it divides into right and left branches, which ramify in the subendocardium of their respective ventricles.

persistent t. arterio'sus, a congenital cardiovascular deformity resulting from failure of development of the bulbar septum and consisting of a common arterial trunk opening out of both ventricles, the pulmonary arteries being given off from the ascending common trunk.

trunk [L. *truncus*] Truncus.

atrioventricular t., *truncus* atrioventricularis.

truss [Fr. *trousser*, to tie up, to pack]. An appliance designed to prevent the return of a reduced hernia or the increase in size of an irreducible hernia.

trypan'ocide [trypanosome + L. *caedo*, to kill] An agent that kills trypanosomes.

Trypanoso'ma [G. *trypanon*, an anger, + *sōma*, body] A genus of asexual, digenetic, protozoan flagellates (family Trypanosomatidae) that are parasitic in the blood plasma of many vertebrates and have an intermediate host, a bloodsucking invertebrate, such as a leech, tick, or insect; pathogenic species cause trypanosomiasis in man.

T. cru'zi, a species that causes South American trypanosomiasis.

T. gambien'se, a species that causes Gambian or chronic trypanosomiasis (West African sleeping sickness); transmitted by several species of tsetse flies, particularly *Glossina palpalis.*

T. rhodesien'se, a species that causes Rhodesian or acute trypanosomiasis (East African sleeping sickness); chief vector is the tsetse fly, *Glossina morsitans.*

trypan'osome Any member of the genus *Trypanosoma* or its family Trypanosomatidae.

trypan'osomi'asis Any disease caused by a trypanosome.

Gambian t., chronic sleeping sickness; t. caused by *Trypanosoma gambiense*, transmitted to man by tsetse flies, chiefly *Glossina palpalis;* symptoms are erythematous patches and local oedemas; neuralgic pains, cramps, tremors, and paraesthesia; enlargement of the lymph glands, spleen, and liver; emaciation; and an evening elevation of temperature; in later stages (after invasion of trypanosomes into the CNS) there is lethargy,

with somnolence deepening to coma in the terminal stage.

Rhodesian t., acute sleeping sickness; t. caused by *Trypanosoma rhodesiense*, transmitted by tsetse flies of the species *Glossina morsitans*, and similar to Gambian t. but running a far more rapid, acute course.

South American t., Chagas or Chagas-Cruz disease; t. caused by *Trypanosoma cruzi* and transmitted by certain species of reduviid bugs in its acute form, there is swelling of the skin at the site of entry, most often the face with regional lymph node enlargement; in its chronic form it assumes several aspects (cardiac, nervous, or myxoedematous) according to the predominating symptoms.

tryp'sin A proteolytic enzyme formed in the small intestine from trypsinogen; a serine proteinase that hydrolyses peptides, amides, esters, etc.

trypsin'ogen, tryp'sogen An inactive substance secreted by the pancreas that is converted into trypsin by the action of enterokinase.

tryp'tophan (TRP) A component of proteins.

tse'tse [S. African native name] See Glossina.

tu'bal Relating to a tube, especially the uterine tube.

tube [L. *tubua*, straight trumpet] **1.** A hollow cylinder or pipe. **2.** A canal or tubular organ.

auditory t., eustachian t., a t. from the tympanic cavity of the ear to the nasopharynx.

endotracheal t., a catheter inserted into the trachea to provide an airway.

feeding t., a flexible t. passed through oral pharynx and into the oesophagus and stomach, through which liquid food is fed.

nasogastric t., a stomach tube passed through the nose.

stomach t., a flexible t. passed into the stomach for lavage or feeding.

tracheotomy t., a curved t. used to keep the stoma free after tracheotomy.

uterine t., fallopian t., a t. from each ovary to the side of the fundus of the uterus, through which the ova pass.

tu'ber, pl. **tu'bera** [L. protuberance, swelling] [NA] A localized swelling; a knob, tuberosity, or eminence.

t. cine′reum [NA], a prominence of the base of the hypothalamus, extending ventrally into the infundibulum and hypophyseal stalk.

tu′bercle [L. *tuberculum*, dim. of *tuber*, a swelling] **1.** In anatomy, tuberculum. **2.** In dentistry, a small elevation arising on the surface of a tooth. **3.** A granulomatous lesion due to infection by *Mycobacterium tuberculosis*, although morphologically indistinguishable lesions may occur in diseases caused by other agents.

tuber′cular, tuber′culate, tuber′culated Pertaining to or characterized by tubercles or small nodules.

tuber′culid A lesion of the skin or mucous membrane resulting from specific sensitization to the tubercle bacillus.

tuber′culin A liquid culture of *Mycobacterium tuberculosis* used chiefly for diagnostic tests; originally known as Koch's old t. (OT).

tuberculo-, tubercul- Combining forms denoting a tubercle, tuberculosis.

tuber′culoid [tuberculo- + G. *eidos*, resemblance] Resembling tuberculosis, or a tubercle.

tuber′culo′sis [tuberculo- + G. *-osis*, condition] A specific disease caused by the presence of *Mycobacterium tuberculosis*, the most common seat being the lungs, which produces a tubercle that undergoes caseation; general symptoms are those of sepsis: fever, sweats, and emaciation.

acute t., acute miliary t., a rapidly fatal disease due to the general dissemination of tubercle bacilli in the blood, resulting in the formation of miliary tubercles in various organs and tissues, and producing symptoms of profound toxaemia.

cutaneous t., pathologic lesions of the skin caused by *Mycobacterium tuberculosis*.

open t., pulmonary t., tuberculous ulceration, or other form in which the bacilli are present in the excretions or secretions.

tuberculostat′ic [tuberculo- + G. *statikos*, causing to stand] Denoting an agent that inhibits the growth of tubercle bacilli.

tuber′culous Relating to or affected by tuberculosis.

tuber′culum, pl. **tuber′cula** [L. dim. of a *tuber*, a knob, swelling, tumour] [NA] **1.** An anatomical nodule. **2.** A circumscribed, rounded, solid elevation on the skin, mucous membrane, or surface of an organ. **3.** A slight elevation from the surface of a bone giving attachment to a muscle or ligament.

tuberos′ity [L. *tuberosus*, full of lumps] A large tubercle or rounded elevation, as from the surface of a bone for attachment of a ligament or tendon.

tu′berous [L. *tuberosus*] Knobby, lumpy, or nodular; presenting many tubers or tuberosities.

tubo- Combining form denoting tubular or a tube. See also salpingo-.

tu′bocurar′ine chloride An alkaloid (from the stems of *Chondodendron tomentosum*) that raises the threshold for acetylcholine at the myoneural junction by occupying the receptors competitively, and that also blocks ganglionic tranmission and releases histamine; used to produce muscular relaxation during surgical operations.

tu′bo-ova′rian Relating to the uterine tube and the ovary.

tu′botympan′ic, tubotym′panal Relating to the auditory tube and the tympanic cavity of the ear.

tu′bule [L. *tubulus*, dim. of *tubus*, tube] A small tube.

collecting t., one of the straight t.'s of the kidney, present in the medulla and pars radiata of the cortex.

convoluted t., the first, proximal, or primary leads from the capsule of the kidney; the second or distal lead is formed from the ascending limb of Henle's loop which enters the labyrinth and ends in a collecting t.

seminiferous t., one of two or three twisted curved t.'s in each lobule of the testis, in which spermatogenesis occurs, which becomes straight just before entering the mediastinum to form the rete testis.

tularae′mia [*Tulare*, California, + G. *haima*, blood] A disease caused by *Francisella tularensis* and transmitted to man from rodents through the bite of a deer fly, *Chrysops discalis*, and other bloodsucking insects, and can also be acquired directly through the bite of or handling of an infected animal; symptoms are similar to those of undulant fever and plague.

tumefa′cient [L. *tume-facio*, to cause to swell] Causing or tending to cause swelling.

tumefac′tion [see tumefacient] **1.** A swelling. **2.** Tumescence.

tumes'cence [L. *tumesco*, to begin to swell] The condition of being or becoming tumid.

tu'mid [L. *tumidus*] Swollen, as by congestion, oedema, hyperaemia.

tu'mor [L.] A swelling; one of the four signs of inflammation (t., calor, dolor, rubor) enunciated by Celsus.

tu'mour [L. *tumor*, a swelling] **1.** Any swelling or tumefaction. **2.** Neoplasm.

benign t., a t. that does not form metastases and does not invade and destroy adjacent normal tissue.

carcinoid t., a small slow-growing neoplasm composed of islands of rounded cells of medium size, with moderately small vesicular nuclei, which can occur in the gastrointestinal tract, lungs, and other sites.

embryonal t., embryonic t., embryoma; a neoplasm, usually malignant, that arises during intrauterine or early postnatal development from an organ rudiment or immature tissue, forms immature structures characteristic of the part from which it arises, and may form other tissues.

Ewing's t., a malignant neoplasm which occurs usually before the age of 20 years, about twice as frequently in males, and mostly involves bones of the extremities including the shoulder girdle, with a predilection for the metaphysis.

giant cell t. of bone, a sometimes malignant osteolytic t. composed of multinucleated giant cells and ovoid or spindle-shaped cells, occurring most frequently in an end of a long tubular bone.

granulosa cell t., a benign or malignant t. of the ovary arising from the granular layer of the graafian follicle and frequently secreting oestrogen.

malignant t., a t. that invades surrounding tissues, is usually capable of producing metastases, may recur after attempted removal, and is likely to cause death unless adequately treated.

mixed t., a t. composed of two or more varieties of tissue.

Sertoli cell t., androblastoma (1).

Wilms t., nephroblastoma; a malignant renal mixed t. of young children, composed of small spindle cells and various other types of tissue.

Tun'ga pen'etrans A member of the flea family, Tungidae, commonly known as chigger flea, sand flea, chigoe, or jiggers; the female penetrates the skin, frequently under the toenails, and as she becomes distended with eggs a painful ulcer with inflammation develops.

tu'nic [L. *tunica*] Tunica.

tu'nica, pl. **tu'nicae** [L. a coat] [NA] One of the enveloping layers or coats of a part, as of a blood vessel or other tubular structure.

t. adventi'tia [NA], the outermost fibrous coat of a vessel or an organ that is derived from the surrounding connective tissue.

t. albugin'ea [NA], a dense, white, collagenous sheath surrounding a structure.

t. in'tima [NA], the innermost coat of a blood or lymphatic vessel, consisting of endothelium, usually a thin fibroelastic subendothelial layer, and an inner elastic membrane or longitudinal fibres.

t. me'dia [NA], the middle, usually muscular, coat of an artery or other tubular structure.

t. muco'sa [NA], mucous membrane; a lining of epithelium, lamina propria, and (in the digestive tract) a layer of smooth muscle which secretes mucus.

t. sero'sa [NA], the outermost coat of a visceral structure that lies in a body cavity, consists of a surface layer of mesothelium reinforced by irregular fibroelastic connective tissue.

tun'nel An elongated enclosed passageway, usually open at both ends.

carpal t., canalis carpi.

tur'bid [L. *turbidus*, confused, disordered] Cloudy.

tur'binated [L. *tubinatus*, shaped like a top] Scroll-shaped.

turbinec'tomy [turbinate + G. *ektome*, excision] Surgical removal of a turbinated bone.

tur'gid [L. *turgidus*, swollen] Tumid.

tur'gor [L. fr. *turgeo*, to swell] Fullness.

tus'sis [L.] A cough.

tus'sive [L. *tussis*, a cough] Relating to a cough.

twin [A.S. *getwin*, double] **1.** One of two children born at one birth. **2.** Double; growing in pairs.

conjoined t.'s, monozygotic t.'s with varying extent of union and different degrees of residual duplication.

dizygotic t.'s, fraternal t.'s, t.'s derived from two separate zygotes.

monozygotic t.'s, identical t.'s, t.'s resulting from a single fertilized ovum that at an early stage of development becomes separated into independently growing cell aggregations giving rise to two individuals of the same sex and identical genetic constitution.

twin'ning The production of equivalent structure by division; the tendency of divided parts to assume symmetrical relations.

twitch [A.S. *twiccian*] **1.** To jerk spasmodically. **2.** A momentary spasmodic contraction of a muscle fibre.

tylec'tomy [G. *tylē*, lump, + *ektomē*, excision] Lumpectomy; surgical removal of a tumour from the breast.

tylo'ma [G. a callus] Callosity.

tylo'sis, pl. **tylo'ses** [G. a becoming callous] Formation of a callosity (tyloma).

tympanec'tomy [tympan- + G. *ektomē*, excision] Excision of the tympanic membrane.

tympan'ic 1. Relating to the tympanic cavity or membrane. **2.** Resonant.

tympani'tes [L. fr. G. *tympanitēs*, dropsy in which the belly is stretched like a drum, *tympanon*] Abdominal distension from gas in the intestinal or peritoneal cavity.

tympani'tis Myringitis.

tympano-, tympan-, tympani- [G. *tympanon*, drum] Combining forms denoting tympanum or tympanites.

tym'panomas'toidi'tis Inflammation of the middle ear and the mastoid cells.

tym'panoplasty [tympano- + G. *plassō*, to form] Operative correction of a damaged middle ear.

tympanot'omy [tympano- + G. *tomē*, incision] Myringotomy.

tym'panum, pl. **tym'panums, tym'pana** [L. fr. G. *tympanon*, a drum] *Cavitas tympan-*ica.

ty'phoid [typhus + G. *eidos*, resemblance] **1.** Resembling typhus. **2.** Typhoid *fever*.

ty'phus [G. *typhos*, smoke, stupor] An acute infectious and contagious disease, caused by rickettsiae, and occurring in two chief forms; epidemic t. and murine t.

epidemic t., t. caused by *Rickettsia prowazekii* and spread by body lice; marked by high fever, mental and physical depression, and a macular and papular eruption.

murine t., caused by *Rickettsia typhi* and transmitted to man by rat or mouse fleas; milder than epidemic t., but otherwise similar.

tick t., collective term for tick-borne rickettsial diseases, involving many strains (or species) of the subgenus *Dermacentroxenus;* identified by their immunological reactions and, in some cases, pathogenicity.

typ'ing Classification according to type.

blood t., blood grouping. See under B.

ty'ramine A sympathomimetic amine having an action resembling that of adrenaline.

ty'rosine (Tyr) An α-amino acid present in most proteins.

tyrosino'sis [tyrosine + G. *-osis*, condition] A rare, possibly heritable disorder of tyrosine metabolism characterized by enhanced urinary excretion of tyrosyl metabolites upon ingestion of tyrosine.

tyrosylu'ria Enhanced urinary excretion of certain metabolites of tyrosine, as in tyrosinosis, scurvy, pernicious anaemia.

U

ul'cer [L. *ulcus*, a sore] A lesion on the skin or a mucous surface caused by superficial loss of tissue, usually with necrosis and inflammation.

Curling's u., u. of the duodenum in a patient with extensive superficial burns or severe bodily injury.

decubitus u., bedsore; pressure sore; a chronic u. that appears in pressure areas in debilitated patients confined to bed or otherwise immobilized, due to a circulatory defect in the area under pressure.

peptic u., an u. of the alimentary mucosa, usually in the stomach or duodenum, exposed to acid gastric secretion.

perforated u., an u. extending through the wall of an organ.

rodent u., a slowly enlarging ulcerated basal cell carcinoma, usually on the face.

varicose u., loss of skin surface in the drainage area of a varicose vein, usually in the leg, resulting from stasis and infection.

ul'cerative Relating to, causing, or marked by an ulcer or ulcers.

ulcera'tion 1. The formation of an ulcer. **2.** An ulcer or aggregation of ulcers.

ul'na, pl. **ul'nae** [L. elbow, arm] [NA] Elbow bone; the medial and larger of the two bones of the forearm.

ul'nar Relating to the ulna, or to any of the structures named from it.

ultra- [L. beyond] Prefix denoting excess, exaggeration, beyond.

ultrason'ic [ultra- + L. sonus, sound] Relating to energy waves similar to those of sound but of higher frequencies (above (30,000 Hz).

ul'trasonog'raphy [ultra- + L. sonus, sound, + G. graphō, to write] Echography; sonography; location, measurement, or delineation of deep structures by measuring the reflection or transmission of high frequency or ultrasonic waves.

ul'trasound Sound having a frequency greater than 30,000 Hz.

　diagnostic u., use of u. to obtain images for medical diagnostic purposes, employing frequencies ranging from 1.6 to about 10 MHz.

ultravi'olet Denoting the electromagnetic rays beyond the violet end of the visible spectrum.

umbil'ical Relating to the umbilicus.

umbil'icate, umbil'icated [L. umbilicatus] Of navel shape; pitlike.

umbil'icus, pl. **umbil'ici** [L. navel] [NA] Navel; the pit in the centre of the abdominal wall marking the point where the umbilical cord entered the fetus.

un'cinate [L. uncinatus] Unciform; hooklike or hook-shaped.

uncon'scious **1.** Insensible; not conscious. **2.** In psychoanalysis, the psychic structure comprising the drives and feelings of which one is unaware.

uncon'sciousness A state of impaired consciousness in which one shows a total lack of responsiveness to environmental stimuli, but may respond to deep pain with involuntary movements.

undifferen'tiated Primitive, embryonic, immature, or having no special structure or function.

un'gual, un'guinal [L. unguis, nail] Relating to a nail or the nails.

un'guis, pl. **un'gues** [L.] [NA] Nail; one of the thin, horny, translucent plates covering the dorsal surface at the distal end of each finger and toe; consists of a visible corpus or body and a radix or root concealed under a fold of skin.

uni- [L. unus, one] Prefix denoting one, single, not paired; equivalent to mono-.

unicel'lular Composed of but one cell, as the protozoons.

unilat'eral Confined to one side only.

uniloc'ular [uni- + L. loculus, compartment] Having but one compartment or cavity, as in a fat cell.

u'nion [L. unus, one] **1.** The joining or amalgamation of two or more bodies. **2.** The structural adhesion or growing together of the edges of a wound.

uniov'ular Relating to or formed from a single ovum.

u'nit [L. unus, one] **1.** One; a single entity. **2.** (U) A standard of measure, weight, or any other quality, by multiplications or fractions of which a scale or system is formed. **3.** A group of persons or things considered as a whole because of mutual activities or functions.

　base u.'s, the fundamental u.'s of length (metre), mass (kilogram), time (second), electric current (ampere), thermodynamic temperature (kelvin), amount of substance (mole), and luminous intensity (candela) in the International System of Units (SI).

　intensive care u. (ICU), a hospital facility for provision of intensive care of critically ill patients, characterized by high quality and quantity of continuous nursing and medical supervision and by use of sophisticated monitoring and resuscitative equipment.

　international u. (IU), a u. of biological material or of a drug as accepted by an international body.

　International System of Units (SI), see under I.

unmy'elinated Denoting nerve fibres (axons) lacking a myelin sheath.

unstri'ated Without striations, denoting the structure of the smooth or involuntary muscles.

u'rachus [G. ourachos, the urinary canal of a fetus] That portion of the reduced allantoic stalk between the apex of the bladder and the umbilicus.

u'racil A pyrimidine (base) present in ribonucleic acid.

urae'mia [G. ouron, urine, + haima, blood] **1.** Excess of urea and other nitrogenous waste in the blood. **2.** The complex of symptoms due to severe persisting renal failure that can be relieved by dialysis.

urae'mic Relating to uraemia.

urano- [G. *ouranos*, vault of sky; *ouraniskos*, roof of mouth] Combining form relating to the hard palate.

uranor'rhaphy [urano- + G. *raphē*, suture] Palatorrhaphy.

uranos'chisis [urano- + G. *schisis*, fissure] Cleft of the hard palate.

urarthri'tis [urate + arthritis] Gouty inflammation of a joint.

uratae'mia [urate + G. *haima*, blood] Presence of urates, especially sodium urate, in the blood.

u'rate A salt of uric acid.

uratu'ria [urate + G. *ouron*, urine] Passage of an increased amount of urates in the urine.

ur-defences Fundamental beliefs essential for man's psychological integrity.

ure-, urea-, ureo- [G. *ouron*, urine] Combining forms denoting urea or urine. See also urin-; uro-.

ure'a [G. *ouron*, urine] The chief end product of nitrogen metabolism in mammals, formed in the liver and excreted in the urine.

Ureaplas'ma A genus of nonmotile Gram-negative bacteria (family Mycoplasmataceae) that require urea and cholesterol for growth; in males, associated with nongonococcal urethritis and prostatitis and, in females, with genitourinary tract infections and reproductive failure. The type species is *U. urealyticum*.

urec'chysis [G. *ouron*, urine, + *ekchysis*, a pouring out] Extravasation of urine into the tissues.

ure'sis [G. *ourēsis*] Urination.

ure'ter [G. *ourētēr*, urinary canal] [NA] The tube conducting urine from the renal pelvis of the kidney to the bladder.

ure'teral Relating to the ureter.

uretercys'toscope A cystoscope with an attachment for catheterization of the ureters.

ureterec'tomy [ureter + G. *ektomē*, excision] Excision of a segment or all of a ureter.

ureter'ic Ureteral.

ureteri'tis Inflammation of a ureter.

uretero- [G. *ourētēr*, urinary canal] Combining form denoting the ureter.

ure'terocele [utero- + G. *kēlē*, hernia] Saccular dilatation of the terminal portion of the ureter which protrudes into the lumen of the urinary bladder, due to a congenital stenosis of the ureteral meatus.

ure'terocolos'tomy [uretero- + G. *kolon*, colon, + *stoma*, mouth] Implanting of the ureter into the colon.

ure'teroenteros'tomy [uretero- + G. *enteron*, intestine, + *stoma*, mouth] Surgical formation of an opening between a ureter and the intestine.

ureterog'raphy [uretero- + G. *graphē*, a writing] Radiography of the ureter after injection of contrast media.

ure'teroileos'tomy [uretero- + ileum + G. *stoma*, mouth] Implantation of a ureter into an isolated segment of ileum which drains through an abdominal stoma.

ure'terolith [uretero- + G. *lithos*, stone] A calculus in the ureter.

ure'terolithi'asis [ureterolith + G. *-iasis*, condition] Formation or presence of a calculus or calculi in one or both ureters.

ure'terolithot'omy [ureterolith + G. *tomē*, incision] Surgical removal of a stone lodged in a ureter.

ure'teronephrec'tomy [uretero- + G. *nephros*, kidney, + *ektomē*, excision] Removal of a kidney with its ureter.

ure'teroplasty [uretero- + G. *plassō*, to form] Reparative or plastic surgery of the ureters.

ure'teropyeli'tis [uretero- + G. *pyelos*, pelvis, + *-itis*, inflammation] Inflammation of the pelvis of a kidney and its ureter.

ure'terosigmoidos'tomy Implantation of the ureters into the sigmoid colon.

ureteros'tomy [uretero- + G. *stoma*, mouth] Surgical establishment of an external opening into the ureter.

ure'terovesicos'tomy [uretero- + L. *vesico*, bladder, + *stoma*, mouth] Surgical joining of a ureter to the bladder.

ure'thra [G. *ourēthra*] A canal leading from the bladder, discharging the urine externally; in the male, it also conducts spermatic fluid.

urethral'gia [urethr- + G. *algos*, pain] Pain in the urethra.

urethri'tis [ureth- + G. *-itis*, inflammation] Inflammation of the urethra.

> **nonspecific u.,** u. not resulting from gonococcal or other specific infectious agents.

> **specific u.,** gonorrhoea.

urethro-, urethr- Combining forms denoting urethra.

ure'throcele [urethro- + G. *kēlē*, tumour, hernia] A prolapse of the female urethra.

ure'throcysti'tis [urethro- + G. *kystis*, bladder, + -*itis*, inflammation] Inflammation of the urethra and bladder.

ure'throplasty [urethro- + G. *plassō*, to form] Reparative or plastic surgery of the urethra.

ure'throscope [urethro- + G. *skopeō*, to view] An instrument for viewing the interior of the urethra.

ure'throsteno'sis [urethro + G. *stenōsis*, a narrowing] Stricture of the urethra.

urethrot'omy [urethro- + G. *tomē*, incision] Surgical incision of a stricture of the urethra.

-uretic [G. *ourētikos*, relating to the urine] Combining form denoting urine.

urhidro'sis Uridrosis.

uri-, uric-, urico- [G. *ouron*, urine] Combining forms relating to uric acid.

u'ric acid 2,6,8-Trioxypurine; white crystals, poorly soluble, contained in solution in urine; with sodium and other bases it forms urates.

uricosu'ria [urico- + G. *ouron*, urine] Excessive amounts of uric acid in the urine.

u'ridine (URD) Uracil ribonucleoside; one of the major nucleosides in RNA; as the pyrophosphate (UDP), it is active in sugar metabolism.

uridro'sis [uri- + G. *hidrōs*, sweat] Excretion of urea or uric acid in the sweat.

urin-, urino- Combining forms denoting urine. See also uri-, uro-.

urinal'ysis Analysis of the urine.

u'rinary Relating to urine.

urina'tion Micturition; the passing of urine.

u'rine [L. *urina*; G. *ouron*] The fluid and dissolved substances excreted by the kidney.

   residual u., u. remaining in the bladder at the end of micturition in cases of prostatic obstruction, bladder atony, etc.

urinom'etry Determination of the specific gravity of urine.

uro- [G. *ouron*, urine] Combining form relating to urine. See also ure- and urin-.

urobi'lin One of the natural breakdown products of haemoglobin; a urinary pigment that gives a varying orange-red coloration to urine according to its degree of oxidation.

u'robilin'ogen Precursor of urobilin.

u'robilinu'ria Presence in the urine of excess urobilins.

u'rochrome The principal pigment of urine, a compound of urobilin and a peptide.

urocysti'tis [uro- + G. *kystis*, bladder, + -*itis*, inflammation] Inflammation of the urinary bladder. See also cystitis.

urodyn'ia [uro- + G. *odynē*, pain] Pain on urination.

urogen'ital Genitourinary.

urog'raphy [uro- + G. *graphō*, to write] Radiography of any part of the urinary tract.

uroki'nase A proteinase found in urine, with the same action (cleaving plasminogen to plasmin) as streptokinase or staphylokinase.

u'rolith [uro- + G. *lithos*, stone] A calculus in the kidney, ureter, bladder, or urethra.

urolog'ic, urolog'ical Relating to urology.

urol'ogy [uro- + G. *logos*, study] The medial specialty concerned with the study, diagnosis, and treatment of diseases of the urinary tract in females and the genitourinary tract in males.

urop'athy [uro- + G. *pathos*, suffering] Any disorder involving the urinary tract.

uropoie'sis [uro- + G. *poiēsis*, a making] Production or secretion and excretion of urine.

u'ropor'phyrin A porphyrin excreted in the urine; *e.g.*, urobilin.

uros'copy [uro- + G. *skopeō*, to view] Examination of the urine, usually with a microscope.

ur'ticant [L. *urtica*, nettle] Producing a weal or other similar itching lesion.

urticar'ia [L. *urtica*, nettle] Hives; an eruption of itching weals, usually of systemic origin; may be due to a state of hypersensitivity to foods or drugs, foci of infection, physical agents, or psychic stimuli.

u'terine Relating to the uterus.

utero-, uter- Combining forms relating to the uterus. See also hystero-; metra-; metro-.

u'terofixa'tion Hysteropexy.

u'teroplasty [utero- + G. *plassō*, to form] A plastic operation upon the uterus.

u'terus, pl. **u'teri** [L.] [NA] Womb; the hollow muscular organ in which the impregnated ovum is developed into the fetus. It consists of a main portion (corpus) with an elongated lower part (cervix), at the extremity of which is the opening (os); the upper-rounded portion of the u., opposite the os, is the fundus, at each extremity of which is the cornu marking the part where the uterine tube joins the u.

bicornate u., u. bicor'nis, a u. that is divided into two lateral horns, as a result of imperfect fusion of the paramesonephric ducts; the cervix may be single or double.

u. didel'phys [G. *di-*, two, + *delphys*, womb] double u. with double cervix and double vagina; due to failure of the paramesonephric ducts to unite.

u'tricle Utriculus.

utric'ulus, pl. **utric'uli** [L. dim. of *uter*, leather bag] [NA] The larger of the two membranous sacs in the vestibule of the labyrinth from which arise the semicircular ducts.

u'vea [L. *uva*, grape] The vascular, pigmentary, or middle coat of the eye comprising the choroid, ciliary body, and iris.

uvei'tis [uvea + G. *-itis*, inflammation] Inflammation of the uvea.

uvul-, uvulo- Combining forms denoting the uvula, usually the uvula palatina. See also staphylo-.

u'vula, pl. **u'vuli** [dim. of L. *uva*, a grape] [NA] A pendant fleshy mass, especially the u. palatina.

u. palati'na [NA], a conical projection hanging from the posterior edge of the middle of the soft palate.

u'vular Relating to the uvula.

uvulec'tomy [uvul- + G. *ektomē*, excision] Excision of the uvula.

uvuli'tis Inflammation of the uvula.

uvulot'omy [uvulo- + G. *tomē*, a cutting] Incision of the uvula.

V

vaccina'tion 1. Inoculation with the virus of cowpox as a means of producing immunity against smallpox. 2. The injection of a killed culture of a specific microbe as a means of prophylaxis or cure of the disease caused by that microorganism.

vac'cine [L. *vaccinus*, relating to a cow] Originally, the live cowpox virus inoculated in the skin as prophylaxis against smallpox; now, extended to include any preparation intended for active immunological prophylaxis.

BCG v., bacillus Calmette-Guérin v.; tuberculosis v.; a suspension of an attenuated strain of *Mycobacterium tuberculosis*, bovine type, inoculated into the skin for tuberculosis prophylaxis.

diphtheria and tetanus toxoids and pertussis v., a v. available in three forms; diphtheria and tetanus toxoids plus pertussis vaccine (DTP), tetanus and diphtheria toxoids, adult type (Td), tetanus toxoid (T); used for active immunization against diphtheria, tetanus, and whooping cough.

influenza virus v.'s, influenza virus grown in embryonate eggs and inactivated; because of the marked and progressive antigenic variation of the influenza viruses, strains included are regularly changed following various outbreaks of influenza in order to include most recently isolated epidemic strains of both type A and B influenza.

live v., prepared from living attenuated organisms.

poliovirus or **poliomyelitis v.'s, (1) inactivated poliovirus v. (IPV),** an aqueous suspension of inactivated strains of poliomyelitis virus given by injection; largely replaced by the oral v.; **(2) oral poliovirus v. (OPV),** an aqueous suspension of live attenuated strains of poliomyelitis virus given orally for active immunization against poliomyelitis.

polyvalent v., a v. prepared from cultures of two or more strains of the same species or microorganism.

rabies v., a v. introduced by Pasteur as a method of treatment for the bite of a rabid animal, utilizing daily injections of virus that increased serially from noninfective to fully infective "fixed" virus; largely replaced by rabies v. of duck embryo origin (DEV), prepared from embryonate duck eggs infected with inactivated "fixed" virus.

Sabin v., an orally administered v. containing live attenuated strains of poliovirus.

Salk v., the original poliovirus v., composed of virus propagated in monkey kidney tissue culture and inactivated.

smallpox v., vaccinia virus suspensions prepared from cutaneous vaccinial lesions of calves and inoculated subcutaneously.

vaccin'ia [L. *vaccinus*, relating to a cow] 1. A contagious eruptive disease occurring in cattle, involving chiefly the skin and teats, and caused by the vaccine (vaccinia) virus; lesions are similar to those of smallpox in man, but much milder. 2. An infection, primarily local and limited to the site of inoculation, induced in man by inoculation with the vaccinia virus in order to confer resistance to smallpox.

vac'uolate, vac'uolated Having vacuoles.

vac'uole [fr. L. *vacuum*, an empty space] **1.** A minute space in any tissue. **2.** A clear space in the substance of a cell, sometimes degenerative in character, sometimes surrounding an englobed foreign body and serving to digest the body.

vac'uum [L. *vacuus*, empty] An empty space, one practically exhausted of air or gas.

va'gal Relating to the vagus nerve.

vagi'na, pl. **vagi'nae** [L. sheath, the vagina] [NA] **1.** Any sheathlike structure. **2.** The genital canal in the female, extending from the uterus to the vulva.

vag'inal [Mod. L. *vaginalis*] Relating to the vagina or to any sheath.

vaginec'tomy [vagina + G. *oktomē*, excision] Colpectomy; excision of the vagina, or a segment thereof.

vaginis'mus [vagina + L. *-ismus*, action, condition] Painful involuntary spasm of the vagina preventing intercourse.

vagini'tis, pl. **vaginit'ides** [vagina + G. *-itis*, inflammation] Inflammation of the vagina.

  v. adhesi'va, inflammation of vaginal mucosa with adhesion of the vagina walls to each other.

  atrophic v., thinning and atrophy of the vaginal epithelium usually resulting from diminished endocrine stimulation.

vagino-, vagin- Combining forms denoting the vagina. See also colpo-.

vaginodyn'ia Vaginal pain.

vaginot'omy Colpotomy; a cutting operation in the vagina.

vago- Combining form denoting the vagus nerve.

vagot'omy [vago- + G. *tomē*, incision] Surgical division of the vagus nerve.

vagoto'nia [vago- + G. *tonos*, strain] Irritability of the vagus nerve, often marked by excessive peristalsis and loss of the pharyngeal reflex.

va'gus, pl. **va'gi** [L. wandering, because of its wide distribution] *Nervus* vagus.

va'lency, va'lence [L. *valentia*, strength] The combining power of one atom of an element (or a radical), that of the hydrogen atom being the unit of comparison, deter-

mined by the number of electrons in the outer shell of the atom.

val'gus [Mod. L. turned outward, fr. L. bowlegged] Bent or twisted outward; modern accepted usage, particularly in orthopaedics, erroneously transposes the meaning of varus (*q.v.*) to v., as in *genu* valgum (knock-knee).

val'ine (Val) 2-Aminoisovaleric acid; a constituent of most proteins.

vallec'ula, pl. **vallec'ulae** [L. dim. of *vallis*, valley] [NA] A crevice or depression on any surface; *e.g.*, v. cerebelli, a deep hollow on the inferior surface of the cerebellum, between the hemispheres, in which the medulla oblongata rests.

valve [L. *valva*] **1.** A fold of the lining membrane of a canal or other hollow organ serving to retard or prevent a reflux of fluid. **2.** Any reduplication of tissue or flaplike structure resembling a v.

  aortic v., the v between the left ventricle and the ascending aorta, consisting of three semilunar cusps.

  atrioventricular v.'s, (1) right, the v. closing the orifice between the right atrium and the right ventricle of the heart; **(2) left,** mitral v.; the v. closing the orifice between the left atrium and the left ventricle of the heart.

  bicuspid v., left atrioventricular v

  mitral v., left atrioventricular v.

  pulmonary v., a v. with semilunar cusps at the entrance to the pulmonary trunk from the right ventricle.

  pyloric v., a fold of mucous membrane at the gastroduodenal junction enclosing the pylorus.

  semilunar v., one of three semilunar segments serving as the cusps of a v. preventing regurgitation at the beginning of the aorta; a similar v. is the pulmonary v.

  tricuspid v., right atrioventricular v.

val'voplasty [valve + G. *plassō*, to form] Surgical reconstruction of a deformed cardiac valve.

valvot'omy [valve + G. *tomē*, incision] **1.** Cutting through a stenosed cardiac valve to relieve obstruction. **2.** Incision of a valvular structure.

valvuli'tis [L. *valvula*, valve, + G. *-itis*, inflammation] Inflammation of a valve, especially a heart valve.

val'vuloplasty Valvoplasty.

valvulot'omy Valvotomy (1).

vanil'lism   **1.** Symptoms of irritation of the skin, nasal mucous membrane, and conjunctivae from which workers handling vanilla sometimes suffer. **2.** Infestation of the skin by sarcoptiform mites found in vanilla pods.

vanil'lylmandel'ic acid (VMA) The major urinary metabolite of adrenal and sympathetic catecholamines.

va'porizer   An apparatus for reducing medicated liquids to a state of vapour fit for inhalation or application to accessible mucous membranes.

varicel'la   [L. dim. of *variola*] Chickenpox; an acute contagious disease, occurring usually in children, caused by the varicella-zoster virus and marked by a sparse eruption of papules, becoming vesicles and then pustules, like that of smallpox although less severe.

varicel'liform   Resembling varicella.

varico-   Combining form denoting a varix or varicosity.

var'icocele   [varico- + G. *kēlē*, tumour, hernia] Abnormal dilation of the veins of the spermatic cord, caused by incompetency of valves in the internal spermatic vein and resulting in downward reflux of blood into the spermatic cord veins when the patient assumes the upright position.

var'icocelec'tomy   [varicocele + G. *ektomē*, excision] Ligature and excision and ligation of the dilated veins of a varicocele.

var'icose   Relating to, affected with, or characterized by varices or varicosis.

varico'sis, pl. **varico'ses** [varico- + G. *-osis*, condition] A dilated or varicose state of a vein.

varicos'ity   A varix or varicose condition.

varicot'omy   [varico- + G. *tomē*, a cutting] An operation for varicose veins by subcutaneous incision.

vario'la   [dim. of L. *varius*, spotted] Smallpox.

var'ix, pl. **var'ices** [L. dilated vein] **1.** A dilated vein. **2.** An enlarged and tortuous vein, artery, or lymphatic vessel.

va'rus   [Mod. L. bent inward, fr. L. knock-kneed] Bent or twisted inward; modern accepted usage, particularly in orthopaedics, erroneously transposes the meaning of valgus (*q.v.*) to v., as in *genu* varum (bowleg).

vas, pl. **va'sa** [L. vessel, dish] [NA] A vessel; a duct or canal conveying a liquid.

   v. af'ferens, pl. **va'sa affer'entia** [NA], **(1)** any artery conveying blood to a part; **(2)** the arteriole that enters a renal glomerulus; **(3)** a lymphatic vessel entering a lymph node.

   v. def'erens, pl. **va'sa deferen'tia,** *ductus* deferens.

   v. ef'ferens, pl. **va'sa efferen'tia** [NA], **(1)** a vein carrying blood away from a part; **(2)** the arteriole that carries blood out of a renal glomerulus; **(3)** a lymphatic vessel leaving a lymph node.

   va'sa vaso'rum [NA], small arteries distributed to the outer and middle coats of the larger blood vessels, and their corresponding veins.

va'sal   Relating to a vas or to vasa.

vas'cular   [L. *vasculum*, a small vessel] Relating to or containing blood vessels.

vas'culariza'tion   Formation of new blood vessels in a part.

vasculi'tis   Angiitis.

vasculo-   [L. *vasculum*, a small vessel] Combining form denoting a blood vessel. See also vas-; vaso-.

vasec'tomy   [vas- + G. *ektomē*, excision] Excision of a segment of the vas deferens, performed in association with prostatectomy, or to produce sterility.

vaso-, vas-   Combining forms denoting a vas or blood vessel. See also vasculo-.

vasoac'tive   Influencing the tone and calibre of blood vessels.

va'soconstric'tor   **1.** An agent that causes narrowing of the blood vessels. **2.** A nerve, stimulation of which causes vascular constriction.

va'sodepress'or   An agent that lowers blood pressure through reduction in peripheral resistance.

va'sodila'tor.   **1.** An agent that causes dilation of the blood vessels. **2.** A nerve, stimulation of which results in dilation of the blood vessels.

va'soinhib'itor   An agent that restricts or prevents the functioning of the vasomotor nerves.

vasomo'tor   Causing dilation or constriction of the blood vessels.

vasopres'sin (VP)   Antidiuretic hormone; a nonapeptide hormone, related to oxytocin, synthetically prepared or obtained from the neurohypophysis of healthy food animals; acts as a vasopressor and stimulates intestinal motility.

vasopres′sor Producing vasoconstriction and a rise in blood pressure.

va′sospasm Angiospasm; contraction or hypertonia of the muscular coats of the blood vessels.

vasova′gal Relating to the action of the vagus nerve upon the blood vessels.

vec′tion [L. *vectio*, conveyance] Transference of agents of disease from the sick to the well by a vector.

vec′tor [L. *vector*, a carrier] **1.** An invertebrate animal capable of transmitting an infectious agent among vertebrates. **2.** Anything having magnitude, direction, and sense which can be represented by a straight line of appropriate length and direction.

vectorcar′diogram A graphic representation of the magnitude and direction of the heart's action currents in the form of a vector loop.

vec′torcardiog′raphy 1. A variant of electrocardiography in which the heart's activation currents are represented by vector loops. **2.** The study and interpretation of vectorcardiograms.

vegeta′tion [Mod. L. *vegetatio*, growth] A growth or excrescence of any sort; specifically, a clot, composed largely of fused blood platelets, fibrin, and sometimes bacteria, adherent to a diseased heart valve.

veg′etative 1. Growing or functioning involuntarily or unconsciously, after the assumed manner of vegetable life. **2.** Not active; denoting the resting stage of a cell or its nucleus.

ve′hicle [L. *vehiculum*, a conveyance] A substance, usually without therapeutic action, used as a medium, to give bulk, for the administration of medicines.

Veillonel′la [A. *Veillon*] A genus of Gram-negative bacteria (family Veillonellaceae) that are parasitic in the mouth and the intestinal and respiratory tracts of man and other animals. The type species is *V. parvula*.

vein [L. *vena*] Vena.

  azygos v., vena azygos.

  capillary v., venule.

  hepatic v.'s, venae hepaticae.

  jugular v., vena jugularis.

  portal v., vena portae.

  pulmonary v.'s, venae pulmonalis inferior and superior.

  thoracic v., vena thoracica.

varicose v.'s, permanent dilation and tortuosity of v.'s most commonly seen in the legs.

velamen′tous Expanded in the form of a sheet or veil.

ve′lar Relating to any velum.

ve′lum, pl. **ve′la** [L. veil, sail] **1.** [NA] Any structure resembling a veil or curtain. **2.** Any serous membrane or membranous envelope or covering.

  v. palati′num, soft *palate.*

ve′nacavog′raphy Angiography of a vena cava

ve′na, pl. **ve′nae** [L.] [NA] Vein; a blood vessel carrying blood toward the heart; all veins except the pulmonary carry dark unaerated blood.

  v. az′ygos [NA], azygos vein; arises from the right ascending lumbar vein or the inferior v. cava, ascends through aortic orifice of the diaphragm, lies in the posterior mediastinum, and terminates in the superior v. cava.

  v. ca′va [NA], **(1)** inferior, postcava; receives blood from lower limbs and greater part of the pelvic and abdominal organs, and empties into the posterior part of the right atrium of the heart; **(2)** superior, precava; returns blood from the head and neck, upper limbs, and thorax; formed by union of the two brachiocephalic veins and the azygos vein.

  ve′nae hepat′icae [NA], hapatic veins; collect blood from the central veins and terminate in three large veins (right, middle, left) opening into the inferior vena cava below the diaphragm and several small inconstant veins entering the vena cava lower down.

  v. jugula′ris [NA], jugular vein: **(1)** anterior, arises below the chin from veins draining the lower lip and mental region, descends the anterior portion of the neck superficially, and terminates in the external jugular at the lateral border of the scalenus anterior muscle; **(2)** external, formed below the parotid gland by junction of the posterior auricular and the retromandibular veins, passes down the side of the neck superficial to the sternocleidomastoid muscle, and empties into the subclavian vein; **(3)** internal, continuation of the sigmoid sinus of the dura mater, uniting, behind the cartilage of the first rib, with the subclavian to form the brachiocephalic vein.

  v. por′tae [NA], portal vein; formed by the superior mesenteric and splenic veins behind the pancreas, ascends in front of the inferior v. cava, and divides at the right end of the transverse fissure of the liver into right and left branches, which ramify within the liver.

v. pulmona'lis infe'rior [NA], inferior pulmonary vein; **(1)** right, vein returning blood from the inferior lobe of the right lung to the left atrium; **(2)** left, vein returning blood from the inferior lobe of the left lung to the left atrium.

v. pulmona'lis supe'rior [NA], superior pulmonary vein; **(1)** right, returns blood from the superior and middle lobes of the right lung to the left atrium; **(2)** left, returns blood from the left superior lobe of the lung to the left atrium.

superior v. cava, see v. cava.

v. thora'cica [NA], thoracic vein; **(1)** internal, usually two veins accompany each artery of the same name, fusing into one at the upper part of the thorax and emptying into the brachiocephalic vein; **(2)** lateral, tributary of the axillary vein that drains the lateral thoracic wall and communicates with the thoracoepigastric and intercostal veins.

vene- **1.** [L. *vena*, vein] Combining form denoting the veins. See also veno-. **2.** [L. *venenum*, poison] Combining form relating to venom.

vene'real [L. *Venus*, goddess of love] Relating to or resulting from sexual intercourse.

venesec'tion [L. *vena*, vein, + *sectio*, a cutting] Phlebotomy.

ve'nipuncture Puncture of a vein, usually to withdraw blood or inject a solution.

veno-, veni- Combining forms denoting the veins. See also vene- (1).

venog'raphy [veno- + G. *grapho*, to write] Radiographic visualization of a vein, after injection of a radiopaque substance.

ven'om [L. *venenum*, poison] A poisonous fluid secreted by snakes, insects, etc.

Russell's viper v., a v. used as a coagulant in the arrest of haemorrhage from accessible sites in haemophilia.

ve'nous [L. *venosus*] Relating to a vein or to the veins.

venous return The blood returning to the heart via the great veins.

ven'ter [L. *venter*, belly] **1.** Abdomen. **2.** [NA] Belly; the wide swelling part of a muscle. **3.** One of the great cavities of the body. **4.** Uterus.

ventila'tion [L. *ventilo*, pp. *-atus*, to fan, fr. *ventus*, the wind] **1.** Replacement of the air or other gas in a space by fresh air or gas. **2.** Respiration; movement of gas(es) into and out of the lungs. **3.** In physiology, tidal exchange of air between the lungs and the atmosphere that occurs in breathing.

artificial v., artificial respiration; application of mechanically or manually generated pressures, usually positive, to gas(es) in or about the airway as a means of producing gas exchange between the lungs and surrounding atmosphere.

pulmonary v., the total volume of gas per minute inspired (V_I) or expired (V_E) expressed in litres per minute.

ven'tral [L. *ventralis*] **1.** Pertaining to the abdomen or to any venter. **2.** Anterior (2). **3.** In veterinary anatomy, situated nearer the undersurface of an animal body.

ven'tricle [L. *ventriculus*, dim. of *venter*, belly] A normal cavity, as of the brain or heart.

left v., the cavity on the left side of the heart that receives the arterial blood from the left atrium and drives it by the contraction of its walls into the aorta.

right v., the cavity on the right side of the heart which receives the venous blood from the right atrium and drives it by the contraction of its walls into the pulmonary artery.

ventric'ular Relating to a ventricle.

ventriculi'tis [ventricle + G. *-itis*, inflammation] Inflammation of the ventricles of the brain.

ventriculo- Combining form denoting a ventricle.

ventric'uloa'trial (V-A) Relating to both ventricles and atria, especially to the passage of conduction.

ventric'ulocisternos'tomy [ventriculo- + L. *cisterna*, cistern, + G. *stoma*, mouth] A surgical opening between the ventricles of the brain and the cisterna magna.

ventriculog'raphy [ventriculo- + G. *graphē*, a writing] Radiographic visualization of the ventricular system by direct injection of a contrast or radiopaque agent.

ventric'ulopuncture Insertion of a needle into a ventricle.

ventriculos'copy [ventriculo- + G. *skopeō*, to view] Direct instrumental inspection of a ventricle.

ventriculot'omy [ventriculo- + G. *tomē*, incision] Incision into a ventricle.

ventriculus, pl. **ventriculi** [L. dim. of *venter*, belly] **1.** [NA] Stomach. **2.** [NA] Ventricle.

ventro- [L. *venter*, belly] Combining form meaning ventral.

ven'ule Capillary vein; a minute vein; a venous radicle continuous with a capillary.

ver'gence [L. *vergo*, to incline, to turn] Disjunctive movement of the eyes in which the fixation axes are not parallel, as in convergence or divergence.

vermi- [L. *vermis*, worm] Combining form denoting a worm or wormlike.

ver'micide [vermi- + L. *caedo*, to kill] An agent that kills intestinal parasitic worms.

vermic'ular [L. *vermiculus*, dim. of *vermis*, worm] Relating to, resembling, or moving like a worm.

vermicula'tion A wormlike movement, as in peristalsis.

ver'miform [vermi- + L. *forma*, form] Worm-shaped.

ver'mifuge [vermi- + L. *fugo*, to chase away] Anthelmintic (1).

ver'minous [L. *verminosus*, wormy] Relating to, caused by, or infested with worms, larvae, or vermin.

ver'mis, pl. **ver'mes** [L. worm] [NA] The narrow middle zone between the two hemispheres of the cerebellum.

ver'nix caseo'sa The fatty substance, consisting of desquamated epithelial cells and sebaceous matter, which covers the skin of the fetus.

verru'ca, pl. **verru'cae** [L.] Wart; a flesh-coloured growth characterized by circumscribed hypertrophy of the papillae of the corium, with thickening of the malpighian, granular, and keratin layers of the epidermis, and caused by papilloma virus; also applied to epidermal verrucous tumours of nonviral aetiology.

    v. acumina'ta, *condyloma* acuminatum.

    v. pla'na, a small, smooth, flat, flesh-coloured wart, occurring in groups, seen especially on the face of the young.

    v. planta'ris, plantar *wart*.

verru'ga [Sp.] Verruca.

    v. perua'na, v. peruvia'na, a stage or cutaneous form of Oroya fever, character-

ized by an eruption of soft conical or pedunculated papules.

ver'sion [L. *verto*, pp. *versus*, to turn] **1.** Displacement of the uterus, with a tilting of the entire organ without bending upon itself. **2.** Change of position of the fetus in the uterus, occurring spontaneously or effected by manipulation. **3.** Inclination. **4.** Conjugate rotation of the eyes in the same direction.

ver'tebra, pl. **ver'tebrae** [L. joint, fr. *verto*, to turn] [NA] One of the segments of the spinal column, usually 33: 7 cervical, 12 thoracic, 5 lumbar, 5 fused sacral (sacrum), and 4 fused coccygeal (coccyx).

ver'tebral Relating to a vertebra or the vertebrae.

Vertebra'ta [L. *vertebratus*, jointed] The vertebrates, a major division of the phylum Chordata, consisting of those animals with a dorsal nerve cord enclosed in a cartilaginous or bony spinal column; includes several classes of fishes, and the amphibians, reptiles, birds, and mammals.

ver'tebrate 1. Having a vertebral column. **2.** A member of the *Vertebrata*.

ver'tex, pl. **ver'tices** [L. whirl, whorl] **1.** [NA] The crown of the head; the topmost point of the vault of the skull. **2.** In obstetrics, the portion of the fetal head bounded by the planes of the trachelobregmatic and biparietal diameters, with the posterior fontanel at the apex.

vertig'inous Relating to or suffering from vertigo.

ver'tigo [L. *vertigo*, dizziness fr. *verto*, to turn] A sensation of irregular or whirling motion, either of oneself (subjective), or of external objects (objective).

    auditory v., labyrinthine v., Ménière's *disease*.

    postural v., v. which occurs with change of position, usually from lying or sitting to standing position.

ves'ica, pl. **ves'icae** [L.] **1.** [NA] A bladder; a distensible musculomembranous organ serving as a receptacle for fluid. **2.** Any hollow structure or sac, normal or pathologic, containing a serous fluid.

    v. fel'lea [NA], gallbladder; a pear-shaped receptacle, on the inferior surface of the liver between the right and the quadrate lobes, which serves as a storage reservoir for bile.

v. urina'ria [NA], urinary bladder; a musculomembranous elastic receptacle serving as a storage place for the urine.

ves'ical Relating to any bladder, especially the urinary bladder.

ves'icant An agent that produces blisters.

ves'icle [L. *vesicula*, a blister, dim. of *vesica*, bladder] **1.** A small bladder-like structure. **2.** A small, circumscribed elevation of the skin, containing serum. See also bleb; blister; bulla. **3.** A small sac containing liquid or gas.

    seminal v., one of two glandular structures that is a diverticulum of the ductus deferens and secretes a component of semen.

vesico-, vesic- Combining forms denoting a vesica or vesicle. See also vesiculo-.

vesicospi'nal Denoting the spinal neural mechanisms that control retention and evacuation of urine by the bladder.

vesic'ula, pl. **vesic'ulae** [L.] [NA] Vesicle (1).

vesic'ular 1. Relating to a vesicle. **2.** Characterized by or containing vesicles.

vesiculi'tis [L. *vesicula*, vesicle, + G. *-itis*, inflammation] Inflammation of any vesicle; especially of a seminal vesicle.

vesiculo- Combining form denoting vesicle.

vesic'ulopap'ular Pertaining to or consisting of a combination of vesicles and papules.

vesic'uloprostati'tis [vesiculo- + prostate + G. *-itis*, inflammation] Inflammation of the bladder and prostate.

vesic'ulopus'tular Pertaining to a mixed eruption of vesicles and pustules.

vesiculot'omy [vesiculo- + G. *tomē*, incision] Surgical division of the seminal vesicles.

ves'sel [O. Fr. fr. L. *vascellum*, dim. of *vas*] A duct or canal conveying any liquid, such as blood, lymph, chyle, or semen.

    afferent v., *vas* afferens.

    blood v., see under B.

    efferent v., *vas* efferens.

vestib'ular Relating to a vestibule, especially of the ear.

ves'tibule [L. *vestibulum*, antechamber] **1.** A small cavity or space at the entrance of a canal. **2.** Specifically, of the ear, the central cavity of the osseous labyrinth that communicates with the semicircular canals and the cochlea.

vestibulo- Combining form denoting vestibule, vestibulum.

vestib'ulococh'lear Relating to the vestibulum and cochlea of the ear.

vestib'ulum, pl. **vestib'ula** [L.] [NA] Vestibule.

ves'tige [L. *vestigium*, footprint (trace)] A rudimentary structure, the degenerated remains of which occurs as an entity in the embryo or fetus.

vestig'ial Relating to a vestige.

viabil'ity [Fr. *viabilité* fr. L. *vita*, life] Capability of living; the state of being viable.

vi'able [Fr. fr. *vie*, life, fr. L. *vita*] Capable of living; denoting a fetus sufficiently developed to live outside of the uterus.

Vib'rio [L. *vibro*, to vibrate] A genus of Gram-negative bacteria (family Spirillaceae) that are saprophytes in salt and fresh water and in soil; others are parasites or pathogens. Type species is *V. cholerae*.

    V. chol'erae, a species that produces a soluble exotoxin (permeability factor) that seems to be the cause of Asiatic cholera in human beings.

    V. fe'tus, *Campylobacter fetus*.

    V. parahaemolyt'icus, a marine species which may contaminate shellfish and cause human gastroenteritis.

vibris'sa, pl. **vibris'sae** [L. *vibrissae*, fr. *vibro*, to quiver] [NA] One of the hairs growing at the anterior nares.

vicar'ious [L. *vicarius*, fr. *vicis*, supplying place of] Acting as a substitute; occurring in an abnormal situation.

vidar'abine A purine nucleoside obtained from *Streptomyces antibioticus* and used to treat herpes simplex infections.

vil'lous 1. Relating to villi. **2.** Covered with villi.

vil'lus, pl. **vil'li** [L. shaggy hair (of beasts)] **1.** [NA] A projection from the surface, especially of a mucous membrane. See also microvillus. **2.** An elongated dermal papilla projecting into an intraepidermal vesicle or cleft.

    chorionic villi, vascular processes of the chorion of the embryo entering into the formation of the placenta.

    intestinal villi, projections of the mucous membrane of the intestine that are leaf-shaped in the duodenum and become shorter, more finger-shaped, and sparser in the ileum; serve as sites of adsorption.

vinblas'tine sulphate An alkaloid obtained from *Vinca rosea* that arrests mitosis in metaphase and exhibits antimetabolic activity; used in the treatment of Hodgkin's disease, choriocarcinoma, acute and chronic leukaemias, and other neoplastic diseases.

vincris'tine sulphate An alkaloid obtained from *Vinca rosea*, with antineoplastic activity is similar to that of vinblastine sulphate, but more useful in treating lymphocytic lymphosarcoma and acute leukaemia.

virae'mia [virus + G. *haima*, blood] Presence of a virus in the bloodstream.

vi'ral Pertaining to or caused by a virus.

-viridae Suffix denoting a virus family.

vir'ilism [L. *virilis*, masculine] Possession of mature masculine somatic characteristics by a female.

vi'rion An elementary virus particle composed of a central core (nucleoid) containing either DNA or RNA, surrounded by a protein covering (capsid); this nucleic acid-protein complex (nucleocapsid) may be the complete v. (as in adenoviruses and picornaviruses) or may be surrounded by an "envelope" (as in herpetroviruses and myxoviruses).

virol'ogy [virus + G. *logos*, study] The study of viruses and of virus disease.

vi'rucide [virus + L. *caedo*, to kill] An agent active against virus infections.

vir'ulence [L. *virulentus*, poisonous] The quality of being poisonous; the disease-evoking power of a microorganism in a given host.

vir'ulent [L. *virulentus*, poisonous] Extremely poisonous; denoting a markedly pathogenic microorganism.

vi'rus, pl. **vi'ruses** [L. poison] **1.** Formerly, the specific agent of an infectious disease. **2.** Filtrable v.; specifically, a term for a group of microbes which with few exceptions are capable of passing through fine filters that retain most bacteria, and are incapable of growth or reproduction apart from living cells. Classification of v.'s depends upon characteristics of virions as well as upon mode of transmission, host range, symptomatology, and other factors. **3.** Relating to or caused by a v.; *e.g.*, virus disease.

 attenuated v., a variant strain of a pathogenic v., so modified as to excite the production of protective antibodies, yet not producing the specific disease.

 ECHO v. [enteric *c*ytopathogenic *human orphan*], echovirus; an enterovirus belonging to the Picornaviridae, associated with fever and aseptic meningitis; some serotypes appear to cause mild respiratory disease.

 Epstein-Barr v., EB v., a herpetovirus found in cell cultures of Burkitt's lymphoma; antibodies reactive with this v. have been reported in cases of infectious mononucleosis.

 filtrable v., virus (2).

 herpes simplex v., herpesvirus (type 1 or 2).

 herpes zoster v., varicella-zoster v.

 human immunodeficiency v. (HIV), a retrovirus that is the aetiologic agent of acquired immunodeficiency syndrome (AIDS).

 influenza v.'s, v.'s (family Orthomyxoviridae) that cause influenza and influenza-like infections; v.'s included are types A and B (genus *Influenzavirus*) causing influenza A and B, and type C, which probably belongs to a separate genus and causes influenza C.

 poliomyelitis v., the picornavirus (genus *Enterovirus*) causing poliomyelitis; serologic types 1, 2, and 3 are recognized, type 1 being responsible for most paralytic poliomyelitis and most epidemics.

 rabies v., a rather large bullet-shaped v. of the genus *Lyssavirus* that causes rabies.

 slow v., a v., or virus-like agent, aetiologically associated with a slow virus disease.

vis'cera Plural of viscus.

vis'ceral Relating to the viscera.

viscero- [L. *viscera*, internal organs] Combining form denoting the viscera. See also splanchno-.

vis'ceropto'sis [viscero- + G. *ptōsis*, a falling] Descent of the viscera from their normal positions.

vis'ceroskel'eton 1. Any bony formation in an organ; may also include the cartilaginous rings of the trachea and bronchi. **2.** That part of the skeleton protecting the viscera.

vis'cid [L. *viscidus*, sticky] Adhesive; sticky; glutinous.

viscos'ity [L. *viscositas*, fr. *viscosus*, viscous] Resistance to flow or alteration of shape by a substance as a result of molecular cohesion.

vis'cus, pl. **vis'cera** [L. the soft parts, internal organs] An organ of the digestive, respiratory, urogenital, and endocrine systems as well as the spleen, the heart, and great vessels.

vi'sion [L. *visio*, to see] The act of seeing.

    binocular v., v. with a single image, by both eyes simultaneously.

    double v., diplopia.

    peripheral v., indirect v.; resulting from retinal stimulation beyond the macula.

    tunnel v., a narrowing of the visual field, as though one were looking through a hollow cylinder or tube.

vi'tal [L. *vitalis*, fr. *vita*, life] Relating or necessary to life.

vit'amin [L. *vita*, life, + amine] One of a group of organic substances, present in minute amount in natural foodstuffs, that are essential to normal metabolism.

    v. A, any β-ionone derivative, except provitamin A carotenoids, possessing qualitatively the biological activity of retinol; deficiency interferes with the production and resynthesis of rhodopsin, thereby causing a night blindness, and produces a keratinizing metaplasia of epithelial cells that may result in xerophthalmia, keratosis, susceptibility to infections, and retarded growth.

    v. B_1, thiamine.

    v. B_6, pyridoxine and related compounds.

    v. B_{12}, generic descriptor for compounds exhibiting the biological activity of cyanocobalamin.

    v. B complex, a pharmaceutical term applied to drug products containing a mixture of the B v.'s usually thiamine, riboflavin, nicotinamide, pantothenic acid, and pyridoxine.

    v. C, ascorbic acid.

    v. D, generic descriptor for all steroids exhibiting the biological activity of ergocalciferol (or cholecalciferol); promote the proper utilization of calcium and phosphorus, thereby producing growth in young children together with proper bone and tooth formation.

    v. D_2, ergocalciferol.

    v. D_3, cholecalciferol.

    v. E, (1) α-tocopherol; **(2)** generic descriptor of tocol and tocotrienol derivatives possessing the biological acitivity of α-tocopherol; contained in various oils, whole grain cereals (constitutes the nonsaponifiable fraction) certain animal tissue, and lettuce.

    v. K, generic descriptor for fat-soluble, thermostable compounds essential for formation of normal amounts of prothrombin; found in alfalfa, hog liver, fish meal, and vegetable oils.

    v. P, a mixture of bioflavonoids extracted from plants (especially citrus fruits) that reduces the permeability and fragility of capillaries.

vitili'go, pl. **vitilig'ines** [L. a skin eruption, fr. *vitium*, blemish, vice] The appearance, on otherwise normal skin, of loss of melanin with white patches of varied sizes, often symmetrically distributed.

vitrec'tomy [vitreous + G. *ektomē*, excision] Removal of the vitreous by means of an instrument which simultaneously removes it by suction and cutting, and replaces it with saline or some other fluid.

vitreo- Combining form denoting vitreous.

vit'reous [L. *vitreus*, glassy, fr. *vitrum*, glass] **1.** Glassy; resembling glass. **2.** Corpus vitreum.

vit'reum [L. ntr. of *vitreus*, glassy] Corpus vitreum.

vivi- [L. *vivus*, alive] Combining form denoting living, alive.

vivisec'tion [vivi- + section] Any cutting operation on a living animal for purposes of experimentation; often extended to denote any form of animal experimentation.

vo'cal [L. *vocalis*] Pertaining to the voice or the organs of speech.

vo'lar Referring to the vola, the palm of the hand or sole of the foot.

vol'atile 1. Tending to evaporate rapidly. **2.** Tending toward violence, explosiveness, or rapid change.

voli'tion [L. *volo*, fut. p. *voliturus*, to wish] The conscious impulse to perform or not perform an act.

vol'ley [Fr. *volée*, fr. L. *volo*, to fly] A synchronous group of impulses induced simultaneously by artificial stimulation of either nerve fibres or muscle fibres.

volume (V) The space occupied by any form of matter, expressed usually in cubic millimetres, cubic centimetres, litres, etc.

    expiratory reserve v. (ERV), the maximal v. of air (about 1000 ml) that can be expelled from the lungs after a normal expiration.

    inspiratory reserve v. (IRV), the maximal v. of air that can be inspired after a normal inspiration; inspiratory capacity less tidal v.

mean cell v. (MCV), the average v. of red cells, calculated from the haematocrit and the red cell count, in erythrocyte indices.

packed cell v., the v. of the blood cells in a sample of blood after it has been centrifuged in a haematocrit.

residual v. (RV), the v. of air remaining in the lungs after a maximal expiratory effort.

tidal v. (V_T), the v. of air inspired or expired in a single breath during regular breathing.

volumet'ric Relating to measurement by volume.

vol'untary [L. *voluntarius*, fr. *voluntas*, will] Relating to or acting in obedience to the will.

vol'vulus [L. *volvo*, to roll] A twisting of the intestine causing obstruction.

vo'mer [L. ploughshare] [NA] A flat bone of trapezoidal shape forming the inferior and posterior portion of the nasal septum; articulates with the sphenoid, ethmoid, two maxillae, and two palatine bones.

vo'merine Relating to the vomer.

vom'it [L. *vomo*, pp. *vomitus*, to vomit] **1.** To eject matter from the stomach through the mouth. **2.** The matter so ejected.

vom'iting Emesis; ejection of matter from the stomach through the oesophagus and mouth.

faecal v., stercoraceous v., ejection of faecal matter aspirated into the stomach from the intestine by repeated spasmodic contractions of the gastric muscles.

v. of pregnancy, v. occurring in the early months of pregnancy, as in morning sickness.

projectile v., expulsion of the contents of the stomach with great force.

voy'eurism [Fr. *voir*, to see] The practice of obtaining sexual pleasure by looking the naked body or genitals of another or at erotic acts between others.

vul'va, pl. **vul'vae** [L. a wrapper or covering] Pudendum; the external genitalia of the female, comprising the mons pubis, labia majora and minora, clitoris, vestibule of the vagina, and the opening of the urethra and of the vagina.

vulvec'tomy [vulva + G. *ektomē*, excision] Excision of the vulva.

vulvi'tis [vulva + G. *-itis*, inflammation] Inflammation of the vulva.

vul'vovagini'tis Inflammation of both vulva and vagina, or of the vulvovaginal glands.

W

wall [L. *vallum*] An investing part enclosing a cavity, chamber, or any anatomical unit.

cell w., the outer layer or membrane of some animal and plant cells.

chest w., in respiratory physiology, the total system of structures outside the lungs that move as a part of breathing; it includes the rib cage, diaphragm, abdominal w. and abdominal contents.

wall-eye **1.** Extropia. **2.** Absence of colour in the iris, or leucoma of the cornea.

war'farin sodium An anticoagulant with the same actions as dicoumarol.

wart Verruca.

genital w., venereal w., *condyloma* acuminatum.

plantar w., a w. on the sole, often painful.

Was'sermann-fast A term used to designate a case in which the Wassermann test remains positive despite all treatment.

water [A.S. *waeter*] **1.** H_2O; a clear, odourless, tasteless liquid, solidifying at 32°F (0°C) and boiling at 212°F (100°C) that is present in all animal and vegetable tissues. **2.** Euphemism for urine. **3.** A pharmacopoeial preparation: clear, saturated aqueous solutions of volatile oils or other aromatic or volatile substances.

waters Colloquialism for amniotic *fluid*.

bag of w., colloquialism for the amniotic sac and contained amniotic fluid.

false w., a leakage of fluid prior to or in beginning labour, before the rupture of the amnion.

wave'length The distance from one point on a wave to the next point in the same phase; *i.e.*, from peak to peak or from trough to trough.

weal [A.S. *hwēle*] A circumscribed evanescent area of oedema of the skin, appearing as an urticarial lesion, slightly reddened, and usually accompanied by intense itching.

wean [A.S. *wenian*] **1.** To take from the breast; to deprive permanently of breast milk and to begin to nourish with other food. **2.** To gradually withdraw from a life support system.

web'bing A congenital condition apparent when adjacent structures are joined by a broad band of tissue not normally present to such a degree.

weight [A.S. *gewiht*] The product of the force of gravity, defined internationally as 980.665 cm/s^2, times the mass of the body.

   birth w., in humans, the first w. of an infant obtained within less than the first 60 completed minutes after birth; a full-size infant is one weighing 2500 g or more.

welt [O.E. *waelt*] Weal.

wen [A.S.] Sebaceous *cyst*.

wheeze [A.S. *hwēsan*] **1.** To breathe with difficulty and noisily. **2.** A squeaking or puffing sound made in difficult breathing.

whip'lash See whiplash *injury*.

whip'worm See *Trichuris*.

white'head Milium.

whit'low [M.E. *whitflawe*] Felon.

   herpetic w., painful herpes simplex virus infection of a finger, often accompanied by lymphangitis and regional adenopathy.

   melanotic w., a melanoma beginning in the skin at the border of or beneath the nail.

whoop'ing cough Pertussis.

wind'burn Erythema of face due to exposure to wind.

win'dow Fenestra.

   oval w., *fenestra* vestibuli.

wind'pipe Trachea.

wink [A.S. *wincian*] **1.** To close and open the eyes rapidly. **2.** An involuntary act by which the tears are spread over the conjunctiva, keeping it moist.

wi'ring Fastening together the ends of a broken bone by wire sutures.

withdraw'al 1. The act of removal or retreating. **2.** A psychological and/or physical syndrome caused by abrupt cessation of the use of a drug in an habituated individual. **3.** The therapeutic process of discontinuing a drug so as to avoid w. (2). **4.** A pattern of behaviour, observed in schizophrenia and depression, characterized by a pathological retreat from interpersonal contact and social involvement, and leading to self-preoccupation.

Wohlfahr'tia [P. *Wohlfahrt*] A genus of dipterous fleshflies (family Sarcophagidae); larvae of some species breed in ulcerated surfaces and flesh wounds.

womb [A.S. belly] Uterus.

word salad A jumble of meaningless and unrelated words, as emitted by persons with certain kinds of schizophrenia.

worm [A.S. *wyrm*] Any member of the phyla Annelida (segmented or true worms), the Aschelminthes (roundworms), and the Platyhelminthes (flatworms).

wound 1. Trauma to any of the tissues of the body, especially that caused by physical means and with interruption of continuity. **2.** A surgical incision.

   gutter w., a tangential w. that makes a furrow without perforating the skin.

   open w., a w. in which the tissues are exposed to the air.

   penetrating w., a w. with disruption of the body surface that extends into underlying tissue or into a body cavity.

   perforating w., a w. with an entrance and exit opening.

   puncture w., a w. in which the opening is relatively small as compared to the depth, as produced by a narrow pointed object.

wrist [A.S. wrist joint, ankle joint] Carpus (1).

wrist-drop Paralysis of the extensors of the wrist and fingers.

wry'neck Torticollis.

Wucherer'ia A genus of filarial nematodes (family Onchocercidae, superfamily Filarioidea) characterized by adult forms that live chiefly in lymphatic vessels and produce large numbers of embryos or microfilariae that circulate in the bloodstream, often appearing in the peripheral blood at regular intervals; the extreme form of this infection (wuchereriasis or filariasis) is elephantiasis.

   W. bancrof'ti, a species transmitted to man by mosquitoes (*Culex, Aëdes, Anopheles,* and *Mansonia*); adult worms inhabit the larger lymphatic vessels and the sinuses of lymph nodes where they sometimes cause temporary obstruction to the flow of lymph and slight or moderate degrees of inflammation.

wuchereri'asis Infestation with worms of the genus *Wuchereria*. See also filariasis.

X

xan'thine Oxidation product of guanine and hypoxanthine; a precursor of uric acid that occurs in many organs and in the urine.

xanthinu'ria [xanthine + G. *ouron*, urine] **1.** Excretion of abnormally large amounts of xanthine in the urine. **2.** A disorder resulting from defective synthesis of xanthine oxidase, characterized by urinary excretion of xanthine in place of uric acid, and by hypouricaemia; autosomal recessive inheritance.

xantho-, xanth- [G. *xanthos*, yellow] Combining forms denoting yellow or yellowish.

xantho'ma [xantho- + G. *-oma*, tumour] A yellow nodule or plaque, especially of the skin, composed of lipid-laden histiocytes.

eruptive x., sudden appearance of groups of waxy yellow or yellowish-brown lesions, especially over extensors of the elbows and knees, and on the back and buttocks, on patients with severe hyperlipaemia.

x. palpebra'rum, soft yellow-orange plaques found about the eyes; the most common type of x.

xan'thomato'sis Widespread xanthomas, especially on the elbows and knees, and sometimes the mucous membranes.

xanthom'atous Relating to xanthoma.

xanthop'sia [xantho- + G. *opsis*, vision] Chromatopsia in which all objects appear yellow.

xantho'sis [xantho- + G. *-osis*, condition] A yellowish discoloration of degenerating tissues, especially seen in malignant neoplasms.

xeno- [G. *xenos*, stranger, foreign] Combining form denoting strange or relationship to foreign material.

xenobiot'ic A pharmacologically, endorminologically, or toxicologically active substance not endogenously produced.

xenogene'ic Heterologous, with respect to tissue grafts, especially when donor and recipient belong to widely separated species.

xenogen'ic, xenog'enous [xeno- + G. *-gen*, producing] **1.** Originating outside of the organism, or from a foreign substance introduced into the organism. **2.** Xenogeneic.

xen'ograft Heterograft.

Xenopsyl'la [xeno- + G. *psylla*, flea] The rat flea, a genus of fleas parasitic on the rat and involved in the transmission of bubonic plague; *X. cheopis* is a vector of *Yersinia pestis*.

xero- [G. *xeros*, dry] Combining form meaning dry.

xeroder'ma [xero- + G. *derma*, skin] A mild form of ichthyosis characterized by excessive dryness of the skin due to a slight increase of the horny layer and diminished cutaneous secretion.

x. pigmento'sum, an eruption of exposed skin occurring in childhood and characterized by numerous pigmented spots resembling freckles, larger atrophic lesions eventually resulting in glossy white thinning of the skin surrounded by telangiectases, and multiple solar keratoses which undergo malignant change; results from a single-gene autosomal recessive disorder in which DNA repair processes are defective, with consequent hypersensitivity to the carcinogenic effect of ultraviolet light.

xerophthal'mia [xero- + G. *ophthalmos*, eye] Extreme dryness of the conjunctiva, due to local disease or to a systemic deficiency of vitamin A.

xero'sis [xero- + G. *-osis*, condition] **1.** Pathologic dryness of the skin, conjunctiva, or mucous membranes. **2.** The normal evolutionary sclerosis of the tissues in old age.

xerosto'mia [xero- + G. *stoma*, mouth] Dryness of the mouth, resulting from diminished or arrested salivary secretion.

x-ray 1. Electromagnetic radiation emitted from a highly evacuated tube excited by the bombardment of the target anode with a stream of electrons from a heated cathode. **2.** Electromagnetic radiation produced by excitation of the inner orbital electrons of an atom.

xy'lose An aldopentose, isomeric with ribose, obtained by fermentation or hydrolysis of naturally occurring carbohydrate substances.

Y

yaw An individual lesion of yaws.

mother y., a large granulomatous lesion, considered to be the initial lesion in yaws, most commonly present on the hand, leg, or foot.

yawn [A.S. *gānian*] An involuntary opening of the mouth, usually accompanied by a movement of respiration.

yaws [African, *yaw*, a raspberry] Framboesia; an infectious tropical disease caused by *Treponema pertenue*, characterized by the development of crusted granulomatous ulcers on extremities which may involve bone.

yeast [A.S. *gyst*] General term denoting true fungi of the family Saccharomycetaceae that are widely distributed in substrates that contain sugars, and in soil, animal excreta, vegetative parts of plants, etc.

Yersin'ia [A. J. E. *Yersin*] A genus of Gramnegative bacteria (family Enterobacteriaceae) that are parasitic on man and other animals; type species is *Y. pestis*.

Y. enterocolit'ica, a species that causes yersiniosis.

Y. pes'tis, A species causing plague; transmitted from rat to man by the rat flea.

Y. pseudotuberculo'sis, a species causing pseudotuberculosis in rodents (rarely in man) and some cases of acute mesenteric lymphadenitis.

yersinio'sis An infectious disease caused by *Yersinia enterocolitica* and marked by diarrhoea, enteritis, pseudoappendicitis, ileitis, erythema nodosum, and sometimes septicaemia or acute arthritis.

Z

zinc [Ger. *zink*] A metallic element, symbol Zn, atomic no. 30, atomic weight 65.38; a number of its salts are used in medicine.

zo'na, pl. **zo'nae** [L. fr. G. *zōnē*, a girdle] **1.** [NA] Zone; a segment; any encircling or belt-like structure. **2.** *Herpes* zoster.

z. arcua'ta, the inner third of the basilar membrane of the cochlear duct, from the tympanic lip of the osseous spiral lamina to the outer pillar cell of the spiral organ (of Corti).

z. pellu'cida, a layer consisting of microvilli of the oocyte, cellular processes of follicular cells, and an intervening substance rich in glycoprotein.

z. vasculo'sa, an area in the external acoustic meatus where a number of minute blood vessels enter from the mastoid bone.

zonaesthe'sia [G. *zōnē*, girdle, + *aisthēsis*, sensation] Girdle sensation; a sensation as if a cord were drawn around the body, constricting it.

zone [L. *zona*] Zona (1).

erogenous z., a part of the body, stimulation of which excites sexual feelings.

pupillary z., the central region of the anterior surface of the iris.

trigger z., the area which when stimulated by touch or pressure excites an attack of neurologic pain.

vascular z., *zona* vasculosa.

zo'nula, pl. **zo'nulae** [L. dim. of *zona*, zone] [NA] Zonule.

zo'nule Zonula; a small zone.

ciliary z., Zinn's z., suspensory ligament of lens; a series of delicate meridional fibres arising from the inner surface of the orbiculus ciliaris and diverge into two groups that are attached to the capsule on the anterior and posterior surfaces of the lens close to the equator.

zonuli'tis [zonule + G. *-itis*, inflammation] Assumed inflammation of the ciliary zonule.

zonulol'ysis [zonule + G. *lysis*, dissolution] Disintegration of the ciliary zonule by enzymes instilled into the anterior chamber in selected cases of cataract extraction to facilitate surgical removal.

zoo- [G. *zōon*, animal] Combining form denoting an animal or animal life.

zoono'sis [zoo- + G. *nosos*, disease] An infection or infestation shared in nature by man and lower vertebrate animals.

zootox'in A substance, resembling the bacterial toxins in its antigenic properties, found in the fluids of certain animals.

zos'ter [G. *zōstēr*, a girdle] *Herpes* zoster.

zoster'iform, zos'teroid Resembling herpes zoster.

Z-plasty. A procedure to elongate a contracted scar, or to rotate tension 90°; the middle line of the Z-shaped incision is made along the line of greatest tension or contraction, and triangular flaps are raised on opposite sides of the two ends and transposed.

zygo-, zyg- [G. *zygon*, yoke, *zygōsis*, a joining] Combining forms denoting yoke, a joining.

zygo'ma [G. a bar, bolt] *Os* zygomaticum.

zygomat'ic Relating to the os zygomaticum.

zygos'ity The nature of the zygotes from which individuals are derived.

zy'gote [G. *zygōtos*, yoked] **1.** The diploid cell resulting from union of a sperm and an ovum. **2.** The individual that develops from a fertilized ovum.

zymo-, zym- [G. *zymē*, leaven] Combining forms denoting fermentation, enzymes.

zymogen'ic Causing fermentation.

APPENDICES

COMPARATIVE TEMPERATURE SCALES

To convert Celsius, Fahrenheit, or Réaumur to Kelvin:

C to K: add 273.16
10°C to K: 10 + 273.16 = 283.16 K

F to K: convert to C, add 273.16
63°F = 17.2°C + 273.16 = 290.36 K

R to K: convert to C, add 273.16
34°R = 42.5°C + 273.16 = 315.66 K

To convert Fahrenheit to Celsius or Réaumur, Celsius to Fahrenheit or Réaumur, or Réaumur to Fahrenheit or Celsius:

Above 0°C and R, or 32°F

F to C: subtract 32, multiply by 5, divide by 9
63°F to C: 63 − 32 = 31 × 5 = 155 ÷ 9 = 17.2°C

F to R: subtract 32, multiply by 4, divide by 9
63°F to R: 63 − 32 = 31 × 4 = 124 ÷ 9 = 13.8°R

C to F: multiply by 9, divide by 5, add 32
37°C to F: 37 × 9 = 333 ÷ 5 = 66.6 + 32 = 98.6°F

C to R: multiply by 4, divide by 5
37°C to R: 37 × 4 = 148 ÷ 5 = 29.6°R

R to F: multiply by 9, divide by 4, add 32
34°R to F: 34 × 9 = 306 ÷ 4 = 76.5 + 32 = 108.5°F

R to C: multiply by 5, divide by 4
34°R to C: 34 × 5 = 170 ÷ 4 = 42.5°C

Between 0° and 32°F, −17.77° and 0°C, or −14.22° and 0°R

F to C: subtract from 32, multiply by 5, divide by 9
10°F to C: 32 − 10 = 22 × 5 = 110 ÷ 9 = −12.2°C

F to R: subtract from 32, multiply by 4, divide by 9
10°F to R: 32 − 10 = 22 × 4 = 88 ÷ 9 = −9.8°R

C to F: multiply by 9, divide by 5, subtract from 32
−12°C to F: 12 × 9 = 108 ÷ 5 = 21.6;
32 − 21.6 = 10.4°F

C to R: multiply by 4, divide by 5
−12°C to R: 12 × 4 = 48 ÷ 5 = 9.6°R

R to F: multiply by 9, divide by 4, subtract from 32
−12°R to F: 12 × 9 = 108 ÷ 4 = 27; 32 − 27 = 5°F

R to C: multiply by 5, divide by 4
−12°R to C: 12 × 5 = 60 ÷ 4 = 15°C

Below 0°F, −17.77°C, or −14.22°R

F to C: add 32, multiply by 5, divide by 9
−10°F to C: 10 + 32 = 42 × 5 = 210 ÷ 9 = −23.3°C

F to R: add 32, multiply by 4, divide by 9
−10°F to R: 10 + 32 = 42 × 4 = 168 ÷ 9 = −18.7°R

C to F: multiply by 9, divide by 5, subtract 32
−18°C to F: 18 × 9 = 162 ÷ 5 = 32.4 − 32 = 0.4°F

C to R: multiply by 4, divide by 5
−18°C to R: 18 × 4 = 72 ÷ 5 = 14.4°R

R to F: multiply by 9, divide by 4, subtract 32
18°R to F: 18 × 9 = 162 ÷ 4 = 40.5 − 32 = −8.5°F

R to C: multiply by 5, divide by 4
18°R to C: 18 × 5 = 90 ÷ 4 = 22.5° C

COMPARATIVE TEMPERATURE SCALES

Celsius °C	Fahrenheit °F	Réaumur °R	Kelvin K
100	220	80	370
90	210	70	360
80	200	60	350
70	190	50	340
60	180	40	330
50	170	30	320
40	160	20	310
30	150	10	300
20	140	0	290
10	130	10	280
0	120	20	270
10	110		260
20	100		250
	90		
	80		
	70		
	60		
	50		
	40		
	30		
	20		
	10		
	0		
	10		

TEMPERATURE EQUIVALENTS

				Celsius to Fahrenheit			
°C	°F	°C	°F	°C	°F	°C	°F
−50	−58.0	20	68.0	49	120.2	78	172.4
−40	−40.0	21	69.8	50	122.0	79	174.2
−35	−31.0	22	71.6	51	123.8	80	176.0
−30	−22.0	23	73.4	52	125.6	81	177.8
−25	−13.0	24	75.2	53	127.4	82	179.6
−20	−4.0	25	77.0	54	129.2	83	181.4
−15	5.0	26	78.8	55	131.0	84	183.2
−10	14.0	27	80.6	56	132.8	85	185.0
−5	23.0	28	82.4	57	134.6	86	186.8
0	32.0	29	84.2	58	136.4	87	188.6
1	33.8	30	86.0	59	138.2	88	190.4
2	35.6	31	87.8	60	140.0	89	192.2
3	37.4	32	89.6	61	141.8	90	194.0
4	39.2	33	91.4	62	143.6	91	195.8
5	41.0	34	93.2	63	145.4	92	197.6
6	42.8	35	95.0	64	147.2	93	199.4
7	44.6	36	96.8	65	149.0	94	201.2
8	46.4	37	98.6	66	150.8	95	203.0
9	48.2	38	100.4	67	152.6	96	204.8
10	50.0	39	102.2	68	154.4	97	206.6
11	51.8	40	104.0	69	156.2	98	208.4
12	53.6	41	105.8	70	158.0	99	210.2
13	55.4	42	107.6	71	159.8	100	212.0
14	57.2	43	109.4	72	161.6	101	213.8
15	59.0	44	111.2	73	163.4	102	215.6
16	60.8	45	113.0	74	165.2	103	217.4
17	62.6	46	114.8	75	167.0	104	219.2
18	64.4	47	116.6	76	168.8	105	221.0
19	66.2	48	118.4	77	170.6	106	222.8

				Fahrenheit to Celsius			
°F	°C	°F	°C	°F	°C	°F	°C
−50	−46.7	1	−17.2	34	1.1	44	6.6
−40	−40.0	5	−15.0	35	1.6	45	7.2
−35	−37.2	10	−12.2	36	2.2	46	7.7
−30	−34.4	15	−9.4	37	2.7	47	8.3
−25	−31.7	20	−6.6	38	3.3	48	8.8
−20	−28.9	25	−3.8	39	3.8	49	9.4
−15	−26.6	30	−1.1	40	4.4	50	10.0
−10	−23.3	31	−0.5	41	5.0	55	12.7
−5	−20.6	32	0	42	5.5	60	15.5
0	−17.7	33	0.5	43	6.1	65	18.3

(continued)

Fahrenheit to Celsius *(continued)*

°F	°C	°F	°C	°F	°C	°F	°C
70	21.1	115	46.1	148	64.4	182	83.3
75	23.8	116	46.6	149	65.0	183	83.8
80	26.6	117	47.2	150	65.5	184	84.4
85	29.4	118	47.7	151	66.1	185	85.0
86	30.0	119	48.3	152	66.6	186	85.5
87	30.5	120	48.8	153	67.2	187	86.1
88	31.0	121	49.4	154	67.7	188	86.6
89	31.6	122	50.0	155	68.3	189	87.2
90	32.2	123	50.5	156	68.8	190	87.7
91	32.7	124	51.1	157	69.4	191	88.3
92	33.3	125	51.6	158	70.0	192	88.8
93	33.8	126	52.2	159	70.5	193	89.4
94	34.4	127	52.7	160	71.1	194	90.0
95	35.0	128	53.3	161	71.6	195	90.5
96	35.5	129	53.8	162	72.2	196	91.1
97	36.1	130	54.4	163	72.7	197	91.6
98	36.6	131	55.0	164	73.3	198	92.2
98.6	**37.0**	132	55.5	165	73.8	199	92.7
99	37.2	133	56.1	166	74.4	200	93.3
100	37.7	134	56.6	167	75.0	201	93.8
101	38.3	135	57.2	168	75.5	202	94.4
102	38.8	136	57.7	169	76.1	203	95.0
103	39.4	137	58.3	170	76.6	204	95.5
104	40.0	138	58.8	171	77.2	205	96.1
105	40.5	139	59.4	172	77.7	206	96.6
106	41.1	140	60.0	173	78.3	207	97.2
107	41.6	141	60.5	174	78.8	208	97.7
108	42.2	142	61.1	175	79.4	209	98.3
109	42.7	143	61.6	176	80.0	210	98.8
110	43.3	144	62.2	177	80.5	211	99.4
111	43.8	145	62.7	178	81.1	**212**	**100.0**
112	44.4	146	63.3	179	81.6	213	100.5
113	45.0	147	63.8	180	82.2	214	101.1
114	45.5			181	82.7		

WEIGHTS AND MEASURES

SI Base Units

Quantity	Name	Symbol
length	metre	m
mass*	kilogram†	kg
time	second	s
electric current	ampere	A
thermodynamic temperature	kelvin‡	K
luminous intensity	candela	cd
amount of substance	mole	mol

*In commercial and everyday use, "weight" usually means mass, e.g., when speaking of a person's weight, the quantity referred to is mass.

†For historic reasons, kilogram is the only base unit with a prefix. Multiples and submultiples of the kilogram are formed by attaching the appropriate prefix to the stem word "gram" (e.g., milligram) and the appropriate prefix symbol to the symbol "g" (e g , mg)

‡The degree Celsius (°C) is still widely accepted usage for expressing temperature and temperature intervals. Celsius (formerly centigrade) *temperature* is converted to kelvin (K) thermodynamic temperature by adding 273.16 to the Celsius scale. For *temperature interval*, 1°C equals 1 K.

Some SI Derived Units
Expressed in Terms of Base Units

Quantity	Name	Symbol
area	square metre	m^2
volume*	cubic metre	m^3
specific volume	cubic metre per kilogram	m^3/kg
speed, velocity	metre per second	m/s
acceleration	metre per second squared	m/s^2
mass density	kilogram per cubic metre	kg/m^3
concentration	mole per cubic metre	mol/m^3
luminance	candela per square metre	cd/m^2

*Litre (L, l), 10^{-3} m^3, is regarded as a special name for the cubic decimetre which is preferred for high accuracy measurement.

Some SI Derived Units with Special Names

Quantity	Name	Symbol	Expression
frequency	hertz	Hz	s^{-1}
force	newton	N	$m \, kg \, s^{-2}$
pressure, stress	pascal	Pa	$m^{-1} \, kg \, s^{-2}$
energy	joule	J	$m^2 \, kg \, s^{-2}$
power	watt	W	$m^2 \, kg \, s^{-3}$
quantity of electricity, electric charge	coulomb	C	$s \, A$
electric potential, electromotive force	volt	V	$m^2 \, kg \, s^{-3} \, A^{-1}$
capacitance	farad	F	$m^{-2} \, kg^{-1} \, s^4 \, A^2$
electric resistance	ohm	Ω	$m^2 \, kg \, s^{-2} \, A^{-2}$
electric conductance	siemens	S	$m^{-2} \, kg^{-1} \, s^3 \, A^2$
magnetic flux	weber	Wb	$m^2 \, kg \, s^{-2} \, A^{-1}$
magnetic flux density	tesla	T	$kg \, s^{-2} \, A^{-1}$
activity of radionuclide	becquerel*	Bq	s^{-1}
absorbed dose of radiation	gray†	Gy	$m^2 \, s^{-2}$
exposure (x and γ radiation)	coulomb per kilogram‡	C kg	$kg^{-1} \, s \, A$

* Replacing the curie (Ci), $3.7 \times 10^{10} \, s^{-1}$.
†Replacing the rad (rad), $10^{-2} \, J \, kg^{-1}$.
‡Replacing the roentgen (R), $2.58 \times 10^{-4} \, C \, kg^{-1}$.

Measures of Length

Micrometres	Millimetres	Centimetres	Metres	Kilometres	Miles	Yards	Feet	Inches
1	0.001	10^{-4}						0.000039
10^3	**1**	10^{-1}					0.00328	0.03937
10^4	10	**1**	0.01			0.0109	0.03281	0.3937
254,000	25.4	2.54	0.0254			0.0278	0.0833	**1**
	304.8	30.48	0.3048			0.333	**1**	12
10^6	10^3	10^2	**1**	0.001	0.0006213	1.0936	3.2808	39.37
914,400	914.40	91.44	0.9144	0.009	0.0005681	**1**	3	36
10^9	10^6	10^5	10^3	**1**	0.6215	1093.6121	3280.8	
			1609.0	1.609	**1**	1760.0	5280.0	

To convert:
Millimetres to inches: multiply by 10, divide by 254
Inches to millimetres: multiply by 254, divide by 10
Centimetres to feet: multiply by 10, divide by 307
Feet to centimetres: multiply by 307, divide by 10
Metres to yards: multiply by 70, divide by 64
Yards to metres: multiply by 64, divide by 70
Kilometres to miles: multiply by 5, divide by 8
Miles to kilometres: multiply by 8, divide by 5

Measures of Mass (Weight)
Avoirdupois Weights

				Metric Equivalents		
Grains	Drams	Ounces	Pounds	Milligrams	Grams	Kilograms
1	0.0366	0.0023	0.00014	64.8	0.0648	0.000065
27.34	**1**	0.0625	0.0039		1.772	0.001772
437.5	16	**1**	0.0625		28.350	0.028350
7,000	256	16	**1**		453.5924	0.453592
0.0154				**1**	0.001	
15.4324	0.5648	0.0353	0.002205	1000	**1**	0.001
15,432.358	564.32	35.27	2.2046		1000	**1**

To convert (approximately):
Kilograms to pounds: multiply by 1000, divide by 454
Pounds to kilograms: multiply by 454, divide by 1000
Grams to ounces: multiply by 20, divide by 567
Ounces to grams: multiply by 567, divide by 20

Apothecaries' Weight

					Metric Equivalents		
Grains	Scruples	Drams	Ounces	Pounds	Milligrams	Grams	Kilograms
1	0.05	0.0167	0.0021	0.00017	64.8	0.0648	0.000065
20	**1**	0.333	0.042	0.0035		1.296	0.001296
60	3	**1**	0.125	0.0104		3.888	0.000389
480	24	8	**1**	0.0833		31.103	0.031103
5,760	288	96	12	**1**		373.2418	0.373242
0.0154					**1**	0.001	
15.4324		0.2576	0.0322	0.0027	1000	**1**	0.001
15,432.358		257.2	32.15	2.6792		1000	**1**

Measures of Capacity
Apothecaries' Measures

Minims	Fluid Drams	Fluid Ounces	Pints	Quarts	Gallons	Metric Equivalents	
						Litres	Millilitres
1	0.0166	0.002	0.00013			0.0006	0.06161
60	1	0.125	0.0078	0.0039		0.0037	3.6967
480	8	1	0.0625	0.0312	0.0078	0.0296	29.5737
7,680	128	16	1	0.5	0.125	0.4732	473.166
15,360	256	32	2	1	0.25	0.9464	946.358
61,440	1024	128	8	4	1	3.7854	3785.434
16,230	270.52	33.8418	2.1134	1.0567	0.2642	1	1000
16.23	0.2705	0.0338	0.00212	0.00106	0.000265	0.001	1

To convert (approximately):
Litres to gallons: multiply by 264, divide by 1000
Gallons to litres: divide by 264, multiply by 1000
Litres to pints: multiply by 21, divide by 10
Pints to litres: multiply by 10, divide by 21

Approximate Household Measures and Weights[*]

Grams	Millilitres	Fluid Ounces	Drams	Teaspoons	Tablespoons	Cups or Glasses
5	5	0.125	1	1		
15	15	0.50	4	3	1	
240	237	8	64	48	16	1

[*]A drop is a measure of uncertain quantity, depending on the nature of the liquid as well as the shape of the container and of the opening from which the liquid falls. One drop of water is roughly equivalent to 1 minim.

LABORATORY REFERENCE RANGE VALUES

Thomas R. Koch, Ph.D., D.A.B.C.C., Department of Pathology,
  University of Maryland School of Medicine
Show-Hong Duh, Ph.D., Department of Pathology, University of
  Maryland School of Medicine

Reference range values are for apparently healthy individuals
and often overlap significantly with values for persons who are
sick. Actual values may vary significantly due to differences in
assay methodologies and standardization. Institutions may also
set up their own reference ranges based on the particular populations that they serve, thus there can be regional differences.
Consequently, values reported by individual laboratories may
differ from those listed in this appendix.

All values are given in conventional and SI units. However, where
the SI units have not been widely accepted, conventional units
are used. In case of the heterogenous nature of the materials
measured or uncertainty of the exact molecular weight of the
compounds, the SI system cannot be followed, and mass per
volume is used as the unit of concentration.

Abbreviations:
ACD, acid-citrate-dextrose; **CHF**, congestive heart failure; **Cit**,
citrate; **CNS**, central nervous system; **CSF**, cerebrospinal fluid;
cyclic AMP, adenosine 3′ : 5′-cyclic phosphate; **EDTA**, ethylene-
diaminetetraacetic acid; **HDL**, high-density lipoprotein; **Hep**,
heparin; **LDL-C**, low-density lipoprotein-cholesterol; **Ox**, oxalate; **RBC**, red blood cell(s); **RIA**, radioimmunoassay; **SD**, standard deviation

References:
Conn, R.B.: Laboratory values of clinical importance. In *Conn's Current Therapy
    1988*. R.E. Rakel, Ed. Philadelphia, W.B. Saunders Co., 1988.
Tietz, N.W., and Logan, N.M. Reference ranges. In *Textbook of Clinical Chemistry*.
    N.W. Tietz, Ed. Philadelphia, W.B. Saunders Co., 1986.
National Cholesterol Education Program: Report of the expert panel on detection,
    evaluation, and treatment of high blood cholesterol in adults. *Arch. Intern. Med.*
    1988;148:36–69.
Clinical Chemistry Laboratory: *Reference Range Values in Clinical Chemistry*.
    Professional services manual. Baltimore, Department of Pathology, University
    of Maryland Medical System, 1988.

Tests	Conventional Units	SI Units
Acetaminophen, serum or plasma (Hep or EDTA)		
Therapeutic	10–30 µg/mL	66–199 µmol/L
Toxic	>200 µg/mL	>1324 µmol/L
Acetoacetate plus acetone		
Serum		
Qualitative	Negative	Negative
Quantitative	0.3–2.0 mg/dL	3–20 mg/L
Urine		
Qualitative	Negative	Negative
Acid haemolysis test (Ham)	No haemolysis	No haemolysis
Adrenocorticotropin (ACTH), plasma		
6 AM	10–80 pg/mL	10–80 ng/L
6 PM	<50 pg/mL	<50 ng/L
Alanine aminotransferase (see Transaminase)		
Albumin		
Serum		
Adult	3.5–5.0 g/dL	35–50 g/L
>60 y	3.4–4.8 g/dL	34–48 g/L
	Avg. of 0.3 g/dL higher in upright individuals	Avg. of 3 g/L higher in upright individuals
Urine		
Qualitative	Negative	Negative
Quantitative	10–100 mg/24 h	10–100 mg/24 h
CSF	10–30 mg/dL	100–300 mg/L
* Aldolase, serum	0–11 mIU/mL (30°C)	0–11 U/L (30°C)
Aldosterone		
Serum		
Supine	3–10 ng/dL	0.08–0.3 nmol/L
Standing		
Male	6–22 ng/dL	0.17–0.61 nmol/L
Female	5–30 ng/dL	0.14–0.8 nmol/L
Urine	3–20 µg/24 h	8.3–55 nmol/24 h
Alpha amino nitrogen		
Serum	3.0–5.5 mg/dL	2.1–3.9 mmol/L
Urine	50–200 mg/24 h	3.6–14.3 nmol/24 h
Amikacin, serum or plasma (EDTA)		
Therapeutic		
Peak	25–35 µg/mL	43–60 µmol/L
Trough		
Less severe infection	1–4 µg/mL	1.7–6.8 µmol/L
Life-threatening infection	4–8 µg/mL	6.8–13.7 µmol/L
Toxic		
Peak	>35–40 µg/mL	>60–68 µmol/L
Trough	>10–15 µg/mL	>17–26 µmol/L

*Test values are method dependent.　　　　　　　　　　　　　(continued)

Tests	Conventional Units	SI Units
δ-Aminolevulinic acid, urine	1.3–7.0 mg/24 h	10–53 μmol/24 h
Amitriptyline, serum or plasma (Hep or EDTA); trough (≥12 h after dose)		
Therapeutic	120–250 ng/mL	433–903 nmol/L
Toxic	>500 ng/mL	>1805 nmol/L
Ammonia nitrogen		
Plasma	15–49 μg/dL	11–35 μmol/L
Urine	20–70 mEq/24 h	20–70 nmol/24 h
* Amylase		
Serum	25–125 mIU/mL	25–125 U/L
Urine	1–17 U/h	1–17 U/h
Amylase/creatinine clearance ratio	1–4%	0.01–0.04
Anion gap	8–16 mEq/L	8–16 mmol/L
Arsenic		
Whole blood (Hep)	0.2–6.2 μg/dL	0.03–0.83 μmol/L
Chronic poisoning	10–50 μg/dL	1.33–6.65 μmol/L
Acute poisoning	60–930 μg/dL	7.98–124 μmol/L
Urine, 24 h	5–50 μg/dL	0.07–0.67 μmol/dL
Ascorbic acid, blood	0.4–1.5 mg/dL	23–85 μmol/L
Aspartate aminotransferase (see Transaminase)		
Base excess, blood	0 ± 2 mEq/L	0 ± 2 mmol/L
Bicarbonate, serum	23–29 mEq/L	23–29 mmol/L
Bile acids, serum	0.3–3.0 mg/dL	3.0–30.0 mg/L
* Bilirubin		
Serum		
Adults		
Conjugated	0.0–0.3 mg/dL	0–5 μmol/L
Unconjugated	0.01–1.1 mg/dL	0–19 μmol/L
Delta	0–0.2 mg/dL	0–5 μmol/L
Total	0.2–1.3 mg/L	3–22 μmol/L
Neonates		
Conjugated	0–0.6 mg/dL	0–10 μmol/L
Unconjugated	0.6–10.5 mg/dL	10–180 μmol/L
Total	1.0–10.5 mg/dL	1.7–180 μmol/L
Urine, qualitative	Negative	Negative

Bone marrow, differential cell count	Range (%)	Average (%)	Range	Average
Myeloblasts	0.3–5.0	2.0	0.003–0.05	0.02
Promyelocytes	1.0–8.0	5.0	0.01–0.08	0.05
Myelocytes				
Neutrophilic	5.0–19.0	12.0	0.05–0.19	0.12
Eosinophilic	0.5–3.0	1.5	0.005–0.03	0.015
Basophilic	0.0–0.5	0.3	0.00–0.005	0.003
Metamyelocytes	13.0–32.0	22.0	0.13–0.32	0.22
Polymorphonuclear neutrophils	7.0–30.0	20.0	0.07–0.30	0.20

*Test values are method dependent.

(continued)

Tests	Conventional Units		SI Units	
Polymorphonuclear eosinophils	0.5–4.0	2.0	0.005–0.04	0.02
Polymorphonuclear basophils	0.0–0.7	0.2	0.00–0.007	0.002
Lymphocytes	3.0–17.0	10.0	0.03–0.17	0.10
Plasma cells	0.0–2.0	0.4	0.00–0.02	0.004
Monocytes	0.5–5.0	2.0	0.005–0.05	0.02
Reticulum cells	0.1–2.0	0.2	0.001–0.02	0.002
Megakaryocytes	0.3–3.0	0.4	0.003–0.03	0.004
Pronormoblasts	1.0–8.0	4.0	0.01–0.08	0.04
Normoblasts	7.0–32.0	18.0	0.07–0.32	0.18
Cadmium, whole blood (Hep)	0.1–0.5 μg/dL		0.89–4.45 nmol/L	
Toxic	10–300 μg/dL		0.89–26.70 μmol/L	
Cadmium, urine, 24 h	<15 μg/dL		<0.13 μmol/dL	
Calcium, serum	4.5–5.5 mEq/dL 9.0–11.0 mg/dL (Slightly higher in children) (Varies with protein concentration)		2.25–2.75 mmol/L (Slightly higher in children) (Varies with protein concentration)	
Calcium, ionized, serum	2.1–2.6 mEq/L 4.25–5.25 mg/dL		1.05–1.30 mmol/L	
Calcium, urine				
Low calcium diet	<150 mg/24 h		<3.8 nmol/24 h	
Usual diet (Hep or EDTA); trough	<250 mg/24 h		<6.3 nmol/24 h	
Therapeutic	8–12 μg/mL		34–51 μmol/L	
Toxic	>15 μg/mL		>63 μmol/L	
Carbon dioxide, total, serum/plasma (Hep)	22–29 mmol/L (lower in children)		Same	
Carbon dioxide tension (PCO₂), blood	35–45 mm Hg		35–45 mm Hg	
Carbon monoxide, as carboxyhaemoglobin (HbCO), whole blood (EDTA)				
Nonsmokers	0.5–1.5% total Hb		0.005–0.015 HbCO fraction	
Smokers				
1–2 packs/d	4–5% total Hb		0.04–0.05 HbCO fraction	
>2 packs/d	8–9% total Hb		0.08–0.09 HbCO fraction	
Toxic	>20% total Hb		>0.20 HbCO fraction	
Lethal	>50% total Hb		>0.5 HbCO fraction	
Carotene, serum	40–200 μg/dL		0.74–3.72 μmol/L	
* Catecholamines, urine				
Adrenaline	<10 μg/24 h		<55 nmol/24 h	
Noradrenaline	<100 μg/24 h		<590 nmol/24 h	
Total free catecholamines	4–126 μg/24 h		24–745 nmol/24 h (as noradrenaline)	
Total metanephrines	0.1–1.6 mg/24 h		0.5–8.1 μmol/24 h (as metanephrine)	

*Test values are method dependent.

(continued)

Tests	Conventional Units	SI Units
Cell counts		
Erythrocytes		
Males	4.0–0.2 million/mm³	4.6–6.2 × 10¹²/L
Females	4.2–5.4 million/mm³	4.2–5.4 × 10¹²/L
Children (varies with age)	4.5–5.1 million/mm³	4.5–5.1 × 10¹²/L
Leucocytes		
Total	4500–11,000/mm³	4.5–11.0 × 10⁹/L
Differential	*Percentage* *Absolute*	
Myelocytes	0 0/mm³	0/L
Band neutrophils	3–5 150–400 mm	150–400 × 10⁶/L
Segmented neutrophils	54–62 3000–5800/mm³	3000–5800 × 10⁶/L
Lymphocytes	25–33 1500–3000/mm³	1500–3000 × 10⁶/L
Monocytes	3–7 300–500/mm³	300–500 × 10⁶/L
Eosinophils	1–3 50–250/mm³	50–250 × 10⁶/L
Basophils	0–0.75 15–50/mm³	15–50 × 10⁶/L
Platelets	150,000–350,000/mm³	150–350 × 10⁶/L
Reticulocytes	25,000–75,000/mm³	25–75 × 10⁹/L
	0.5–1.5% of erythrocytes	
Cells, CSF	<5/mm³ (all mononucleocytes)	Same
Ceruloplasmin, serum	23–44 mg/dL	230–440 mg/L
Chloramphenicol, serum or plasma (Hep or EDTA); trough		
Therapeutic	10–25 µg/mL	31–77 µmol/L
Toxic	>25 µg/mL	>77 µmol/L
Chloride		
Serum	96–106 mEq/L	06–106 mmol/L
Sweat		
Normal	0–30 mmol/L	Same
Cystic fibrosis	60–200 mmol/L	Same
Urine, 24 h (vary greatly with Cl intake)		
Infant	2–10 mmol/d	Same
Child	14–50 mmol/d	Same
Adults	110–250 mmol/d	Same
CSF	120–130 mEq/L (20 mEq/L higher than serum)	120–130 mmol/L (20 mmol/L higher than serum)
Cholesterol, serum	Recommended desirable range: <200 mg/dL	Recommended desirable range: <5.2 mmol/L
	Borderline range: 200–230 mg/dL	Borderline range: 5.2–6.0 mmol/L
Cholinesterase		
Serum	0.5–1.3 pH units	0.5–1.3 pH units
Erythrocytes	0.5–1.0 pH unit	0.5–1.0 pH unit

(continued)

Tests	Conventional Units	SI Units
Chorionic gonadotropin β-subunit (β-hCG)		
Serum or plasma (EDTA)		
Male and nonpregnant female	<3.0 mU/mL	<3.0 U/L
Female, post-conception		
7–10 d	>3.0 mU/mL	>3.0 U/L
30 d	100–5000 mU/mL	100–5000 U/L
40 d	>2000 mU/mL	>2000 U/L
10 wk	50,000–140,000 mU/mL	50,000–140,000 U/L
14 wk	10,000–50,000 mU/mL	10,000–50,000 U/L
Trophoblastic disease	>100,000 mU/mL	>100,000 U/L
Urine, 24 h		
Male and nonpregnant female	0 U/d	Same
Pregnancy (wk)		
6th	13,000 U/d (mean)	Same
8th	30,000 U/d (mean)	Same
12–14th	105,000 U/d (mean)	Same
16th	46,000 U/d (mean)	Same
Thereafter	5,000–20,000 U/d (mean)	Same
Clonazepam, serum or plasma (Hep or EDTA); trough		
Therapeutic	15–60 ng/mL	48–190 nmol/L
Toxic	>80 ng/mL	>254 nmol/L
Coagulation tests		
Antithrombin III (synthetic substrate)	80–120% of normal	0.8–1.2 of normal
Bleeding time (Duke)	1–5 min	1–5 min
Bleeding time (Ivy)	<5 min	<5 min
Bleeding time (template)	2.5–9.5 min	2.5–9.5 min
Clot retraction, qualitative	Begins in 30–60 min Complete in 24 h	Begins in 30–60 min Complete in 24 h
Coagulation time (Lee-White)	5–15 min (glass tubes) 19–60 min (siliconized tubes)	5–15 min (glass tubes) 19–60 min (siliconized tubes)
Cold haemolysin test (Donath-Landsteiner)	No haemolysis	No haemolysis
Complement components		
Total haemolytic complement activity, plasma (EDTA)	75–160 U/mL or >33% of plasma CH50	75–160 kU/L Fraction of CH50: >0.33

(continued)

Tests	Conventional Units	SI Units
Total complement decay rate (functional), plasma (EDTA)	10–20%	Fraction decay rate: 0.10–0.20
	Deficiency: >50%	>0.50
$C1_q$, serum	6.5 ± 0.7 mg/dL (SD)	65 ± 7 mg/L (SD)
$C1_r$, serum	2.5–3.8 mg/dL	25–38 mg/L
$C1_s$ (C1 esterase), serum	2.5–3.8 mg/dL	25–38 mg/L
C2, serum	2.8 ± 0.6 mg/dL (SD)	28 ± 6 mg/L (SD)
C3, serum	80–155 mg/dL	800–1550 mg/L
C4, serum	13–37 mg/dL	130–370 mg/L
C5, serum	6.4 ± 1.3 mg/dL (SD)	64 ± 13 mg/L (SD)
C6, serum	5.6 ± 0.80 mg/dL (SD)	56 ± 8.0 mg/L (SD)
C7, serum	4.9–7.0 mg/dL	49–70 mg/L
C8, serum	4.3–6.3 mg/dL	43–63 mg/L
C9, serum	4.7–6.9 mg/dL	47–69 mg/L
Coombs' test		
Direct	Negative	Negative
Indirect	Negative	Negative
Copper		
Serum		
Males	70–140 μg/dL	11–22 μmol/L
Females	85–155 μg/dL	13–24 μmol/L
Urine	0–50 μg/24 h	0–0.80 μmol/24 h
Corpuscular values of erythrocytes (values are for adults; in children, values vary with age)		
Mean corpuscular haemoglobin (MCH)	27–31 pg	0.42–0.48 fmol
Mean corpuscular haemoglobin concentration (MCHC)	32–36%	0.32–0.36
Mean corpuscular volume (MCV)	80–96 μ³	80–96 fL
Cortisol		
Plasma		
8 AM	6–23 μg/dL	170–635 nmol/L
4 PM	3–15 μg/dL	82–413 nmol/L
10 PM	<50% of 8 AM value	<0.5 of 8 AM value
Free, urine	10–100 μg/24 h	27.6–276 mmol/24 h
Creatine		
Serum	0.2–0.8 mg/dL	15–61 μmol/L
Urine		
Males	0–40 mg/24 h	0–0.30 mmol/24 h
Females	0–100 mg/24 h	0–0.76 mmol/24 h
	(Higher in children and pregnant women)	(Higher in children and pregnant women)

(continued)

Tests	Conventional Units	SI Units
*† Creatine kinase, serum (CK, CPK)		
White		
Male	60–320 mU/mL (37°C)	60–320 U/L (37°C)
Female	50–200 mU/mL (37°C)	50–200 U/L (37°C)
Black		
Male	130–450 mU/mL (37°C)	130–450 U/L (37°C)
Female	60–270 mU/mL (37°C)	60–270 U/L (37°C)
* Creatine kinase MB isoenzyme, serum	<15 U/L (37°C)	Same
Creatinine, enzymatic		
Serum or plasma, adult		
Male	0.8–1.5 mg/dL	71–133 µmol/L
Female	0.7–1.2 mg/dL	62–106 µmol/L
Urine	15–25 mg/kg body weight/24 h	0.13–0.22 mmol/kg body weight/24 h
* Creatinine clearance, enzymatic		
Males	110–150 mL/min	110–150 mL/min
Females	105–132 mL/min (1.73 m² surface area)	105–132 mL/min (1.73 m² surface area)
Cryoglobulins, serum	0	0
Cyanide		
Serum		
Nonsmokers	0.004 mg/L	0.15 µmol/L
Smokers	0.006 mg/L	0.23 µmol/L
Nitroprusside therapy	0.01–0.06 mg/L	0.38–2.30 µmol/L
Toxic	>0.1 mg/L	>3.84 µmol
Whole blood (Ox)		
Nonsmokers	0.016 mg/L	0.61 µmol/L
Smokers	0.041 mg/L	1.57 µmol/L
Nitroprusside therapy	0.05–0.5 mg/L	1.92–19.20 µmol/L
Toxic	>1 mg/L	>38.40 µmol/L
Cyclic AMP		
Plasma (EDTA)		
Males	5.6–10.9 ng/mL	17–33 nmol/L
Females	3.6–8.9 ng/mL	11–27 nmol/L
Urine, 24 h	<3.3 mg/d or <1.64 mg/g creatinine	<10 µmol/d or <565 µmol/mol creatinine
Cystine or cysteine, urine, qualitative	Negative	Negative
C-Peptide, serum		
Adult	4.0 ng/mL	4.0 µg/L
>60 y, male	1.5–5.0 ng/mL	1.5–5.0 µg/L
>60 y, female	1.4–5.5 ng/mL	1.4–5.5 µg/L
C-Reactive protein, serum		
Cord blood	1–35 µg/dL	10–350 µg/L
Adult	6.8–820 µg/dL	68–8200 µg/L

*Test values are method dependent.
†Test values are race dependent.

(continued)

Tests	Conventional Units	SI Units
Dehydroepiandrosterone, urine	<15% of total 17-ketosteroids	<0.15 of total 17-ketosteroids
Males	0.2–2.0 mg/24 h	0.7–6.9 μm/24 h
Females	0.2–1.8 mg/24 h	0.7–6.2 μm/24 h
Desipramine, serum or plasma (Hep or EDTA); trough (12 h after dose)		
Therapeutic	75–160 ng/mL	281–600 nmol/L
Toxic	>1000 ng/mL	>3750 nmol/L
Diazepam, serum or plasma (Hep or EDTA); trough		
Therapeutic	100–1000 ng/mL	0.35–3.51 μmol/L
Toxic	>5000 ng/ml	>17.55 μmol/L
Digitoxin, serum or plasma (Hep or EDTA); 6 h after dose		
Therapeutic	20–35 ng/mL	26–46 nmol/L
Toxic	>45 ng/mL	>59 nmol/L
Digoxin, serum or plasma (Hep or EDTA); 12 h after dose		
Therapeutic		
CHF	0.8–1.5 ng/mL	1.0–1.9 nmol/L
Arrhythmias	1.5–2.0 ng/mL	1.9–2.6 nmol/L
Toxic		
Adult	>2.5 ng/mL	>3.2 nmol/L
Child	>3.0 ng/mL	>3.8 nmol/L
Disopyramide, serum or plasma (Hep or EDTA); trough		
Therapeutic arrhythmias		
Atrial	2.8–3.2 μg/mL	8.3–9.4 μmol/L
Ventricular	3.3–7.5 μg/mL	9.7–22 μmol/L
Toxic	>7 μg/mL	>20.7 μmol/l
Doxepin, serum or plasma (Hep or EDTA); trough (≥12 h after dose)		
Therapeutic	00–150 ng/mL	107–537 nmol/L
Toxic	>500 ng/mL	>1790 nmol/L
Electrophoresis, CSF	Predominantly albumin	Predominantly albumin
Ethanol, whole blood (Ox) or serum		
Depression of CNS	>100 mg/dL	>21.7 mmol/L
Fatalities reported	>400 mg/dL	>86.8 mmol/L
Ethosuximide, serum or plasma (Hep or EDTA); trough		
Therapeutic	40–100 μg/mL	283–708 μmol/L
Toxic	>150 μg/mL	>1062 μmol/L

(continued)

Tests	Conventional Units	SI Units
Euglobulin lysis time	2–6 at 37°C	2–6 h at 37°C
Factor VIII and other coagulation factors	50–150% of normal	0.50–1.5 or normal
Fibrin split products (Thrombo-Wellco test)	<10 µg/mL	<10 mg/L
Fibrinogen	200–400 mg/dL	5.9–11.7 µmol/L
Fibrinolysins	0	0
Partial thromboplastin time, activated (APTT)	20–35 sec	20–35 sec
Prothrombin consumption	Over 80% consumed in 1 h	Over 0.80 consumed in 1 h
Prothrombin content	100% (calculated from prothrombin time)	1.0 (calculated from prothrombin time)
Prothrombin time (one stage)	12.0–14.0 sec	12.0–14.0 sec
Tourniquet test	Ten or fewer petechiae in a 2.5 cm circle after 5 min	Ten or fewer petechiae in a 2.5 cm circle after 5 min
Fat, Faecal, F, 72 h		
Infant, breast-fed	<1 g/d	Same
0–6 y	<2 g/d	Same
Adult	<7 g/d	Same
Adult (fat-free diet)	<4 g/d	Same
‡ Fatty acids, total, serum	190–420 mg/dL	7–15 mmol/L
Nonesterified, serum	8–25 mg/dL	0.30–0.90 mmol/L
Ferritin, serum		
Males	27–270 ng/mL	27–270 µg/L
Females	9–180 ng/mL (higher if postmenopausal)	9–180 µg/L (higher if postmenopausal)
Ferritin values of <20 ng/mL (20 µg/L) have been reported to be generally associated with depleted iron stores		
Fibrinogen, plasma	200–400 mg/dL	5.9–11.7 µmol/L
Fluoride		
Plasma (Hep)	0.01–0.2 µg/mL	0.5–10.5 µmol/L
Urine	0.2–1.1 µg/mL	10.5–57.9 µmol/L
Urine, occupational exposure	4–5 µg/mL	210–263 µmol/L
Folate, serum	2.2–17.3 ng/mL	5.0–39.2 nmol/L
Erythrocytes	169–707 ng/mL	451–1602 nmol/L
Follicle-stimulating hormone (FSH), plasma		
Males	4–25 mU/mL	4–25 U/L
Females	4–30 mU/mL	4–30 U/L
Postmenopausal females	40–250 mU/mL	40–250 U/L
Gastrin, serum	0–200 pg/mL	0–200 ng/L
Gentamicin, serum or plasma (EDTA)		

‡"Fatty acids" include a mixture of different aliphatic acids of varying molecular weight: a mean molecular weight of 284 daltons has been assumed. (continued)

Tests	Conventional Units	SI Units
Therapeutic		
Peak		
Less severe infection	5–8 μg/mL	10.4–16.7 μmol/L
Severe infection	8–10 μg/mL	16.7–20.9 μmol/L
Trough		
Less severe infection	<1 μg/mL	<2.1 μmol/L
Moderate infection	<2 μg/mL	<4.2 μmol/L
Severe infection	<2–4 μg/mL	<4.2–8.4 μmol/L
Toxic		
Peak	>10–12 μg/mL	>21–25 μmol/L
Trough	>2–4 μg/mL	>4.2–8.4 μmol/L
Glucose (fasting)		
Blood	60–100 mg/dL	3.33–5.55 mmol/L
Plasma or serum	70–115 mg/dL	3.89–6.38 mmol/L
Glucose, 2 h postprandial, serum	<120 mg/dL	<6.7 mmol/L
Glucose, urine		
Quantitative	<500 mg/24 h	<2.8 mmol/24 h
Qualitative	Negative	Negative
Glucose, CSF	50–75 mg/dL (20 mg/dL less than serum)	2.8–4.2 mmol/L (1.1 mmol/L less than serum)
* Glucose-6-phosphate dehydrogenase (G-6-PD) in erythrocytes, whole blood (ACD, EDTA, or Hep)	12.1 ± 2.9 U/g Hb (SD) 351 ± 60.6 U/10¹² RBC 4.11 ± 0.71 U/mL RBC	0.78 ± 0.13 mU/mol Hb 0.35 ± 0.06 nU/RBC 4.11 ± 0.71 kU/L RBC
* γ-Glutamyltransferase		
Males	6–32 mU/mL (30°C)	6–32 U/L (30°C)
Females	4–18 mU/mL (30°C)	4–18 U/L (30°C)
Glutethimide, serum		
Therapeutic	2–6 μg/mL	9–28 μmol/L
Toxic	>5 μg/mL	>20 μmol/L
Growth hormone, serum	0–10 ng/mL	0–10 μg/L
Haematocrit		
Males	40–54 mL/dL	0.40–0.54
Females	37–47 mL/dL	0.37–0.47
Newborn	49–54 mL/dL	0.49–0.54
Children (varies with age)	35–49 mL/dL	0.35–0.49
Haemoglobin (Hb)		
Males	14.0–18.0 g/dL	2.17–2.79 mmol/L
Females	12.0–16.0 g/dL	1.86–2.48 mmol/L
Newborn	16.5–19.5 g/dL	2.56–3.20 mmol/L
Children (varies with age)	11.2–16.5 g/dL	1.74–2.56 mmol/L
Haemoglobin, fetal	≥1 y old: <2% of total Hb	≥1 y old: <2% of total Hb
Haemoglobin, plasma	0–5.0 mg/dL	0–0.8 μmol/L
Haemoglobin and myoglobin, urine, qualitative	Negative	Negative

*Test values are method dependent.   (continued)

Tests	Conventional Units	SI Units
Haemoglobin electrophoresis, whole blood (EDTA, Cit, or Hep)		
HbA	>95%	>0.95 Hb fraction
HbA$_{1c}$	5.6–7.5%	0.056–0.075 Hb fraction
HbA$_2$	1.5–3.5%	0.015–0.035 Hb fraction
HbF	<2%	<0.02 Hb fraction
Haptoglobin, serum	100–200 mg/dL (As haemoglobin binding capacity)	16–31 μmol/L (As haemoglobin binding capacity)
Haptoglobin (as haemoglobin binding capacity)	100–200 mg/dL	16–31 μmol/L
HDL-cholesterol (HDL-C), serum or plasma (EDTA)	Recommended desirable range: >35 mg/dL	Recommended desirable range: >0.91 mmol/L
Homogentisic acid, urine, qualitative	Negative	Negative
* Hydroxybutyric dehydrogenase serum (HBD)	0–180 mU/mL (30°C)	0–180 U/L (30°C)
17-Hydroxycortico-steroids, urine		
Males	3–9 mg/24 h	8.3–25 μmol/24 h (as cortisol)
Females	2–8 mg/24 h	5.5–22 μmol/24 h (as cortisol)
5-Hydroxyindoleacetic acid, urine		
Qualitative	Negative	Negative
Quantitative	<9 mg/24 h	<47 μmol/24 h
Imipramine, serum or plasma (Hep or EDTA); trough (≥12 h after dose)		
Therapeutic	125–250 ng/mL	446–893 nmol/L
Toxic	>500 ng/mL	>1785 nmol/L
Immunoglobulins, serum		
IgG	550–1900 mg/dL	5.5–19.0 g/L
IgA	60–333 mg/dL	0.60–3.3 g/L
IgM	45–145 mg/dL	0.45–1.5 g/L
IgD	0.5–3.0 mg/dL	5–30 mg/L
IgE	<500 ng/mL (Varies with age in children)	<500 μg/L (Varies with age in children)
Immunoglobulin G (IgG), CSF		
Children under 14	<8% of total protein	<0.08 of total protein
Adults	<14% of total protein	<0.14 of total protein
Insulin, plasma (fasting)	5–25 μU/mL	36–179 pmol/L
Iron, serum	75–175 μg/dL	13–31 μmol/L

*Test values are method dependent.

(continued)

Tests	Conventional Units	SI Units
Iron binding capacity, serum		
Total	250–410 μg/dL	45–73 μmol/L
Saturation	20–55%	0.20–0.55
Ketosteroids, urine		
Males	6–18 mg/24 h	21–62 μmol/24 h
Females	4–13 mg/24 h (decrease with age)	14–45 μmol/24 h (decrease with age)
l-Lactate		
Plasma (NaF)		
Venous	4.5–19.8 mg/dL	0.5–2.2 mmol/L
Arterial	4.5–14.4 mg/dL	0.5–1.6 mmol/L
Whole blood (Hep), at bed rest		
Venous	8.1–15.3 mg/dL	0.9–1.7 mmol/L
Arterial	<11.3 mg/dL	<1.25 mmol/L
Urine, 24 h	496–1982 mg/d	5.5–22 mmol/d
CSF	<25.2 mg/dL	<2.8 mmol/L
* Lactate dehydrogenase (LDH)		
Total (L→P), 30°C, serum		
Newborn	160–450 U/L	Same
Neonate	300–1500 U/L	Same
Infant	100–250 U/L	Same
Child	60–170 U/L	Same
Adult	45–90 U/L	Same
>60 y	55–100 U/L	Same
* Isoenzymes, serum by agarose gel electrophoresis		
Fraction 1	14–26% of total	0.14–0.26 fraction of total
Fraction 2	29–39% of total	0.29–0.39 fraction of total
Fraction 3	20–26% of total	0.20–0.26 fraction of total
Fraction 4	8–16% of total	0.08–0.16 fraction of total
Fraction 5	6–16% of total	0.06–0.16 fraction of total
* Lactate dehydrogenase, CSF	10% of serum value	0.10 fraction of serum value
LDL-cholesterol (LDL-C), calculated, serum or plasma (EDTA)	Recommended desirable range for adults: <130 mg/dL	<3.37 mmol/L
Lead		
Whole blood (Hep)		
Child	<25 μg/dL	<1.21 μmol/L
Adult	<25 μg/dL	<1.21 μmol/L
Toxic	≥60 μg/dL	≥2.90 μmol/L
Urine, 24 h	<80 μg/d	<0.39 μmol/d
Lecithin-sphingomyelin (L/S) ratio, amniotic fluid	2.0–5.0 indicates probable fetal lung maturity: >3.0 in diabetics	Same
* Leucine aminopeptidase, serum	14–40 mU/mL (30°C)	14–40 U/L (30°C)

*Test values are method dependent.   (continued)

Tests	Conventional Units	SI Units
Lidocaine, serum or plasma (Hep or EDTA); 45 min after bolus dose		
Therapeutic	1.5–6.0 µg/mL	6.4–26 µmol/L
Toxic		
CNS, cardiovascular depression	6–8 µg/mL	26–34.2 µmol/L
Seizures, obtundation, decreased cardiac output	>8 µg/mL	>34.2 µmol/L
* Lipase, serum	0–1.5 units (Cherry-Crandall)	0–1.5 units (Cherry-Crandall)
Lithium, serum or plasma (Hep or EDTA); 12 h after last dose		
Therapeutic	0.6–1.2 mEq/L	0.6–1.2 mmol/L
Toxic	>2 mEq/L	>2 mmol/L
Lorazepam, serum or plasma (Hep or EDTA), therapeutic	50–240 ng/mL	156–746 nmol/L
Luteinizing hormone (LH), serum		
Males	6–18 mU/mL	6–18 U/L
Females		
Premenopausal	5–22 mU/mL	5–22 U/L
Midcycle	3 times baseline	3 times baseline
Postmenopausal	>30 mU/mL	>30 U/L
Magnesium		
Serum	1.5–2.5 mEq/L	0.75–1.25 mmol/L
	1.8–3.0 mg/dL	
Urine	6.0–8.5 mEq/24 h	3.0–4.3 mmol/24 h
Mercury		
Whole blood (EDTA)	1–3 µg/dL	0.05–0.15 µmol/L
Urine, 24 h	<20 µg/d	<0.1 µmol/d
Toxic	>150 µg/d	>0.75 µmol/d
Metanephrines (see Catecholamines)		
Methemoglobin (MetHb, hemiglobin), whole blood (EDTA, Hep, or ACD)	0.06–0.24 g/dL or 0.78 ± 0.37% of total Hb (SD)	9.3–37.2 µmol/L or Mass fraction of total Hb: 0.008 ± 0.0037 (SD)
Methotrexate, serum or plasma (Hep or EDTA)		
Therapeutic	Variable	Variable
Toxic		
1–2 wk after low-dose therapy	>9.1 ng/mL	>20 nmol/L
48 h after high-dose therapy	454 ng/mL	>1000 nmol/L
Myelin basic protein, CSF	<4 ng/mL	<4 µg/L

---

*Test values are method dependent.

(continued)

Tests	Conventional Units	SI Units
Nitroprusside, serum or plasma (EDTA), as thiocyanate, therapeutic	6–29 µg/mL	103–499 µmol/L
Nortriptyline, serum or plasma (Hep or EDTA); trough (≥12 h after dose)		
Therapeutic	50–150 ng/mL	190–570 nmol/L
Toxic	>500 ng/mL	>1900 nmol/L
* 5'-Nucleotidase, serum	3.5–12.7 mU/mL (37°C)	3.5–12.5 U/L (37°C)
N-Acetylprocainamide, serum or plasma (Hep or EDTA); trough		
Therapeutic	5–30 µg/mL	18–108 µmol/L
Toxic	>40 µg/mL	>144 µmol/L
Occult blood, faeces, random	Negative (<2 mL blood/ 150 g stool/d)	Negative (13.3 mL blood/ kg stool/d)
Qualitative, urine, random	Negative	Negative
Oestrogens, urine		
Males		
Oestrone	3–8 µg/24 h	11–30 nmol/24 h
Oestradiol	0–6 µg/24 h	0–22 nmol/24 h
Oestriol	1–11 µg/24 h	3–38 nmol/24 h
§Total	4–25 µg/24 h	14–90 nmol/24 h
Females		
Oestrone	4–31 µg/24 h	15–115 nmol/24 h
Oestradiol	0–14 µg/24 h	0–51 nmol/24 h
Oestriol	0–72 µg/24 h	0–250 nmol/24 h
§Total	5–100 µg/24 h	18–360 nmol/24 h
	(Markedly increased during pregnancy)	(Markedly increased during pregnancy)
Osmolality		
Serum	285–295 mOsm/kg serum water	285–295 mmol/kg serum water
Urine	38–1400 mOsm/kg water	38–1400 mmol/kg water
Ratio, urine/serum	1.0–3.0	Same
	>3.0 after 12 h fluid restriction	
Osmotic fragility of erythrocytes	Begins in 0.45–0.39% NaCl	Begins in 77–67 mmol/L NaCl
	Complete in 0.33–0.30% NaCl	Complete in 56–51 mmol/ L NaCl
Oxazepam, serum or plasma (Hep or EDTA), therapeutic	0.2–1.4 µg/mL	0.70–4.9 µmol/L
Oxygen, blood		
Capacity	16–24 vol% (varies with hemoglobin)	7.14–10.7 mmol/L (varies with hemoglobin)

*Test values are method dependent.
§Assuming a mixture of oestrone, oestradioles, and oestriol in a molecular proportion of 2:1:2.

(continued)

Tests	Conventional Units	SI Units
Content		
Arterial	15–23 vol%	6.69–10.3 mmol/L
Venous	10–16 vol%	4.46–7.14 mmol/L
Saturation		
Arterial	94–100% of capacity	0.94–1.00 of capacity
Venous	60–85% of capacity	0.60–0.85 of capacity
Tension, pO_2 arterial	75–100 mm Hg	75–100 mm Hg
P50, blood	26–27 mm Hg	27–27 mm Hg
Pentobarbital, serum or plasma (Hep or EDTA); trough		
Therapeutic		
Hypnotic	1–5 μg/mL	4–22 μmol/L
Therapeutic coma	20–50 μg/mL	88–221 μmol/L
Toxic	>10 μg/mL	>44 μmol/L
pH		
Blood, arterial	7.35–7.45	7.35–7.45
Urine	4.6–8.0 (depends on diet)	Same
Phenacetin, plasma (EDTA)		
Therapeutic	1–20 μg/mL	6–112 μmol/L
Toxic	50–250 μg/mL	279–1395 μmol/L
Phenobarbital, serum or plasma (Hep or EDTA); trough		
Therapeutic	15–40 μg/mL	65–170 μmol/L
Toxic		
Slowness, ataxia, nystagmus	35–80 μg/mL	151–345 μmol/L
Coma with reflexes	65–117 μg/mL	280–504 μmol/L
Coma without reflexes	>100 μg/mL	>430 μmol/L
Phenolsulphonphthalein exretion (PSP), urine	25% or more in 15 min	0.25 or more in 15 min
	40% or more in 30 min	0.40 or more in 30 min
	55% or more in 2 h	0.55 or more in 2 h
	(After injection of 1 mL PSP intravenously)	(After injection of 1 mL PSP intravenously)
Phenylalanine, serum	<3 mg/dL	<0.18 mmol/L
Phenylpyruvic acid, urine, qualitative	Negative	Negative
Phenytoin, serum or plasma (Hep or EDTA); trough		
Therapeutic	10–20 μg/mL	40–79 μmol/L
Toxic	>20 μg/mL	>79 μmol/L
* Phosphatase, acid, prostatic, serum		
RIA	<3.0 ng/mL	<3.0 μg/L
Enzymatic, 37°C	0.11–0.60 U/L (Roy, Brower, Hayden)	0.11–0.60 U/L
* Phosphatase, alkaline		
Leucocyte	Total score: 14–100	Total score: 14–100

*Test values are method dependent.

(continued)

Tests	Conventional Units	SI Units
Serum (ALP)	20–90 mU/mL (30°C) (Values are higher in children)	20–90 U/L (30°C) (Values are higher in children)
Phosphate, inorganic, serum		
Adults	3.0–4.5 mg/dL	1.0–1.5 mmol/L
Children	4.0–7.0 mg/dL	1.3–2.3 mmol/L
Phosphatidylglycerol (PG), amniotic fluid		
Absent	Fetal immaturity	Same
Present	Fetal maturity	Same
Phospholipids, serum	6–12 mg/dL (As lipid phosphorus)	1.9–3.9 mmol/L (As lipid phosphorus)
Phosphorus, urine	0.4–1.3 g/24 h	12.9–42 mmol/24 h
Phorphobilinogen, urine		
Qualitative	Negative	Negative
Quantitative	0–0.2 mg/dL <2.0 mg/24 h	0–0.9 μmol/L <9 μmol/24 h
Porphyrins, urine		
Coproporphyrin	50–250 μg/24 h	77–380 nmol/24 h
Uroporphyrin	10–30 μg/24 h	12–36 nmol/24 h
Potassium, plasma (Hep)		
Males	3.5–4.5 mEq/L	3.5–4.5 mmol/L
Females	3.4–4.4 mEq/L	3.4–4.4 mmol/L
Potassium		
Serum		
Premature		
Cord	5.0–10.2 mEq/L	5.0–10.2 mmol/L
48 h	3.0–6.0 mEq/l	3.0–6.0 mmol/L
Newborn, cord	5.6–12.0 mEq/L	5.6–12.0 mmol/L
Newborn	3.7–5.9 mEq/L	3.7–5.9 mmol/L
Infant	4.1–5.3 mEq/L	4.1–5.3 mmol/L
Child	3.4–4.7 mEq/L	3.4–4.7 mmol/L
Adult	3.5–5.1 mEq/L	3.5–5.1 mmol/L
Urine, 24 h	25–125 mEq/d, varies with diet	25–125 mmol/d; varies with diet
CSF	70% of plasma level or 2.5–3.2 mEq/L, rises with plasma hyperosmolality	0.70 of plasma level or 2.5–3.2 mmol/L; rises with plasma hyperosmolality
Pregnanediol, urine		
Males	0.4–1.4 mg/24 h	1.2–4.4 μmol/24 h
Females		
Proliferative phase	0.5–1.5 mg/24 h	1.6–4.7 μmol/24 h
Luteal phase	2.0–7.0 mg/24 h	6.2–22 μmol/24 h
Postmenopausal phase	0.2–1.0 mg/24 h	0.6–3.1 μmol/24 h
Pregnanetriol, urine	<2.5 mg/24 h in adults	<7.4 μmol/24 h in adults
Pressure, CSF	70–180 mm H$_2$O	Same
Primidone, serum or plasma (Hep or EDTA); trough		
Therapeutic	5–12 μg/mL	23–55 μmol/L

(continued)

Tests	Conventional Units	SI Units
Toxic	>15 μg/mL	>69 μmol/L
Procainamide, serum or plasma (Hep or EDTA); trough		
Therapeutic	4–10 μg/mL	17–42 μmol/L
Toxic (also consider effect of metabolite (NAPA))	>10–12 μg/mL	>42–51 μmol/L
Prolactin, serum		
Males	1–20 ng/mL	1–20 μg/L
Females	1–25 ng/mL	1–25 μg/L
Propoxyphene, plasma (EDTA)		
Therapeutic	0.1–0.4 μg/mL	0.3–1.2 μmol/L
Toxic	>0.5 μg/mL	>1.5 μmol/L
Propranolol, serum or plasma (Hep or EDTA); trough		
Therapeutic	50–100 ng/mL	193–386 nmol/L
* Protein, serum		
Total	6.0–8.0 g/dL	60–80 g/L
Albumin	3.5–5.0 g/dL	35–50 g/L
	52–68% of total	0.52–0.68 of total
Globulin		
α_1	0.2–0.4 g/dL	2–4 g/L
	2–5% of total	0.02–0.05 of total
α_2	0.5–0.9 g/dL	5–9 g/L
	7–14% of total	0.07–0.14 of total
β	0.6–1.1 g/dL	6–11 g/L
	9–15% of total	0.09–0.15 of total
γ	0.7–1.7 g/dL	7–17 g/L
	11–21% of total	0.11–0.21 of total
Protein		
Urine		
Qualitative	Negative	Negative
Quantitative	10–150 mg/24 h	10–150 mg/24 h
CSF, total	15–45 mg/dL (higher, up to 70 mg/dL in the elderly and children)	0.150–0.450 g/L (higher, up to 0.70 g/L in the elderly and children)
Protoporphyrin, free, erythrocyte	27–61 μg/dL packed RBC	0.48–1.09 μmol/L packed RBC
Pyruvate, blood	0.3–0.9 mg/dL	0.03–0.10 mmol/L
Quinidine, serum or plasma (Hep or EDTA); trough		
Therapeutic	2–5 μg/mL	6–15 μmol/L
Toxic	>6 μg/mL	>18 μmol/L
Salicylates, serum or plasma (Hep or EDTA); trough		
Therapeutic	150–300 μg/mL	1086–2172 μmol/L
Toxic	>300 μg/mL	>2172 μmol/L

*Test values are method dependent.

(continued)

Tests	Conventional Units	SI Units
Sedimentation rate		
Wintrobe		
Males	0–5 mm in 1 h	0–5 mm/h
Females	0–15 mm in 1 h	0–15 mm/h
Westergren		
Males	0–15 mm in 1 h	0–15 mm/h
Females	0–20 mm in 1 h	0–20 mm/h
Sodium		
Serum or plasma (Hep)		
Premature		
Cord	116–140 mEq/L	116–140 mmol/L
48 h	128–148 mEq/L	128–148 mmol/L
Newborn, cord	126–166 mEq/L	126–166 mmol/L
Newborn	134–144 mEq/L	134–144 mmol/L
Infant	139–146 mEq/L	139–146 mmol/L
Child	138–145 mEq/L	138–145 mmol/L
Adult	136–146 mEq/L	136–146 mmol/L
Urine, 24 h	40–220 mEq/d (diet dependent)	40–220 mmol/d (diet dependent)
Sweat		
Normal	10–40 mEq/L	10–40 mmol/L
Cystic fibrosis	>70 mEq/L	>70 mmol/L
Specific gravity	1.003–1.030	1.003–1.030
Sulphates, inorganic, serum	0.8–1.2 mg/dL	83–125 μmol/l
Testosterone, plasma		
Males	275–875 ng/dL	9.5–30 nmol/L
Females	23–75 ng/dL	0.8–2.6 nmol/L
Pregnant females	38–190 ng/dL	1.3–6.6 nmol/L
Theophylline, serum or plasma (Hep or EDTA)		
Therapeutic		
Bronchodilator	8–20 μg/mL	44–111 μmol/L
Prem. apnea	6–13 μg/mL	33–72 μmol/L
Toxic	>20 μg/mL	>110 μmol/l
Thiocyanate		
Serum or plasma (EDTA)		
Nonsmoker	1–4 μg/mL	17–69 μmol/L
Smoker	3–12 μg/mL	52–206 μmol/L
Therapeutic after nitroprusside infusion	6–29 μg/mL	103–499 μmol/L
Urine		
Nonsmoker	1–4 mg/d	17–69 μmol/d
Smoker	7–17 mg/d	120–292 μmol/d
Thiopental, serum or plasma (Hep or EDTA); trough		
Hypnotic	1.0–5.0 μg/mL	4.1–20.7 μmol/L
Coma	30–100 μg/mL	124–413 μmol/L
Anaesthesia	7–130 μg/mL	29–536 μmol/L
Toxic concentration	>10 μg/mL	>41 μmol/L

(continued)

Tests	Conventional Units	SI Units
Thyroid-stimulating hormone (TSH), serum	0.35–7 μU/mL	0.35–7 mU/L
Thyroxine (T₄) serum	5–12 μg/dL (varies with age, higher in children and pregnant women)	66–155 nmol/L (varies with age, higher in children and pregnant women)
Thyroxine, free, serum	1.0–2.1 ng/dL	13–27 pmol/L
Thyroxine binding globulin (TBG), serum (as thyroxine)	10–26 μg/dL	129–335 nmol/L
Titratable acidity, urine	20–40 mEq/24 h	20–40 mmol/24 h
Tobramycin, serum or plasma (Hep or EDTA)		
Therapeutic		
Peak		
Less severe infection	5–8 μg/mL	11–17 μmol/L
Severe infection	8–10 μg/mL	17–21 μmol/L
Trough		
Less severe infection	<1 μg/mL	<2 μmol/L
Moderate infection	<2 μg/mL	<4 μmol/L
Severe infection	<2–4 μg/mL	<4–9 μmol/L
Toxic		
Peak	>10–12 μg/mL	>21–26 μmol/L
Trough	>2–4 μg/mL	>4–9 μmol/L
* Transaminase, serum		
AST (asparate aminotransferase, SGOT)	7–40 mU/mL (37°C)	7–40 U/L (37°C)
ALT (alanine aminotransferase, SGPT)	5–35 mU/mL (37°C)	5–35 U/L (37°C)
Transferrin, serum		
Newborn	130–275 mg/dL	1.30–2.75 g/L
Adult	220–400 mg/dL	2.20–4.00 g/L
>60 y	180–380 mg/dL	1.80–3.80 g/L
Triglycerides, serum, fasting	40–150 mg/dL	0.4–1.5 g/L 0.45–1.71 mmol/L
Triiodothyronine (T₃), serum	150–250 ng/dL	2.3–3.9 nmol/L
* Triiodothyronine (T₃) uptake, resin (T3RU)	25–38% uptake	0.25–0.38 uptake
Uric acid		
Serum, enzymatic		
Male	3.5–7.2 mg/dL	0.21–0.42 mmol/L
Female	2.6–6.0 mg/dL	0.15–0.35 mmol/L
Child	2.0–5.5 mg/dL	0.12–0.32 mmol/L
* Urine	250–750 mg/24 h (with normal diet)	1.48–4.43 mmol/24 h (with normal diet)
Urea nitrogen, plasma or serum	11–23 mg/dL	7.9–16.4 mmol/L

*Test values are method dependent.

(continued)

Tests	Conventional Units	SI Units
Urea nitrogen/creatinine ratio, serum	12:1 to 20:1	12:1 to 20:1
Urobilinogen, urine	Up to 1.0 Ehrlich unit/2 h (1–3 PM) 0–4.0 mg/24 h	Up to 1.0 Ehrlich unit/2 h (1–3 PM) 0–6.8 μmol/24 h
Valproic acid, serum or plasma (Hep or EDTA); trough		
Therapeutic	50–100 μg/mL	347–693 μmol/L
Toxic	>100 μg/mL	>693 μmol/L
Vancomycin, serum or plasma (Hep or EDTA); trough		
Therapeutic	Not well established	
Toxic	>80–100 μg/mL	>80–100 mg/L
Vanillylmandelic acid (VMA), urine (4-hydroxy-3-methoxymandelic acid)	1–8 mg/24 h	5–40 μmol/24 h
Viscosity, serum	1.4–1.8 times water	1.4–1.8 times water
Vitamin A, serum	20–80 μg/dL	0.70–2.8 μmol/L
Vitamin B$_{12}$, serum	180–900 pg/mL	133–664 pmol/L
Vitamin E, serum		
Normal	7–20 μg/mL	16.2–46.4 μmol/L
Therapeutic	30–50 μg/mL	69.6–116 μmol/L
Zinc, serum	70–150 μg/dL	10.7–22.9 μmol/L

*Test values are method dependent.

BLOOD GROUPS

In this appendix, and in related terms defined in the dictionary proper, the term "blood group" is used to refer to an entire blood group system consisting of erythrocyte antigens whose specificity is controlled by a series of allelic genes or by a series of genes so closely linked on a single chromosome that they cannot be distinguished from alleles by available genetic methods. The terms "blood type" and "phenotype" are used to refer to a specific reaction pattern to testing antisera within a system. This usage is not universal. It should be noted that in current literature a single system may be referred to in the plural (*i.e.*, ABO blood groups) and the term "blood group" may be assigned to a single phenotype (*i.e.*, blood group A).

Each blood group is defined in terms of reaction to the original antiserum with which the system was discovered, with modification or extension as required by the discovery of additional antisera proved to be related to the same system. A "new" blood group antigen can be defined by showing that it is detected by an antiserum with reactions different from those of previously known antisera. If it can be shown that the "new" antigen is genetically independent of known blood group systems, it may qualify as the prototype antigen of a new blood group. If it can be shown that the "new" antigen is controlled by a gene allelic to one or more known blood group genes, it is assigned to the blood group of its alleles. Many known antigens have not been shown to be either genetically independent or related to certain other known antigens, and their status remains in doubt.

In the blood group definitions, emphasis has been placed on identification of symbols for genes, antigens, antisera, and phenotypes. These often appear in the literature without specification that they refer to a blood group. Attention is called to the general convention, followed here, that symbols for genes and genotypes are set in italics, whereas symbols for gene products or antigens, antisera, and phenotypes are set in Roman type. In the Rh-Hr terminology for the Rh blood group, Roman type is used to designate antigenic substances, and boldface type is used to designate serologic factors and their corresponding antibodies.

These conventions are in wide usage but are not consistently followed by all authors.

ABO blood group

This classical blood group system is defined by the agglutination reactions of erythrocytes to the natural isoantibodies anti-A and anti-B and related antisera (Landsteiner, 1900). In normal human blood there is a reciprocal relationship between the ABO antigens or agglutinogens on the surface of the erythrocyte and the natural antibodies or isoagglutinins found in serum. Individuals of type O do not have either A or B antigens on the erythrocytes, but their serum contains both anti-A and anti-B agglutinins. Individuals of type A have antigen A on the erythrocytes and anti-B in the serum. Individuals of type B have antigen B on the erythrocytes and anti-A in the serum. Individuals of type AB have both A and B antigens on the erythrocytes but no isoagglutinins in the serum. Types A and AB may be subdivided by anti-A_1 serum into types A_1 and A_2, and A_1B and A_2B. The A_2 antigen is weaker in reaction than the A_1, but their difference is also qualitative. Production of ABO antigens is controlled by a series of allelic genes A_1, A_2, B, and O (sometimes designated I^{A_1}, I^{A_2}, I^B, and i; i^{A_1}, i^{A_2}, i^B, and i; or A_1, A_2, a^B, and a). A_1 is dominant to A_2, and both are dominant to O; there is no dominance between A_1 and B or A_2 and B.

In the usual typing method a strong anti-A serum that agglutinates cells containing A_1 or A_2 antigen is used; cells agglutinated by this serum but not by anti-B are of type A but may be of genotype A_1A_1, A_1A_2, A_1O, A_2A_2, or A_2O. Cells of persons of type A that are agglutinated by anti-A_1 are of type A_1 and may be of genotype A_1A_1, A_1A_2, or A_1O; type A cells not agglutinated by anti-A_1 are of type A_2 and may be of genotype A_2A_2 or A_2O. Cells agglutinated by anti-B but not anti-A are of type B and may be of genotype BB or BO. Cells agglutinated by both anti-A and anti-B are of type AB and can be divided into types A_1B (genotype A_1B) and A_2B (genotype A_2B) by anti-A_1. Cells not agglutinated by either anti-A or anti-B are of type O and genotype OO. Cells of type O do not simply lack antigenic substance; the vast majority possess an antigen called H that is chemically similar to antigens

A and B and is probably the precursor antigen that is modified under the influence of genes A_1, A_2, and B into their corresponding antigens.

Rare individuals fail to form H antigen and, regardless of ABO genotype, do not produce A, B, or H antigens; such persons seem to be homozygous for a recessive gene called h or x. The postulated allele H or X is apparently necessary to convert a mucopolysaccharide precursor into H antigen. The term "Bombay" phenotype was assigned to such persons whose cells lack A, B, and H antigen and whose serum contains anti-A, anti-B, and anti-H; they are also referred to as the "Oh" phenotype. In addition, weak variants of antigen A have been described with phenotypes designated A_3, A_4, A_5, A_x, and A_z; more rarely, weak variants of B have been found. The ABO types are of prime importance with respect to blood transfusion, and maternal-fetal incompatibility is a frequent cause of fetal death and erythroblastosis fetalis.

Auberger blood group

This erythrocyte antigen is defined by reaction to an antibody designated anti-Au^a, originally found in the serum of a Madame Auberger who had received many transfusions (Salmon, Salmon, Liberge, Andre, Tippett, and Sanger, 1961). The Au^a antigen is inherited as a dominant trait and occurs in about 80 percent of whites and blacks.

Diego blood group

The erythrocyte antigen defined by anti-Di^a antibody was first found in Venezuela where it had been the cause of erthroblastosis fetalis (Layrisse, Arends, and Dominguez, 1955). An antibody with antithetical reactions, anti-Di^b, was discovered in 1967. The antigen system is controlled by two alleles, Di^a and Di^b. The Di^a antigen is common in American Indians and in Asiatics but is apparently absent in whites. This distribution is considered strong anthropological evidence to support the thesis that American Indians are derived from Mongolian or Asiatic ancestors.

Dombrock blood group

This erythrocyte antigen is defined by reaction to anti-Do^a antibody (Swanson, Polesky, Tippett, and Sanger, 1965). The Do^a antigen exhibits autosomal dominant inheritance and is found in about 65 to 66 percent of Northern Europeans, U.S. whites, and Israelis, in about 45 to 55 percent of U.S. blacks and American Indians, and in about 13 percent of Thais.

Duffy blood group

These erythrocyte antigens are defined by reactions to an immune serum called anti-Fy^a, first found in a haemophilic patient named Duffy who had received many transfusions (Cutbush, Mollison, and Parkin, 1950), and a serum with antithetical reactions, anti-Fy^b (Ikin, Mourant, Peffenkofer, and Blumenthal, 1951). The bloods of practically all whites are agglutinated by one, the other, or both of these antisera, but bloods of the majority of blacks and some Yemenite Jews give negative reactions to both antisera. It is therefore assumed that the production of Duffy antigens is controlled by a series of at least three allelic genes, Fy^a, Fy^b, and Fy, with antibodies specific for only the first two of the series being now known. Persons with blood reacting positively to anti-Fy^a and negatively to anti-Fy^b are of phenotype Fy(a+b−), and their genotype may be either Fy^aFy^a or Fy^aFy. Persons of phenotype Fy(a+b+) are of genotype Fy^aFy^b. Those of phenotype Fy(a−b+) may be of genotype Fy^bFy^b or Fy^bFy. Those of phenotype Fy(a−b−) are of genotype $FyFy$. Duffy antibodies occasionally cause transfusion reactions or erythroblastosis fetalis.

High frequency blood groups

This group of antigens is found in almost all individuals but is absent in members of a very few families. Because of very high frequency they are often called "public" antigens. The antibodies usually have been found in the serum of a patient lacking the antigen who has become immunized by transfusion or pregnancy. Names or symbols applied to public antigens include: Vel, Yt^a, Ge, Lan, and Sm. See also low frequency blood groups.

I blood group

These erythrocyte antigens are defined by reactions to antibodies designated anti-I (Wiener, Unger, Cohen, and Feldman, 1956) and anti-i. Antigen I differs from other blood group antigens in the slowness of its development and in its wide range of strength in different individuals; the range approximates a normal distribution curve. Anti-I occurs in a wide range of strength and in two forms: autoanti-I is the antibody usually found in the serum of patients with acquired haemolytic anaemia of the "cold agglutinin" type and in sera described as containing "non-specific complete cold autoagglutinin"; natural anti-I or isoanti-I occurs regularly in the serum of persons of phenotype i. Phenotype i may be divided into types i_1 and i_2, both rare in adults.

Kell blood group

These erythrocyte antigens are defined by an immune antibody, anti-K, first found in the serum of a Mrs. Kell (Coombs, Mourant, and Race, 1946), and by anti-k (Levine, Backer, Wigod, and Ponder, 1949). Anti-k was known as anti-Cellano until its antithetical reactions to anti-K were established. An antiserum originally designated anti-Si was found to be identical to anti-K. The antigens K and k are controlled by a pair of allelic genes without dominance, hence three genotypes (*KK, Kk, kk*) may be recognized by agglutination of erythrocytes by anti-K alone, both anti-K and anti-k, or anti-k alone. Variant antigens of this system detected by human sera have been designated Kp^a and Kp^b. Very rare families have been found in which erythrocytes of certain persons give negative reactions with all antisera of the Kell group; this phenotype is designated K-k-Kp(a−b−). As a cause of transfusion reactions and erythroblastosis fetalis, the Kell blood group is next in clinical importance after the ABO and Rh blood groups.

Kidd blood group

These erythrocyte antigens are defined by reactions to an antibody designated anti-Jk^a, discovered in the serum of a Mrs. Kidd who had delivered an infant with erythroblastosis (Allen, Diamond, and Niedziela, 1951), and by reactions to its antithetical serum, anti-Jk^b (Plaut, Ikin, Mourant, Sanger, and Race, 1953). The antigens are controlled by a pair of genes without dominance, Jk^a and Jk^b, that are genetically independent of other blood group genes. Persons with erythrocytes that are agglutinated by anti-Jk^a but not by anti-Jk^b are of phenotype Jk(a+b−) and genotype Jk^aJk^a; agglutination by both antisera indicates phenotype Jk(a+b+) and genotype Jk^aJk^b; agglutination by only anti-Jk^b indicates phenotype Jk(a−b+) and genotype Jk^bJk^b. The possibility that there may be a third allele at this locus or a modifier capable of suppressing the action of genes at this locus or a modifier capable of suppressing the action of genes at this locus has been raised by the discovery of rare individuals (usually of Asiatic or South American Indian ancestry) whose erythrocytes give negative reactions to both antisera. Kidd antibodies occasionally cause transfusion reactions or erythroblastosis fetalis.

Lewis blood group

These antigens of erythrocytes, saliva, and certain other body fluids are defined by reactions to anti-Le^a antibody, first found in the serum of a Mrs. Lewis (Mourant, 1946), by reactions to related sera particularly anti-Le^b, and by interactions with the secretor factor. The Lewis antigens are formed in tissue under control of genes designated Le and le (Le dominant to le) and released into body fluids where they may be absorbed onto the surface of erythrocytes and determine the reactions of erythrocytes to antisera. The Lewis erythrocyte types of children may not develop fully until about age six years. The Lewis genes are genetically independent of those controlling the secretor factor (Se and se), but their products interact in certain phenotypic effects. Several theories have been proposed to account for the complex immunologic and genetic observations. The theory of Grubb and Ceppellini was summarized by Race and Sanger (1962) as shown in Table 1.

Variant antibodies of this system include: anti-Le^x (originally called anti-X), which seems to be anti-Le^a plus anti-Le^b; anti-Le^c, an immune rabbit serum that agglutinates Le(a−b−) cells; the

Table 1. Secretor-Lewis Interactions*

Genotypes	Antigens				
	Of Saliva				Of Erythrocytes
	ABH	Le^a	Le^{bL}	Le^{bH}	
SeSe LeLe SeSe Lele Sese LeLe Sese Lele	+	+	+	+	Le(a−b+)
sese LeLe sese Lele	−	+	−	−	Le(a+b−)
SeSe lele Sese lele	+	−	−	+	Le(a−b−)
sese lele	−	−	−	−	Le(a−b−)

*From Race, R.R., and Sanger, R.: *Blood Groups in Man*, Ed. 4. Oxford, England, Blackwell Scientific Publications, Ltd., 1962.

Magard antiserum, obtained from a patient with carcinoma of the stomach, that agglutinates strongly the cells of A$_1$ Le(a−b−) secretors and less strongly those of A$_2$ Le(a−b−) secretors. Lewis antibodies have occasionally been implicated as a cause of transfusion reactions.

Low frequency blood groups

In this group of erythrocyte antigens, each is defined by a specific antiserum, and each is found only in members of a very few families. Because of their rarity they are often referred to as "private" antigens. The antibodies usually have been found in the sera of patients who have received transfusions or in mothers of erythroblastotic infants. They are often named for the family in which they were first discovered. The names or symbols assigned to some private antigens are: Levay, Jobbins, Becker, Ven, Chr^a, Wright or Wr^a, Be^a, By, Swann or Sw^a, Good, Biles or Bi, Tr^a, Stobo, Ot, Ho, and Webb. See also high frequency blood groups.

Lutheran blood group

These blood group antigens are defined by reactions to an antibody designated anti-Lu^a, first found in serum of a patient who had received many transfusions (Callender, Race, and Paykoc, 1945), and its reciprocal, anti-Lu^b (Cutbush and Chanarin, 1956). Production of the antigens is controlled by a pair of allelic genes, Lu^a and Lu^b, without dominance. The erythrocytes of persons with genotype Lu^aLu^a are agglutinated by anti-Lu^a but not by anti-Lu^b, those of genotype Lu^aLu^b are agglutinated by both antisera, and those of genotype Lu^bLu^b are agglutinated by anti-Lu^b but not by anti-Lu^a. These antibodies are an uncommon cause of transfusion reactions.

MNSs blood group

This system of erythrocyte antigens was originally defined by reactions to immune rabbit sera designated anti-M and anti-N (Landsteiner and Levine, 1927) and has since been extended by reactions to sera anti-S, anti-s, and certain others. When tested with the readily available anti-M and anti-N sera only, the erythrocytes of all individuals may be assigned to one of three classes, M, N or MN, depending on whether they are agglutinated by one, the other, or both antisera. Production of M and N antigens is controlled by two allelic genes, *M* and *N*; persons of genotype *MM* are type M, those of genotype *NN* are type N, and those of the heterozygous genotype *MN* are type MN. As anti-M and anti-N sera are commercially available and the reactions are simple and reliable, they are widely used for medicolegal blood testing in disputed paternity actions and for genetic linkage and population studies. The *MN* locus is not genetically linked to loci of other major blood group systems. The MNSs antigens are only rarely the cause of haemolytic reactions to transfusion.

With the discovery of anti-S serum (1947) and its reciprocal anti-s (1951), it was shown that the MNS group is complex and that nine phenotypes representing ten genotypes may be defined by the four antisera (Table 2). In addition, nearly 1 percent of blood samples of blacks lack both S and s. An antibody designated as anti-U has been found that reacts with both S and s antigens. Weak variants of the M and N antigens that react with some anti-M

Table 2. MNSs Phenotypes and Genotypes

Antisera				Genotypes
M	N	S	s	
+	−	+	−	MS/MS
+	−	+	+	MS/Ms
+	−	−	+	Ms/Ms
+	+	+	−	MS/Ns
+	+	+	+	MS/Ns or Ms/NS
+	+	−	+	Ms/Ns
−	+	+	−	NS/Ns
−	+	+	+	NS/Ns
−	+	−	+	Ns/Ns

or anti-N sera but not with others have been designated M_2 and N_2. A qualitative variant of M has been designated M_1. An antigen that gives intermediate reactions has been designated M^c. An extremely rare variant of M detected with a special serum has been designated M^g. Antigens designated Hu and He are detected by sera obtained from rabbits immunized with blood of certain blacks and are found almost entirely in persons of African ancestry; anti-Hu gives distinct reactions only with cells that also contain N, and most positives to anti-He possess both N and S. Other rare antigens that are associated with or are variants of the MNS group have been designated Mi_2, Vw (identical with Gr), and Mu.

P blood group

This system of erythrocyte antigens was originally defined by reaction to immune rabbit serum designated anti-P (Landsteiner

Table 3. P Blood Group*

Phenotypes		Phenotype Symbol	Genotypes
anti-P + P_1 (Tj^a)	anti-P_1 (P)		
+	+	P_1	P_1P_1; P_1P_2; P_1p
+	−	P_2	P_2P_2; P_2p
−	−	p	pp

*From Race, R.R., and Sanger, R.: Blood Groups in Man, Ed. 4. Oxford, England, Blackwell Scientific Publications, Ltd., 1962.

and Levine, 1927) but has since been extended to include related antigens. An antibody previously known as anti-Tj[a] was shown to be related to anti-P in 1955, and the terminology presented in Table 3 was proposed by Sanger. In this terminology, P_1 is the phenotype previously called P+, P_2 is the phenotype previously called P−, and p is the phenotype previously called Tj(a−). A rare variant designated P^k has also been found.

Rh blood group

This complex system of erythrocyte antigens was originally defined by reactions to serum from rabbits or guinea pigs immunized with blood of the rhesus monkey (Landsteiner and Wiener, 1940) but is now defined by reactions to a series of human antisera usually obtained from persons immunized by transfusion or pregnancy. The nomenclature of genes, antigens, and antisera of this system has undergone an evolution reflecting the acquisition of new knowledge since 1940, and conflicting systems of nomenclature have been in use. The most widely used nomenclatures are those proposed by Wiener (Rh-Hr system) and by Fisher and Race (CDE system), both of which have been frequently modified and extended, and that proposed in 1962 by Rosenfield, Allen, Swisher, and Kochwa (numerical system). Certain differences of theoretic interpretations of both immunology and genetics are associated with the different nomenclatures. It is agreed that production of Rh antigens is controlled by a complex series of genes located on a single chromosome, that there are eight major genes or gene complexes that control production of qualitatively different antigens, that the paired arrangements of these eight genes give rise to 18 qualitative phenotypes or erythrocyte patterns that can be recognized by reactions with five standard antisera that are commercially available, and that many more antigens or antigen combinations exist, with both qualitative and quantitative differences that can be recognized by a series of other antisera not generally available with reaction specificities that reflect wide immunologic and genetic variation. The Rh-Hr nomenclature implies that all Rh genes constitute a single set of multiple alleles located at a single chromosome locus and that a single gene may control production of an erythrocyte antigen or agglutinogen possessing many factors each of different antibody specificity. The CDE nomenclature implies that there are three contiguous chromosome loci or areas of genetic information, each with a series of two major and probably several minor alleles, each controlling production of a specific erythrocyte antigen. The numerical system assigns an arbitrary number to each known anti-serum, using numbers 1 through 5 for the five standard antisera and higher numbers for others, and classifies individuals by positive or negative reactions to the antisera used. The correspondence of the three nomenclatures with respect to designations for genes, phenotypes, and antisera are given in Tables 4, 5, and 6.

The symbol D^u is used in the CDE nomenclature to designate antigens that are agglutinated by some anti-D sera and not by others, and these apparently represent weak or incomplete forms of the D antigen. Many varieties of D^u exist. Individuals possessing D^u may be mistyped as D-negative (d), but D^u blood may stimulate the formation of anti-D if transfused to a D-negative recipient. Some D^u persons have made anti-D when transfused with D-positive blood. In the Rh-Hr nomenclature, weak variants are indicated by using Germanic type (*e.g.*, $\mathfrak{Rh}_o$). The Rh-Hr nomenclature also designates the extremely rare phenotypes that lack the factor pairs rh'-hr' and rh''-hr'' by placing a double

Table 4. Rh Gene Designations in Three Nomenclature Systems[*]

Rh-Hr (Wiener)	CDE (Fisher-Race)	Numerical (Rosenfield *et al.*)
r	cde	$R^{-1, -2, -3, 4, 5}$
R^1	CDe	$R^{1, 2, -3, -4, 5}$
R^2	cDE	$R^{1, -2, 3, 4, -5}$
R^0	cDe	$R^{1, -2, -3, 4, 5}$
r'	Cde	$R^{-1, 2, -3, -4, 5}$
r''	cdE	$R^{-1, -2, 3, 4, -5}$
R^z	CDE	$R^{1, 2, 3, -4, -5}$
r^y	CdE	$r^{-1, 2, 3, -4, -5}$
(Paired combinations of the above give rise to 36 genotypes)		

[*]Tables 4 and 5 are modified from Rosenfield, R.E., Allen, F.H., Jr., Swisher, S.N., and Kochwa, S.: A review of Rh serology and presentation of a new terminology. *Transfusion* **2**:287, 1962 (official journal of the American Association of Blood Banks, J.B. Lippincott Co., publisher).

Table 5. Rh Antiserum Designations in Three Nomenclature Systems

Rh-Hr (Wiener)	CDE (Fisher-Race)	Numerical (Rosenfield et al.)
Standard antisera		
Rh₀	D	Rh1
rh'	C	Rh2
rh''	E	Rh3
hr'	c	Rh4
hr''	e	Rh5
Other antisera		
hr	f, ce	Rh6
rh	Ce	Rh7
rhʷ¹	Cʷ	Rh8
rhˣ	Cˣ	Rh9
hrᵛ	V, ce⁵	Rh10
rhʷ²	Eʷ	Rh11
rhᵍ	G	Rh12
Rhᴬ	No term	Rh13
Rhᴮ	No term	Rh14
Rhᶜ	No term	Rh15
Rhᴰ	No term	Rh16
Hr₀	No term	Rh17
Hr	No term	Rh18
hrˢ	No term	Rh19
Hrᴴ plus hrᵛ	VS, e⁵	Rh20
No term	Cᴳ	Rh21

bar above the appropriate symbol ($\overline{\overline{R}}h_o$; $\overline{\overline{R}}h^w$); the corresponding phenotype in the CDE nomenclature is designated —D—.

Sutter blood group

This erythrocyte antigen is defined by reaction to an antibody designated anti-Js^a, first found in the serum of a Mr. Sutter who had been previously transfused (Giblett, 1958). The Js^a antigen is inherited as a dominant trait. It occurs in about 20 percent of American blacks but is rare in other ethnic groups.

Xg blood group

This erythrocyte antigen is defined by reaction to an antibody designated anti-Xg^a (Mann, Cahan, Gelb, Fisher, Hamper, Tippett, Sanger, and Race, 1962) which was found in the serum of a

Table 6. Rh Phenotypes Defined by Five Standard Antisera

Antiserum Reactions					Phenotypes		
Rh₀ D Rh1	**rh'** C Rh2	**rh''** E Rh3	**hr'** c Rh4	**hr''** e Rh5	Rh-Hr	CDE	Numerical
−	−	−	+	+	rh	cde/cde	Rh: −1, −2, −3, 4, 5
+	+	−	+	+	Rh_1rh	CDe/cde*	Rh: 1, 2, −3, 4, 5
+	+	−	−	+	Rh_1Rh_1	CDe/CDe*	Rh: 1, 2, −3, −4, 5
+	+	+	+	+	Rh_2Rh_0	CDe/cDE*	Rh: 1, 2, 3, 4, 5
+	−	+	+	+	Rh_2rh	cDE/cde*	Rh: 1, −2, 3, 4, 5
+	−	−	+	+	Rh_0	cDe/cde*	Rh: 1, −2, −3, 4, 5
+	−	+	+	−	Rh_2Rh_2	cDE/cDE*	Rh: 1, −2, 3, 4, −5
−	+	−	+	+	rh'rh	Cde/cde	Rh: −1, 2, −3, 4, 5
−	−	+	+	+	rh''rh	cdE/cde	Rh: −1, −2, 3, 4, 5
+	+	+	−	+	Rh_zRh_1	CDE/CDe*	Rh: 1, 2, 3, −4, 5
+	+	+	+	−	Rh_zRh_2	CDE/cDE*	Rh: 1, 2, 3, 4, −5
−	+	+	+	+	rh_yrh	Cde/cdE*	Rh: −1, 2, 3, 4, 5
−	+	−	−	+	rh'rh'	Cde/Cde	Rh: −1, 2, −3, −4, 5
−	−	+	+	−	rh''rh''	cdE/cdE	Rh: −1, −2, 3, 4, −5
−	+	+	−	+	rh_yrh'	CdE/Cde	Rh: −1, 2, 3, −4, 5
−	+	+	+	−	rh_yrh''	CdE/cdE	Rh: −1, 2, 3, 4, −5
+	+	+	−	−	Rh_zRh_z	CDE/CDE*	Rh: 1, 2, 3, −4, −5
−	+	+	−	−	rh_yrh_y	CdE/CdE	Rh: −1, 2, 3, −4, −5

*Expressed as most common of two or more genotypes of this phenotype.

patient who had received many transfusions. In contrast to all other known blood group antigens, Xg^a proved to be controlled by a gene located on the X chromosome and is thus the only known sex-linked blood group. Anti-Xg^a has been used for genetic linkage studies of diseases caused by sex-linked genes.

PHYSIOLOGICAL VALUES DURING PREGNANCY

Haematological Functions	Prepregnancy	Weeks of pregnancy		
		20	30	40
Total Blood Volume (ml)	4000	4600	5500	5700
Erythrocyte Volume (ml)	1400	1500	1650	1800
Red Blood Cells (10^{12}/L)	4.5	4.0	3.7	4.0
White Blood Cells (10^9/L)	7.2	9.4	10.7	10.4
Haemoglobin (g/dL)	13.5	12.0	11.5	12.0
Serum Iron (mg/L)	1.2	1.0	0.9	0.9
Serum Folate (μg/L)	10	7	6	6
Total Iron Binding Capacity (μmol/L)	50	40	60	70

Biochemical Functions	Prepregnancy	Weeks of pregnancy		
		20	30	40
Sodium (mmol/L)	138	136	137	136
Potassium (mmol/L)	4.26	4.00	4.10	4.21
Calcium (mEq/L)	5.00	4.90	4.55	4.60
Colloid Osmotic Pressure (cm H_2O)	37	32	31	31
Albumin (g/L)	35	28	26	25
Total Protein (g/L)	70	60	61	62
Plasma Osmolality (mmol/kg)	281	283	280	280

Biochemical Functions	Prepregnancy	Weeks of pregnancy		
		20	30	40
Total Bilirubin (μmol/L)	4–16	0.5–16	0.5–16	0.5–16
Cholesterol (mmol/L)	4–8	6–8	7–9	8–10
Alkaline Phosphatase (I.U./L)	16–24	16–44	16–60	20–100

Hytten, F. & Chamberlain, G. (1990) *Clinical Physiology in Pregnancy*, 2nd edition, Blackwells, Medical Publishers, Oxford.
Reprinted with permission

SYMBOLS AND ABBREVIATIONS

α Alpha, first letter of the Greek alphabet; used to denote the first in a series, as in chemistry to designate the order of components of isomeric compounds or of carbon atoms.

A Ampere; adenosine or adenylic acid in polynucleotides; absorbance (usually capitalized italic); alveolar *gas* (subscript).

Å Angstrom.

a Total acidity; area; asymmetric; atto-; specific absorption coefficient (usually italic); systemic arterial blood (subscript).

AA Amino acids or aminoacyl.

Ac Actinium; acetate.

a.c. L. *ante cibum,* before meals.

AC/A Accommodative convergence-accommodation ratio.

AcG, ac-g Accelerator globulin.

Ach Acetylcholine.

ACP Acyl carrier protein.

ADH Antidiuretic hormone.

Ado Adenosine.

ADP Adenosine diphosphate.

AFP α-Fetoprotein.

Ag Silver (L. *argentum*); antigen.

AHF Antihaemophilic factor.

AHG Antihaemophilic globulin.

AID Donor of heterologous (artificial) insemination.

AIH Homologous (artificial) insemination.

Al Aluminium.

Ala Alanine or its mono- or diradical.

ALD Adrenoleucodystrophy.

ALL Acute lymphocytic leukaemia.

ALS Antilymphocyte serum.

Am Americium.

AML Acute myelogenous leukaemia.

AMP Adenosine monophosphate (adenylic acid).

amu Atomic mass unit.

ANF Antinuclear factor.

Ar Argon.

ARDS Adult respiratory distress syndrome.

Arg Arginine or its mono- or diradical.

As Arsenic.

ASC Alterered state of consciousness.

Asn Asparagine, or its mono- or diradical.

Asp Aspartic acid or its radical forms.

AST Aspartate aminotransferase.

At Astatine.

atm Standard atmosphere.

ATP Adenosine 5'-triphosphate

ATPase Adenosine triphosphatase.

at wt Atomic weight.

Au Gold (L. *aurum*).

A-V Arteriovenous; atrioventricular.

AVP Antiviral protein.

AW Atomic weight.

Ax Axis.

β Beta, second letter of the Greek alphabet; used to denote the second in a series, as in chemistry to designate the order of components of isomeric compounds or of carbon atoms.

B Boron; as a subscript, refers to barometric pressure.

b As a subscript refers to blood.

BA Bachelor of Arts.

Ba Barium.

BAL British anti-Lewisite.

BCG Bacille biliède Calmette-Guérin; ballistocardiograph.

BDA British Dental Association.

Be Beryllium

Bi Bismuth.

b.i.d. L. *bis in die*, twice a day.

Bk Berkelium.

BMA British Medical Association.

BMR Basal metabolic rate.

BNF British National Formulary.

BP British Pharmacopoeia; blood pressure.

bp Boiling point.

BPharm Bachelor of Pharmacy.

Br Bromine

BSP Bromosulphophthalein.

BTU British thermal unit.

BUN Blood urea nitrogen.

C Large calorie; carbon; Celsius; centigrade; cylindrical lens; cytidine; when followed by a subscript, indicates renal clearance of a substance; compliance, or concentration.

c Small calorie; centi-; as a subscript, refers to blood capillary.

CA Cancer; carcinoma; cytosine arabinoside.

Ca Calcium; cathode; cathodal.

ca About, approximately (L. *circa*).

Cal Large calorie.

cal Small calorie.

cAMP Adenosine 3':5'-cyclic phosphate (cyclic AMP).

CAT Computerized axial tomography.

CBC Complete blood count.

CBG Corticosteroid-binding globulin.

cc Cubic centimetre.

Cd Cadmium.

cd Candela.

cDNA Complementary DNA.

CDP Cytidine 5'-diphosphate.

Ce Cerium.

CEA Carcinoembryonic antigen.

Cf Californium.

CG Chorionic gonadotropin.

CGS, cgs Centimetre-gram-second.

ChB Bachelor of Surgery (*Chirurgiae Baccalaureus*).

Ch.D. Doctor of Surgery (*Chirurgiae Doctor*).

Ci Curie.

CI Colour Index.

Cl Chlorine.

CLL Chronic lymphocytic leukaemia.

CM Master in Surgery (*Chirurgiae Magister*).

Cm Curium.

cM Centimorgan.

cm Centimetre.

CMI Cell-mediated immunity.

CML Chronic myelogenous leukaemia.

CMP Cytidine 5'-phosphate (or for any cytidine monophosphate).

CNS Central nervous system.

Co Cobalt.

CoA Coenzyme A.

CPAP Constant positive airway pressure.

CPH Certificate in Public Health.

CPPB Constant positive pressure breathing.

CPR Cardiopulmonary resuscitation.

cps Cycles per second.

CR Conditioned reflex; crown-rump length.

Cr Chromium; creatinine.

CRD Chronic respiratory disease.

CRH Corticotropin-releasing hormone.

CRL Crown-rump length.

CRP Cross-reacting protein.

Cs Caesium.

CSF Cerebrospinal fluid.

CT Computed tomography.

CTP Cytidine 5′-triphosphate.

Cu Copper (L. *cuprum*).

CVA Cerebrovascular accident, older classical term for stroke.

CVP Central venous pressure.

Cyd Cytidine.

Cys Cysteine.

Cyt Cytosine.

δ, Δ Delta.

D Vitamin D potency of cod liver oil; deuterium; in optics, dioptre and dexter (right); dihydrouridine in nucleic acids; diffusing capacity; as a subscript, refers to dead space.

D-. Prefix indicating a chemical compound to be sterically related to D-glyceraldehyde, the basis of stereochemical nomenclature.

2,4-D (2,4-Dichlorophenoxy)acetic acid.

d Deci-.

DA Diploma in Anaesthetics.

dAMP Deoxyadenylic acid.

db, dB Decibel.

D & C Dilation and curettage.

dCMP Deoxycytidylic acid.

DDS Doctor of Dental Surgery.

DDT Dicophane (Dichlorodiphenyltrichloroethane).

D & E Dilation and evacuation.

def, DEF *Decayed*, extraction indicated due to caries, or filled; designation used in dental examinations of deciduous (lower case letters) or permanent (capital letters) teeth, to describe the caries history.

DET Diethyltryptamine.

dGMP Deoxyguanylic acid.

DIC Disseminated intravascular coagulation.

DipPharmMed Diploma in Pharmaceutical Medicine.

dk Deca-.

DL-. Chemical prefix denoting a substance consisting of equal quantities of the two enantionmorphs, D and L; replaces the older *dl-* as a more exact definition of structure.

dM Decimorgan.

DMD Doctor of Dental Medicine.

dmf, DMF *D*ecayed, *m*issing, or *f*illed; a designation used in dental examinations of deciduous (lower case letters) or permanent (capital letters) teeth, to describe the caries history.

DMR Diploma in Medical Radiology.

DMSO Dimethyl sulphoxide.

DMT Dimethyltryptamine.

DN Dibucaine number.

DNAse, DNAse, DNase Deoxyribonuclease.

DNP 1. 2,4-Dinitrophenol. **2.** Deoxyribonucleoprotein.

Dnp DNP (1).

DNR Do not resuscitate.

DO Diploma in Ophthalmology.

DOA Dead on admission (arrival).

DPH Diploma in Public Health.

DPM Doctor of Psychological Medicine.

DR Reaction of degeneration.

dr Drachm(s).

dT Thymidine.

Dt Duration tetany.

dTDP Thymidine 5'-diphosphate.

dThd Thymidine.

dTMP Deoxythymidylic acid.

DTPA Diethylenetriamine pentaacetic acid.

dTTP Thymidine 5'-triphosphate.

Dy Dysprosium.

ECF-A Eosinophil chaemotactic factor of anaphylaxis.

ECG Electrocardiogram.

ECS Electrocerebral silence.

ECT Electroconvulsive (electroshock) therapy.

ED Effective dose.

EDTA Ethylenediaminetetra-acetic acid.

EEG Electroencephalogram.

EKG Electrocardiogram.

EKY Electrokymogram.

EMF Electromotive force.

EMG Electromyogram.

ENG Electronystagmography.

ENT Ear, nose, and throat.

EOG Electro-oculography.

ER Endoplasmic reticulum.

Er Erbium.

ERBF Effective renal blood flow.

ERCP Endoscopic retrograde cholangiopancreatography.

ERG Electroretinogram.

ERPF Effective renal plasma flow.

ERV Expiratory reserve volume.

Es Einsteinium.

ESP Extrasensory perception.

ESR Erythrocyte sedimentation rate; electron spin resonance.

Eu Europium.

eV, ev Electron-volt.

F Fractional concentration, followed by subscripts indicating location and chemical species; free energy; Fahrenheit; faraday; visual field; fluorine; force; filial generation.

f Respiratory frequency; femto-.

FACP Fellow of the American College of Physicians.

FACS Fellow of the American College of Surgeons.

FAD Flavin adenine dinucleotide.

Fe Iron (L. *ferrum*).

FEV Forced expiratory volume.

FF Filtration fraction.

FIGLU Formiminoglutamic acid.

Fm Fermium.

FMN Flavin mononucleotide.

FPS, fps Foot-pound-second.

Fr Francium; French scale.

FRC Functional residual capacity.

FRCP Fellow of the Royal College of Physicians.

FRCS Fellow of the Royal College of Surgeons.

FRF Follicle-stimulating hormone-releasing factor.

FRS First rank symptoms.

FRS Fellow of the Royal Society.

Fru Fructose.

FSH Follicle-stimulating hormone.

FSH-RF Follicle-stimulating hormone-releasing factor.

FSH-RH Follicle-stimulating hormone-releasing hormone.

FUO Fever of unknown origin.

γ Gamma, third letter in the Greek alphabet; used as a symbol to denote the third in a series, fourth carbon in an aliphatic acid, or position 2 removed from the α position in the benzene ring.

G Newtonian constant of gravitation; giga-; glucose, as in UDPG; guanosine (or guanylic acid) residues in polynucleotides, as in poly(G).

g Gram.

g A unit of acceleration based on the acceleration produced by the earth's gravitational attraction, where $1\,g = 980.6$ cm (about 32 ft./sec), per second.

Ga Gallium.

GABA γ-Aminobutyric acid.

Gal Galactose.

Gd Gadolinium.

Ge Germanium.

GFR Glomerular filtration rate.

GH Growth hormone.

GHRF, GH-RF Growth hormone-releasing factor.

GHRH, GH-RH Growth hormone-releasing hormone.

GI Gastrointestinal; Gingival Index.

GLC Gas-liquid chromatography.

Gln Glutamine or glutaminyl.

Glu Glutamic acid or glutamyl.

Gly Glycine or glycyl.

gm Former abbreviation for gram.

GMP Guanylic acid.

GnRH Gonadotropin-releasing hormone.

GOT Glutamic oxaloacetic transaminase, now known as aspartate aminotransferase.

GP General Practitioner.

GPI Gingival-Periodontal Index.

GPT Glutamic pyruvic transaminase, now known as alanine aminotransferase.

gr Grain.

GSH Reduced glutathione.

GSR Galvanic skin response.

GSSG Oxidized glutathione.

GTP Guanosine 5′-triphosphate.

GU Genitourinary.

Guo Guanosine.

H Henry; hydrogen; hyperopia or hyperopic.

H$^+$ Hydrogen ion.

h Hecto-.

h Planck's constant.

HAA Hepatitis-associated antigen.

HAV Hepatitis A virus.

Hb Haemoglobin.

HB$_c$Ag Hepatitis B core antigen.

HB₅Ag Hepatitis B surface antigen.

Hb AS Heterozygosity for haemoglobin A and haemoglobin S, the sickle cell trait.

HBe, HB₅Ag Heptitis B e antigen.

Hb S Sickle cell haemoglobin.

HBV Hepatitis B virus.

HCG Human chorionic gonadotropin.

HCS Human chorionic somatomammotropic hormone; human chorionic somatomammotropin.

Hct Haematocrit.

HDL High density lipoprotein.

He Helium.

Hf Hafnium.

Hg Mercury (*hydrargyrum*).

His Histidine or histidyl.

HIV Human immunodeficiency virus.

Hl Latent hyperopia.

HLA Human lymphocyte antigens.

Hm Manifest hyperopia.

HMG Human menopausal gonadotropin.

Ho Holmium.

HPL Human placental lactogen.

Ht Total hyperopia.

HTLV Human T-cell lymphocytotrophic virus.

HVL Half-value layer.

Hz Hertz.

I Iodine; as a subscript, inspired gas; I blood group.

ICD International Classification of Diseases of the World Health Organization.

ICP Intracranial pressure.

ICSH Interstitial cell-stimulating hormone.

ICU Intensive care unit.

IFN Interferon(s).

Ig Immunoglobulin.

IH Infectious hepatitis.

ILA Insulin-like activity.

Ile Isoleucine or its radical isoleucyl.

I.M., i.m. Intramuscular, or intramuscularly.

IMP Inosine monophosphate.

In Indium.

Ino Inosine.

IP, ip, Intraperitoneal, or intraperitoneally.

IPPB Intermittent positive pressure breathing.
IQ Intelligence quotient.
Ir Iridium.
IRV Inspiratory reserve volume.
ITP Idiopathic thrombocytopenic purpura; inosine 5'-triphosphate.
ITyr Monoiodotyrosine.
IU International unit.
IUCD Intrauterine contraceptive device.
IUD Intrauterine device.
I-V Intraventricular.
I.V., i.v. Intravenous or intravenously.

J Joule.
J Flux.

K Potassium (L. *kalium*); kelvin.
k Kilo-.
k Rate or velocity constant.
kc Kilocycle.
kcal Kilogram calorie or kilocalorie.
kg Kilogram.
Kr Krypton.
kv Kilovolt.

λ The 11th letter of the Greek alphabet, lambda, used as a symbol for
   wavelength, Ostwald's solubility coefficient, and radioactive con-
   stant.
L Left; litre; inductance; limes, used with a lower case letter or a plus sign
   (or a subscript letter or plus sign) as a symbol for various doses of
   toxin.
l Litre.
La Lanthanum.
LATS Long-acting thyroid stimulator.
LBT Lupus band test.
LD Lethal dose.
LDH Lactate dehydrogenase.
LDL Low density lipoprotein.
L.E. Left eye; lupus erythematosus.
LETS Large external transformation-sensitive fibronectin.
LH Luteinizing hormone.
LH/FSH-RF Luteinizing hormone/follicle-stimulating hormone-releas-
   ing factor.
LH-RF Luteinizing hormone-releasing factor.

LH-RH Luteinizing hormone-releasing hormone.
Li Lithium.
LM Licentiate in Midwifery.
LMA Left mentoanterior position.
LMP Left mentoposterior position.
LNPF Lymph node permeability factor.
Lr Lawrencium.
LRCP Licentiate of the Royal College of Physicians.
LRCS Licentiate of the Royal College of Surgeons.
LRH Luteinizing hormone-releasing hormone.
LSA Left sacroanterior position.
LSA Licentiate of the Society of Apothecaries.
LSD Lysergic acid diethylamide.
LSH Lutein-stimulating hormone.
LSP Left sacroposterior position.
LTH Luteotropic hormone.
LTM Long term memory.
Lu Lutetium.
LVET Left ventricular ejection time.
Lys Lysine or its radicals in peptides.

μ Mu, 12th letter of the Greek alphabet; micro-; micron.
$\mu\mu$ Micromicro- (pico-).
μm Micrometre.
M Myopia or myopic; mega-; morgan.
M Moles per litre.
m Metre; minim; milli-; mass.
m- meta-.
mμ Millimicron.
ma Milliampere.
MAA Macroaggregated albumin.
MAO Monoamine oxidase.
MAOI Monoamine oxidase inhibitor.
MBC Maximum breathing capacity.
Mb, MbCO, MbO$_2$ Myoglobin and its combinations with CO and O_2.
MC Master of Surgery (*Magister Chirurgiae*); Medical Corps.
MCH Mean cell haemoglobin.
MCh Master of Surgery (*Magister Chirurgiae*).
MCHC Mean cell haemoglobin concentration.
mCi Millicurie.
MCV Mean cell volume.
Md Mendelevium.
MD *Medicinae Doctor*, Doctor of Medicine.

mEq, meq Milliequivalent.
MET Metabolic equivalent.
Met Methionine or its radicals in peptides.
metHb Methaemoglobin.
metMb Metmyoglobin.
Mg Magnesium.
mg Milligram.
mho [*ohm* reversed]. Siemens.
mHz Megahertz.
MID Minimal infecting dose.
MK Menaquinone.
MKS, mks Metre-kilogram-second.
ml Millilitre.
MLD, mld Minimal lethal dose.
mm Millimetre.
mmol Millimole.
Mn Manganese.
MO Medical Officer.
Mo Molybdenum.
mol Mole.
mol wt Molecular weight.
MPD Maximal permissible dose.
M$_r$ Molecular weight ratio.
MRCP Member of the Royal College of Physicians.
MRCS Member of the Royal College of Surgeons.
MRD, mrd Minimal reacting dose.
mRNA Messenger RNA.
MS Multiple sclerosis.
ms Millisecond.
MSc Master of Science.
msec Millisecond.
MSH Melanocyte-stimulating hormone.
Mu Mache unit.
mV Millivolt.
MVV Maximum voluntary *ventilation*.
MW Molecular weight.
my Myopia.

v Nu, thirteenth letter of the Greek alphabet; kinematic viscosity.
N Newton; nitrogen.
N Normal concentration.
n Nano-; refractive index.
NA Nomina Anatomica.

Na Sodium (L. *natrium*).

NAD Nicotinamide adenine dinucleotide.

NAD$^+$ Nicotinamide adenine dinucleotide (oxidized form).

NADH Nicotinamide adenine dinucleotide (reduced form).

NADP Nicotinamide adenine dinucleotide phosphate.

NADP$^+$ Nicotinamide adenine dinucleotide phosphate (oxidized form).

NADPH Nicotinamide adenine dinucleotide phosphate (reduced form).

Nb Niobium.

Nd Neodymium.

Ne Neon.

NEEP Negative end-expiratory pressure.

ng Nanogram.

NHS National Health Service.

Ni Nickel.

nm Nanometre.

NMN Nicotinamide mononucleotide.

NMR Nuclear magnetic resonance.

NPN Nonprotein nitrogen.

nRNA Nuclear RNA.

NUG Necrotizing ulcerative gingivitis.

O Oxygen; opening (in formulas for electrical reactions); oculus; a blood group in the ABO system.

OB/GYN Obstetrics and gynaecology.

OD Right eye (L. *oculus dexter*); overdose.

ORD Optical rotatory dispersion.

Oro Orotic acid or orotate.

OS Left eye (L. *oculus sinister*).

Os Osmium.

OT Occupational therapist, Koch's old tuberculin.

OTC Over the counter; denoting a drug available without a prescription.

OU Each eye (L. oculus uterque); both eyes.

OXT Oxytocin.

oz Ounce.

P Phosphorus; in nucleic acid terminology, symbol for phosphoric residue; followed by a subscript, refers to the plasma concentration of the substance indicated by the subscript; pressure or partial *pressure*, frequently with subscripts indicating location and chemical species.

P$_1$ Parental generation.

p Pupil; optic papilla; phosphoric ester or phosphate in polynucleotide symbolism; pico-.

Pa Protactinium; pascal.

PABA *p*-Aminobenzoic acid.

PAF Platelet-aggregating (or -activating) factor.

PAH *p*-Aminohippuric acid.

PAS *p*-Aminosalicylic acid; periodic acid-Schiff (stain).

PASA *p*-Aminosalicyclic acid.

Pb Lead (L. *plumbum*).

PBG Porphobilinogen.

PBI Protein-bound iodine.

p.c. L. *post cibum,* after meals.

PCB Polychlorinated biphenyl, an industrial carcinogen.

PCO_2, pCO_2 Partial pressure (tension) of carbon dioxide.

PCP Phencyclidine.

Pd Palladium.

pd Prism dioptre.

PDLL Poorly differentiated lymphocytic lymphoma.

PEEP Positive end-expiratory pressure.

PET Positron emission tomography.

pg Picogram.

PGA, PGB, PGE, PGF. Abbreviations, with numerical subscripts according to structure, often used for prostaglandins.

Ph Phenyl.

pH [p (power) of [H^+]] Symbol for the logarithm of the reciprocal of the H ion concentration; a solution with pH 7.00 is neutral, one with a pH of more than 7.0 is alkaline, one with a pH lower than 7.00 is acid.

PHA Phytohaemagglutinin.

PhC Pharmaceutical Chemist.

PhD Doctor of Philosophy.

Phe Phenylalanine or its radical.

pI The pH value for the isoelectric point of a given substance.

PID Pelvic inflammatory disease.

PIF Prolactin-inhibiting factor.

pK Negative logarithm of the ionization constant (K_a) of an acid; the pH at which equal concentrations of the acid and basic forms of a substance (usually a buffer) are present.

PKU Phenylketonuria.

Pm Promethium.

pm Picometre.

PNPB Positive-negative pressure breathing.

Po Polonium.

PO_2 or **pO_{2+s}** Partial pressure (tension) of oxygen.

PP Pyrophosphate.

PPCA Proserum prothrombin conversion accelerator.

PPD Purified protein derivative of tuberculin.

PPLO Pleuropneumonia-like organisms.

Pr Presbyopia; praseodymium.

PRA Plasma renin activity.

PRL Prolactin.

p.r.n. L. *pro re nata,* as needed.

Pro Proline or its radicals.

PSP Phenolsulphonphthalein.

Pt Platinum.

PT Physical therapy.

PTA Plasma thromboplastin antecedent.

PTH Parathyroid hormone.

PUO Pyrexia of unknown (or uncertain) origin, applied to febrile illness before diagnosis has been established.

PUVA Oral administration of psoralen and subsequent exposure to long wavelength ultraviolet light (*uv-a*); used to treat psoriasis.

PVC Polyvinyl chloride.

PVP Polyvinylpyrrolidone.

Q Coulomb.

$\dot{Q}$ [quantity + an overdot denoting the time derivative]. Symbol for blood *flow.*

QCO_2 Microlitres of CO_2 given off per milligram of tissue per hour.

q.d. L. *quaque die,* every day.

q.h. L. *quaque hora,* every hour.

q.i.d. L. *quater in die,* four times a day.

QO or **QO_2** Oxygen consumption.

R Gas constant; electrical resistance; radical (usually an alkyl or aryl group); Réaumur scale; L. *recipe;* respiration; respiratory exchange ratio; roentgen; unit of resistance in the cardiovascular system.

℞ L. *recipe,* prescription.

r Roentgen; "racemic," occasionally used in naming compounds in place of the more common "*dl.*"

Ra Radium.

RAS Reticular activating system.

RAST Radioallergosorbent test.

RAV Rous-associated virus.

Rb Rubidium.

rbc, RBC Red blood cell; red blood count.

RBF Renal blood flow.

RCP Royal College of Physicians.

RCS Royal College of Surgeons.
RD Reaction of degeneration.
RE Right eye.
Re Rhenium.
REM Rapid eye movement.
rem Roentgen-equivalent-man.
rep Roentgen-equivalent-physical.
RF Releasing factor; rheumatoid factors.
RFP Right frontoposterior position.
RH Releasing hormone.
Rh 1. Rhodium. **2.** Rh blood group.
Rib Ribose.
RMA Right mentoanterior position.
RMP Right mentoposterior position.
Rn Radon.
RNase Ribonuclease.
RNP Ribonucleoprotein.
ROA Right occipitoanterior position.
RPF Renal plasma flow.
rpm Revolutions per minute.
RQ Respiratory quotient.
rRNA Ribosomal RNA.
RSA Right sacroanterior position.
RSP Right sacroposterior position.
RSV Rous sarcoma virus.
Ru Ruthenium.
RV Residual volume.

σ Sigma, 18th letter of the Greek alphabet; reflection coefficient; standard deviation.
S Spherical; spherical lens; Svedberg unit; siemens; sulphur; percentage saturation of haemoglobin, when followed by subscript O_2 or CO_2.
S$_f$ Flotation constant.
s L. *sinister*, left; L. *semis*, half; as a subscript, denotes steady state.
S-A Sinoatrial.
SAN Sinoatrial node.
sat. Saturated.
sat. sol. Saturated solution.
Sb Antimony (L. *stibium*).
Sc Scandium
s.c. Subcutaneous or subcutaneously.
SD Streptodornase; standard deviation.

SDA Specific dynamic action.

Se Selenium.

SEN State Enrolled Nurse.

Ser Serine.

SH Serum hepatitis.

SI International System of Units.

Si Silicon.

SIDS Sudden infant death syndrome.

SK Streptokinase.

SLE Systemic lupus erythematosus.

Sm Samarium.

Sn Tin (L. *stannum*).

s.o.s. L. *sit opus sit,* if needed.

SPCA Serum prothrombin conversion accelerator.

sp gr Specific gravity.

sph Spherical; spherical lens.

Sr Strontium.

SRF Somatotropin-releasing factor.

SRF-A Slow-reacting factor of anaphylaxis.

SRIF Somatotropin release-inhibiting factor.

SRN State Registered Nurse.

sRNA Soluble RNA; now known as transfer RNA (tRNA).

SRS, SRS-A Slow-reacting *substance* or slow-reacting *substance* of
    anaphylaxis.

STD Sexually transmitted disease.

STH Somatotropic hormome.

STM Short term memory.

STPD A gas volume expressed as if it were at standard temperature
    ($0°C$), standard pressure (760 mm Hg absolute), dry.

T Tension (T+, increased tension; T-, diminished tension); tera-; tritium;
    as a subscript, refers to tidal *volume;* tocopherol.

T Absolute temperature.

T$_3$ 3,5,3'-Triiodothyronine.

T$_4$ Thyroxine.

T$_m$ Temperature midpoint (Kelvin).

t Metric ton.

t Temperature on the Celsius scale, and for tritium.

t$_m$ Temperature midpoint (Celsius).

Ta Tantalum.

TAF Tumour angiogenic factor.

Tb Terbium.

tb Tuberculosis; tubercle bacillus.

TBP Thyroxine-binding protein.

Tc Technetium.

TDP Ribothymidine 5′-diphosphate.

Te Tellurium.

TEN Toxic epidermal necrolysis.

Th Thorium.

Thr Threonine, or its radicals.

Ti Titanium.

TIA Transient ischaemic attack.

t.i.d. L. *ter in die,* three times a day.

Tl Thallium.

TLC Thin-layer chromatography; total lung *capacity*.

TLV Threshold limit value.

Tm Thulium; transport or tubular maximum.

TMP Ribothymidine 5′-phosphate.

Tn Intraocular tension.

TPI *Treponema pallidum* immobilization test.

TPN Total parenteral nutrition.

tr. Tincture.

TRH Thyrotropin-releasing hormone.

TRIC Trachoma and inclusion conjunctivitis.

tRNA Transfer RNA.

Trp Tryptophan and its radicals.

TSH Thyroid-stimulating hormone.

TSTA Tumour-specific transplantation antigens.

TU Toxic or toxin unit.

Tyr Tyrosine and its radicals.

U Unit; uranium; uridine in polymers; urinary concentration, followed by subscripts indicating location and chemical species.

UDP Uridine diphosphate.

UMP Uridine phosphate.

ung. L. *unguentum,* ointment.

Urd Uridine.

UTP Uridine triphosphate.

V Vision or visual acuity; volt; with subscript 1, 2, 3, etc., the unipolar chest electrocardiogram leads; vanadium; volume, frequently with subscripts denoting location, chemical species, and conditions.

V_{max} Maximum velocity in an enzymic reaction and of shortening of a contractile element.

$\dot{V}$ Gas flow, frequently with subscripts indicating location and chemical species; ventilation.

$\dot{V}CO_2$ Carbon dioxide elimination.

$\dot{V}O_2$ Oxygen consumption.

v Volt; as a subscript, venous *blood*.

V-A Ventriculoatrial.

Val Valine and its radicals.

VC Colour vision; vital capacity.

VDRL Venereal Disease Research Laboratories.

VLDL Very low density lipoprotein.

VMA Vanillylmandelic acid.

VP Vasopressin.

VR Vocal resonance.

VS Volumetric solution.

W Tungsten; watt.

WBC White blood cell or blood count.

WDLL Well differentiated lymphocytic lymphoma.

WHO World Health Organization.

Wr Wassermann reaction.

X Xanthosine.

Xao Xanthosine.

Xe Xenon.

Y Yttrium.

Yb Ytterbium.

Zn Zinc.

Zr Zirconium.

DRUG NAMES

The drugs in this appendix are grouped according to categories as listed in the British National Formulary. Generic names are shown in bold face type, followed by trade names in standard type. The categories, together with their BNF group number, are as follows:

Anaesthesia (BNF 15)
Cardiovascular System (BNF 2)
Central Nervous System (BNF 4)
Ear, Nose & Oropharynx (BNF 12)
Endocrine System (BNF 6)
Eye (BNF 11)
Gastro-Intestinal System (BNF 1)
Immunological Products & Vaccines (BNF 14)
Infections (BNF 5)
Malignant Disease & Immunosuppression (BNF 8)
Musculoskeletal & Joint Diseases (BNF 10)
Nutrition & Blood (BNF 9)
Obstetrics, Gynaecology & Urinary-Tract Disorders (BNF 7)
Respiratory System (BNF 3)
Skin (BNF 13)

DRUG NAMES

ANAESTHESIA

Atropine sulfate
  Isopto Atropine
  Lomotil
  Minims Atropine
Bupivacaine hydrochloride
  Marcain
Lignocaine hydrochloride
  Betnovate Rectal
  Bradosol Plus
  Calgel
  Depo-Medrone with Lidocaine
  Emla Cream
  Instillagel
  Lignostab
  Mimims Lignocaine &
    Fluorescein
  Pensacaine 2% with
    Adrenaline
  Xylocaine
  Xylocard
  Xyloproct
  Xylotox
Mepivacaine hydrochloride
  Estradurin
Methohexitone sodium
  Brietal Sodium
Midazolam
  Hypnovel
Papaveretum
  Aspav
  Omnopon
Prilocaine hydrochloride
  Citanest
  Emla Cream
Propofol
  Diprivan

CARDIOVASCULAR SYSTEM

Aspirin
  Angettes 75
  Nu-Seals Aspirin
  Platet

Atenolol
  Antipressan
  Beta-Adalat
  Kalten
  Tenif
  Tenoret 50
  Tenoretic
  Tenormin
  Totamol
Bendrofluazide
  Aprinox
  Berkozide
  Centyl
  Centyl-K
  Corgaretic
  Inderetic
  Inderex
  Neo-Naclex
  Neo-Naclex-K
  Prestim
Captopril
  Acepril
  Acezide
  Capoten
  Capozide
Co-amilofruse (amiloride
    HCL/frusemide)
  Frumil
  Lasoride
Co-amilozide (amiloride
    HCL/hydchloroth)
  Amilco
  Hypertane
  Moduret 25
  Moduretic
Co-tenidone (amiloride
    HCL/chlorthalidone)
  Atenixco
  Tenoret 50
  Tenoretic
Digoxin
  Lanoxin
Enalapril maleate
  Innovace
  Innozide

449

Frusemide
  Diumide-K Continus
  Dryptal
  Frumil
  Frusene
  Lasikal
  Lasilactone
  Lasipressin
  Lasix
  Lasix + K
  Lasoride
  Rusyde
Glyceryl trinitrate
  Coro-Nitro Spray
  Deponit
  Glytrin
  GTN
  Nitrocine
  Nitrocontin Continus
  Nitro-Dur
  Nitrolingual
  Nitronal
  Percutol
  Suscard Buccal
  Sustac
  Transiderm-Nitro
  Tridil
Isosorbide mononitrate
  Elantan
  Elantan LA
  Imdur
  Ismo
  Isotrate
  MCR-50
  Monit
  Mono-Cedocard
Nifedipine
  Adalat
  Adalat Retard
  Beta-Adalat
  Coracten
  Nifensar XL
  Tenif
Propranolol hydrochloride
  Apsolol
  Berkolol
  Cardinol
  Half-Betadur

  Inderal
  Inderal LA
  Inderetic
  Inderex
Triamterene
  Dyazide
  Dytac
  Dytide
  Frusene
  Kalspare

CENTRAL NERVOUS SYSTEM

Amitriptyline hydrochloride
  Lentizol
  Limbitrol
  Triptafen
  Triptafen-M
  Tryptizol
Aspirin
  Caprin
  Nu-Seals Aspirin
  Solprin 75 mg
Carbamazepine
  Tegretol
Co-codamol (codeine phos &
      paracetamol)
  Panadeine
  Paracodol
  Parake
  Solpadeine
Co-dydramol (dihydrocodeine &
      paracet)
  Galake
  Paramol
Co-proxamol (dextroprop HCL
      & paracet)
  Cosalgesic
  Distalgesic
Diazepam
  Diazemuls
  Stesolid
  Valium Roche
Dihydrocodeine tartrate
  DF118
  DHC Continus
  Paramol
  Remedeine

Dothiepin hydrochloride
  Prothiaden
Nitrazepam
  Mogadon
  Somnite
Paracetamol
  Calpol
  Disprol Paediatric
  Lobak
  Midrid
  Migraleve
  Panadol
  Panadol Soluble
  Propain
  Solpadol
  Tylex
Phenytoin
  Epanutin
Prochlorperazine maleate
  Buccastem
  Stemetil
  Vertigon
Temazepam
  Normison

EAR, NOSE & OROPHARYNX

Beclomethasone dipropionate
  Beconase
Benzydamine hydrochloride
  Difflam Spray
Budesonide
  Preferid
  Pulmicort
  Rhinocort
Chlorhexidine gluconate
  Chlorhexitulle
  Corsodyl
  Hibidil
  Hibiscrub
  Hibisol
  Hibitane
  Naseptin
  Nystaform
  Nystaform-HC
  pHiso-Med
  Savloclens
  Savlodil

  Savlon
  Xylocaine Antiseptic Gel
Clioquinol
  Barquinol HC
  Betnovate-C
  Haelen-C
  Locorten-Vioform
  Oralcer
  Synalar C
  Vioform Hydrocortisone
Ephedrine hydrochloride
  C.A.M.
  Franol
  Franol Plus
  Haymine
Flunisolide
  Syntaris
Gentamicin sulphate
  Cidomycin
  Garamycin
  Genticin
  Gentisone HC
Hydrocortisone
  Neo-Cortef
  Otosporin
  Terra-Cortril
Miconazole nitrate
  Daktarin
Neomycin sulphate
  Adcortyl with Graneodin
  Audicort
  Betnesol-N
  Betnovate-N
  Cicatrin
  Dermovate NN
  Dexa-Rhinaspray
  Eumovate-N
  FML-Neo
  Graneodin
  Gregoderm
  Maxitrol
  Minims Neomycin
  Naseptin
  Neo-Cortef
  Neo-Medrone Cream
  Neosporin
  Nivemycin
  Otomize

Otosporin
Polybactrin
Predsol-N
Stiedex LPN
Synalar N
Tri-Adcortyl
Tribiotic
Tricicatrin
Vibrocil
Vista-Methasone N
Nystatin
Dermovate-NN
Flagyl Compak
Gregoderm
Mysteclin
Nystadermal
Nystaform
Nystaform-HC
Nystan
Terra-Cortril Nystatin
Timodine
Tinaderm-M
Tri-Adcortyl
Tri-Adcortyl Otic
Tricicatrin
Trimovate
Ear-Wax Removal
Audinorm
Cerumol
Dioctyl
Exterol
Molcer
Waxsol
Triamcinolone acetonide
Adcortyl
Adcortyl in Orabase
Adcortyl with Graneodin
Audicort
Aureocort
Kenalog
Ledercort
Ledermix
Lederspan
Nystadermal
Pevaryl TC
Tri-Adcortyl
Tri-Adcortyl Otic

Xylometazoline hydrochloride
Otrivine
Otrivine-Antistin Eye Drops
Rynacrom Compound

ENDOCRINE SYSTEM

Chlorpropamide
Diabinese
Glibenclamide
Calabren
Daonil
Euglucon
Semi-Daonil
Gliclazide
Diamicron
Hydrocortisone
Solu-Cortef
Insulin
Human Actraphane
Human Actrapid
Human Initard
Human Insulatard
Human Mixtard
Human Monotard
Human Protaphane
Human Ultratard
Human Velosulin
Humulin I
Humulin Lente
Humulin M
Humulin S
Humulin Zn
Hypurin Isophane
Hypurin Lente
Hypurin Neutral
Hypurin Protamine Zinc
Initard
Insulatard
Lentard MC
Mixtard
Penmix
Pur-In Isophane
Pur-In Mix
Pur-In Neutral
Rapitard MC
Semitard MC
Velosulin

Velosulin Cartridge
Oestradiol
Climaval
Cyclo Progynova
Estraderm TTS
Estrapak
Hormonin
Implants (Organon)
Progynova
Vagifem
Zumenon
Oestradiol with progestogen
Cyclo Progynova
Estracomrbi
Estrapak 50
Nuvelle
Syntex Menopause
Trisequins
Trisequins Forte
Oestrogens, conjugated
Premarin
Oestrogens conjugated with progestogen
Prempak C
Prednisolone
Deltacortril Enteric
Deltastab
Minims Prednisolone Sodium Phosphate
Precortisyl
Predenema
Predfoam
Pred Forte
Prednesol
Predsol
Predsol-N
Scheriproct
Sintisone
Thyroxine sodium
Eltroxin
Tolbutamide
Rastinon

EYE

Antazoline
Otrivine-Antistin Eye Drops
RBC

Vasocon-A
Betamethasone sodium phosphate
Betnesol
Betnesol-N
Vista-Methasone
Vista-Methasone N
Betaxolol hydrochloride
Betoptic
Kerlone
Chloramphenicol
Actinac
Chloromycetin
Chloromycetin Hydrocortisone
Kemicetine
Minims Chloramphenicol
Sno Phenicol
Tanderil Chloramphenicol
Dexamethasone
Decadron
Dexa-Rhinaspray
Maxidex
Maxitrol
Otomize
Sofradex
Dipivefrine hydrochloride
Propine
Fusidic acid (sodium fusidate)
Fucidin Intertulle
Fucithalmic
Gentamicin sulphate
Cidomycin
Garamycin
Genticin
Minims Gentamicin
Hydrocortisone
Chloromycetin-Hydrocortisone Ophthalmic Ointment
Neo-Cortef
Hypromellose
Ilube
Isopto Alkaline
Isopto Atropine
Isopto Carbachol
Isopto Carpine
Isopto Frin
Isopto Plain
Tears Naturale

Levobunolol hydrochloride
  Betagan
Paraffin, liquid
  Agarol
  Lacrilube
Pilocarpine hydrochloride
  Isopto Carpine
  Minims Pilocarpine
  Ocusert Pilo
  Sno Pilo
Polyvinyl alcohol
  Hypotears
  Liquifilm Tears
  Sno Tears
Sodium cromoglycate
  Opticrom
Timolol maleate
  Betim
  Blocadren
  Moducren
  Prestim
  Timoptol

GASTRO-INTESTINAL SYSTEM

Aluminium hydroxide with magnesium
  Aludrox
  Maalox
  Mucagel
Aluminium & magnesium & ACT dimethicone
  Maalox Plus
  Polycrol Tablets
  Simeco
Aluminium & magnesium & alginates
  Algicon
  Gastrocote
  Gastron
  Topal
Aluminium & magnesium & oxethazaine
  Mucaine
Cimetidine
  Algitec
  Dyspamet
  Tagamet

Gentamicin sulphate
  Septopal Chains
Hydrocortisone
  Anugesic-HC Cream
  Anusol HC
  Colifoam
  Corlan
  Hydrocortone
  Proctofoam HC
  Proctosedyl
  Solu-Cortef
  Xyloproct
Ispaghula
  Colven
  Fybogel
  Isogel
  Metamucil
  Regulan
Lactulose
  Duphalac
Loperamide hydrochloride
  Imodium
Mebeverine hydrochloride
  Colofac
  Colven
Omeprazole
  Losec
Ranitidine
  Zantac
Senna
  Manevac
  Pripsen
  Senokot
  X-Prep
Sulphasalazine
  Salazopyrin

IMMUNOLOGICAL PRODUCTS & VACCINES

Diphtheria vaccine
  Trivax
Hepatitis A vaccine
  Havrix
Hepatitis B vaccine
  Engerix B

**Immunoglobulin, human
    normal** (gamma globulin)
  Endobulin
  Gamimune N
  Gammabulin
  Kabiglobulin
  Sandoglobulin
  Venoglobulin
Influenza vaccine
  Fluzone
  Influvac
  MFV-Ject
**Measles, mumps & rubella
    vaccine**
  Immravax
  M-M-R$_{II}$
  Pluserix MMR
Meningitis vaccine
  AC Vax
  Mengivac (A & C)
Pneumococcal vaccine
  Pneumovax
Rabies vaccine
  Merieux Inactivated Rabies
    Vaccine
Rubella vaccine
  Almevax
  Ervevax
  Rubavax
Tetanus vaccine
  Clostet
  Tetavax
Typhoid vaccine
  Typhim VI
  Vivotif
Yellow fever vaccine
  Arilvax

INFECTIONS

Amoxycillin
  Almodan
  Amoxil
  Augmentin
  Flemoxin
Ampicillin
  Amfipen
  Ampiclox
  Dicapen
  Magnapen
  Penbritin
  Vidopen
Cefaclor
  Distaclor
Cephalexin
  Ceporex
  Keflex
Co-amoxiclav
    (amoxycillin/clavul acid)
  Augmentin
Co-trimoxazole
  Bactrim
  Septrin
Doxycycline
  Nordox
  Vibramycin
Erythromycin
  Erycen
  Erymax
  Erythrocin
  Erythromid
  Erythroped
  Ilosone
  Stiemycin
  Zineryt
Flucloxacillin sodium
  Floxapen
  Ladropen
  Magnapen
  Stafoxil
  Staphlipen
Metronidazole
  Flagyl
  Flagyl Compak
  Motrogol
  Metrolyl
  Metrotop
  Zadstat
Oxytetracycline
  Berkmycen
  Imperacin
  Terra-Cortril
  Terra-Cortril Nystatin
  Terramycin
  Trimovate

Phenoxymethylpenicillin
(penicillin V)
Apsin VK
Distaquaine V-K
Stabilin V-K
V-Cil-K
Trimethoprim
Ipral
Monotrim
Trimopan

MALIGNANT DISEASE &
IMMUNOSUPPRESSION

Aminoglutethimide
Orimeten
Azathioprine
Imuran
Buserelin acetate
Suprecur
Suprefact
Chlorambucil
Leukeran
Cyclophosphamide
Endoxana
Cyclosporin
Sandimmun
Cyproterone acetate
Androcur
Cyprostat
Dianette
Goserelin
Zoladex
Hydroxyurea
Hydrea
Medroxyprogesterone acetate
Depo-Provera
Farlutal
Provera
Megestrol acetate
Megace
Methotrexate
Maxtrex
Stilboestrol
Apstil
Tampovagan Stilboestrol and
Lactic Acid

Tamoxifen
Emblon
Noltam
Nolvadex
Tamofen

MUSCULOSKELETAL & JOINT
DISEASES

Allopurinol
Caplenal
Hamarin
Zyloric
Benzydamine hydrochloride
Difflam
Diclofenac sodium
Voltarol
Voltarol Emulgel
Felbinac
Traxam
Fenbufen
Lederfen
Flurbiprofen
Froben
Ocufen
Gentamicin sulphate
Palacos R with Gentamicin
Septopal Chains
Heparinoid
Anacal
Bayolin
Hirudoid
Lasonil
Movelat
Hydrocortisone
Hydrocortistab
Ibuprofen
Brufen
Codafen Continus
Fenbid Spansule
Ibugel
Junifen
Proflex
Indomethacin
Flexin Continus
Imbrilon
Indocid
Indocid PDA

Indolar
Indomod
Ketoprofen
Alrheumat
Orudis
Oruvail
Oruvail Gel
Mefenamic acid
Ponstan
Naproxen
Anthroxen
Napratec
Naprosyn
Nycopren
Synflex
Nicotine Products
Nicabate
Nicorette
Nicorette Plus
Nicotinell TTS
Piroxicam
Feldene
Feldene Gel
Tiaprofenic acid
Surgam

NUTRITION & BLOOD

Ascorbic acid
Parentrovite
Redoxon
Ferrous gluconate
Fergon
Ferrous sulphate
Feospan
Ferrograd
Pregnavite Forte F
Slow-Fe
Hydroxocobalamin
Cobalin-H
Neo-Cytamen
Iron & folic acid
Fefol
Fefol-Vit
Fefol Z
Ferfolic SV
Ferrocap-F 350
Ferrocontin Folic

Ferrograd Folic
Folex-350
Folicin
Galfer F.A.
Givitol
Ketovite Tablets
Lexpec with Iron
Lexpec with Iron-M
Metrefolic
Pregaday
Pregnavite Forte F
Slow-Fe Folic
Solivito N
Oral rehydration salts
Dext
Dioralyte
Rehydrat
Potassium chloride
Glandosane
Kay-Cee-L
Kloref
Kloref-S
Leo K
Luborant
Nu-K
Potassium Chloride Solution
  BP Strong (15%)
Sando-K
Sandostatin
Slow-K
Pyridoxine hydrochloride
Benadon
Complement Continus
Parentrovite
Vitamin B compound
Becosym
Benerva Compound
Viaranon B
Vitamins caps
Abidec
Albee with C
BC 500
Calcimax
Concavit
Dalavit
Forceval
Ketovite
Orovite

Orovite 7
Surbext

OBSTETRICS, GYNAECOLOGY, & URINARY-TRACT DISORDERS

Clotrimazole
  Canesten
Dienoestrol
  Ortho Dienoestrol
Econazole nitrate
  Econacort
  Ecostatin
  Gyno-Pevaryl
  Pevaryl
  Pevaryl TC
Ethinyloestradiol
  BiNovum
  Brevinor
  Cilest
  Conova 30
  Dianette
  Eugynon 30
  Femodene
  Femodene ED
  Loestrin 20
  Loestrin 30
  Logynon
  Logynon ED
  Marvelon
  Mercilon
  Microgynon 30
  Minulet
  Neocon 1/35
  Norimin
  Ovran
  Ovran 30
  Ovranette
  Ovysmen
  Schering PC4
  Synphase
  Triadene
  Tri-Minulet
  Trinordiol
  TriNovum
  TriNovum ED
Ethynodiol diacetate
  Conova 30

Femulen
Miconazole nitrate
  Acnidazil
  Daktacort
  Dermonistat
  Gynodaktarin
  Monistat
Nonoxynol-9
  C-film
  Delfen
  Double Check
  Duracreme
  Duragel
  Gynol II
  Ortho-Creme
  Orthoforms
  Staycept Pessaries
Norethisterone
  BiNovum
  Brevinor
  Estrapak
  Loestrin 20
  Loestrin 30
  Menzol
  Micronor
  Neocon 1/35
  Noriday
  Norimin
  Norinyl-1
  Noristerat
  Ortho-Novin 1/50
  Ovysmen
  Primolut N
  SH420
  Synphase
  Syntex Menophase
  TriNovum
  TriNovum ED
  Utovlan
Oxybutynin hydrochloride
  Cystrin
  Ditropan

RESPIRATORY SYSTEM

Aminophylline
  Pecram
  Phyllocontin

Theodrox
Beclomethasone dipropionate
AeroBec
Becloforte
Becodisks
Becotide
Ventide
Chlorpheniramine maleate
Galpseud Plus
Haymine
Piriton
Codeine phosphate
Codafen Continus
Diarrest
Formulix
Galcodine
Hypon
Kaodene
Migraleve
Paracodol
Parahypon
Propain
Solpadol
Syndol
Terpoin Antitussive
Tylox
Choline Theophyllinate
Choledyl
Sabidal SR 270
Hydrocortisone
Solu-Cortef
Ipratropium bromide
Atrovent
Duovent
Rinatec
Pholcodine
Copholco
Galenphol
Pavacol-D
Pholcomed
Promethazine hydrochloride
Avomine
Pamergan P100
Phenergan
Phensedyl
Sominex

Pseudoephedrine hydrochloride
Actifed
Congesteze
Dimotane Co
Dimotane Expect.
Dimotane Plus
Galpseud
Galpseud Plus
Sudafed
Sudafed Co
Sudafed Plus
Sudafed SA
Salbutamol
Aerolin Autohaler
Asmaven
Salbulin
Salbutamol Cyclocaps
Salbuvent
Steri-neb Salamol
Ventide
Ventodisks
Ventolin
Volmax
Sodium cromoglycate
Cromogen
Intal
Intal Compound
Nalcrom
Rynacrom
Terbutaline sulphate
Bricanyl
Bricanyl SA
Terfenadine
Triludan
Theophylline
Biophylline
Franol
Franol Plus
Labophylline Injection
Lasma
Nuelin
Pro-Vent
Slo-Phyllin
Theo-Dur
Uniphyllin Continus

SKIN

Acyclovir
  Zovirax
Beclomethasone dipropionate
  Propaderm
  Propaderm-A
Betamethasone sodium phosphate
  Betnelan
  Betnovate
  Betnovate-C
  Betnovate-N
  Betnovate Rectal
  Diprosalic
  Diprosone
  Fucibet
  Lotriderm
Clobetasol propionate
  Dermovate
  Dermovate-NN
Clobetasone butyrate
  Eumovate
  Eumovate-N
  Trimovate
Clotrimazole
  Canesten-HC
  Lotriderm
Fluocinolone acetonide
  Synalar
  Synalar C
  Synalar N
  Synandone
Fusidic acid (sodium fusidate)
  Fucibet
  Fucidin
Hydrocortisone
  Actinac
  Alphaderm
  Alphosyl HC
  Barquinol HC
  Calmurid HC
  Canesten-HC
  Carbo-Cort
  Cobadex
  Daktacort
  Dioderm
  Econacort

Efcortelan
Efcortesol
Epifoam
Eurax-Hydrocortisone
Fucidin H
Gentisone HC
Gregoderm
Hydrocal
Hydrocortisyl
Mildison Lipocream
Nystaform-HC
Quinocort
Quinoderm with
  Hydrocortisone
Sential HC
Solu-Cortef
Tarcortin
Terra-Cortril
Terra-Cortril Nystatin
Timodine
Tricicatrin
Uniroid HC
Vioform Hydrocortisone
Hydrocortisone-17-butyrate
  Locoid
  Locoid C
Mupirocin
  Bactroban
  Bactroban Nasal
Salicylic acid
  Aserbine
  Capasal Shampoo
  Cuplex
  Diprosalic
  Dithrolan
  Duofilm
  Gelcosal
  Ionil T
  Monphytol
  Movelat
  Phytex
  Phytocil
  Posalfilin
  Pragmatar
  Psorin
  Pyralvex
  Salactol
  Salatac Gel

Stiedex Lotion
Verrugon
Sodium chloride
Alcon BSS
Glandosane
Minims Artificial Tears
Minims Sodium Chloride
Normasol

Sential
Sential E
Sential HC
Slow-Sodium
Sodium Chloride 0.9%
 Intravenous Infusion BP
Sterac Saline
Steripod Blue